Aromatherapy for Health Professionals

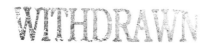

For Churchill Livingstone

Commissioning Editor: Inta Ozols
Project Editor: Dinah Thom
Project Manager: Ewan Halley
Design Direction: Judith Wright

Aromatherapy for Health Professionals

Shirley Price FISPA MIFA LIAM
Practitioner and Lecturer in Aromatherapy, Hinckley, Leicestershire

Len Price MIT FISPA LIAM
Lecturer in Aromatherapy, Hinckley, Leicestershire

Foreword by

Dr Daniel Pénoël
International Lecturer in, and Medical Practitioner of, Integrated Aromatic
Medicine, Aouste-sur-Sye, Drôme, France

SECOND EDITION

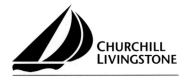

CHURCHILL
LIVINGSTONE

EDINBURGH LONDON NEW YORK PHILADELPHIA ST LOUIS SYDNEY TORONTO 1999

CHURCHILL LIVINGSTONE
An imprint of Harcourt Brace and Company Limited

© Pearson Professional Limited 1995
© Harcourt Publishers Limited 1999

✍ is a registered trade mark of Harcourt Publishers Limited

First Edition 1995
Second Edition 1999

ISBN 0 443 06210 2

British Library of Cataloguing in Publication Data
A catalogue record for this book is available from the British Library.

Library of Congress Cataloging in Publication Data
A catalogue record for this book is available from the Library of Congress.

Note
Medical knowledge is constantly changing. As new information becomes available,
changes in treatment, procedures, equipment and the use of drugs become necessary.
The authors and publishers have, as far as it is possible, taken care to ensure that the
information given in this text is accurate and up to date. However, readers are strongly advised to confirm that the information, especially with regard to drug usage, com-
plies with the latest legislation and standards of practice.

The
publisher's
policy is to use
**paper manufactured
from sustainable forests**

Printed in China

Contents

Foreword to the Second Edition

The first edition of *Aromatherapy for Health Professionals* has had well deserved success, not only among aromatherapists but also among a great variety of health practitioners throughout the world.

After three years it was obvious, with the rapid acceleration of progress in theoretical knowledge and development of the technical and practical applications of essential oils, that a new enlarged, revised edition had become desirable. During these years, Shirley and Len Price have not ceased to take part in major events to learn and to teach (even in French for Shirley Price!) everywhere with the same enthusiasm and the same dedication. They have extracted and 'distilled' the best of the new harvest of information and included this in the new edition of a book which has now become a standard for the serious student—and for all therapists open to natural and alternative answers.

Aromatic plants have been used for thousands of years in every part of the world by numerous civilizations which, driven by their intuition and sense of observation, were able to find answers to their health problems in the plant environment. Fortunately, the progress of analytical chemistry enables us to begin to understand the extraordinary laboratory which exists inside the aromatic plant cell; we can only be spellbound when we realize the amazing complexity of this biochemical manufacture and the harmonious and powerful results produced by the aromatic substance inside plants. Essential oils made up of natural aromatic molecules are endowed with so many physiological and pharmacological properties that they find applications in almost every field of curative and prophylactic medicine.

Len and Shirley rightly insist upon the importance of using whole essential oils, each from a single, named botanical plant. Having created strong links with growers and distillers, in particular in the Drôme area, which is the foremost region in France for the production of aromatic and medicinal plants, they know that excellent therapeutic results can only be obtained by the use of top quality products and that poor quality or adulteration will lead to disappointment and eventually to discarding the whole method.

Provided that the practitioner has relevant information and has undergone the appropriate training and that the aromatic extracts used are neither standardized nor otherwise adulterated, aromatherapy and aromatology can bring real therapeutic help to many patients, far beyond the antistress massage approach.

The aromatology course that Shirley and Len have created, including the module concerning the intensive application and internal use of essential oils—which is so necessary in order to make full use of the essential oils' potential—enables properly trained aromatherapists to extend and deepen their field of understanding and their capacity for efficacious treatment interventions. The launching of such a training was not achieved without overcoming obstacles and countervailing severe critical opinions! However, the one-time critics now realize that it is much better to provide sound and clear information than to leave a void which opens the door to wrong ideas and inadequate, ill-informed actions (what people do with this information is another question).

Therapists from the UK and from many other countries who have had the opportunity of receiving precise theoretical information and practical training have significantly increased their potential for aromatic healing. Many have said how wonderful it felt for them to obtain therapeutic results that were previously beyond their scope, restricted, as they were in the main, to basic, diluted aromatic massage. From a legal viewpoint, Shirley Price has made it possible for newly qualified aromatologists (and students) to obtain comprehensive professional liability insurance so that they can work openly and with a clear and peaceful mind.

Meanwhile, in my country, English books are translated and published in French (including books by Shirley Price), and this paves the way for a future 'Aromatic European Country' which is one of our main purposes. Step by step, by joining our efforts, the dream is beginning to turn into reality on both sides of the Channel and, hopefully, by the first years of the next century we will have succeeded in building the 'Aromatic Eurochunnel'.

In France, a major success was achieved by the pharmacists' union over the government—the rescinding of the law, voted in 1990 and applied since 1991, that suppressed the reimbursement of phytotherapeutic preparations (see Chapter 17, France).

This new spirit of close international collaboration and the determination to cooperate and create strong links and efficacious networking systems, was felt by all the participants at 'Aroma 97', organized by the *International Journal of Aromatherapy* and held at Warwick University in July 1997. This was followed in 1998 by the 'First International Symposium on Integrated Aromatic Medicine', which was held in Grasse (initiated by myself and in which the authors took an active part). It was an auspicious sign of our determination to progress towards more global unity (while respecting individual differences) and better exchange of information.

I am convinced that this new edition will have an even greater success and reach an ever increasing number of therapists and health professionals. I offer heartfelt thanks to the authors (and the publisher) for their courageous and continuous involvement in the noble task of spreading accurate 'good news' about essential oils and aromatherapy.

The holding back of information concerning both the science and the art of healing is tantamount to a collective crime. In this way I am confident, after 21 years of practising medical aromatherapy, intensively and extensively, that this book will make a major contribution to the saving of lives and the relief of suffering, and will bring hope and joy to many patients all over our 'little village planet'.

Finally, I would like each reader of this book to realize the importance of personal involvement in this 'aromatic revolution' and to accomplish with full awareness his or her part of the global task. 'An individual success is not a success unless it is transformed into a collective success .'

Drôme, France 1999   Dr Daniel Pénoël

Preface

Twenty-five years ago aromatherapy was very little known, and even when recognized it was usually regarded as a pleasant adjunct to a beauty treatment, or at best a 'rejuvenating' skin treatment; the teaching of aromatherapy reflected this beauty angle, whereas today the health-promoting aspect is more dominant. The majority of training programmes in the past have been notoriously inadequate, and this situation is only now being properly addressed. Aromatherapy as a complement to medical treatment is very young, and while it has made significant progress there remains much to be researched and established. Aromatherapy is complex, involving as it does a wide range of topics, from botany through organic chemistry, essential oil knowledge and massage to client care. Therefore it is not possible for there to be a sole authority on the subject as a whole. A multitude of books on aromatherapy have appeared in recent years, many aimed at the lay public. Such books are of limited use to the health professional wishing to practise aromatherapy, and so it is perhaps advisable to discuss briefly the quality of the information contained in this book.

Since the 1980s standards of training in aromatherapy have greatly improved, guided by leading schools and the professional associations. This prompted Shirley to write *The Aromatherapy Workbook* (Price 1993), which was aimed at helping student aromatherapists acquire an in-depth knowledge of the physiological and psychological effects of essential oils. One of the issues raised in the book was the importance of specifying accurately the essential oils employed, for example by using the botanical name and the part of the plant in preference to the common plant name only.

In addition, because professionals such as physiotherapists, occupational therapists and nurses have become increasingly aware of the possibilities of using essential oils in hospices, hospitals, clinics, day care, residential and community care work, we felt that the time was ripe for a book aimed specifically at health professionals. This feeling was confirmed at the lectures and workshops we gave at hospitals throughout the UK, the Republic of Ireland and Switzerland in the period 1992 to 1995. It became clear that many nurses were introducing essential oils into their hospitals without attending an accredited training course. This may be because much aromatherapy course time is concerned with full-body massage, a treatment which is seldom appropriate and which professionals in healthcare situations rarely have the time to carry out. In response to this, we have introduced aromatic medicine (aromatology) courses into colleges. We also feel that a book which emphasizes the need to obtain extensive knowledge of essential oils before using them on sick people will discourage the incorrect application of these powerful agents, which in some unfortunate cases has led hospitals to forbid their use.

To be able to put together such a book it has been necessary to look at the hundreds of references that exist on the properties and actions of the essential oils. Up until now this research has been carried out principally for the perfume and food industries. There is a large body of information available on some of the antiseptic, antibacterial, antiparasitic and even antiviral properties of some essential oils, and their effects on skin, but the information is by no means complete and much more research with aromatherapy in mind needs to be done. Further progress has been made since the publication of the first edition of this book 4 years ago, and so it was thought desirable to bring out a new edition which, as well as providing updated information on some aspects of essential oils and additional information on carrier oils, gives updated and greatly expanded information on aromatherapy worldwide.

In collecting material for this book, only the writings of eminent practitioners have been used. Without their evidence this book would be quite slim and of little use. Trials and pilot studies, anecdotal evidence and single case studies are mostly what aromatherapy has to rely on at this time; and we thought it better to give this information rather than copy plant properties from herbal books, since the properties of the essential oil and a given plant are not necessarily the same.

The bulk of the research carried out in the past has been in vitro or on animals, and it can be difficult, and often impossible, to extrapolate such results to humans. There is a dearth of evidence on such aspects as, for example, the analgesic and diuretic effects of essential oils, and when it comes to the effects of essential oils on conditions such as rheumatism, arthritis and headaches, there is realistically only anecdotal evidence available. Properly constructed and conducted trials are desperately needed, but many aromatherapists have neither the background nor the appropriate training (nor the necessary finances) to carry out this work, although this situation is now changing. The Research Council for Complementary Medicine has an increasing data bank of research trials using aromatherapy. As for double-blind tests, new thinking will have to be adopted because it is not possible to do this type of test using an aromatic substance, as the presence or absence of an aroma is immediately

obvious to the participants. Double-blind studies, though desirable, can usually be achieved only by internal use, a rarely used method in aromatherapy.

Therefore, while there is a great deal of information in this book, where 'scientific' evidence is not available then anecdotal evidence has been used. In our opinion it is of good quality, having been carefully selected from acknowledged (mainly French) sources—some written by medical doctors—which are in accord with our own experience obtained over more than two decades of practice and teaching. It is the moral duty of aromatherapists to carry out such investigations, as far as they are able, to determine how and whether essential oils work in particular circumstances, and to have a unified system of reporting and sharing information. At the present time this is not in place; many more trials, projects and single case studies are needed to demonstrate unequivocally the efficacy of these holistic medicines before they can be generally accepted. Professionals in the 'orthodox' field generally fall into two categories; either they pitch in and help to design protocols for such studies, or they stand back and criticize our lack of proper research, of which we are already painfully aware.

We realize that the value of anecdotal evidence is questionable because of various factors: many illnesses are self-limiting and spontaneously disappear; others are only in the minds of the sufferers and such people are usually open to suggestion, and in others the sufferer has phases of feeling poorly alternating with phases of feeling well. There are also the unexplained 'miraculous' cures, which do occasionally happen. Obviously false good results can appear to occur; however, it is against common sense to dismiss all anecdotal evidence gathered over the years.

This book contains guidelines on the preparation of a professionally based policy and protocol to present to hospital management when applying for permission to use essential oils in a healthcare setting. In those hospitals where the use of essential oils has already been introduced on a correct footing, many trials and projects have been carried out. Although they do not constitute research in the accepted scientific sense of the word, such studies are extremely valuable for the future acceptance of aromatic medicine. It is hoped that by publicizing some of them here more health professionals will be encouraged to continue the good work.

Why bother with this strange therapy at all? We hope that this book will convince the doubters that there is something of substance to be looked into, something which can be used alongside orthodox treatments, especially in hospitals where, in addition, there may be substantial cash savings to be made. Most general practitioners discuss alternative (complementary) treatments with their patients, and over half of them refer patients to alternative practitioners (Anderson & Anderson 1987, Borkan et al 1994).

Many general practitioners believe that alternative medicine has ideas and methods from which conventional medicine could benefit (Verhoef & Sutherland 1995a), and in a questionnaire 73% of physicians taking part felt that they

should have some knowledge of the most important alternative treatments (Verhoef & Sutherland 1995b)

Wharton & Lewith (1986) found that, although most general practitioners knew little of the techniques of complementary medicine, a majority found that the complementary techniques being assessed were useful to their patients, and most had referred patients for this type of treatment over the past year to their medical colleagues and also to complementary practitioners; but they felt that complementary practitioners needed statutory regulation. Harmonization of training and regulation of practitioners is the urgent requirement in the immediate future (Fisher & Ward 1994).

We trust that this book will prove to be of value to you and your colleagues.

Hinckley 1999   Shirley and Len Price

REFERENCES

Anderson E, Anderson P 1987 General practitioners and alternative medicine. Journal of Royal College of General Practitioners Feb 37(295): 52–55
Borkan J, Neher J O, Anson O, Smoker B 1994 Referrals for alternative therapies. Journal of Family Practice 39(6): 545–550
Fisher P, Ward A 1994 Complementary medicine in Europe. British Medical Journal 309(6947): 107–111
Price S 1993 The Aromatherapy Workbook. Thorsons, London

Verhoef M J, Sutherland L R 1995a Alternative medicine and general practitioners. Opinions and behaviour. Canadian Family Physician 41: 1005–1011
Verhoef M J, Sutherland L R 1995b General practitioners' assessment of and interest in alternative medicine in Canada. Social Science and Medicine 41(4): 511–515
Wharton R, Lewith G 1986 Complementary medicine and the general practitioners. British Medical Journal (Clinical Research) June 7 292(6533): 1498–1500

Acknowledgements

The authors wish to thank the following people, whose understanding and help have been much appreciated: Alan Barker for the interest and support he gave us when preparing the first edition; Inta Ozols for her friendly support during stressful times; Dinah Thom, Michael Dean (who checked our work so thoroughly) and Chris Wyard for their editorial advice; Katya Svoboda, Jane Buckle, Susan Lundie and Maureen Farrell for reading relevant parts of the text at manuscript stage; David Witty for his specialist advice on essential oils; Marie Hélène Grandvoinnet, Doreen Bishop and Harry Thomte for their patient willingness to be photographed for the massage section; Julia Foley for her help with the chapter on Primary Care; and the staff of Shirley Price Aromatherapy—Justine Finney for prompt attention to requests, Sue Minkley (particularly for her patience in collecting information from abroad), Sally Turnidge for help with the references and Ian Smith for his chemistry advice.

The authors are also grateful to the following people for supplying information about the practice of aromatherapy in the different countries listed in Chapter 17.

Australia—Margaret Meyer, Margaret Tozer, Marlene Cadwallader, Marlene Anderson, Therese Wilson, Irma Gol and Margaret O'Brien

Belgium—Michel Vanhove
Canada—Jean-Pierre LeBlanc
France—Dr Daniel Pénoël—thanks too for writing the foreword for both editions
Germany—Margaret Demleiter and Ulrike Rädlein
Republic of Ireland—Mary Kileen, Catherine Pepper, Monica Mackin, Nicola Darrell and Mary Cavanaugh
Israel—Dr Gadi Zilkha and Fern Allen
Japan—Harumi Nara, Oz International
Korea—Dr David Oh
Norway—Margareth Thomte
New Zealand—Anne Bennett, Tracey Fearn, Katrina Lloyd, Wendy Maddocks, Maureen Powell, Trevor Pugh and Sarah Willacy
South Africa—Lucille Bischoff and Karen Ten Velden
Sweden—Anna Hanson
Switzerland—Gian Furrer, Rosemary Mathys, Ueli Morgenthaler, Jan Straub and Eeva Salo
Taiwan—Mr J Y Su
United States of America—Laraine Kyle, Eli Muller, Cheryl Hoard, Jane Buckle and Dorene Petersen

—and last, but not least, our seven grandchildren, for not minding too much the infrequency of their overnight visits.

Introduction

Historical use of essential oils

Plants and their extracts have been used since time immemorial to relieve pain, aid healing, kill bacteria and thus revitalize and maintain good health. Many books have now been written on aromatherapy, its history usually being included in more or less detail. Suffice it to say here that, although the word itself was not coined until this century, the distilled extracts from plants—the essential oils—have been employed by humankind for countless years in religious rites, perfumery and hygiene. Cedarwood oil, known to have been used by the Egyptians for embalming and for hygienic purposes 5000 years ago, was probably the first 'distilled' oil to have been produced although the process used is open to speculation (Ch. 2). Both the lavender plant and its essential oil were used by the abbess Hildegard of Bingen as early as the 12th century, and by the 15th century it is thought that essential oils of turpentine, cinnamon, frankincense, juniper, rose and sage were also known and used (Pignatelli 1991). About 60 oils were known and used in perfumes and medicines by the beginning of the 17th century (Valnet 1980 p. 28).

Modern evidence for the antiseptic powers of essential oils

Towards the end of the 19th century, the first acknowledged research to prove the antiseptic properties of essential oils was that undertaken by Chamberland (1887). This was followed early in the 20th century by Cavel's research into the

1

individual effects of 35 essential oils on microbial cultures in sewage. The most effective oil in terms of the quantity required to render inactive 1000 ml of culture was found to be thyme (0.7 ml). Two other well-known oils showing high efficacy were sweet orange (1.2 ml, 3rd) and peppermint (2.5 ml, 9th) (Cavel 1918). The antiseptic power of several oils has now been proved to be many times greater than that of phenol. Certain essential oils have also been shown to be effective against different bacteria, e.g. lemon, which is one of the best in its antiseptic and bactericidal properties, neutralizing both the typhus bacillus and *Staphylococcus aureus* in a matter of minutes. Cinnamon kills the typhus bacillus even when diluted to 1 part in 300 (Valnet 1980 p. 36).

Professor Griffon, a member of the French Academy of Pharmacy, made up a blend of seven essential oils (cinnamon, clove, lavender, peppermint, pine, rosemary and thyme) to study their antiseptic effect on the surrounding air when sprayed from an aerosol; all the staphylococci and moulds present were destroyed after 30 minutes (Valnet 1980 p. 37). (See Chapter 4 for more recent studies on the antiseptic properties of essential oils.)

The bacteriological approach of aromatherapy is an extremely complex field of the utmost interest, opening the way to the ecological understanding and management of the different colonies and flora that live in cohabitation—or at war—within us. Allopathic medicine has begun to realize that the misuse of antibiotics leads to numerous side-effects and sometimes results in chronic disastrous conditions (i.e. systemic candidosis) that could have been avoided if medical aromatherapy had been implemented in due time (Pénoël 1993 personal communication).

Today, the properties of herb volatile oils are researched in many centres throughout the world. A typical case is the excellent work carried out in Scotland since the early 1980s by Deans & Svoboda at the Scottish Agricultural College, Auchincruive (Ch. 4), assessing antibacterial and antifungal properties of essential oils and their constituents.

Wide-ranging application

Essential oils can be put to a multitude of uses both in general practice and in hospitals, as this quote from Dr J Valnet illustrates:

The doctor who is familiar with essential oils can use them to treat a whole range of infections— pulmonary, hepatic, intestinal, urinary, uterine, rhinopharyngeal and cutaneous (infected wounds and suppurating dermatoses). The use of these oils usually produces satisfactory results, provided they have been prescribed wisely and that, in the case of certain long-standing complaints, the treatment is followed for a long enough period. Aromatic therapy can neutralise enteritis, colitis and putrid fermentations, and can relieve chronic bronchitis and pulmonary tuberculosis. The colon bacillus cannot resist essential oils.

(Valnet 1980 p. 41)

Orthodox medicine currently uses plant material to help cure diseases which previously had a high death rate. Twenty years ago, four out of every five children with leukaemia lost their lives; nowadays four out of five are returned to health with the aid of vincristine and vinblastine, derivatives of the rosy periwinkle—a plant used for hundreds of years by tribal healers as a medicine (Craker 1990). The snakeroot plant from India is now used in the Western world to treat hypertension; digitalis, for heart conditions, is produced from the humble foxglove and the well-known rhododendron is used in the treatment of fatigue. 'Plants are an intrinsic part of natural medicine, and not even the most orthodox doctor can get by without them; indeed they represent the link between the natural and the orthodox, the traditional and the ultra-new' (Pahlow 1980).

Phytotherapy is the name increasingly given to the use of the whole, or part, of the plant for medicinal purposes. Aromatherapy and aromatology (similar to aromatherapy but including intensive and internal uses) are branches of this, utilizing only the essential oils produced by distillation and citrus oils produced by expression. These are simple to use and administer, yet can compete with the steroids and antibiotics used in allopathic medicine today without the body's defence mechanism becoming exhausted or tolerance developing to them.

The basic reason which accounts for the diversity of conception and application of aromatherapy lies in the very nature of the aromatic substance. Lending itself to easy cutaneous penetration, being endowed with the capacity to influence the mind through its powerful impact upon the olfactive sense, and owing multiple and strong pharmacological properties to its highly active molecular components, it was natural for the aromatic substance to find developments in so many areas.

(Pénoël 1993 personal communication)

Powerful healing agents

Many plant extracts used in the production of conventional medicines are, like the foxglove, poisonous and therefore exceptionally low doses are employed. Some essential oils are also toxic when used incorrectly and the most powerful of these are not normally available to aromatherapists (Chs 3 and 4). Essential oils are concentrated and intensely energetic in their effects, so very little is needed (even of those in general use) for successful treatment—dilutions generally being in the range 0.05–3%, depending on the oil used. Apart from the difference in the intensity of the aroma, no apparent benefit is gained from higher concentrations, particularly where the problem is an emotional one, although neat oils are used in certain medical conditions and aromatology.

Their mode of action

It cannot yet be proved exactly *how* they work, but research and extensive anecdotal evidence exists to prove that they *do* work. In the distant past, essences have been used to heal wounds, inhibit the decay of flesh (as in mummification) and reduce the spread of infection (as in the time of the Black Death)—all without anyone knowing how they worked, just as the humble aspirin was in use for many years before anyone knew its mode of action.

Bios is the Greek word for life and essential oils may be classed as probiotic (for life), as opposed to antibiotic (against life). To illustrate this point, antibiotics kill not only harmful bacteria, but also the beneficial flora that we need to keep us healthy, leaving the body in a weakened state.

Carefully selected essential oils kill only the bacteria inimical to the successful functioning of the body (Valnet 1980 p. 45). Some essential oils also possess antiviral and fungicidal qualities. 'A serious condition obviously authorises the use of antibiotics, and in high doses; but one should be aware that the price of a cure may be a permanent disability' (Valnet 1980 p. 54).

User-friendly

Natural, whole essential oils can be used on living tissue with minimal unwanted effects (unlike some synthetic drugs, however successful these may be against their intended targets). Also, the human body accustoms itself to the effects of chemical synthetics, leading to escalating doses. This has not been found to be the case with essential oils, which retain their effectiveness in repeated applications and can in fact strengthen the living tissue while killing off the unwanted bacteria (Valnet 1980 p. 48).

Quantities of essential oils used

Tens of thousands of tonnes of essential oils are used by the food and perfume industries (Verlet 1993), with the food industry being the largest user. It is important to realize that the total amount of essential oil used by the aromatherapy profession is extremely small compared with these industries, and this contributes to the difficulties of obtaining high quality, pure, natural oils (Ch. 2). Some oils which could be beneficial when used in aromatherapy are not generally supplied by distillers because they are not required by the giant users. Fortunately, however, a small number of independent distillers produce essential oils solely for aromatherapy use, although such products tend to be more expensive.

Economy of use

Compared with the very high price of drugs (perhaps due to the tremendous research and development costs) essential oils are extremely inexpensive—a factor which should interest those in charge of public health funds. Not only that, they are pleasant to use for both patient and carer. In many hospitals and hospices they are used not only to improve the quality of a patient's life but in waiting rooms to relieve the anxiety of relatives and friends. More specifically, they can be used in place of secondary drugs, which might be prescribed to counteract iatrogenic effects of the primary drugs being taken. They have been found to aid relaxation effectively, both pre- and post-operatively, to regenerate tissue in cases of severe burns and inflammation, and to relieve pain in cases of rheumatoid arthritis. They have helped to improve the quality of life for the terminally ill, and they have also found important uses in maternity care.

Areas of use

Essential oils are used extensively by aromatherapists and aromatologists to improve or uplift a patient's state of mind. The effect of the attitude of mind on a person's health is being recognized more and more and essential oils can play an important part here. Florence Nightingale said 'what nursing has to do ... is to put the patient in the best condition for nature to act upon him', reinforcing the ancient tag *medicus cura, natura sanat*—the doctor treats, nature cures.

By far the majority of essential oil users are outside the medical profession, some people using them merely on instruction from one of the many books written for the general public on the subject. They are simple to use and it should come as a relief to GPs that minor everyday ailments such as a sore throat or a winter cold, and even some more serious problems like bronchitis, sinusitis and rheumatism, can be treated in the home easily and successfully, leaving the doctor's time free for the cases requiring expert knowledge.

All this is achievable by anyone, without professional medical skills. However, in France (from where aromatherapy was introduced to the UK) doctors prescribe essential oils for internal use in capsules or in drops diluted in alcohol, or in suppositories and pessaries (Ch. 17). They are used externally in dressings, fumigations, inhalations, ointments and in foot, hand or complete baths. The original concept of aromatherapy in England, as introduced by Mme Maury, was to use the essential oils in massage only—suitably diluted in a fixed vegetable oil. This unfortunately led to the belief that this is all there is to aromatherapy, and the authors are actively trying to correct this image. It needs the medical profession not only to take an interest but also to use its professional skills to utilize these precious commodities to their fullest capabilities in order to bring the benefits of this aromatic therapy to the hospitals of the world in the 21st century.

The subject of aromatherapy involves pharmacy and farming, botany and bodies, medicine and chemistry, toxicity and safety—all so intertwined and interconnected that it is scarcely possible to disentangle the ramifications for the purpose of setting them down without some repetition and much cross-referral.

REFERENCES

Cavel L 1918 Sur la valeur antiseptique de quelques huiles essentielles. Comptes Rendus (Académie des Sciences) 166: 827

Chamberland M 1887 Les essences au point du vue de leurs propriétés antiseptiques. Annales Institut Pasteur 1: 153–154

Craker L E 1990 News and commentary. The Herb, Spice and Medicinal Plant Digest 8(4): 5

Pahlow M 1980 Living medicine. Thorsons, Wellingborough, p 9

Pignatelli M F 1991 Viaggio nel mondo della essenze. Muzzio, Padora

Valnet J 1980 The practice of aromatherapy. Daniel, Saffron Walden

Verlet N 1993 Commercial aspects. In: Hay R K M, Waterman P G (eds) Volatile oil crops. Longman, Harlow, ch 8, pp 145–146

SECTION 1

Essential oil science

SECTION CONTENTS

1

The genesis of essential oils

Introduction

Aromatherapy involves the use of essential oils, all of which are derived from plants. Anyone wishing to practise aromatherapy must gain as full an understanding of the plants concerned as possible, so that the oils can be used knowledgeably to their best effect. This chapter enables the practitioner to do this, looking beyond the oil in the little glass bottle to the plant from which it was extracted, its growing environment and the family to which it belongs.

BOTANY FOR AROMATHERAPISTS

Taxonomy

The precise identification of plants was made possible by the Swedish naturalist Carl von Linné or Linnaeus (1707–1778) who developed the system of classifying organisms in groups according to their similarities. Over the years the Linnaean method of classification has been subject to modification but is still at the core of the international taxonomical system used today. Each plant belongs to a family and is given a generic name based on structural characteristics (written in italics with an initial capital), and a specific name (lower-case italics). For example, lavender is classified in the following way:

Kingdom	Plantae
Division	Tracheophyta
Subdivision	Spermatophyta
Class	Dicotyledons
Subclass	Asteridae

Order	Lamiales
Family	Lamiaceae (syn. Labiatae)
Genus	*Lavandula*
Species	*angustifolia*

To identify a plant accurately it is necessary to give at least the generic and the specific name: lavender is therefore referred to as *Lavandula angustifolia*. However, there are further divisions below this level, such as subspecies (often denoting a geographic variation of a species), variety (see below), forma (denoting trivial differences), cultivar, chemotype and hybrid (see below). Therapists prescribing essential oils must take care to identify precisely the plants from which they are derived, and this means giving not only the generic and specific names but also specifying, where necessary, the chemotype, variety, cultivar, etc. as well.

Variety: indicates a rank between subspecies and forma. They are named by adding 'var'. and the italicized variety name, e.g. *Citrus aurantium* var. *amara*. It used to indicate a major subdivision of a species, or a variant of horticultural origin or importance (although these are now labelled cultivar), and many names of horticultural origin reflect the historical use of the variety rank.

Cultivar: indicates a cultivated variety, and a rank known only in horticultural cultivation. These names are non-latinized and in living languages (usually the name of, or chosen by, the originator). They are not italicized, and appear within quotation marks, e.g. *Lavandula angustifolia* 'Maillette'.

Chemotype: indicates visually identical plants with significantly different chemical components, resulting in different therapeutic properties. Chemotypes occur naturally in plants grown in the wild, some species throwing up many chemical variations; they can be propagated by cuttings for cultivation. They are named by the abbreviation 'ct.' followed by the constituent, e.g. *Thymus vulgaris* ct. alcohol, *T. vulgaris* ct. geraniol, etc.

Hybrid: indicates natural or artificially produced crosses between species. They are represented by ×, e.g. *Mentha × piperita*, which is a cross between *M. aquatica* and *M. spicata*.

Metabolism

Each plant is a vibrant chemical factory capable of transforming the electromagnetic rays from the sun into energetic substances which are then available for the plant's use. The plant takes up water and minerals from the soil through its roots and carbon dioxide from the air mainly through its leaves. These supplies are then converted by the energy absorbed from the sun into a simple six-carbon sugar, glucose, which provides food for the plant's growth. The waste product of this chemical change is oxygen. The whole process is called photosynthesis, and because it is essential to the life of the plant it is termed primary metabolism. Secondary metabolism products include alkaloids, bitters, glycosides, gums, mucilages, saponins, steroids, tannins and essential oils, which are not necessary for the vital functions of the plant. Of these secondary metabolites it is the essential oils that have the greatest commercial significance, being used in many industries (Verlet 1993).

The metabolic changes in plants are made possible by the action of protein catalysts known as enzymes. Enzymes are highly specific and assist in only one particular reaction (as they do in humans). To function they need manganese or iron combined with a tiny amount of energy which is to be found stored in phosphate bonds in the plant chemicals. Volatile oil secondary metabolites vary widely in chemical structure and their purpose and function in the plant is little understood. Whatever else they may do, they give the plant its aroma and flavour and often have a significant physiological effect on people.

Why does a plant contain essential oil?

Before seeing how an essential oil comes into being, it is worth reflecting on what value essential oils have for plants. This has been debated for many years and there is as yet no definitive answer. Perhaps there never will be, given that science is much better at answering the question 'how?' than the question 'why?', and that there is no obvious commercial advantage in this knowledge. Most commercial research effort is put into investigating the properties and effects of the oils themselves, and it is left to disinterested investigators at universities to look into what possible use the essential oils may be to the plant. However, conjecture on the subject has thrown up many possible reasons:

• To prevent attack by herbivores: both mono- and sesquiterpenes are involved in various ways, such as acting as insect hormones to interfere with the development of the feeding insects, or having a straightforward repellent action.
• To prevent attack from insects: it has been shown that the number of oil glands in a plant increases when it is under attack by insects (Carlton 1990, Carlton, Gray & Waterman 1992).
• To prevent attack by bacteria, fungi and other microorganisms: there is ample proof available from studies done in vitro on the antifungal and bactericidal properties of herb volatile oils (see section on aromatograms in Ch. 8).
• To aid pollination by attracting bees and other insects such as moths and bats (Harborne 1988).
• To help in the healing of wounds inflicted on the plant itself, and to act as an energy reserve.
• To help survival in difficult growth conditions: for instance by the production of allelopathic compounds, such as 1,8-cineole and camphor, which are freely given off from the plant and find their way to the soil where they prevent other plants from growing (Deans & Waterman 1993).
• To prevent dehydration and afford some degree of protection in hot dry climates by surrounding the plant with a haze of volatile oil, thus helping to prevent water loss from its foliage. One of the oldest plants in the world, the leaves of which can be as much as 10% oil by weight, is the eucalyptus. Living root stock of this plant has been found dating back thousands of years to the Ice Age (Dr Mike Crisp, Australian National Botanic Gardens unpublished information 1986). The free oil vapour emanating from other ancient plants, e.g. pine trees, can be smelt easily when walking in pine forests on a sunny day.

The genesis of essential oils

Plants produce a tremendous variety of chemicals, including a major group of compounds, the terpenes. According to Harborne (1988) more than 1000 monoterpenes and possibly 3000 sesquiterpenes have presently been identified. The phenylpropanoids constitute another much smaller but significant group. In essential oils most of the components belong either to the terpene group, based on the mevalonic acid pathway, or to the phenylpropene group which is based on shikimic acid.

Terpenic structures

The starting point for the terpenes is acetyl coenzyme A (acetyl coA, mentioned also in Ch. 4), from which is formed the six-carbon mevalonic acid. This is then modified to the five-carbon skeleton known as the isoprene unit (Fig. 1.1), which occurs in two forms: IPP (isopentenylpyrophosphate) and DMAPP (dimethylallylpyrophosphate).

Monoterpenes are hydrocarbons (consisting only of carbon and hydrogen atoms) and are formed from two isoprene units; sesquiterpenes are formed from three isoprene units and diterpenes from four isoprene units. Molecules larger than this do not occur in essential oils because the molecular weight would exceed the limit imposed by the distillation process. Monoterpenes constitute the most commonly occurring kind of terpene in plant volatile oils and exist in acyclic (open-ended chain) and cyclic (closed-circle chain) forms. The latter can be either monocyclic or bicyclic. Further complexity arises when double bonds are added (by oxidation) or subtracted (by reduction), and there may also be the addition of various oxygen-containing active groups. Numerous alcohols, ketones, aldehydes and esters are formed by this process.

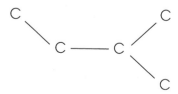

Figure 1.1 Isoprene carbon skeleton.

Phenylpropanoid structures

Precursors (phenylalanine, tyrosine, cinnamic acid) of these molecules act to form compounds that have a six-carbon benzene ring attached to a short (three-carbon) chain to form a phenyl-propene. Even though phenylpropenes occur much less frequently in essential oils than do terpenes, they can have a great impact on the aroma, flavour and therapeutic effect. Examples of phenylpropenes in essential oils are estragole in tarragon oil, cinnamaldehyde in cinnamon bark oil, anethole (Fig. 1.2a) in aniseed oil and apiole (Fig. 1.2b) in fennel seed oil. The chemistry of essential oils is discussed further in Chapter 2.

Secretory structures

Essential oils are synthesized and stored in different sites, which are broadly dependent on the plant family. Oils may be found, for instance, in the leaves, seeds, petals, roots, bark, etc. Sometimes different oils occur in more than one site in a plant; for example two different oils are produced by the cinnamon tree (bark, leaf), and three different oils by the orange tree (leaf, blossom, peel).

Essential oils and their mixtures with resins and gums are commonly found in special secre-tory structures. The type of structure is one of the characteristics of a family, as shown below.

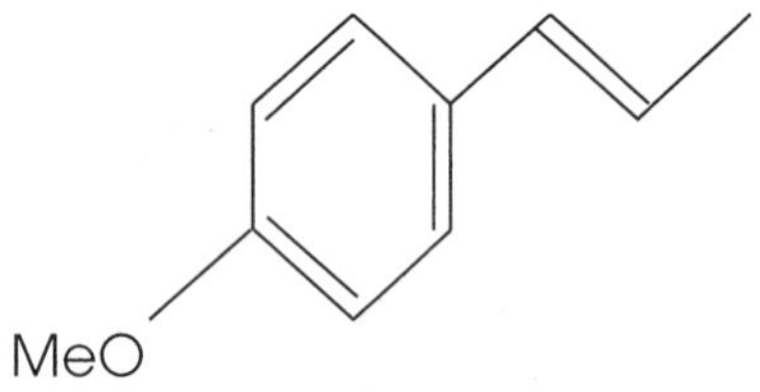

* Oil cells and resin cells
  — Lauraceae (e.g. cinnamon)
  — Zingiberaceae (e.g. cardamom, ginger, turmeric)
  — Piperaceae (e.g. black pepper)
  — Myristicaceae (e.g. nutmeg)
* Cavities, sacs, oil reservoirs (schizolysigenous)
  — Rutaceae (e.g. orange)
  — Myrtaceae (e.g. clove, eucalyptus)
* Oil or resin canals
  — Apiaceae or Umbelliferae (e.g. dill)
  — Pinaceae (e.g. pine, cedarwood)
  — Burseraceae (e.g. myrrh)
* Oil ducts
  — Compositae or Asteraceae (e.g. tarragon)
* Glandular hairs
  — Labiatae or Lamiaceae (e.g. lavender, rosemary)
* Internal hairs
  — Orchidaceae (e.g. vanilla).

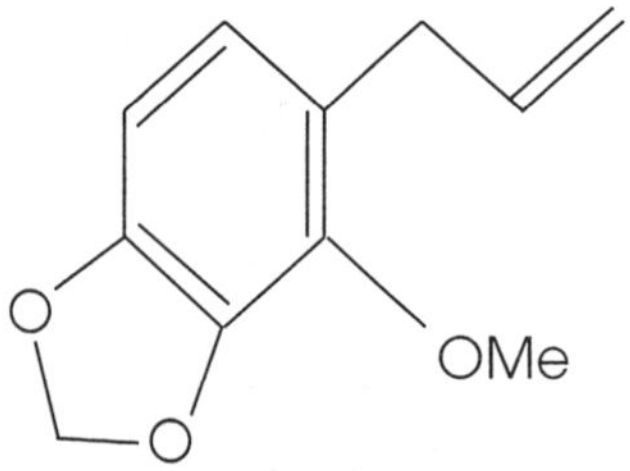

Stereochemistry

The word 'stereo' comes from the Greek meaning solid, and here refers to the spatial arrangement of atoms within a molecule. The same atoms in a molecule may have different relative positions, which has an influence on the chemical activity, and this influence may be slight or very great. In the phenylpropenes the short carbon chain may be attached to the benzene ring at three different locations, known as ortho(o-), meta(m-) and para(p-). A molecule may adopt a different shape with side chains differently orientated. These isomers are known as cis and trans forms.

Some molecules are dextrorotatory (+) and others laevorotatory (−), which indicates their capability to rotate light. The stereochemical form of the molecule will determine the odour and flavour attributes of the oil (Craker 1990). For example, carvone is present as (−)-carvone in spearmint, where it has the aroma of spearmint (Fig. 1.3a), and as (+)-carvone in caraway, where it has the aroma of caraway (Fig. 1.3b). Clearly, a small change in spatial arrangement can have a significant effect.

Figure 1.2a   Anethole.

Figure 1.2b   Apiole.

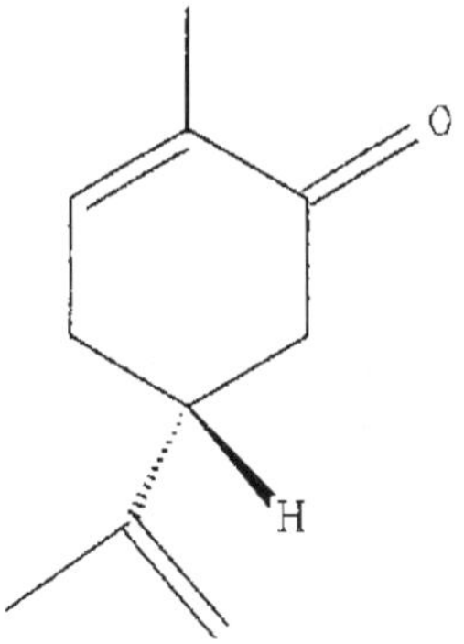

Figure 1.3a   (–)-Carvone.

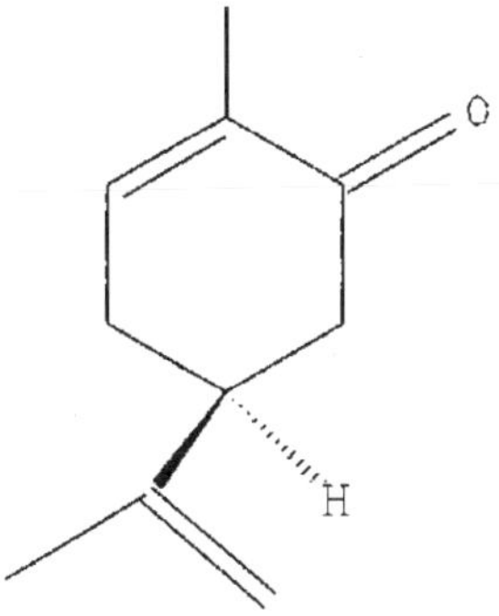

Figure 1.3b   (+)-Carvone.

CHEMICAL VARIATION WITHIN SPECIES

Chemotype is a term applied to plants of the same genus and species, which have the same external appearance but differ, sometimes considerably, in their internal chemical composition. These chemotypes usually occur naturally in plants growing in the wild, and can result partly from cross-pollination. The place and manner of a plant's growing will also promote internal changes; many essential-oil-bearing plants, e.g. rosemary and thyme, are prone to this kind of change owing to genetic and environmental factors. They become resistant to local pests and diseases and have adapted to make the best use of the soil and other surrounding conditions. Such plants are termed 'landrace', and strains which yield specified chemical constituents are sought and selected for propagation by cloning. Cuttings are taken and then cultivated to produce the specific oils required. Included in this category are the thymes and lavenders flourishing wild on the sunny dry hills of Provence.

Thyme chemotypes

The thyme plant is particularly prolific in spontaneously producing strains bearing essential oils of different compositions. Some of these are described below:

• *Thymus vulgaris* ct. thymol. The thymol-bearing thyme is strongly antiseptic and aggressive to the skin owing to the presence of the phenol thymol. Cut in the spring the essential oil contains 30% thymol (Fig. 1.4) plus para-cymene (*p*-cymene) (a monoterpene hydrocarbon). When the same plant is cut in the autumn the essential oil may be found on analysis to contain 60–70% thymol and less *p*-cymene (Table 1.1)

• *Thymus vulgaris* ct. carvacrol. This variant behaves in the same way as the thymol chemotype of thyme, but the phenol involved is carvacrol (Fig. 1.5). In the spring the essential oil contains 30% carvacrol, which increases to 60–80% in the autumn (Table 1.1).

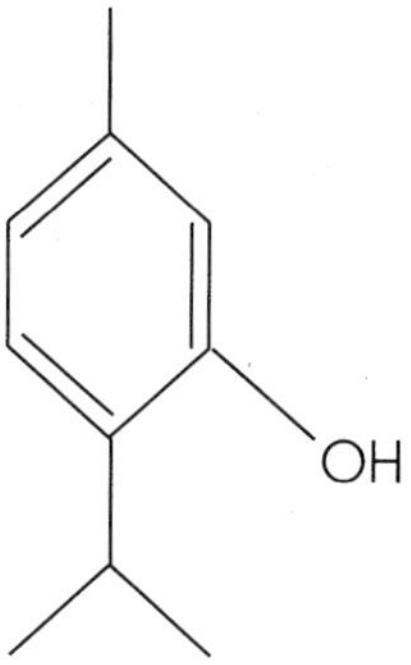

Figure 1.4   Thymol.

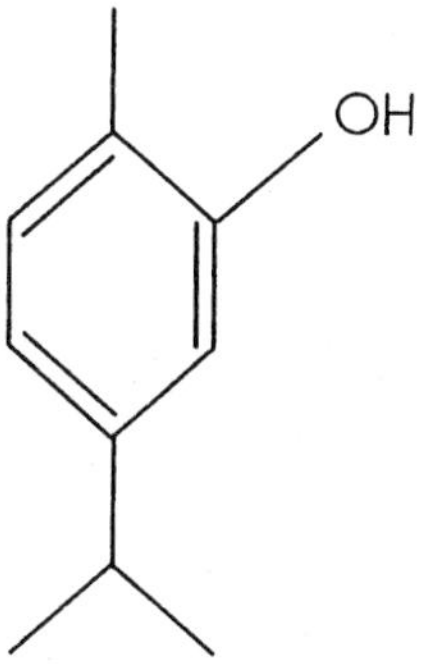

Figure 1.5   Carvacrol.

The thymol and the carvacrol chemotypes do not flourish at high altitudes but are cultivated in the valleys. Both of these phenolic chemotypes are often, although inaccurately, referred to as red thymes, and they are major antiinfective agents with a wide range of action (Belaiche 1979).

The alcohol-containing chemotypes below are commonly referred to as yellow or sweet thymes. These chemotypes, do not have the aggressive effects of the red thymes (thymol and carvacrol) and can be used safely on children, sensitive skins and mucous surfaces (Roulier 1990 p. 305).

• *Thymus vulgaris* ct. linalool. The linalool-bearing thyme has a herbaceous smell and (like the thujanol and terpineol thymes) is grown at high altitudes. It contains the alcohol linalool (Fig. 1.6) and the ester linalyl acetate, therefore the essential oil from the linalool thyme is gentle in action. This chemotype is antibacterial, fungicidal (e.g. against *Candida albicans*), viricidal, parasiticidal and vermifugal, also neurotonic and uterotonic (Franchomme & Pénoël 1990 p. 403).

• *Thymus vulgaris* ct. thujanol-4. In contrast to all the other chemotypes of thyme, the thujanol-4 type does not show seasonal variation in the constitution of the essential oil, but is the same all year round with a content of 50% of the alcohol *trans*-thujanol-4 (Fig. 1.7), 15% approximately of terpinen-4-ol and 15% approximately of *cis*-myrcenol-8. It is found only in the wild because it has so far resisted all attempts to cultivate it—cloning has not yet been successful, except on a very small scale. It is hoped that a new clone currently being grown in southern France will succeed. It has a floral smell. The oil is antiinfective, bactericidal (against *Chlamydia*), and a powerful viricide. It stimulates the immune system (by augmenting IgA) and the circulation. It is described as neurotonic, balancing to the ner-

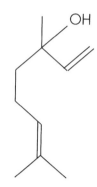

Figure 1.6   Linalool.

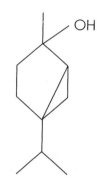

Figure 1.7   Thujanol-4.

vous system, hormone like and antidiabetic (Franchomme & Pénoël 1990 p. 403). According to Roulier (1990 p. 305) this oil is a notable hepatic regenerant, and is non-irritant.

• *Thymus vulgaris* ct. α-terpineol. The oil from this chemotype contains the ester terpenyl acetate (more so in the spring) and the alcohol α-terpineol (Fig. 1.8) (80–90% free and esterified). The smell is slightly peppery.

• *Thymus vulgaris* ct. geraniol. The geraniol thyme grows at high altitude and the oil contains the ester geranyl acetate and the alcohol geraniol (80–90% in free and esterified forms) (Fig. 1.9); again there is a seasonal variation, the thyme chemotype which produces geraniol in the autumn contains geranyl acetate in the spring and geraniol in the autumn (see Table 1.1). This thyme is very assertive and when grown in a field of mixed thymes it gradually comes to predominate. It has a lemony smell. (It is interesting

Table 1.1   Variation in chemotypes of *Thymus vulgaris* with season

Chemotype	Spring	Autumn
Thymol	γ-terpinene + *p*-cymene	thymol
Carvacrol	γ-terpinene + *p*-cymene	carvacrol
Geraniol	geranyl acetate	geraniol

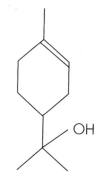

Figure 1.8   α-Terpineol.

Table 1.2   Variation in chemotypes of *Thymus vulgaris* with stage of growth

	Stage of growth		
	Bud	Flower	End of flowering
Carvacrol	22.8	35.9	53.7
Thymol	5	10.7	13.7
p-cymene	32.1	22.4	17.8
γ-terpinene	13.5	7.4	0.9

to note that the creeping wild thyme (*Thymus serpyllum*), which is found everywhere in the hills, also has a somewhat lemony smell because the geraniol chemotype is dominant and is gradually taking over.) The properties are antiviral, antifungal and antibacterial, also uterotonic, neurotonic and cardiotonic (Franchomme & Pénoël 1990 p. 402).

Other *Thymus vulgaris* chemotypes also exist. The cineole-bearing plant has 80–90% 1,8-cineole. According to Franchomme and Pénoël (1990 p. 403), the *p*-cymene chemotype is analgesic when applied to the skin, a notable antiinfective agent and useful for rheumatism and arthritis.

For the thyme chemotypes, the harvesting time is crucial in order to obtain the required composition of an essential oil, as the internal chemistry of the plant changes with the seasons (see also Fig 1.12). Concerning the thymol and carvacrol chemotypes, *p*-cymene is the precursor of both thymol and carvacrol (see Table 1.2); at the beginning of the season, in the spring, the

plants contain γ-terpinene (Fig. 1.10a) and *p*-cymene (Fig. 1.10b), but as the season progresses these precursors are transformed into either carvacrol or thymol, so that plants harvested in the autumn yield essential oils containing the phenols.

Altitude and light

The lower the altitude at which the thyme plant is grown the more pronounced are the following effects:

- the essential oil becomes more aggressive—more phenolic and antiseptic
- the colour of the essential oil also changes, from a light straw to a deeper hue
- the structure of the main component molecule changes from an open chain to a monocyclic chain to an aromatic ring base.

These effects are due in part to the quality of light available to the plant. At high altitudes (above 1000 metres) there is a relatively high amount of free ultraviolet, while at low altitudes there is less ultraviolet and a proportional increase in the more penetrating infrared frequencies. The plant

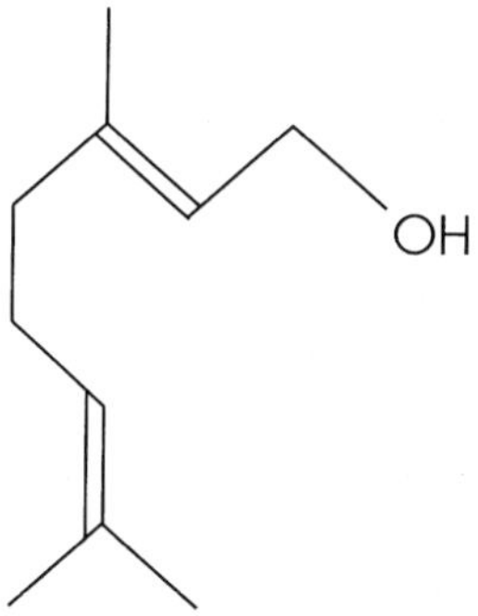

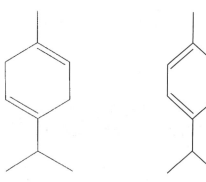

Figure 1.9   Geraniol.

Figure 1.10a   γ-Terpinene.

Figure 1.10b   *p*-cymene.

responds to the quality of light falling on it (and to other growing conditions) and produces different chemicals accordingly. Another influencing factor is the latitude of the country of origin. The further north the plant grows, the more phenols are produced—for instance *Thymus vulgaris* grown in Finland produces up to 89% phenol (von Schantz et al 1987).

More changes may be expected in oil-bearing plants in the future because of chlorofluorocarbon damage to the ozone layer. Higher levels of ultraviolet radiation are expected to reach the surface of the earth, and research carried out to test the possible effects of this on plant growth suggests that alpine species will be least affected by increased ultraviolet radiation. These tests involved *Aquilegia canadensis* and *A. caerulea*. The first normally grows at low altitude, and showed less growth during the test, but the second, alpine, plant was not affected in this way: it even grew extra leaves (Gates 1991).

Rosemary chemotypes

Rosemary has three chemotypes, all of which are used in aromatherapy.

• *Rosmarinus officinalis* ct. camphor (camphor 30%) (Fig. 1.11b) with the properties: mucolytic, cholagogic, diuretic, circulatory decongestant/stimulant (vein), emmenagogic (non-hormonal), muscle relaxant.

• *Rosmarinus officinalis* ct. cineole (1,8-cineole 40–55%) whose properties are anticatarrhal, mucolytic, expectorant, fungicidal (e.g. *Candida albicans*), bactericidal (*Staphylococcus aureus* and *S. alba*).

• *Rosmarinus officinalis* ct. verbenone (Fig. 1.11a) (verbenone 15–40%, α-pinene 15–35%). It is anticatarrhal, expectorant, mucolytic (Roulier 1990 p. 298) and antispasmodic (which Roulier attributes to the cineole and camphor chemotypes—this has been our experience also), cicatrizant and an endocrine system regulator (Franchomme & Pénoël 1990 p. 393).

Roulier (1990) classes the camphor and cineole chemotypes together as having similar effects, as the authors have done in this book, because

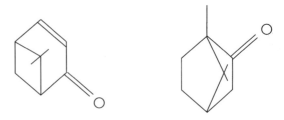

Figure 1.11a Verbenone.   **Figure 1.11b** Camphor.

often rosemary oil contains similar quantities of cineole and camphor.

Other chemotypes

Some further examples of plants with different chemotype forms are:

• *Artemisia dracunculus* [TARRAGON] ct. estragole, ct. sabinene (Tucker & Maciarello 1987)
• *Ocimum basilicum* [BASIL] ct. linalool, ct. estragole, ct. eugenol (Sobti et al 1978)
• *Salvia officinalis* [SAGE] ct. thujone, ct. cineole (there is also a thujone-free chemotype) Tegel 1984, Tucker & Maciarello 1990)
• *Valeriana officinalis* [VALERIAN] ct. valeranone, ct. valeranal, ct. cryptofouranol (Bos, van Putten & Hendri 1986).
• *Melissa officinalis* [LEMON BALM] ct. citral, ct. citronellal (Lawrence 1989).

Clones of lavender and lavandin

True lavender grown from seed is properly called *Lavandula angustifolia* Miller (syn. *L. officinalis*, *L. vera*). However, many cultivated lavender plants are cloned (i.e. grown from cuttings taken from the hardiest, healthiest, most colourful and biggest plants with a high yield of good quality oil), the name of probably the most popular clone being *L. angustifolia* 'Maillette'. Clones contain only the constituents found in the source plant.

Three lavenders are described below:

• *L. angustifolia* contains mainly alcohols and esters. It is a calming oil recommended to induce sleep. However, an overdose has the opposite effect—another pointer to the importance of using these potent oils correctly. It has been recommended for respiratory ailments, asthma, spasmodic cough (whooping cough), influenza, bronchitis, tuberculosis and pneumonia (Valnet 1980) on account of its antiinflammatory properties.

• *Lavandula latifolia* [SPIKE LAVENDER] (syn. *L. spica*) is a much bigger plant, with larger florets than true lavender. It contains very few esters and is slightly lower in alcohol content also, containing instead about 30% of the oxide 1,8-cineole and about 15% of the ketone camphor. It is an efficient expectorant and is also indicated for severe burns (Franchomme & Pénoël 1990 p. 365) because it is well tolerated on all parts of the skin surface. It is especially useful in chest and throat infections, whether for children or adults (Roulier 1990 p. 276).

• *Lavandula stoechas* contains about 75% ketones, of which almost two-thirds is fenchone. It shares some properties with the previous two, being anticatarrhal, antiinflammatory and cicatrizant. This plant, which is believed to be the one used by the Romans in their baths and gave rise to the name lavender, has never been cultivated commercially (Meunier 1985) and is not easily available, which is perhaps fortunate because it is sometimes confused with true lavender, which is almost free of ketones. Its effects can be found in many other, safer oils.

Lavandins

Lavandin is the natural hybrid between *L. angustifolia* Miller and *L. latifolia* Medicus. The resulting plant has been given many taxonomical classifications, such as *Lavandula × burnatii* 'Briq.', *Lavandula spica-latifolia* 'Albert', *Lavandula × hortensis* 'Hy', *Lavandula × leptostachya* 'Pau', etc. All these are in common use along with other names—Duraffourd (1982 p. 77) calls it *Lavandula fragrans*. This confused state of affairs prompted Tucker (1981) to research the situation and he reported that the correct name for lavandin is *Lavandula × intermedia* 'Emeric' ex 'Loiseleur', which covers all the lavandin cultivars, and is the name used in this book.

The '×' in the names above indicates that the plant is a hybrid or cross-pollinated plant and should not be mistaken for a variety of true lavender. Lavandin plants occur naturally, but

cultivators have attempted for many years to find a plant that combines the oil yield of *L. latifolia* with the aromatic quality of *L. angustifolia*. As a result there are many cultivars currently grown, including *L. × intermedia* 'Abrialis', *L. × intermedia* 'Super', *L. × intermedia* 'Grosso' and *L. × intermedia* 'Reydovan'. Although the Abrialis clone is deteriorating after long use, other cultivars are now producing large quantities of lavandin oil. All cultivated lavandin plants are grown from cuttings—they are all clones.

When lavandin is used, especially in clinical trials, it is imperative to specify the particular clone. The two clones of lavandin most used in aromatherapy are:

• *L. × intermedia* 'Reydovan': principally antibacterial, antifungal and antiviral, it is also a nerve tonic and expectorant.

• *L. × intermedia* 'Super' (sometimes known under other names): this on the other hand, is calming and sedative and antiinflammatory. In fact, it seems to have most of the properties of its mother plant, true lavender (Franchomme & Pénoël 1990 p. 364), and its production is on the increase. It was this oil which was used by Buckle (1993) along with true lavender in tests on cardiac patients; the oil from this cultivar of lavandin was found to be more effective than oil of lavender in this instance.

Other factors in plant change

It is not only nature which brings about changes in the chemicals produced in a plant: farmers have an influence too. The use of chemicals in the form of artificial fertilizers influences some of the plant's secondary metabolites, but has little effect on the essential oils. These are composed in the main of carbon, hydrogen and oxygen, whereas fertilizers are made up of nitrogen, phosphates and potassium. However, as fertilizers cause an increase in plant growth, there may be an overall gain in the yield of essential oil.

Herbicides, pesticides and heavy metals are absorbed by the plant, and the more pesticides are absorbed, the more they appear as residue. A safe level of residue may be regarded as 2 mg (per) 1 kg of dry material. Some safe herbicides are decomposed in the plant, but still add to the residue levels. In Europe, toxic pesticides are prohibited, but unfortunately they are still manufactured and sent to third world countries (Wabner 1993). Heavy metals do not pass over in the steam distillation process.

Toxic residues are easily transferred to expressed oils, absolutes and vegetable oils, which makes it necessary to know the source and the manner of growing of such oils before using them therapeutically. Although many pesticides contain volatile molecules, it is not clear how many of these are taken into a distilled oil. Wabner (1993) concludes that 'aromatherapy is much safer than eating' because 'no clear cut correlation has been established between pesticide residues in oils and detrimental effects on the human organism' and 'essential oils are used in much smaller quantities and much less frequently than food products'. This article emphasizes the fact that health professionals should purchase their oils for therapeutic use from a trusted supplier, who knows where to procure high quality, pesticide-free, unadulterated essential oils and fixed vegetable oils, especially as the latter normally make up 95% or more of any oil prepared for application to the skin.

Yield of essential oils

Many factors affect the yield, in terms of both quantity and quality, of an essential oil. Some are under the control of the farmer, e.g. time of harvest, chemicals used and plant selection, and others are more or less beyond control, e.g. available light, altitude, temperature and rain (although drought can be remedied by use of a watering system).

Essential oils are not spread equally throughout all parts of the plant, and the quantity of essential oil varies throughout the growing season to such a degree that the time of harvesting, even to the time of day, can have a critical effect on the quantity and quality of the essential oil derived (Fig. 1.12).

The farmer may have to face the fact that the time of maximum yield of essential oil may not coincide with the quality required. This is

especially so when the oils are intended for therapeutic use, when compromise on quantity against quality cannot be accepted.

SOME ESSENTIAL-OIL-PRODUCING FAMILIES

Plants are divided into families, and it is generally recognized that familial therapeutic characteristics may be ascribed to many of the individual plants in a particular family, e.g. the beneficial influence on the digestive system of

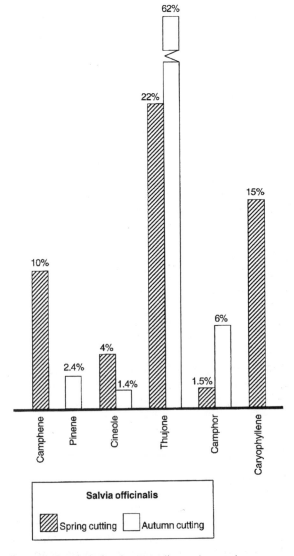

Figure 1.12 Variation in sage oil constituents between spring and autumn cuttings (Lamy 1985, 1988).

the citrus oils or the warming action of oils from the ginger family. There can also be toxic familial effects as with the Solanaceae and Apiaceae. Several hundred plant essential oils have been identified worldwide. Many are not commercially available, either because the yield of distilled oil is so small that the cost is prohibitive (as in the case of lime blossom oil) or because there is no commercial demand for them. Between 40 and 60 essential oils are normally used by the professional aromatherapist, and most suppliers offer in the region of 70–80. These oils generally belong to just a few of the many plant families, and the families dealt with below include the majority of plants utilized in the production of essential oils.

In the text below, the common names have been used, since to name each species or variety is not necessary when giving general familial characteristics. The botanical name will be used when talking about a specific essential oil. Where only one oil from a family is used in aromatherapy, no family characteristics will be given, only the therapeutic properties of that individual oil. Where there are several oils in a family, only the family properties will be given. Individual properties of selected individual oils can be found in Appendix A (p. 313). The lists are not comprehensive, since reference can be made to the many books written on the properties of essential oils for details of oils not mentioned here. Neither will every essential oil appear in the lists—the main purpose of this book is to make health professionals aware of the principal beneficial essential oils.

Reference sources for the properties and effects of the essential oils below are as follows: Bardeau (1976), Bernadet (1983), Duraffourd (1982), Franchomme & Pénoël (1990), Lautié & Passebecq (1984), Mailhebiau (1989), Roulier (1990). Other references will be mentioned individually.

Angiospermae

Because they bear seeds, all the plants used to obtain essential oils belong to the Spermatophyta subdivision. The vast majority also belong to the class Angiospermae, or flowering plants.

Anonaceae

This family consists of only one species, *Cananga odorata*, with two varieties, of which ylang ylang is one (*C. odorata* forma *genuina*). Distillation is carried out in several stages, and the resulting oils (superior, extra and grades one, two and three) each have a slightly different aroma. It is not easy to procure the complete oil, which would be preferable for the holistic aspect of aromatherapy (Price 1993). *C. odorata* is antiinflammatory, antispasmodic, hypotensive, sedative and a tonic to the pancreas.

Apiaceae (or Umbelliferae)

Examples include aniseed, caraway, coriander, dill and fennel. In this family the oils are usually extracted from the seeds, which are renowned for their digestive properties. They have been used in digestive and aperitif drinks and consumed for centuries with bread, and as an accompaniment with cheeses such as Munster. Umbellifer therapeutic qualities are aromatic, carminative, stimulating, tonic and warming when they are grown naturally in dry regions. It should be noted that this family is also known as the hemlocks. If grown in the shade or humid regions a narcotic principle can develop (particularly so for green anise), and many of the oils in this family are neurotoxic because of the presence of particular ketones or phenolic ethers.

Asteraceae (or Compositae)

Examples include calendula (only available in a fixed oil), the chamomiles, tagetes and tarragon. The essential oils from plants in the Asteraceae are taken from the flowerheads. In the case of calendula they are macerated in a fixed oil—not distilled, so the fixed oil also contains larger non-volatile plant molecules, e.g. some coloured molecules. Two of the main characteristics of essential oils in this family are their antiinflammatory and antiseptic action on the skin and digestive tract, notably oils from the chamomiles. Many toxic oils come from this family, e.g. the artemisias, which contain a high percentage of ketones or phenolic ethers. *Tagetes glandulifera* also contains a ketone (tagetone) at 50% and should be used with caution.

Burseraceae

Examples include frankincense (olibanum) and myrrh. These two are available as distilled oils and as resinoids, but the distilled oils are required for therapeutic use. The family has cicatrizant properties, indicating their use for scar tissue, ulcers and wounds. They are also expectorant, and useful in catarrhal conditions. *Boswellia carteri* [FRANKINCENSE] is also indicated in the treatment of depression, immune system deficiency and perhaps cancer (Franchomme & Pénoël 1990 p. 328).

Geranaceae

The oil utilized from this small family comes from one or two species belonging to the *Pelargonium* genus. The essential oil of *Pelargonium graveolens* [GERANIUM] has anti-inflammatory, astringent, cicatrizant and haemostatic properties and is antidiabetic (Valnet 1980 p. 133).

Lamiaceae (or Labiatae)

This is by far the biggest family from which essential oils are gained; examples include basil, clary, hyssop, lavandin, lavender, marjoram, melissa, origanum, patchouli, peppermint, rosemary, sage, savory and thyme. Of all the families in the plant kingdom none offers a greater array of healing aromatic plants than the Lamiaceae. These plants are strongly aromatic owing to the volatile essence stored in special glandular trichomes, which are found principally on the leaves. In general the Lamiaceae produce aromatic and stimulating essential oils, which bring vigour and energy to the whole body (or sometimes to just one system in particular, e.g. the respiratory system). They have remarkable antiseptic and antispasmodic properties and some are also emmenagogic and sudorific. Oils derived from the Lamiaceae are generally safe, with one or two exceptions such as *Salvia*

officinalis [SAGE] and *Hyssopus officinalis* [HYSSOP], both of which contain ketones (thujone and pinocamphone respectively), which could be neurotoxic in overdose. Ingestion of large quantities of these oils can lead to serious disorders, as pointed out by the Centre Anti-poisons de Marseille (Rouvière & Meyer 1983 p. 6).

Many of the plants in this family have been in constant culinary use for thousands of years, not only to add flavour but for their preservative and health-giving properties as well. The use and ingestion of herbs and their essential oils in small doses over such a long period of time proves their fundamental safety.

Lauraceae

Examples include cinnamon and camphor. Members of this family generally have a pleasant aroma, sometimes strong and penetrating, a warm pungency, and are sometimes bitter. All the oils are considered to be uplifting in their effects (Rouvière & Meyer 1983 p. 7). However, the majority of the family are highly toxic (e.g. cassia, laurel and sassafras), and they will not be recommended in this book because similar therapeutic properties can be found in other safer oils. Even when they are not actually dangerous, these oils still need extra care in use.

Myrtaceae

Examples include cajuput, eucalyptus, niaouli, clove and tea tree. The essential oils from this family are contained in cells in the body of the leaf. They are powerful antiseptics (especially to the respiratory system) as well as being antiviral (see Table 4.6), astringent, stimulant and tonic.

It is advisable to use them with caution as they can be irritant. This is particularly so of clove and adulterated niaouli. It is worth mentioning that the latter oil is adulterated more often than not and will not have the desired therapeutic effect. Care should be taken to obtain the genuine oil. Rectified *Eucalyptus globulus* [TASMANIAN BLUE GUM] is irritant because the natural balance has been destroyed. It can be identified because the rectification process renders it clear, and unfortunately very little of the eucalyptus oil harvest escapes this fate.

Oleaceae

Jasminum officinale is a well-loved oil, but a steam-distilled essential oil does not exist and the absolute is subject to the most deplorable adulteration. 'A large number of synthetic materials, some of them chemically related to the jasmones … are of great help … to reproduce the much wanted jasmine effect at a much lower cost. … Jasmine absolute is frequently adulterated. Its high cost seems to tempt certain suppliers and producers beyond their moral resistance' (Arctander 1960 pp. 310–311). If it is to be used therapeutically at all, only the finest quality should be sought and purchased. It is often used as a relaxant on account of its aroma.

Piperaceae

Examples include black pepper and cubeb. *Piper nigrum* is the most used of the two oils and possesses analgesic, anticatarrhal, expectorant, stimulant and tonic properties.

Poaceae or Gramineae

Examples include citronella, lemongrass, palmarosa and vetiver. Most of this family have antiinflammatory and tonic properties, *Vetivera zizanioides* [VETIVER] also being stimulating to the immune system (Franchomme & Pénoël 1990 p. 405). Oils from this family, together with lemon and/or grapefruit oil, are used to make a cheap 'melissa' oil.

Rosaceae

The only essential oil utilized from this family is rose otto, whose aroma is less sweet than the absolute oil obtained by solvent extraction. Strictly speaking, only the distilled oil should be used by health professionals (see *J. officinale* above). Rose otto has astringent, antihaemorrhagic, cicatrizant, hormonal and neurotonic properties.

Rutaceae

Citrus oils are derived from three different sites in the plant. Examples are:

- peel: bergamot, grapefruit, lemon, mandarin and orange
- leaf: petitgrain oils, mainly from the bitter orange, but occasionally from other citrus trees
- flower: neroli, mainly from the bitter orange tree for therapeutic purposes

To obtain citrus peel oils for aromatherapy the rinds are not distilled, but mechanically squeezed by a method called expression. They are therefore not strictly essential oils and contain many large molecules, which would not come over in distillation. These include colour and waxes, and the latter can precipitate if the oils are stored incorrectly or kept for a long time. In storage these oils are especially susceptible to oxidation and the precious active aldehydes may degrade into acids. To help prevent this, nitrogen gas is used to displace the air as the oil is decanted. For small bottles, the air can be displaced with tiny glass beads as the level of the oil goes down with use.

Expressed oils from the citrus family have a refreshing aroma and are antiseptic, stimulating and tonic, having significant effects on the whole of the digestive tract. This is especially true of bergamot and bitter orange, which are stomach antispasmodics. These two are also sedative to the nervous system.

Both leaf and flower oils from *Citrus aurantium* [ORANGE] are obtained by distillation and their aroma is sweeter and more floral than that of the peel oils. The best leaf and flower oils are obtained from the bitter orange, *C. aurantium* var. *amara*: both of these oils are effective on the nervous system, relieving irritability and promoting sleep (Mailhebiau 1989 pp. 269–270). Petitgrain bigarade from the bitter orange tree (bigarade means 'bitter') is indicated for infected acne, whereas neroli bigarade is indicated for varicose veins and haemorrhoids, and is also a hypotensor.

Styraceae

The only extracts from this family which are of interest to aromatherapists are the resinoids from *Styrax tonkinensis* and *S. benzoin* (both have the common name benzoin). This resinoid is anticatarrhal and expectorant. It is also cicatrizant, promoting healing on cracked and dry skin. Care should be taken when purchasing this oil: some sources abroad still use benzene as a solvent (forbidden in Europe), and a high proportion of benzene may remain in the final product.

Valerianaceae

Examples include valerian and spikenard. The general family effects are calming and sedative, and they are helpful in the reduction of varicose veins and haemorrhoids. The true oil is very difficult to obtain.

Verbenaceae

Aloysia triphylla (= *Lippia citriodora*) [LEMON VERBENA] is rarely obtainable; like jasmine it is frequently grossly adulterated and *Thymus hiemalis* is often sold in its place as Spanish verbena (Arctander 1960 pp. 648–649).

Gymnospermae

The Gymnospermae display their seeds directly, rather than hiding them within a structure of petals. The important oil-bearing plants of this class belong to the order Coniferae (cone-bearing plants).

Cupressaceae and Pinaceae

Examples include cypress, juniper (Cupressaceae), pine and cedar (Abietaceae). The chief common characteristics of essential oils derived from plants in these two families of the conifer order are their good general hygienic qualities, particularly in the air and on the skin. Cedar, cypress and juniper also have specific individual properties for urinary tract infections, the circulatory system and scalp maladies (Rouvière & Meyer 1983 p. 7). Thuja belongs to the Pinaceae, but is not used in aromatherapy because of its toxic high ketone content. These two families are noted for their beneficial effects on the respiratory system.

Summary

Traditionally, plants have been the main source of materials to maintain health and prevent ill health, and it is only comparatively recently that they have been replaced by synthetics. The study of plant structure and function should not be regarded as an interesting but inessential requirement for aromatherapy. The more knowledgeable the therapist is about the exact botanical derivation of the oils used, the more effective he can be in practice.

REFERENCES

Arctander S 1960 Perfume and flavour materials of natural origin. Published by the author, Elizabeth, New Jersey
Bardeau F 1976 La médecine aromatique. Laffont, Paris
Belaiche P 1979 Traité de phytothérapie et d'aromathérapie, vol 1. Maloine, Paris p 93
Bernadet M 1983 La phyto-aromathérapie pratique. Dangles, St-Jean-de-Braye
Bos R, van Putten F M S, Hendriks H 1986 Variations in the essential oil content and composition in individual plants obtained after breeding experiments with a *Valeriana*

officinalis strain. In: Brunke E J (ed) Progress in essential oil research. W de Gruyter, Hamburg, pp 223–230
Buckle J 1993 Does it matter which lavender essential oil is used? Nursing Times 89(20): 32–35
Carlton R R 1990 An investigation into the rapidly induced responses of *Myrica gale* to insect herbivory. Unpublished PhD Thesis, University of Strathclyde
Carlton R R, Gray A I, Waterman P G 1992 The antifungal activity of the leaf gland oil of sweet gale (*Myrica gale*). Chemecology 3: 55–59

Craker L E 1990 Herbs and volatile oils. Herb, Spice and Medicinal Plant Digest 8(4): 1–5

Deans S G, Waterman P G 1993 Biological activity of volatile oils. In: Hay R K M, Waterman P G (eds) Volatile oil crops. Longman, Harlow pp 100–101

Duraffourd P 1982 En forme tous les jours. La Vie Claire, Périgny

Franchomme P, Pénoël D 1990 L'aromathérapie exactement. Jollois, Limoges

Gates P 1991 Gardening in tomorrow's world. Gardener's World July: 4

Harborne J B 1988 Introduction to ecological biochemistry. Academic Press, London

Lamy J 1985 De la culture à la distilleries. Quelques facteurs influant sur la composition des huiles essentielles. Chambre d'Agriculture de la Drôme, Valence

Lamy J 1988 Présentation de 30 huiles essentielles typées produites dans la Drôme. Congress des Parfumeurs Allemandes: 23–25

Lautié R, Passebecq A 1984 Aromatherapy. Thorsons, Wellingborough

Lawrence B M 1989 Progress in essential oils. Perfumer and Flavorist 14(3): 71

Mailhebiau P 1989 La nouvelle aromathérapie. Vie Nouvelle, Toulouse

Meunier C 1985 Lavandes et lavandins. Edisud, Aix-en-Provence

Price S 1993 The aromatherapy workbook. Thorsons, London, p 116,117

Roulier G 1990 Les huiles essentielles pour votre santé. Dangles, St-Jean-de-Braye

Rouvière A, Meyer M C 1983 La santé par les huiles essentielles. M A Editions, Paris

Sobti S N, Pushpangadan P, Thapa R K, Aggarwal S G, Vashist V N, Atal C K 1978 Chemical and genetic investigations in essential oils of some Ocimum species, their F1 hybrids and synthesised allopolyploids. Lloydia 41: 50–55

Tegel C 1984 Morphologische und chemische Variabilität sowie Anbau und Verwendung von Salvia sp (Salbei). Unpublished MSc Thesis, Technical University of Munich

Tucker A O 1981 The correct name of lavandin and its cultivars (Labiatae). Baileya 21: 131–133

Tucker A O, Maciarello M J 1987 Plant identification. In: Simon J E, Grant L (eds) Proceedings of the first national herb growing and marketing conference. Purdue University Press, West Lafayette, pp 341–372

Tucker A O, Maciarello M J 1990 Essential oils of cultivars of Dalmation sage (Salvia officinalis L). Journal of Essential Oil Research 2: 139–144

Valnet J 1980 The practice of aromatherapy. Daniel, Saffron Walden

Verlet N 1993 Commercial aspects. In: Hay R K M, Waterman P G (eds) Volatile oil crops. Longman, Harlow, ch 8, p 144

von Schantz M, Holm Y, Hiltunen R, Galambosi B 1987 Arznei- und Gewürzpflanzenversuche zum Anbau in Finnland. Deutsche Apotheke Zeitung 127: 2543–2548

Wabner D 1993 Purity and pesticides. International Journal of Aromatherapy 5(2): 27–29

Chemistry and quality

2

Introduction

The highest possible quality of medicament is always required in therapy. This chapter shows that aromatherapy is no exception to the rule. The main chemical groups found in essential oils are outlined, along with an account of methods of testing for quality.

GENUINE ESSENTIAL OILS

In medicine the quality and wholeness of any essential oils used are of paramount importance, irrespective of the cost, whereas when used in flavours and fragrances the taste and the aroma respectively are the most important considerations. For the food and perfume industries essential oils may be adjusted or changed to suit the particular need of the purchaser or the vendor.

In these commercial enterprises price is an important consideration, and standardized essential oils are necessary to ensure repeatability and consistent quality. It is tacitly accepted that traders in essential oils add other cheaper oils or synthetics to the genuine oils, in order to maintain the same standard taste, aroma and price for successive repeat deliveries to the same customer.

Natural and commercial variations

Wine is a commodity which is expected to have a different taste and character from year to year although harvested, processed and bottled at the same vineyard and from the same vines. The differences are even welcomed and certainly make for conversational one-upmanship! Plants, whether grown to make wine or essential oils, are subject to varying amounts of sunshine, frost, rain, heat or cold each year and it is these factors, plus the composition of the soil, which are responsible for the variations in quality in the plant extracts (and the bouquet in the case of essential oils) occurring naturally from year to year. However, in the essential oil world of perfumery and flavouring, this natural variation cannot be tolerated. Müller et al (1984) outline some contributory factors that lead essential oil merchants to modify the natural product: 'bad harvests, political conflicts, exhaustion of the soil or transportation difficulties are imponderables which make it impossible for the perfumer to rely entirely on Nature's raw materials. Against that background, synthetic fragrance substances appear as *economically indispensable substitutes for Nature's originals*' (Authors' italics).

Most aromatherapy suppliers purchase their essential oils from importers who mainly supply the perfume and food industries, but this is not always a good and reliable source for unadulterated oils for therapeutic use. As Steffen Arctander explains in his book:

The author has nothing in principle against the addition of foreign or 'unnatural' materials to essential oils etc. as long as the intention and the result is an indisputable improvement in respect to perfumery performance and effect. ... However, the above philosophy should not indicate that the author approves of adulteration of natural perfume materials: quite the contrary. But the meaning of the term adulteration should be taken literally: with the intention of acquiring the business (order) through a devaluation of the oil in relation to the labelling of its container. The consumers of perfume oils are buying odor, not physico-chemical data. If the odor and the perfumery (or flavor-) effect is in agreement with the customer's standards, there is no reason to talk about adulteration: the oil is then worth the full price of a true, natural oil and the 'adulteration', if any, has not been a means of direct economical gains.

(Arctander 1960)

In contradistinction to the above, the aromatherapist is buying not merely an odour, but wishes above all to acquire the physicochemical characteristics; however, these may vary from harvest to harvest.

Essential oils are made up of distinct natural chemicals, many of which are found in more than one oil. It is a fairly simple matter for the chemist to remove a desired constituent from a cheap oil and add it to an expensive oil in order to lower the price for a customer, or to sell a modified 'pure' oil to an unsuspecting customer for a high price. Adulteration also takes place when a synthetic isolate is added, especially to one of the costly oils such as rose otto, when synthetic phenyl ethyl alcohol (occurring naturally in rose otto) is used as the adulterant. Alcohol, and occasionally a small amount of vegetable oil, which are both good solvents for essential oils, are also used to adulterate, stretch, or cut Nature's gifts, and many descriptive words are used to justify the standardization sometimes necessary in the fragrance and food industries. 'Certain suppliers with highly developed imagination will even use the term "ennobling" for the disfiguration of an essential oil' (Arctander 1960).

The need for genuine oils

The following case cited by Valnet (1980) illustrates perfectly the need to use genuine essential oils in therapeutic treatments:

A patient being treated for a fistula of the anus by the instillation of pure and natural drops of lavender and who was beginning to recover, had to go on a journey. Having forgotten his essential oil, he purchased a further supply from a chemist. Unfortunately, this essence was neither pure nor natural; one single instillation resulted in such severe inflammation that the patient was unable to sit down for over two weeks.

(Valnet 1980 p. 27)

Essential oils used in the fragrance industry often have their terpenes partly or wholly removed on account of their insolubility in alcohol, which would result in cloudiness—a distinct commercial and aesthetic disadvantage in a perfume! To the therapist, however, a deterpenated oil is incomplete. It then contains a higher percentage of the remaining constituents of the oil. For example, the deterpenation of peppermint increases the content of the possibly hazardous ketone menthone. 'In perfumery, certain essential oils are deterpenised, because too high a degree of terpenes reduces their solubility in alcohol. In aromatherapy, there is no necessity for this, and … it is preferable to avoid interfering with the natural balance of the essence' (Lautié & Passebecq 1984 p. 15).

Some therapists purchase bergapten-free bergamot oil, as this constituent (a furanocoumarin) can be responsible for phototoxicity of the skin in sunlight (see discussion of this in Chapter 3).

Natural wholeness and synergy

It is important also to preserve the wholeness of an essential oil in order to guard its natural synergy (from the Greek *syn* = together, *ergon* = work). The components making up an essential oil cooperate to produce their healing effect and, if these are altered in any way, the natural synergy is upset. When a single active component is removed, not only is the synergy of the remaining constituents diminished, but the isolated component generally needs much greater care when used alone—it may produce side-effects with continued use. However, when present in the whole oil, the other constituents seem to act as 'quenchers' of these unwanted effects, enabling the oil to be used without harm (see Synergy and Quenching in Ch. 3).

It is extremely difficult to judge the probable effects of an essential oil solely by knowing its principal chemical constituent(s), important though this knowledge is. The whole oil has to be considered in all its complexity, with the mixture of possibly hundreds of different types of molecules, their molecular energy and the overall synergy. There is no simple direct relationship between any one of the chemical constituents and the therapeutic effect—or even the hazard— of the whole essential oil (Price 1990).

Ambiguous BP standards

Some essential oils listed in the British Pharmacopoeia (BP) are stocked in hospital pharmacies, but oils prepared to BP standards may not be suitable for use in aromatherapy. One reason for this is that many plants, for example thyme, *Thymus vulgaris*, exist in the wild as many

different chemotypes, some of which are propagated and grown from cuttings, each chemotype producing quite a different essential oil in make-up and therapeutic action (see Ch. 1), but these differences are not reflected in the pharmacopoeia. Another reason is imprecise specification. For instance, a request for lavender may produce *Lavandula angustifolia*, *L. × intermedia* or perhaps *L. spica*, all of which have different properties and indications. According to the BP (1993) eucalyptus essential oil may be any one of four different species, which when unrectified may have different properties and indications, even though the principal constituent in each case is the oxide 1,8-cineole. The same source states that it is not always the whole oil which is used therapeutically—it may be an incomplete oil (e.g. terpeneless), an active constituent, or even prepared synthetically.

CHEMISTRY OF ESSENTIAL OILS

For the safe practice of aromatherapy it is essential to have at least a basic understanding of the chemistry of the essential oils before being able to use them in a meaningful, caring and effective way—not at random, or indiscriminately. Such understanding makes it evident that certain chemicals may have certain effects—'may' because, as stated above, there is no direct link between even the major components of an essential oil and the effects of the complete oil. These complex relationships are little understood at present because hundreds of different chemicals are involved, and many of them are unknown. Suffice it to say that knowledge of the basic composition of each oil contributes to the overall background knowledge of aromatherapy, thus promoting confidence and aiding selection of the oils to be used, until such time as more is discovered about the interaction of the plant chemicals within the human body.

The list of the physiological and pharmacological properties of aromatic molecules encompasses almost all the organs and all the functions of the organism, from skin conditions to psychological disturbances. Chemists have identified more than 3000 different aromatic molecules, and new ones are continually being discovered. Fortunately, these molecules are gathered in main groups or families, with a relationship between the chemical function and the pharmacological activities. Although we use whole essential oils and not isolated molecules, it is necessary to undertake the study not only of the classes of molecules but also a few important individual molecules and possible actions.

Essential oil components

It is not the intention to give a lesson in organic chemistry in this book, but a brief explanation of the building blocks of essential oils will be helpful. Carbon, hydrogen, oxygen are essential to life itself, and all three are contained in every essential oil. They combine in countless mono- and sesquiterpenic families of hydrocarbons, alcohols, aldehydes, ketones, acids, phenols, esters and coumarins (and furanocoumarins).

Hydrocarbons

Terpenic hydrocarbons consist only of hydrogen and carbon atoms, arranged in a chain—which can be either straight or branched. The basic building block for these chains is the isoprene unit—comprising five carbon atoms (Fig. 2.1a). See Chapter 1 page 9; for the basic chemistry leading up to the isoprene unit see Price 1993.

Aliphatic chains

Two isoprene units joined together head to tail form the basis of all monoterpenes (monoterpenic hydrocarbons have 10 carbon atoms) (Figs 2.1b, 2.1c). Three units provide the basic structure for the larger molecules known as sesquiterpenes (sesquiterpenic hydrocarbons have 15 carbon atoms) (Fig. 2.2a). Four isoprene units joined

together are called diterpenes (diterpenic hydrocarbons have 20 carbon atoms) (Fig. 2.2b), and are not often met with in steam-distilled oils because they are almost too heavy to come over in the distillation process—only a few diterpenes manage it. All these chains are known as aliphatic hydrocarbons.

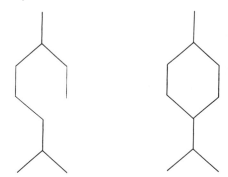

Figure 2.1b   Two isoprene units join to form an acyclic chain.

Figure 2.1c   Two isoprene units join to form a cyclic chain.

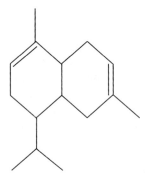

Figure 2.2a   α-Cadinene (15C). Three isoprene units join to form a sesquiterpene.

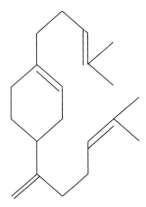

Figure 2.2b   α-Camphorene (20C). Four isoprene units join to form a diterpene.

Figure 2.1a   Carbon skeleton of the isoprene unit.

Terpenic hydrocarbons are generally recognizable from their name: all end in -ene. They are all slightly antiseptic and bactericidal (Franchomme & Pénoël 1990 p. 220, Roulier 1990 p. 51) and may play an important part in the quenching effect mentioned earlier, thus making deterpenated oils unsuitable for aromatherapeutic purposes.

NB. In the chemical families discussed below, the general therapeutic properties attributed to each of the families is based on an unproven theory (set out in detail in Franchomme & Pénoël 1990 pp. 96–114) which associates certain properties with the esters, alcohols, etc., taking into account the electronegative/positive nature of the molecules coupled with their polar/apolar properties. Although this information is a useful general guide to the probable properties of the chemical families discussed, the information given may not hold true for each and every compound (e.g. alcohols are given the familial characteristic of being stimulating, but the alcohol linalool shows as a sedative—see Table 4.9—when tested on mice, although the results obtained in animal testing do not necessarily extrapolate directly to humans). In any case, aromatherapists do not use isolated compounds, but whole essential oils, and while it is interesting to study the effects of single compounds it is worth repeating the statement made above that there is not necessarily any simple direct relationship between the therapeutic effect of any one constituent and that of the whole essential oil.

Explanation of the term 'cyclic'

Sometimes an aliphatic straight chain can, as it were, loop round itself (Fig. 2.1c) and give the *appearance* of an aromatic ring, although it is still a 10-carbon chain. When this looping occurs, the terpene is said to be monocyclic, because one circle has been created, and therefore the complete description is monocyclic monoterpene. More than one circle can arise in a chain, so that it is possible to have a tricyclic sesquiterpenic alcohol. If they do not form a circle at all (i.e. if they form a straight chain) they are said to be acyclic (as in Fig. 2.1b).

To be precise, these terms describing the chains—or the term 'aromatic' (ring-based—see The aromatic ring, below) should be included when describing a particular chemical constituent of an essential oil, e.g.

- geraniol—an acyclic monoterpenic alcohol
- patchoulol—a tricyclic sesquiterpenic alcohol
- citronellal—an acyclic monoterpenic aldehyde
- cinnamic aldehyde—an aromatic aldehyde
- geranic acid—an acyclic monoterpenic acid
- cinnamic acid—an aromatic acid, etc.

Not enough is yet understood about the pharmacological effects of essential oils to know how each type may differ in effect.

Monoterpenes (see Fig. 2.3 for examples) occur to different degrees in almost all essential oils, and in addition to having the antiseptic and bactericidal properties mentioned above they may also be analgesic, expectorant and stimulating (Franchomme & Pénoël 1990 pp. 217–224).

Sesquiterpenes

As well as the antiseptic and bactericidal properties mentioned above, the sesquiterpenes (Figs 2.2a, 2.4) as a class are said to be anti-inflammatory, calming and slight hypotensors; some are analgesic and/or spasmolytic (Franchomme & Pénoël 1990 pp. 217–224).

Diterpenes

Diterpenes (Fig. 2.2b) are believed to have the further properties of being expectorant and purgative and some are antifungal and antiviral. Some appear to have a balancing effect on the hormonal system, e.g. the diterpenic alcohol sclareol in *Salvia sclarea* [CLARY] (and also the sesquiterpenic alcohol viridiflorol in *Melaleuca viridiflora* [NIAOULI]) (Pénoël 1993 personal communication).

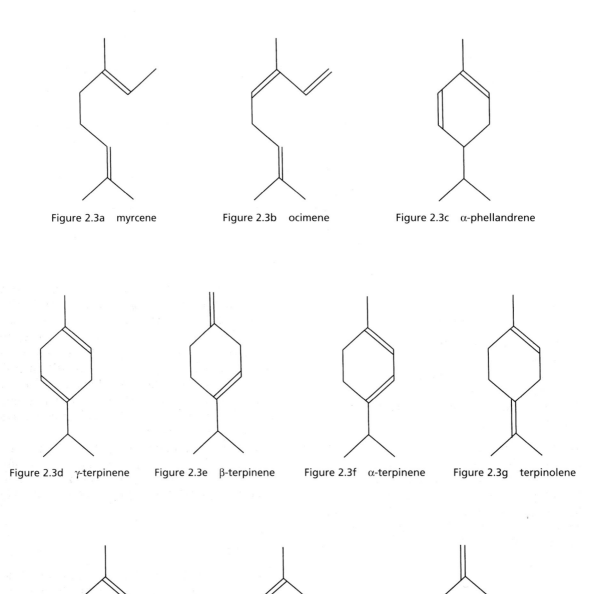

Figure 2.3a   myrcene   Figure 2.3b   ocimene   Figure 2.3c   α-phellandrene

Figure 2.3d   γ-terpinene   Figure 2.3e   β-terpinene   Figure 2.3f   α-terpinene   Figure 2.3g   terpinolene

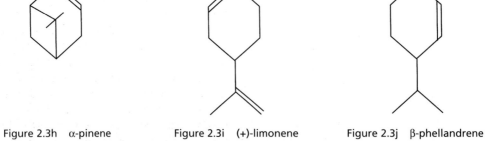

Figure 2.3h   α-pinene   Figure 2.3i   (+)-limonene   Figure 2.3j   β-phellandrene

Figure 2.3   Examples of monoterpenic hydrocarbons.

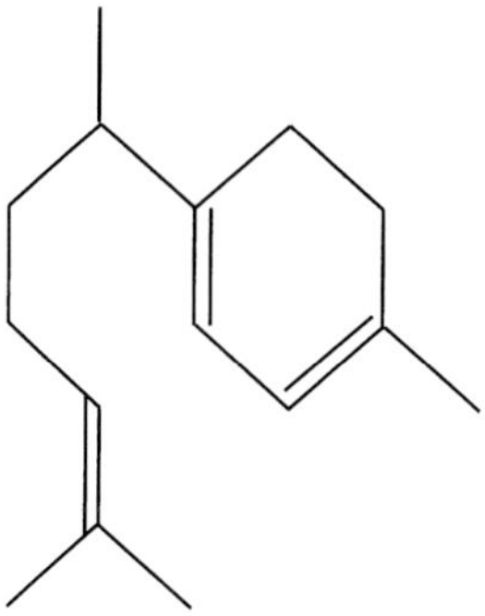

Figure 2.4a γ-curcumene 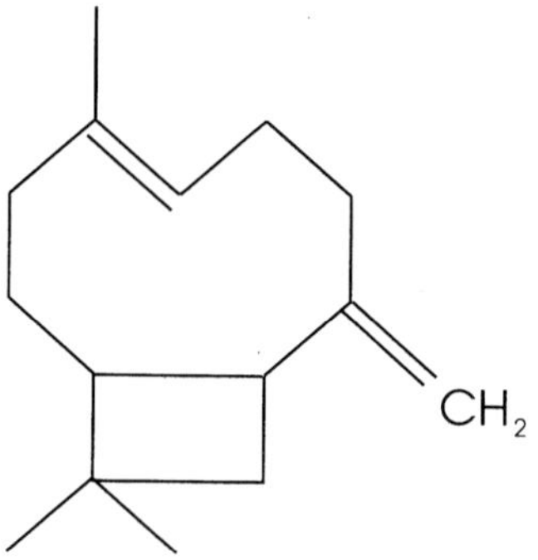   Figure 2.4b caryophyllene 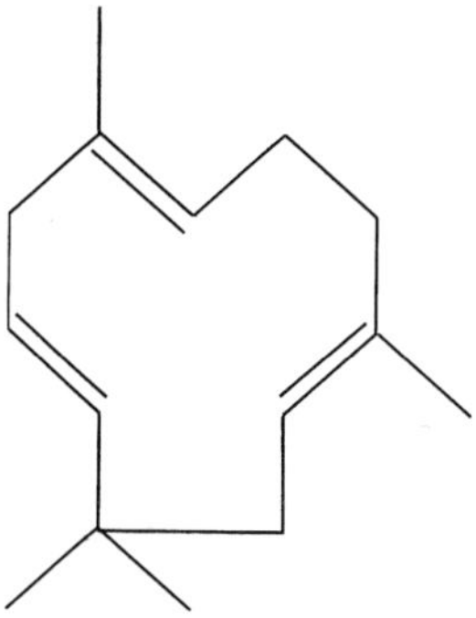   Figure 2.4c humulene

Figure 2.4 Sesquiterpenic hydrocarbons.

The aromatic ring

The second building block occurs when six carbon atoms join together in the form of a ring; this has three names in common use:

1. aromatic ring, because many of the substances based on it are aromatic
2. benzene ring, because the substance so formed is benzene
3. phenyl ring, because phenols are formed from this base.

Thus we find both aliphatic and aromatic aldehydes, ketones and organic acids (involving both chain and ring building blocks) occurring naturally in essential oils. However, when the hydroxyl radical –OH is attached to a chain it is an aliphatic alcohol (Fig. 2.5a); when the same radical is attached to a ring it is an aromatic phenol (Fig. 2.5b).

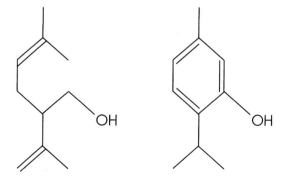

Figure 2.5a Lavandulol (alcohol).

Figure 2.5b Thymol (phenol).

Alcohols

When a hydroxyl radical, consisting of one oxygen atom and one hydrogen atom (–OH), joins on to one of the carbons in an aliphatic chain by displacing one of the hydrogen molecules, an alcohol (Fig. 2.6) is formed: a monoterpenol, sesquiterpenol or diterpenol, depending on whether the chain to which it attaches itself has two, three or four isoprene units. The name of the alcohol so formed always ends in -ol, e.g. geraniol.

Alcohols are antiinfectious, strongly bactericidal, antiviral and stimulating; they are generally non-toxic in use and do not cause skin irritation (Franchomme & Pénoël 1990 p. 115, Roulier 1990 p. 53).

Phenols

When the same hydroxyl group attaches itself to a carbon in an aromatic (or phenyl) ring, the resulting molecule is known as a phenol (Fig. 2.7), which is a kind of alcohol, and has strong effects. Phenols also have names which end in 'ol', e.g. carvacrol; to discriminate between the two classes it is necessary to learn the names of the most important members in each group.

Phenols, like alcohols, are antiseptic and bactericidal. Because they stimulate both the nervous system (making them effective against depressive illness) and the immune system, they activate the body's own healing process. However,

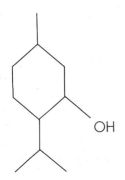

Figure 2.6a   linalool
(aliphatic monoterpenic)

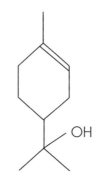

Figure 2.6b   α-terpineol
(monocyclic monoterpenic)

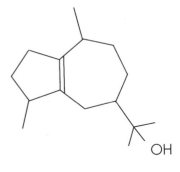

Figure 2.6c   guaiol
(bicyclic sesquiterpenic)

Figure 2.6d   menthol
(monocyclic monoterpenic)

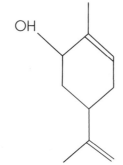

Figure 2.6e   carveol
(monocyclic monoterpenic)

Figure 2.6f   borneol
(bicyclic monoterpenic)

Figure 2.6   Alcohols.

Figure 2.7a   carvacrol

Figure 2.7b   chavicol

Figure 2.7   Phenols.

because the –OH is attached to a ring rather than to a chain molecule, aromatic phenols, unlike the aliphatic alcohols, can be toxic to the liver and irritant to the skin if used in substantial amounts or for too long a time (Roulier 1990 pp. 51–52). 'Some oils—for example, thyme and origanum—owe their value in the pharmaceutical field almost entirely to the antiseptic and germicidal properties of their phenolic content' (Guenther 1949).

A number of phenols appear in essential oils as phenolic ethers (Fig. 2.8). These are more complicated structures than the above phenols and have various forms of names, as seen in the following examples: safrole, methyl chavicol, eugenol methyl ether (as distinct from the straight phenol eugenol) and asarone (which is confusing because of the similarity to the ketone name ending). Some phenolic ethers occur in two forms, as in *trans*-anethole and *cis*-anethole, the latter being the more toxic of the two (Witty 1993 personal communication).

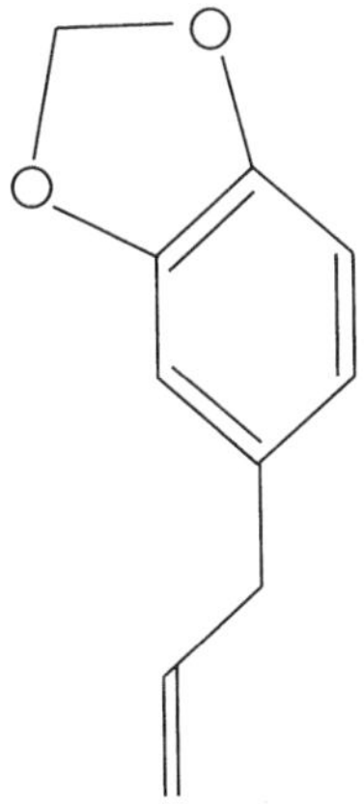

Figure 2.8a   safrole

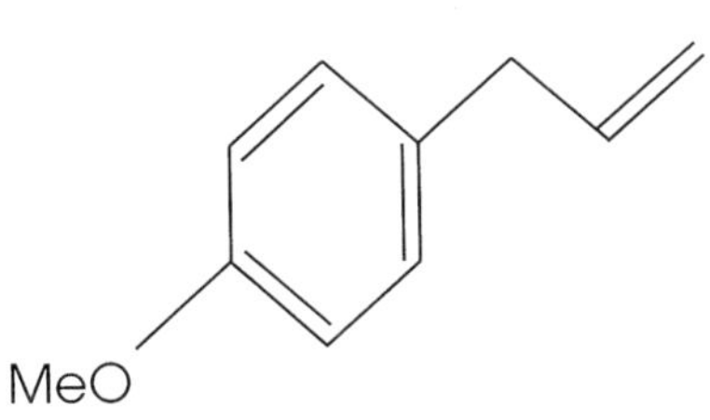

MeO

Figure 2.8b   methyl chavicol

Figure 2.8   Phenolic ethers.

Phenolic ethers have some similar therapeutic effects to those of phenols but, being more powerful, several of them may be neurotoxic if present in large amounts in an essential oil, thus such oils should be used only in the short term and in low concentration.

Ethers rarely, if ever, occur alone in essential oils. Their relationship to phenolic ethers is close, their antidepressant, antispasmodic and sedative properties echoing those of the phenolic ethers, as do those of esters (see below) (Roulier 1990 p. 53).

Aldehydes

An aldehyde is formed when the carbonyl radical (=O) together with a hydrogen atom (–H) attaches itself to one of the carbon atoms in the basic structure, forming a –CHO group (Fig. 2.9). It is easy to recognize an aldehyde from its name, as either aldehydes end in -al, e.g. citral, or the name aldehyde is stated, as in cinnamic aldehyde. They usually have powerful aromas, making them important to the perfumer, and are very reactive, which means that they must be used with care in aromatherapy.

The beneficial properties of aldehydes are that they are antiviral, antiinflammatory, calming to the nervous system, hypotensors, vasodilators and antipyretic; their negative properties—when used incorrectly or inappropriately—include skin irritation and skin sensitivity (Franchomme & Pénoël pp. 211–214, Roulier 1990 p. 53).

Ketones

When the carbonyl group (=O) attaches itself (without a hydrogen atom this time) to a carbon on a chain structure, an aliphatic ketone is formed (aromatic ketones hardly ever occur in essential oils). The ketone names normally end in -one, but look out for false friends like asarone, mentioned above, which is a phenolic ether and not a ketone.

Molecules are not two dimensional, but occupy space. This means that changes in molecular spatial shape can take place. Hence differently shaped molecules made up of the same atoms

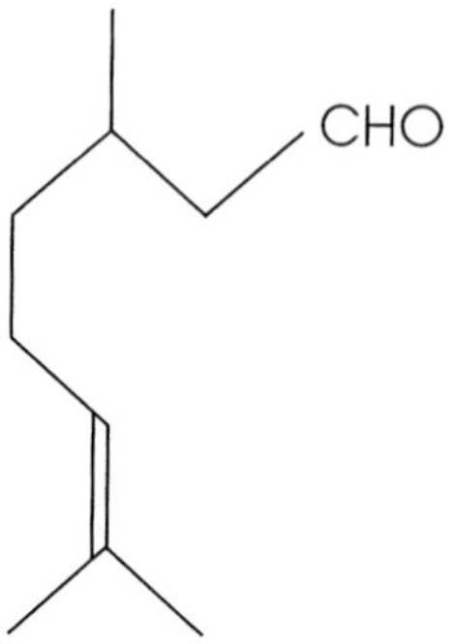

Figure 2.9a   citronellal
(monoterpenic)

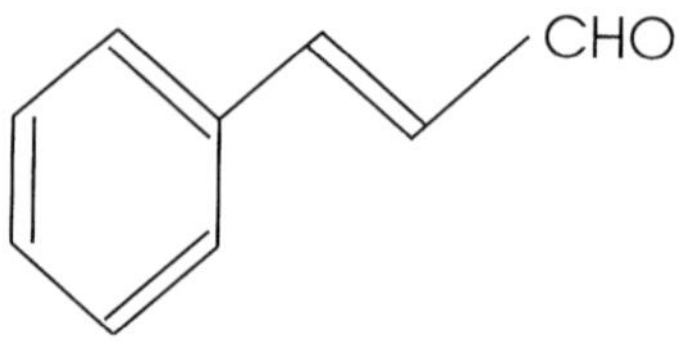

Figure 2.9b   cinnamic aldehyde
(aromatic)

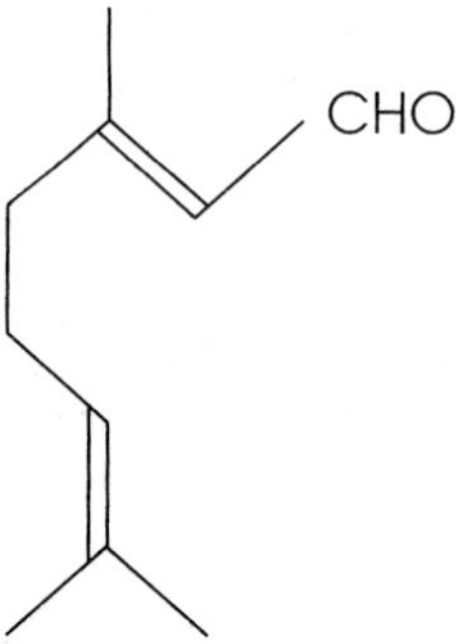

Figure 2.9c   geranial
(monoterpenic)

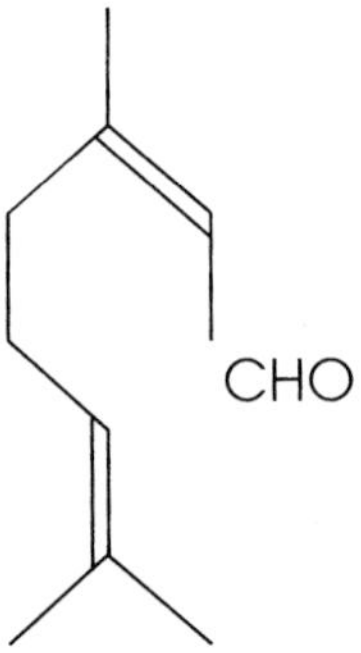

Figure 2.9d   neral
(monoterpenic)

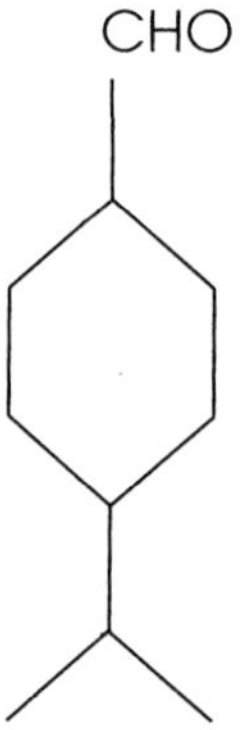

Figure 2.9e   cuminal
(monocyclic monoterpenic)

Figure 2.9   Aldehydes.

do occur and their seemingly insignificant differences can alter the effect that these molecules have on the body. For example, laevo-carvone and dextro-carvone (see Ch. 1 pp. 10–11) are two examples, one being less toxic than the other. Opdyke (1973, 1978) suggests α-thujone and β-thujone may also have differing effects on the body. Time and research alone will tell.

Generally speaking, ketones (Figs 2.10, 2.11) are cicatrizant, lipolytic, mucolytic and sedative; some are also analgesic, anticoagulant, anti-inflammatory, digestive, expectorant or stimulant. They need to be used with care, particularly by pregnant women (Franchomme & Pénoël 1990 p. 193, Roulier 1990 p. 53).

Organic acids and esters

Unlike the above there is no active radical whose presence creates an ester. This compound is formed by the joining together of an organic acid with an alcohol (Fig. 2.12); the formula is:

organic acid + alcohol = ester + water

This chemical reaction is capable of flowing the other way too, which could result in interchanges from acids to esters and back again. Perhaps this is why esters are useful for normalizing some emotional and bodily conditions which are out of balance. There is, however, an acid group (–COOH), which attaches itself to a basic carbon structure and this also plays its part in the formation of an ester. To recognize an ester from its name is not difficult: it usually ends with -ate, e.g. linalyl acetate, or else includes the word ester. Esters generally are believed to be antifungal, antiinflammatory, antispasmodic, cicatrizant and both calming and tonic, especially to the nervous system (Buchbauer, Jirovetz & Jäger 1992, Buchbauer et al 1993) (see Ch. 4). Like alcohols,

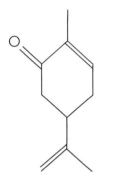

Figure 2.10a   carvone
(monocyclic monoterpenic)

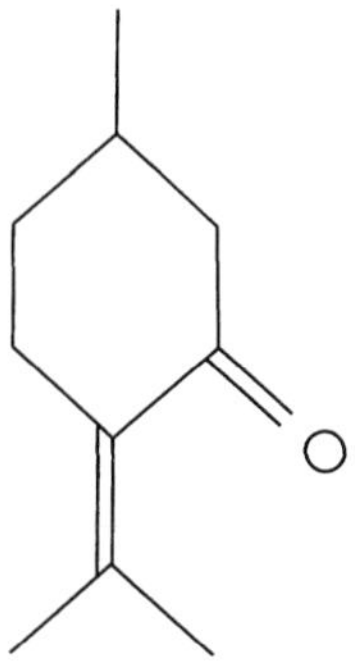

Figure 2.10b   pulegone
(monocyclic monoterpenic)

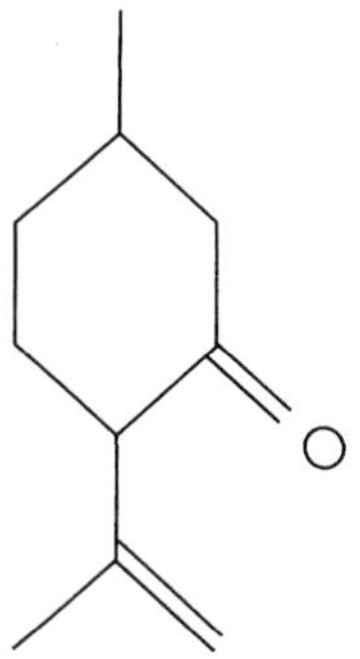

Figure 2.10c   isopulegone
(monocyclic monoterpenic)

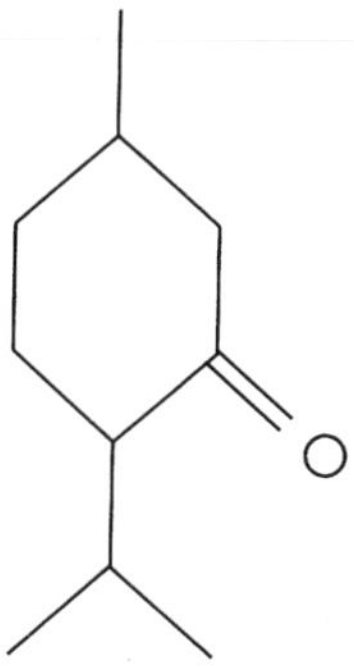

Figure 2.10d   menthone
(monocyclic monoterpenic)

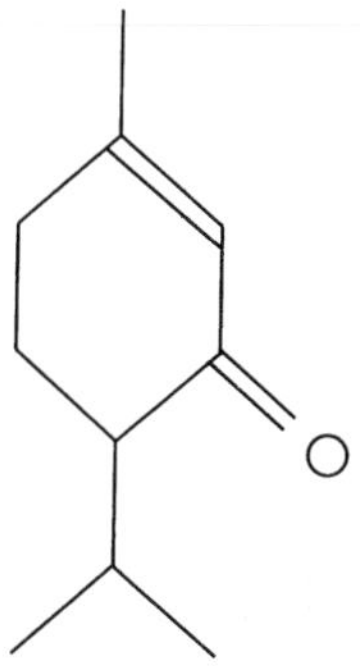

Figure 2.10e   piperitone
(monocyclic monoterpenic)

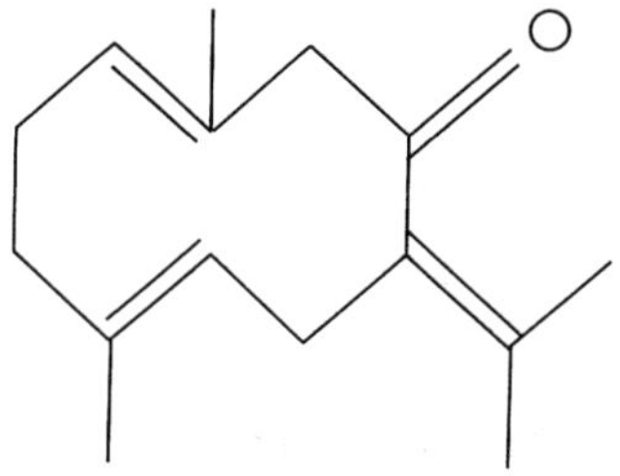

Figure 2.10f   germacrone
(sesquiterpenic)

Figure 2.10   Ketones.

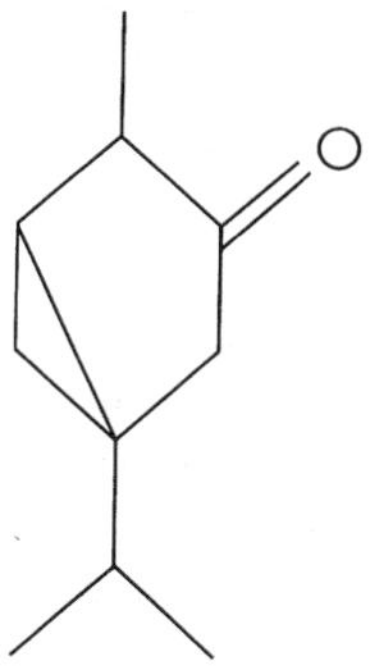

Figure 2.11   Thujone
(bicyclic monoterpenic ketone).

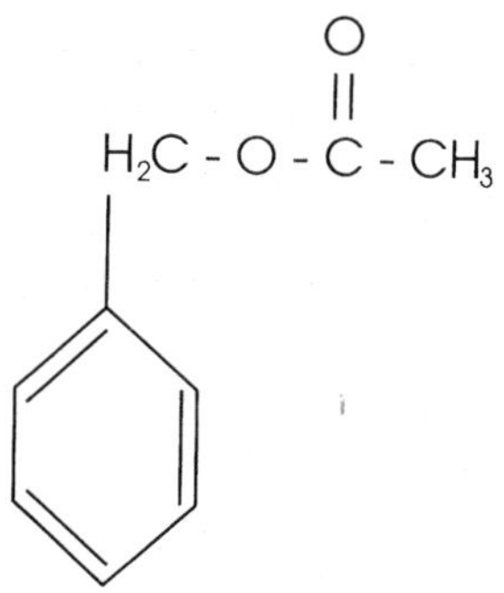

Figure 2.12   Benzyl acetate
(ester).

they are gentle in action, and being free from toxicity they are 'user friendly'. The exception is methyl salicylate, which comprises over 90% of wintergreen and birch oils (neither of which are used in the present British style of aromatherapy).

Oxides

The only oxide known well in aromatherapy is 1,8-cineole, which is otherwise known as eucalyptol (Fig. 2.13); it may also be regarded as a bicyclic ether (Buchbauer 1993). Eucalyptol is expectorant and mucolytic, its unwanted effect being skin irritation, especially on young children.

Lactones

Important members of this family occurring in essences are the coumarins and their derivatives (Fig. 2.14). They occur only in the expressed oils and some absolutes, e.g. jasmine, because the molecular weight is too great to allow distillation.

Lactones are reputed to be mucolytic, expectorant and temperature reducing, their negative aspects being skin sensitization and phototoxicity (Franchomme & Pénoël 1990 p. 202). Coumarins are anticoagulant hypotensors; they are also uplifting and yet sedative (Buchbauer, Jirovetz & Jäger 1992, Franchomme & Pénoël 1990 p. 205). Furanocoumarins are known mainly for their phototoxicity, and oils containing these should not be used immediately prior to sunbathing (or sunbeds) owing to their ability to

Figure 2.14a Coumarin.

OCH3

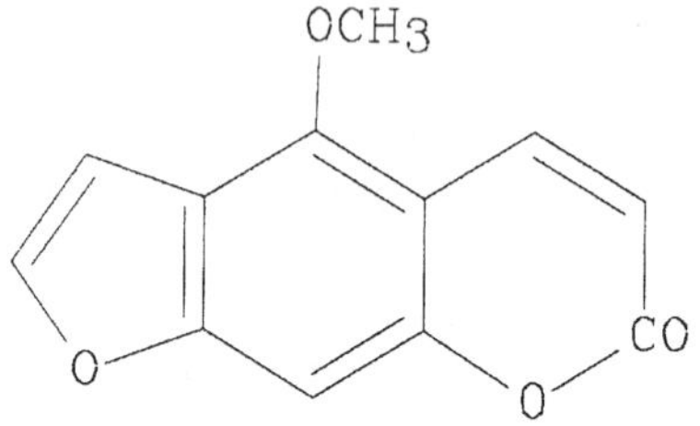

Figure 2.14b Bergaptene (a furanocoumarin).

increase the sensitivity of the skin to the sun. Some are antiviral and antifungal (Franchomme & Pénoël 1990 p. 206).

There are too many individual essential oil components to name here, but knowledge of the different chemical families will aid recognition of new constituents if they are encountered in a listing from a gas chromatograph report (see below).

CHEMICAL VARIABILITY

It is important to recognize that, because of the variability of both climate and soil, no natural chemical will be present in any essential oil in exactly the same proportion at each distillation. Further variations are produced according to the time the plant is harvested. For instance, sage plants cut early in the season contain a much lower percentage of ketones than do those harvested late (Lamy 1985). Constituents can vary sometimes from 20–70% in a genuine oil and suppliers must have obtained an oil from a specific plant grown in the right place and harvested at the right time to ensure the correct proportion of whatever component is required. If this is not the case then the oils may have been adulterated before they reach the buyer, unless bought from source. Even a gas–liquid chromatograph carried out by an independent authority cannot always be relied upon completely. More than one test is needed when checking the purity of an oil, and not all vendors are able to afford such an

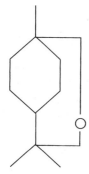

Figure 2.13 Eucalyptol or 1,8-cineole.

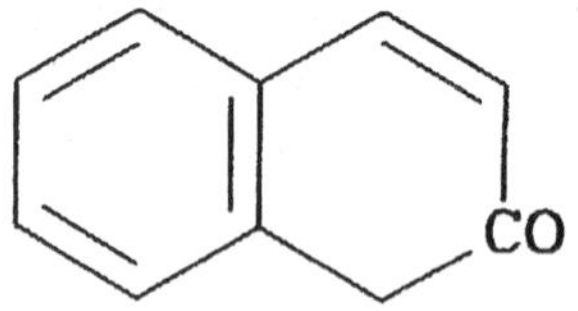

expensive procedure as this for each batch. A certificate showing that an oil is of a required standard is no guarantee unless it refers specifically
to the batch currently being traded.

Testing oils for quality

Gas–liquid chromatography (GLC)

The gas–liquid chromatograph consists of a
coiled, temperature-controlled, tubular column
into which a minute amount (say 1 microlitre) of
essential oil is injected and volatilized. It then
passes through the column, which may itself be
up to 50 m long and contains a liquid phase and
a gas phase. At the other end is a flame ionization
detector and a pen recorder, which plots a trace
(Fig. 2.15) of each component of the essential oil
as it exits the column. The smaller, lighter
molecules have the shortest retention time and
they appear after the shortest time, and so are
recorded first on the trace. These are followed by
successively larger molecules, the heaviest
having the longest retention time and being
recorded last. From the resulting trace the
percentage of each constituent present in the oil
being tested can be calculated. As the reading
will always differ for each batch of any one
essential oil, a trace for each named essential oil
is retained as a standard, to which all future
batches are compared. It can be seen that this test
is comparative rather than absolute, and
although the GLC does not directly identify the
constituents present, this can be done by
comparing the results obtained with a known
standard.

Mass spectrometry

The GLC is a valuable test, but is not the only
one. At the forefront of modern technology is
the gas chromatography–mass spectrometry
(GC–MS), a more expensive process which
is capable of analysing and identifying the
individual components of essential oils. The
mass spectrometer is interfaced to the gas
chromatograph apparatus described above and
as the molecules emerge from the GC column
they are bombarded with high energy electrons,
which fragment them. There is a characteristic
fragmentation pattern for each molecule, and for
identification it is compared by computer with
patterns held in a library. Using this technique it
is possible to identify each component in a
complex mixture such as an essential oil.

Optical rotation

The majority of both mono- and sesquiterpenic
compounds are to be found in one stereochemical form in any given essential oil. This results in
the oils being what is termed 'optically active',
with the ability to bend plane-polarized light
(Table 2.1). The optical activity is measured using
a polarimeter and the angle through which the
light is rotated is an important physical characteristic by which an essential oil may be recognized.

Refractive index

When light passes through a liquid it is refracted,
and this refraction is easily measured to give
consistent figures for a particular oil. This refrac-
tive index (Table 2.1) is quite consistent for a
given oil and is another aid in the authentication
of that oil.

Infrared test

When electromagnetic radiation in the infrared
region is passed through a sample, the spectrum
produced (Fig. 2.16) is a fingerprint from which
the level of some of the oil's components can be
estimated. Some forms of adulteration can readily be seen by this method, depending to some
extent on the skill and knowledge of the person
performing the adulteration.

Essential oils also undergo other checks on
their physical characteristics, which must be
within the accepted tolerances for the given oil.
These checks include specific gravity, solubility
in alcohol, colour, ester content and so on.

The nose

In addition to all this, possibly the finest tool for
some purposes is a well-trained 'nose' (an expert

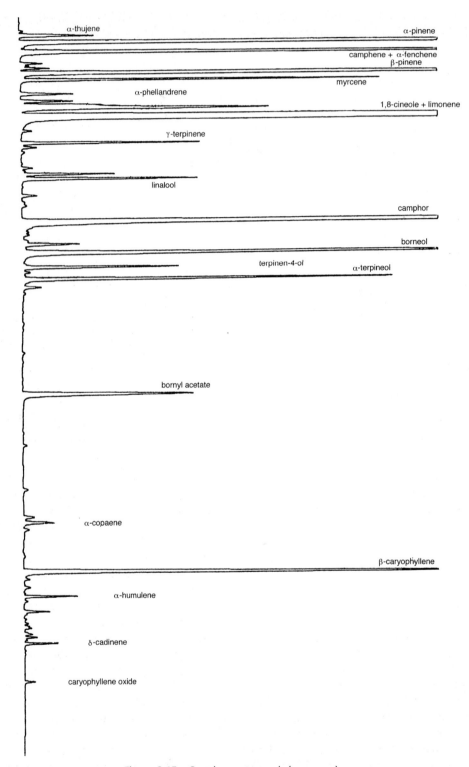

Figure 2.15   Gas chromatograph (rosemary).

Table 2.1 Physical characteristics of some essential oils

Essential oil	Family	Optical rotation	Refractive index	Specific gravity
Cananga odorata (flos) [YLANG YLANG]	Annonaceae	−23.44 to −31.45	1.5041–1.5065	0.960–0.986 (20°)
Carum carvi (fruct.) [CARAWAY]	Umbelliferae	+74 to +80	1.485–1.492	0.902–0.912 (20°)
Cedrus atlantica (lig.) [ATLAS CEDARWOOD]	Pinaceae	+34 to +53.8	1.515–1.523	0.953–0.9756 (20°)
Cinnamomum zeylanicum (cort.) [CINNAMON BARK]	Lauraceae	0 to −2	1.573–1.500	1.000–1.040 (20°)
Citrus limon (per.) [LEMON]	Rutaceae	+57 to +65	1.474–1.476	0.849–0.858 (20°)
Citrus bergamia (per.) [BERGAMOT]	Rutaceae	+8 to +24	1.465–1.4675	0.875–0.880 (20°)
Citrus reticulata (per.) [MANDARIN]	Rutaceae	+65 to +75	1.475–1.478	0.854–0.859 (15°)
Citrus aurantium var. amara (per.) [ORANGE BIGARADE]	Rutaceae	+94 to +99	1.472–1.476	0.842–0.848 (20°)
Coriandrum sativum (fruct.) [CORIANDER]	Umbelliferae	+8 to +12	1.462–1.472	0.863–0.870 (20°)
Cymbopogon flexuosus (fol.) [LEMONGRASS]	Poaceae	−3 to +1	1.485–1.4899	0.889–0.911 (25°)
Eucalyptus globulus (fol.) [TASMANIAN BLUE GUM]	Myrtaceae	0 to +10	1.458–1.470	0.905–0.925 (20°)
Foeniculum vulgare var. dulce (fruct.) [FENNEL]	Umbelliferae	+5 to +16.30	1.5500–1.5519	0.971–0.980 (20°)
Juniperus communis (fruct.) [JUNIPER BERRY]	Cupressaceae	−15 to 0	1.4740–1.4840	0.854–0.871 (20°)
Lavandula angustifolia [LAVENDER]	Labiatae	−5 to −12	1.457–1.464	0.878–0.892 (20°)
Melaleuca leucadendron (fol.) [CAJUPUT]	Myrtaceae	+1 to −4	1.464–1.472	0.910–0.923 (20°)
Melaleuca alternifolia (fol.) [TEA TREE]	Myrtaceae	+6.48 to +9.48	1.4760–1.4810	0.895–0.905 (15°)
Mentha x piperita (fol.) [PEPPERMINT]	Labiatae	−16 to −30	1.460–1.467	0.900–0.912 (20°)
Myristica fragrans (sem.) [NUTMEG EI]*	Myristicaceae	+8 to +25	1.475–1.488	0.883–0.917 (20°)
Myristica fragrans (sem.) [NUTMEG WI]*	Myristicaceae	+25 to +45	1.467–1.477	0.854–0.880 (20°)
Nardostachys jatamansi (rad.) [SPIKENARD]	Valerianaceae	−20	1.5078	0.9649–0.9732 (17°)
Ocimum basilicum (fol.) [BASIL]	Labiatae	−7.24 to −10.36	1.4821–1.4939	0.912–0.935 (20°)
Origanum majorana (fol.) [SWEET MARJORAM]	Labiatae	+14.2 to +19.4	1.4700–1.4750	0.890–0.906 (25°)
Pelargonium graveolens (fol.) [GERANIUM]	Geraniaceae	−7.0 to +13.15	1.461–1.472	0.888–0.896 (20°)
Piper nigrum (fruct.) [BLACK PEPPER]	Piperaceae	−7.2 to +4	1.480–1.492	0.864–0.907 (20°)
Pogostemon patchouli (fol.) [PATCHOULI]	Labiatae	−47 to −70	1.506–1.513	0.955–0.986 (20°)
Santalum album (lig.) [SANDALWOOD]	Santalaceae	−15.58 to −20	1.505–1.510	0.971–0.983 (20°)
Syzygium aromaticum (flos) [CLOVE BUD]	Myrtaceae	−1.5	1.528–1.537	1.041–1.054 (20°)
Vetiveria zizanioides (rad.) [VETIVER]	Poaceae	+19 to +30	1.514–1.519	0.9882–1.0219 (30°)
Zingiber officinale (rad.) [GINGER]	Zingiberaceae	−28 to −45	1.4880–1.440	0.871–0.882 (20°)

*EI = East Indies, WI = West Indies

perfumer) who can make an organoleptic assessment of the oil. The trained nose can identify certain molecules at levels that would be impossibly low for machines.

The distillation process

Distilling as we know it today can involve efficient cooling systems, electronic control gear to regulate the temperature and pressure of the process, energy-saving steam generators and so on. Some thousands of years ago, to obtain the essential oil, cedarwood pieces (for example) would be placed with water in a clay vessel with a lid made of woollen fibres. The vessel would be heated over a wood fire, and as the volatile molecules from the water and the cedarwood escaped they were trapped in the wool. Later they were squeezed out by hand, and the

aromatic water and essential oil, being of different densities, would separate and so could be collected. Over the centuries methods of distillation gradually improved, and 4th century Chinese and 10th century Islamic scientists developed two different methods of obtaining the distillate. Since then, apart from minor improvements, distillation has remained very much the same in principle up to the present day. The availability of modern materials and resources, such as stainless steel and electricity, has permitted much greater control over the whole process and there is a dramatic increase in the quality of the essential oils produced today compared with that in former times. Oils produced in previous centuries, and even during the middle of this century, cannot be compared with some of the very high quality products we have available for aromatherapy today

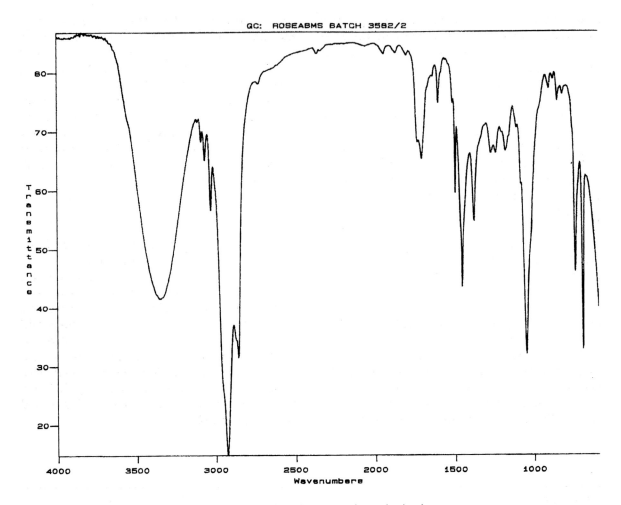

Figure 2.16 Infrared spectrum (rose absolute).

(assuming they are not adulterated after distillation).

Newer methods have been tried in the 20th century, such as percolation (used on a small scale in France), and new solvents such as supercritical CO_2, which can extract, without heat, a wider range of molecules from the plant material than is possible by distillation, thus producing a new material which may well be of use to aromatherapists. The oils produced by any of these newer methods have a different molecular mix and until more is known about them, and research carried out on their possibly different therapeutic (and possible toxic) effects,

aromatherapists may be best advised to use only steam-distilled essential oils and expressed essences for the time being. These have been proven by tradition over a long period of time, as well as by supporting scientific research carried out this century, to be therapeutically effective.

Complexity of essential oils

During the 19th century the first analyses were carried out on essential oils, and attempts made to isolate and identify the various components, some of the terpenes, alcohols and aldehydes being among the first to be named. This was followed by successful attempts to synthesize the individual components; for example, eugenol found naturally in clove bud oil was synthesized in 1822 (Valnet 1980 p. 28).

The complexity of essential oils should be borne in mind when referring to the therapeutic qualities of a given oil; it helps to explain why one oil (lavender) can be listed at the same time as being 'analgesic, anticonvulsive, antidepressant, antimicrobial, antirheumatic, antiseptic, antispasmodic, antitoxic, carminative, cholagogic, choleretic, cicatrizant, cordial, cytophylactic, deodorant, diuretic, emmenagogic, hypotensive, insecticidal, nervine, parasiticidal, rubefacient, sedative, stimulant, sudorific, tonic, vermifuge, vulnerary'. This staggering array of properties (Lawless 1992) perhaps overstates the case, but demonstrates the 'shotgun' holistic approach in contrast to the 'single bullet' symptomatic approach.

This complexity means that only genuine essential oils should be used therapeutically, even though there is natural variation in the oils. It needs emphasizing that for perfectly valid reasons the fragrance industry requires essential oils which are standardized by one means or another and that many (if not most) essential oils in the general market place may have synthetic or natural additions or fractions removed. As well as these already-mentioned cautions, it is also true that some oils are not obtained from plants at all. These laboratory creations are known as reconstructed oils (RCO) and lack many tiny and as yet unidentified components which could well be important to the overall effect of the natural oil.

Summary

The requirements of the food and perfume industries differ dramatically from those of aromatherapy. Essential oils are very complex by nature, and careful selection and extensive testing are needed to obtain oils of therapeutic quality. When altered in any way they will probably not be of a quality suitable for aromatherapy, since the synergy of the natural mix of components in the whole oil will have been destroyed. It goes without saying that they should be obtained only from a reliable and knowledgeable source.

REFERENCES

Arctander S 1960 Perfume and flavor materials of natural origin. Published by the author, Elizabeth New Jersey, p 4
British Pharmacopoeia 1993 HMSO, London, p 273
Buchbauer G 1993 Biological effects of fragrances and essential oils. Perfumer and Flavorist 18: 22
Buchbauer G, Jirovetz L, Jäger W 1992 Passiflora and lime blossoms: motility effects after inhalation of the essential oils and some of the main constituents in animal experiments. Archiva Pharmaceutica (Weinheim) 325: 247–248
Buchbauer G, Jirovetz L, Jäger W, Plank C, Dietrich H 1993 Fragrance compounds and essential oils with sedative effects upon inhalation. Journal of Pharmaceutical Sciences 82(6): 660–664
Franchomme P, Pénoël D 1990 L 'aromathérapie exactement. Jollois, Limoges
Guenther E 1949 The essential oils, vol 2. Van Nostrand, New York, p 499
Lamy J 1985 De la culture à la distillerie: quelques facteurs influant sur la composition des huiles essentielles. Chambre d'Agriculture de la Drôme, Valence, p 5
Lautié R, Passebecq A 1984 Aromatherapy. Thorsons, Wellingborough
Lawless J 1992 The encyclopaedia of essential oils. Element, Shaftesbury, p 118
Müller J, Bräuer H, Mensing J, Beck C 1984 The H&R book of perfumes, vol 1. Johnson, London, p 111
Opdyke D L J 1973 Monographs on fragrance raw materials: laevo-carvone. Food and cosmetics toxicology, vol 11. Pergamon Press, Oxford, p 1057
Opdyke D L J 1978 Monographs on fragrance raw materials: dextro-carvone. Food and cosmetics toxicology, vol. 16. Pergamon Press, Oxford, p 673
Price L 1990 Lecture notes: theory and philosophy of aromatherapy. Shirley Price International College of Aromatherapy Course, Hinckley
Price S 1993 The aromatherapy workbook. Thorsons, London, pp 31–34
Roulier G 1990 Les huiles essentielles pour votre santé. Dangles, St-Jean-de-Braye
Valnet J 1980 The practice of aromatherapy. Daniel, Saffron Walden

3

Power and safety

Introduction

The dangers of essential oils have been greatly exaggerated, usually based on insufficient evidence and inappropriate comparisons. This chapter shows that these powerful substances, used knowledgeably and with due caution, pose no threat to health.

SAFETY

It is necessary to begin this chapter on the safe use of essential oils by making three statements. First, there is no doubt that essential oils are powerful mixtures and have physiological, psychological and pharmacological effects when applied to the body. Secondly, in most countries, including the UK, these oils are freely available and there is no restriction on their sale and use. Thirdly, the majority of people who buy essential oils are members of the general public, who cannot be expected to have expert knowledge of their nature and use. It is remarkable then that their safety record is as good as it undoubtedly is. Despite this record, statements are sometimes made which sensationalize aromatherapy or exaggerate unwanted effects of the oils.

More to the point would be education of both the supplier and the general user in the appropriate and safe use of essential oils. That way lies a safe and sound future for the popular use of aromatherapy.

Tradition, experience and research

On the positive side, centuries of experience of essential oils worldwide has proved they are

41

effective and safe when used knowledgeably and with care. This is true for many oils, e.g.:

- the Egyptians proved the antiseptic powers of aromatics in the mummification process
- Hippocrates fought the plague in Athens by using aromatic essences for fumigation
- St Hildegard of Bingen was using lavender oil in the 12th century
- Hungary water (a lotion scented with rosemary) began its 600 year life in the 14th century
- by the year 1500, oils of benzoin, calamus, cedarwood, cinnamon, frankincense, myrrh, rose, rosemary, sage, spikenard and turpentine were known to the pharmacist.

Essential oils were first mentioned in an official pharmacopoeia around the year 1600 in Germany (Price 1993 p. 6). Borneo camphor (an alcohol) was mentioned in Schröder's pharmacopoeia of 1689 as a 'prodigious alexipharmic' or antidote to poison. For other oils there is little historical evidence, and for almost all essential oils, while there is ample proof of their antiseptic powers, clinical trials are lacking. While this may be due in part to shortage of research funds, it is also attributable to the difficulty (even impossibility) of conducting blind trials with aromatic substances.

There is also a body of knowledge on the use of essential oils on the skin by the perfume industry, based on the impressive work carried out by the independent Research Institute of Fragrant Materials (RIFM) established in 1966. RIFM has now published over 1000 monographs on fragrance materials and almost 200 of these concern natural aromatic materials derived from plants. These include essential oils, absolutes and resins. The International Fragrance Association (IFRA) makes recommendations to the perfume industry for the safe use of such materials based on the published findings of RIFM, and these are useful guides to aromatherapists when applying essential oils to the skin.

Although some tests have been performed on humans, the majority have been carried out on animals—normally rabbits for dermal toxicity and rats for oral toxicity. However, the relevance of animal testing to humans is debatable. For instance, basil and tarragon oils may contain estragole (methyl chavicol) in high amounts and this compound has been implicated by research on animals as being a strong carcinogen. By inference, the use of these oils in aromatherapy might be considered hazardous, but research at St Mary's Hospital in London indicates that the results of animal tests cannot be extended directly to humans. The carcinogenicity is due to the metabolite 1-hydroxyestragole, and the conclusion of the above study was that estragole presented little hazard to humans at normal food usage levels of 1 µg/kg per day (Howes, Chan & Caldwell 1990). The case for skin application of essential oils with a high content of estragole is still undecided. When applied to the skin, not all of the essential oil enters the body, but caution is advisable nevertheless pending investigation of the metabolization of estragole in the transdermal route. It has been found that absorption of chemicals is usually higher through animal skin than through human, but for the aromatic amines the reverse is true: 13% of MDA (methylenedioxyamphetamine) permeated the skin in rats compared with 33% in human skin, while for MbOCA (methylenebis (orthochloroaniline)) the figures were 2 and 6% respectively; for (+)-limonene the figures are 6% (rat) and 3% (human) (Hotchkiss 1994). All this underlines the inadvisability and uncertainty of extrapolating animal experiment results to humans.

Overdosing

When it comes to testing the toxic effects of swallowing essential oils, all studies are carried out using animals. There is currently no viable alternative because testing on humans is considered too hazardous. Occasionally some knowledge is derived from an accident involving a child or a deliberate overdose by an adult. Therefore, many of the opinions offered on this subject in the aromatherapy literature must be regarded as speculative.

Swallowing an overdose

The ingestion of a large quantity of neat essential oil produces a burning sensation in the mouth and throat, and in some serious cases nausea, vomiting and diarrhoea. If the overdose is extreme there may follow lethargy, ataxia and coma or perhaps irritability and convulsions (e.g. pennyroyal—see Ch. 8). The pupils may be dilated (e.g. camphor) or constricted (e.g. eucalyptus).

The effects of molecular shape

Carvone appears in laevo (–) and dextro (+) forms (see Ch. 1, Fig. 1.3b p. 11) in different oils (for example (+)-carvone is present at 48–58% in caraway oil and (–)-carvone is the main constituent of spearmint oil). *Carum carvi* [CARAWAY] is considered to be a safe oil in all respects by Tisserand (1985 p. 19) and by Tisserand & Balacs (1995 p. 204) (who also note that it is a mucous membrane irritant); Winter (1984 pp. 62–63) states both (+)- and (–)-carvone are non-toxic; (–)-carvone has an LD_{50} of 1640 mg/kg in rats (Jenner et al 1964) and (+)-carvone one of 3.71 mg/kg in rats (Levenstein 1976).

Tyman (1990) has suggested that there are probably differences in effect between α- and β-thujone, and others have suggested the same is true for *cis*- and *trans*-anethole.

One frequently repeated statement is that all forms of ketones are neurotoxic, but this is not so (Tisserand 1985 p. 61). Thujone is not to be treated lightly whenever and wherever it occurs; however, the thujone molecule has four possible shapes, and it is not known whether they all have the same toxic potential and should all be avoided (Tyman 1990). The seed oil of *Anethum graveolens* [DILL] contains 40–60% of ketones, with a minimum of 28% (+)-carvone, and is considered neurotoxic by Franchomme & Pénoël (1990 p. 323). On the other hand, Tisserand (1985 p. 62) considers that 'carvone, which occurs in oils of caraway, dill, spearmint … is not present in sufficient quantity in the essential oils to present any risk'. There are many other anomalies such as this to be found in books on aromatherapy, which underlines the complexity of the individual chemicals and the wide variation in percentages present in essential oils and therefore in the overall effect on the human organisms.

Toxicity depends not only on the nature of the main component, but also on the relationships and synergy (see below) between this and some of the smaller (perhaps as yet unidentified) constituents, which are known to ameliorate undesirable effects in some cases.

Essential oils are very complex substances, and it is worth repeating the statement made earlier that there is no simple direct relationship between the effects of any single component of an essential oil and the effects of the complete natural essential oil—essential oils are synergistic mixes (Price 1990). This may illustrate why certain oils high in ketones are not considered toxic, or even why a few oils which are considered toxic by some people do not appear to be so.

The study of essential oils can be a minefield, and to understand them completely would take a lifetime. For the present, it may be preferable in the current state of knowledge to continue to regard aromatherapy as much an art as a science. Nevertheless, it should be remembered that a great deal of good has been done (and no serious harm has so far been recorded) by qualified aromatherapists since the 1960s in the UK.

A nurse practising aromatherapy in a hospice some years ago was concerned to prove the safety of the oils she was administering to patients and took 5 ml of each of about 40 essential oils by mouth (one per week). In a personal communication she stated that she suffered no ill effects apart from dreaming more vividly than usual. The 40 oils included some that are potentially hazardous and it is advisable not to follow this extreme example. Individuals vary greatly in their reaction to different substances and such actions may produce a disastrous result. There is a large safety factor when using the oils in normal aromatherapy quantities, i.e. two or three drops compared with approximately 100 drops that a 5 ml teaspoon will hold.

Synergy

The word synergy is derived from two Greek words which mean 'working together' (see Ch. 2 p. 25). In essential oils this comprises the working together of all the constituents within the whole. The effect of synergy is such that when two or more components are put together there is some extra activity greater than that of the individual components simply added together.

As discussed in Chapter 2, essential oils are complex mixtures, some containing several hundreds of different molecules, some comparatively few. Whole (or complete) essential oils have been found in practice to be more effective than their isolated principal constituent(s) and without side-effects (when used properly) on account of the synergistic effect (Hall 1904). 'It is this principle (synergy) which allows the achievement of strong effects from infinitely small doses of non-toxic products, but judiciously combined by nature herself' (Duraffourd 1982 p. 16). Constituents present in very small amounts (e.g. furanocoumarins) are often found to be as active as or even more active than the principal constituent.

Another complication regarding synergy is illustrated by the case of eucalyptus. Dr Pénoël writes:

Most of the eucalyptus products found on the usual aromatic market have been redistilled, rectified and refined. In reality the residue left behind in the still from the rectification of the crude oils is rich in precious molecules (like the rare phenol australol). Even if their proportion seems low, they work in synergy with the main components and should be kept in order for the essential oil to express its full healing potential.

(Pénoël 1993 personal communication)

Because of this synergistic feature, it can be difficult to assess the contribution made by any one component to the total effect of an essential oil. When tested individually each may behave differently from when in the presence of the other naturally occurring molecules within the make-up of the oil. Tests carried out on individual components from *Eucalyptus citriodora* revealed that they were relatively inactive. However, a combination of the three major components in the same ratio found in the natural oil produced a fourfold increase in antimicrobial activity against *S. aureus* (Low, Rawal & Griffin 1974).

Apart from the synergy produced by the components of a single oil, there is also an enhancement of effect when two or more whole oils are mixed together. For example, the combined bactericidal effect of several oils together is greater than the effect of any of the individual oils.

Quenching

Quenching is another important aspect of synergy, whereby the potential unwanted side-effects of one component are nullified by the presence of other component(s). A good illustration of this is found by comparing the effects of two eucalyptus oils, *Eucalyptus globulus* [TASMANIAN BLUE GUM] and *E. smithii* [GULLY GUM]. Both contain around 65% of 1,8-cineole (an oxide which is a skin irritant), yet the former is contraindicated for use on young children and the latter not (Pénoël 1992/93). This quenching effect is well known in the perfumery industry, which turns it to advantage by adding quenching components to its perfumes to prevent skin irritation. An example is the use of (+)-limonene, which when put together with lemongrass oil quenches the irritating effect of the aldehydes (see below).

To recapitulate, such interactions of components take place between the constituents within one oil and also between two or more essential oils, so that potentially toxic elements may be altered, enhanced or counteracted by other constituents present. It is for this reason that aromatherapists use the whole natural oil rather than an active isolate, e.g. the eucalyptol from eucalyptus, thought to be responsible for the antiseptic, expectorant and contraantigen action. Gattefossé, chemist and perfumer, the man who coined the term aromatherapy, wrote that eucalyptol is 'a substance with no apparent activity' and 'only an excipient' (Gattefossé 1937 pp. 41, 88). Hindsight makes wise men of us all.

Isolates are sometimes used by the medical profession in France, but they need to be used sparingly and with knowledge, and they are not used in aromatherapy as practised in this country.

Tests carried out employing the isolates phenylacetaldehyde, citral and cinnamic aldehyde—found in *Citrus aurantium* (flos) [NEROLI BIGARADE], *Cymbopogon citratus*, *C. flexuosus* [LEMONGRASS] and *Cinnamomum zeylanicum* (cort.) [CINNAMON] oils respectively—showed them to be skin sensitizers. However, the whole essential oils in which the aldehydes are present (at up to 85%) were found not to provoke sensitizing reactions. It appeared that some other component(s) of the natural oil inhibited the induction or expression of sensitization (Opdyke 1976). As a test of this hypothesis, several terpenes and alcohols found along with the particular aldehyde in the natural composition were combined with each of the aldehydes in question. It appears now to be a consistent finding that each of these aldehydes, although producing sensitization reactions when applied alone, produces no sensitization reactions in selected simple mixtures with other compounds (Opdyke 1979) (see Table 3.1). These findings point to the difference between using a single compound and the use of a natural synergistic mix with inbuilt quenching action. The above-mentioned tests contrast with two earlier tests carried out by Kligman in 1971 and 1972 on 25 volunteers using cinnamon bark oil at 8% concentration and producing 18 and 20 sensitization reactions respectively (Kligman & Epstein 1975). Cinnamic aldehyde is not the only component in *C. zeylanicum* (cort.) [CINAMMON BARK] oil acting as a sensitizer, so perhaps this may be a case of synergy enhancing the unwanted effect. IFRA recommend that this oil is used at a maximum 1% concentration in a fragrance compound (IFRA 1992); this is equivalent to 0.2% in an aromatherapy massage oil (i.e. one drop in 25 ml carrier oil), although a lower level of use of 0.1% for the skin has been recommended (Tisserand & Balacs 1995 p. 130).

It is believed that many natural essential oils which have not been tampered with display this quenching effect. Just because an oil contains one or more components which are thought to be hazardous in some way it does not automatically follow that the oil is unsafe, although caution must be observed. This feature can also be made use of when mixing oils. The aldehyde citral is a constituent of *Citrus limon* [LEMON] (5%) which on its own is irritating to the skin, yet the whole oil is not. Essential oil of *C. citratus* and *flexuosus* has a high content of citral (approximately 70%) and the whole oil can therefore be irritant, but this effect can be quenched by adding an oil containing an equal amount of (+)-limonene (a terpene present in some citrus oils to around 80–90%).

The peel oils from *Citrus paradisi* [GRAPEFRUIT] or *Citrus sinensis* [SWEET ORANGE] when added to *C. citratus* in a 50–50 mix successfully quench the

Table 3.1 Results of quenching tests on mixtures of cinnamic aldehyde with other essential oil components. (Reprinted from Opdyke 1979 p. 255, with kind permission from Elsevier Science Ltd, The Boulevard, Langford Lane, Kidlington OX5 1GB, UK)

Second test material	Relative proportions*	Results of sensitization test
Dipropylene glycol	1:1	+
Phenylethyl alcohol	1:1	+
Eugenol	1:1	−
Eugenol	1:1†	−
Eugenol	2.5:1†	+
Cinnamic alcohol	1:1	+
Benzyl salicylate	1:1	+
(+)-limonene	1:1	−

*Ratio (w/w) of cinnamic aldehyde to second test material. Each mixture was tested at an overall concentration of 6% in petrolatum by the maximization procedure (Kligman 1966, Kligman & Epstein 1975).
†Duplicate tests.

irritant properties of the latter (Witty 1992 personal communication).

WHAT ARE WE USING?

Of the many factors involved in the safe use of essential oils, not least is the specification of the oil itself. Knowledge of such factors as where it is grown, whether it is cloned by cuttings or grown from seed, the plant variety, how it is produced (wild, organic or with chemicals), the part of the plant used and the chemotype are important for safe usage.

The importance of knowing what material is being used in a treatment is obvious, therefore it is imperative that the oil is precisely identified. This fact escapes the attention of many people treating others and even of some of those carrying out trials. Before embarking on a trial using essential oils it is of primary importance that a specified oil from a known source is used, and to have as a minimum a GLC analysis of the oil actually used in the test. Oil from the same harvest batch should be used throughout one test because aromatherapy oils are natural products, not standardized, and the actual composition of an oil may vary within wide limits. The botanical name of the plant should always be used (unless talking generally about a species), because common names are imprecise and can cause confusion. The same common name can be given to different plants (such as marjoram, which might be *Origanum majorana* or *Thymus mastichina*), or more than one name may be given to the same plant. An extreme example is cedarwood oil, which may be any one of the following, since all are traded as cedarwood:

- *Cedrus atlantica* [ATLAS CEDARWOOD]
- *Cedrus deodora* [DEODAR OR HIMALAYAN CEDARWOOD]
- *Cedrus libani* [CEDAR OF LEBANON]
- *Chamaecyparis lawsoniana* [WESTERN WHITE CEDAR]
- *Cryptomeria japonica* [JAPANESE CEDAR]
- *Juniperus procera* [EAST AFRICAN CEDARWOOD]
- *Juniperus mexicana* [TEXAS CEDARWOOD]
- *Juniperus virginiana* [RED CEDARWOOD]
- *Thuja occidentalis* [WHITE CEDAR]
- *Thuja plicata* [WESTERN RED CEDAR].

In many cases it is not sufficient merely to specify in Latin the genus and species (and the variety if applicable); it is also necessary to designate the chemotype (explained in Ch. 1) and the part of the plant used for extraction. An example is the cinnamon tree where the oil from the bark consists principally of an aldehyde, while the oil from the leaf is mainly a phenol with different effects and uses. The oil from the thuja or white cedar tree, *Thuja occidentalis* (responsible for the restriction of cedarwood oils in France), is taken from the leaves, but other 'cedarwoods' are taken from the wood. In the umbellifer family, the seed oils can be significantly different from oils extracted from other parts of the same plant, e.g. in the case of *Angelica archangelica* the root oil is phototoxic while that from the seed is not. Therapists need to be aware of this and it is their responsibility to ensure that inappropriate treatment is not given.

Safe quantities

Essential oils may be applied to the body in a variety of ways, and these are discussed in Chapter 5, but usually their use involves inhala-tion, application to the skin or ingestion. Essential oils are powerful, otherwise they would be of no use therapeutically, and this means that they must be employed with care and knowledge to achieve beneficial results. Inappropriate use in whatever way can bring about undesired effects. Dosage, in terms of both quantity and time, is all important since too little may mean little or no result, while too much may (depending on the oils used) have a beneficial effect or create a serious problem. The majority of essential oils may be considered less toxic than the over-the-counter medicines aspirin and paracetamol, and aromatherapy is a safe therapy provided the therapist is suitably trained. If this requirement is observed, there need be no hesitation in introducing these natural aromatic products into a hospital environment. Many substances in common use are toxic in overdose—e.g. carrots are beneficial in moderation, although a surfeit will produce illness, and this is true of many other everyday foods such as tomatoes, saffron and mustard. Valnet (1980) cites the loss of eyebrows and headaches in workers handling vanilla, but vanilla ice cream is produced, eaten and enjoyed without ill effect. An essential oil may be both safe and toxic depending on the amount administered—it all depends on the knowledge, skill and experience of the therapist. For example, we have observed that while lavender is sedative in low dose, a high dose can cause insomnia.

Ingestion of essential oils

NB. This method of using essential oils in the case of pregnant women and very young children may be hazardous. See Chapter 10 for pregnancy and contraindications.

Only genuine natural essential oils, not tampered with by humans (i.e. of therapeutic quality), should be employed for internal use although, as we have seen, it is difficult for anyone to guarantee the purity of an essential oil, given the current state of the market. The ingestion of essential oils should be left in the hands of a competent aromatologist, e.g. an IAM licentiate (see p. 376), or an aromatherapist working under the direction of a doctor; such a therapist should exercise great care and discretion in advising both the use and the procurement of essential oils. Any national legal requirements and any rules of the hospital management board will have to be observed, as also will the ethical considerations of any professional body to which the aromatherapist may belong. The therapist will take into account age, body weight, general state of health, current medication (if any) and the oils to be used.

Nevertheless, some conditions such as enteritis, irritable bowel syndrome and diverticulitis can scarcely be treated in any other way than by ingestion (see Ch. 5). The best medium for diluting the oils for internal use, if a dispersant is not readily available, is a fixed oil because the essential oils will dissolve easily and completely in it (Collin P 1994 personal communication). Runny honey is also a good diluent, with the addition of a little water. Table 3.2 shows the *lethal dose* (LD_{50} is the dose at which 50% of the test subjects die) of some representative oils for a typical adult and a small child. These figures have been extrapolated from figures derived from animal testing and as metabolization in humans is not always the same as in animals their accuracy cannot be guaranteed (as seen above). In the absence of other information we must rely on these figures as a guide, and because the quantities used in aromatherapy are very small, there is normally an extremely high safety factor when comparing the lethal dose with the effective dose. The *effective dose* (ED_{50}) is the term used when some sort of response is being monitored in the experimental animal other than the death of the animal. The *median effective dose* is the dose at which 50% of the test subjects achieve the desired benefit.

Toxicity figures given in aromatherapy literature do not always make it clear that these doses are per *kilogram* of body weight. This could lead to the misunderstanding that the figures given are the effective or lethal doses for a *person*. They are not; it is dependent on their weight. For example the LD_{50} value for the oil from *Salvia officinalis* [SAGE] is 2.6 g/kg, which equates to a fatal dose of approximately 170 ml for a 60 kg person; the equivalent figure for *Chamaemelum nobile* [ROMAN CHAMOMILE] is 570 ml for a 60 kg person. The quantities involved are so great that anyone in their right mind would jib at taking them; however, illness may be caused at a much lower dose.

Health professionals working in hospitals and similar establishments should secure the approval of a consultant or other suitably qualified and responsible person before giving oils by mouth, rectum or vagina. No carer without accredited training should administer oils in these ways unless under the supervision of an aromatologist. It is also important to preserve procedural safety; the prescriber, dispenser and administrator should be separate persons to guard against error.

Only steam-distilled oils and the expressed citrus essences should be employed for ingestion. The following classes of oils should never be administered internally:

- oils obtained from gums (other than by distillation)
- resins (because of the solvent residue)
- absolutes (because of the solvent residue)
- commercial quality oils (i.e. standardized) used by the perfume, food and pharmaceutical industries.

Dispensing and storage precautions

Labelling

As essential oils are freely available in most countries, the supplier needs to ensure that they are properly labelled, with proper cautions regarding children, eyes, pregnancy and skin. In France the sale of a few oils has been restricted since 1986 to the pharmacies; they include: mugwort, wormwood, cedarwood, hyssop, sage, tansy and thuja (botanical names not given). Generally, self-regulation by an industry is to be preferred to governmental regulation and accordingly any oil which may be harmful when used injudiciously should not be offered for sale to anyone lacking adequate aromatherapy training. This would still leave a wide range of safe oils accessible for use by the general public. It is a legal requirement that essential oil containers carry appropriate printed cautions.

Table 3.2   Lethal dose (LD$_{50}$)

Essential oil	*The human lethal doses are extrapolated from animal test results		LD$_{50}$ g/kg (animal)	Lethal dose* 15 k child	Lethal dose* 70 k adult
Latin name	*Common name*			ml	ml
Aniba rosaeodora (lig.)	rosewood		4.3	72	334
Boswellia carteri	frankincense		5	83	389
Cananga odorata (flos)	ylang ylang	more than	5	83	389
Cedrus atlantica (lig.)	atlas cedarwood	more than	5	83	389
Chamaemelum nobile (flos)	roman chamomile		8.56	143	666
Chamomilla recutita (flos)	german chamomile	more than	5	83	389
Cinnamomum zeylanicum (cort.)	cinnamon bark		3.4	57	264
Cinnamomum zeylanicum (fol.)	cinnamon leaf		2.65	44	206
Citrus aurantium var. *amara* (flos)	neroli bigarade	more than	5	83	389
Citrus aurantium var. *amara* (fol.)	petitgrain bigarade	more than	5	83	389
Citrus bergamia (per.)	bergamot	more than	10	167	778
Citrus reticulata (per.)	mandarin	more than	5.00	83	389
Commiphora myrrha	myrrh		1.65	28	128
Coriandrum sativum (fruct.)	coriander		4.13	69	321
Cupressus sempervirens (fol.)	cypress	more than	5	83	389
Eucalyptus citriodora (fol.)	lemon-scented gum	more than	5	83	389
Eucalyptus globulus (fol.)	tasmanian blue gum		4.44	74	345
Foeniculum vulgare var. *dulce* (fruct.)	sweet fennel		3.8	63	296
Hyssopus officinalis	hyssop		1.4	23	109
Juniperus communis (fruct.)	juniper berry		8	133	622
Lavandula angustifolia	lavender	more than	5	83	389
Lavandula x intermedia Super'	lavandin	more than	5	83	389
Melaleuca alternifolia (fol.)	tea tree		1.9	32	148
Melaleuca leucadendron (fol.)	cajuput		3.87	65	301
Mentha x piperita	peppermint		4.5	75	350
Myristica fragrans (sem.)	nutmeg		2.6	43	202
Ocimum basilicum	basil		1.4	23	109
Origanum majorana	marjoram		2.24	37	174
Pelargonium graveolens (fol.)	geranium	more than	5	83	389
Pimpinella anisum (fruct.)	aniseed		2.25	38	175
Pinus sylvestris (fol.)	pine		6.88	115	535
Piper nigrum (fruct.)	black pepper	more than	5	83	389
Pogostemon patchouli (fol.)	patchouli	more than	5	83	389
Rosa damascena, R. centifolia (flos)	rose otto	more than	5	83	389
Rosmarinus officinalis	rosemary		5	83	389
Salvia officinalis	sage		2.52	42	196
Salvia sclarea	clary		5.6	93	436
Santalum album (lig.)	sandalwood		5.58	93	434
Satureia hortensis	summer savory		1.37	23	107
Syzygium aromaticum (flos)	clove bud		2.65	44	206
Thymus mastichina	spanish marjoram	more than	5	83	389
Thymus vulgaris ct. thymol	thyme		4.7	78	366
Vetiveria zizanioides (rad.)	vetiver	more than	5	83	389
Zingiber officinale (rad.)	ginger	more than	5	83	389
Compound	1,8-cineole		2.48	41	193
Compound	carvacrol		0.81	14	63
Compound	carvone		1.64	27	128
Compound	linalool		2.79	47	217
Compound	p-cymene		4.75	79	369
Compound	pulegone		0.4	7	31
Compound	safrole		1.95	33	152
Compound	terpinen-4-ol		4.3	72	334
Compound	thymol		0.98	16	76
			LDLo		
Compound	camphor		0.9	15	70
Compound	borneol		2	33	156

Flammability

One other aspect to be remembered when handling essential oils is that because they are so volatile they are highly inflammable. Flash points for essential oils (Table 3.3) range typically between 32°C for frankincense and about 110°C for atlas cedarwood, though the majority are in the range 43–70°C. They should be stored carefully in a cool, dark area, and working areas for mixing should contain no naked flame. Smoking should not be permitted and the area should be well ventilated. It may be necessary to warn the building insurer if oils are to be stocked in bulk.

UNDESIRED EFFECTS

It is undeniable that, along with the undoubted power of essential oils, there will be some unwanted effects. However, it is safe to say that these are rare, mostly only following an overdose. The general safety of essential oils normally used in aromatherapy may be judged by the health of workers who handle and inhale significant quantities of essential oils in the course of their daily work.

Some members of our own staff have been handling, bottling and breathing a wide range of oils during the whole of their working day for over a decade, with no reported bad effects. There are many therapists (including ourselves) who have been working full time with the oils over an even longer period of time who have experienced nothing but good effects, and it may therefore be inferred that aromatherapy is basically a safe therapy. However, there are one or two therapists who have developed a sensitivity to a few oils; unfortunately if the sensitivity is due to a specific chemical in the oil then wherever that chemical occurs the person may have a reaction. It should be noted, however, that in some cases a reaction may be due to an adulterant rather than a natural essential oil component.

Therapists who do not use perfumes run less risk of developing sensitivities to essential oils, as the overall quantity of synthetics employed in perfumes in day-to-day situations plays a large part in the growing number of people developing allergies and substance sensitivities (Bennett 1990)—quite an alarming fact.

In general, aromatherapists do not use the expression 'side-effects', because of its undesirable connotations. As can be seen from the list of properties of lavender oil given on page 39, most (but not all) of the side-effects of essential oils are desirable. For example, lavender oil may be used

Table 3.3 Flash points of some essential oils

	°C		°C
Boswellia carteri (dist.) [FRANKINCENSE]	32	*Myristica fragrans* (sem.) [NUTMEG]	38
Cananga odorata (flos) [YLANG YLANG]	65	*Nardostachys jatamansi* (rad.) [SPIKENARD]	>74
Cedrus atlantica (lig.) [ATLAS CEDARWOOD]	110	*Ocimum basilicum* var. *basilicum* (fol.) [EXOTIC BASIL]	75
Chamaemelum nobile (flos) [ROMAN CHAMOMILE]	58	*Ocimum basilicum* (fol.) [BASIL]	75
Citrus aurantium var. *amara* (per.) [ORANGE BIGARADE]	43–45	*Origanum majorana* (fol.) [SWEET MARJORAM]	54–59
Citrus aurantium var. *amara* (fol.) [PETITGRAIN BIGARADE]	68	*Pelargonium graveolens* (fol.) [GERANIUM]	77–85
Citrus aurantium var. *amara* (flos) [NEROLI BIGARADE]	59	*Petroselinum sativum* (fol.) [PARSLEY LEAF]	44
Citrus bergamia (per.) [BERGAMOT]	58	*Pimpinella anisum* (fruct.) [ANISEED]	90
Citrus limon (per.) [LEMON]	43–50	*Pinus sylvestris* (fol.) [PINE]	38
Citrus reticulata (per.) [MANDARIN]	43–46	*Piper nigrum* (fruct.) [BLACK PEPPER]	47–58
Cupressus sempervirens (fol.) [CYPRESS]	37	*Pogostemon patchouli* (fol.) [PATCHOULI]	>65
Eucalyptus globulus (fol.) [TASMANIAN BLUE GUM]	38–51	*Rosa damascena, R. centifolia* (flos) [ROSE OTTO]	100
Eucalyptus smithii (fol.) [GULLY GUM]	38–51	*Rosmarinus officinalis* (fol.) [ROSEMARY]	49
Eucalyptus staigeriana (fol.) [LEMON-SCENTED IRON TREE]	38–51	*Salvia officinalis* (fol.) [SAGE]	41
Foeniculum vulgare (fruct.) [FENNEL]	60	*Salvia sclarea* (flos, fol.) [CLARY]	77
Juniperus communis (ram.) [JUNIPER TWIG]	33–41	*Santalum album* (lig.) [SANDALWOOD]	>100
Juniperus communis (fruct.) [JUNIPER BERRY]	33	*Syzygium aromaticum* (flos) [CLOVE BUD]	65–100
Lavandula angustifolia (flos, fol.) [LAVENDER]	75	*Thymus mastichina* (herb.) [SPANISH MARJORAM]	55
Melaleuca alternifolia (fol.) [TEA TREE]	57	*Thymus satureioides* (herb.) [MOROCCAN THYME]	55
Melaleuca leucadendron (fol.) [CAJUPUT]	45	*Thymus vulgaris* (herb.) [THYME]	55
Melaleuca viridiflora (fol.) [NIAOULI]	46	*Valeriana officinalis* (rad.) [VALERIAN]	>74
Melissa officinalis (fol.) [MELISSA]	60	*Vetiveria zizanioides* (rad.) [VETIVER]	>65
Mentha x piperita (fol.) [PEPPERMINT]	67–70	*Zingiber officinale* (rad.) [GINGER]	55

as part of a treatment for depression. If, as a result, there are other beneficial results such as the alleviation of insomnia and relief from rheumatic pain, this is to be welcomed. Undesired side-effects occur usually as a result of the misuse of the oils, e.g. in the attempt to produce an abortion, or by accidental overdose—typically a toddler swallowing essential oils from a bottle. If essential oils are sold only in bottles with integral droppers and sensible precautions are taken to prevent access by children to the essential oils then this can be considered an extremely low risk therapy. In normal aromatherapy or aromatology usage the dose is usually very low, but idiosyncratic reaction is a rare possibility, as with any form of treatment.

In orthodox medicine, as will be explained in Chapter 4, a single molecule 'bullet' is aimed at the symptom. In aromatherapy we point a shotgun at the problem, which sprays all sorts of beneficial shot, together with the very occasional unwanted effect. Many essential oils contain constituents which when isolated are found to be toxic, but it does not automatically follow that the whole essential oil is toxic; many items normally regarded as quite safe also contain substances which, when isolated, could be shown to be toxic—tea, almonds, apples, pears, radishes, mustard, sage and hops, to name but a few (Griggs 1977).

Because of possible harmful effects, some oils are rarely or never used in aromatherapy (a more comprehensive list of such oils can be found in Appendix B.4). Some examples are *Juniperus sabina* [SAVIN], *Gaultheria procumbens* [WINTERGREEN], *Peumus boldus* [BOLDO LEAF], *Sassafras officinale* [SASSAFRAS] and *Thuja occidentalis* [THUJA].

Dermal toxicity

This term includes irritation, phototoxicity and sensitization.

Skin irritation

This is a reaction to an irritant which produces inflammation and itchiness. Some essential oils are irritating to the skin and, usually but not exclusively, these are found to contain high proportions of either aldehydes or phenols. Oils in common use which have been found to be irritant are listed in Appendix B.6. Because there appears to be a wide variation in tolerance between people, a given oil might not cause a reaction in the majority of people yet be irritant to one or two more sensitive individuals. However, dermal irritation produced by essential oils is usually localized and short lived. Assuming that one oil has a 50% presence of an offending component, this is present in the total mix at only 0.5% when the oil is used in a normal massage mix along with two or three other oils at the standard dilution of 3% essential oils in a carrier. When spread over a large area of skin the possibility of irritation is remote; the degree of irritation is proportional to the strength of the mixture applied. Examples of oils containing aldehydes can be found in Appendix B.6. The phenolic oils can also be found there, but are not listed separately. The essential oils which are potentially irritant to the skin include:

- *Cinnamomum verum* (fol.) [CINNAMON LEAF]
- *Origanum vulgare* [OREGANO]
- *Satureia hortensis* [SUMMER SAVORY]
- *Satureia montana* [WINTER SAVORY]
- *Syzygium aromaticum* (flos) [CLOVE BUD]
- *Syzygium aromaticum* (fol.) [CLOVE LEAF]
- *Syzygium aromaticum* (lig.) [CLOVE STEM]
- *Thymus vulgaris* ct. phenol [RED THYME]
- *Thymus capitatus* [SPANISH OREGANO]
- *Thymus serpyllum* [WILD THYME] (depending on chemotype).

Tagetes glandulifera is sometimes cited as being a skin irritant, but we have not found this to be the case in practice, although it is a photosensitizer. Two oils from the Cruciferae family—*Brassica nigra* [MUSTARD] and *Armoracia rusticana* [HORSERADISH]—are not normally recommended for aromatherapy use, because both consist almost entirely of allylisothiocyanate. These oils applied neat to the skin will provoke severe burning and blistering. However, it has been known for them to be recommended at the extremely low concentration of one drop of essential oil in 500 ml of carrier oil for rheumatism.

A Japanese study showed that the skin of men tends to be more than twice as sensitive as that of women, and when in situations of severe stress, lack of sleep, etc., then all skins are rendered more sensitive (Hosokawa & Ogwana 1979)

Mucous membrane irritation

Generally speaking, essential oils with a substantial content of phenols (chiefly thymol, carvacrol and eugenol) can be responsible for irritating a mucous membrane. Oils containing aldehydes may also be implicated. In the past it was believed that the hydrocarbon terpenes caused mucous membrane irritation (Gattefossé 1937 p. 40) but this is now thought not to be the case. Any of the oils listed in Appendix B.6 may cause irritation of the mucous membranes of the alimentary, respiratory and genitourinary tracts. A possible exception is lemon oil, which contains less than 5% aldehyde and consists mainly of hydrocarbon terpenes.

Phototoxicity, photosensitivity

Photosensitization is a process in which reactions to normally ineffective radiation are induced in a system by the introduction of a radiation-absorbing substance: the photosensitizer (Blum 1964, Johnson 1984, Kochevar 1987, Lamola 1974, Spikes 1977). Furanocoumarins (psoralens) appear to be primarily responsible for phytophototoxic reactions in humans (Lovell 1993). Photosensitivity may occur when certain essential oil components, particularly the expressed oils, react with the skin under the influence of ultraviolet rays, and does not occur on skin protected from natural or artificial sunlight. It may result in erythema, hyperpigmentation and perhaps vesicles, depending on the severity of the reaction. Care needs to be taken with the citrus essences, which are expressed from the peel and contain large furanocoumarin molecules: this is particularly so with bergamot. Other oils exhibiting this characteristic at aromatherapeutic doses are *Angelica archangelica* rad. [ANGELICA ROOT], *Juniperus virginiana* [VIRGINIAN CEDARWOOD], *Ruta graveolens* [RUE], *Lippia citriodora* [LEMON VERBENA] and *Cuminum cyminum* [CUMIN]. (See Appendix B.7.)

Factors which influence the phototoxic response to psoralens are the presence of a suntan, natural pigmentation (dark skin), site of application (it is worth mentioning that aromatherapy oils are applied mainly to areas not normally exposed to sunlight), skin hydration and the interval between application of the psoralen and irradiation. A particularly notable culprit is the expressed oil of *Citrus bergamia* [BERGAMOT] (Opdyke 1973), which has been studied by Zaynoun, Johnson & Frain-Bell (1977) and its use in aromatherapy needs consideration; tests by Pathak & Fitzpatrick (1959) have shown the time interval between applying psoralens and the maximal phototoxic effect to be 30–45 min (tested on guinea pig and human skin), and a later test (Arora & Willis 1976) indicated a time interval of up to 75 min.

Tests probably carried out for the benefit of the perfumery trade on bergamot in ethyl alcohol showed no phototoxic responses at a concentration of 0.5%, and at 1.0% no phototoxic response after 8 hours; the tests were carried out on five subjects (Zaynoun, Johnson & Frain-Bell 1977 p. 231) and also showed that intervals of 1 to 2 hours between application and irradiation yielded a maximal phototoxic response. Applying this directly to aromatherapy is questionable as aromatherapists do not use ethyl alcohol as a medium for application, and the flow of psoralen through the horny layer of the skin is dependent on the carrier used (Kaidbey & Kligman 1974, Kammerau et al 1976). It is known that the horny layer is a major barrier to the penetration of psoralens; in tests, 70–90% of topically applied 8-methoxypsoralen (8-MOP, xanthotoxin, which is not present in bergamot oil) did not enter the horny layer and was finally lost through sloughing (Kammerau et al 1976). Bergamot oil itself is resorbed through the skin in 40–60 minutes (Römmelt et al 1974, Valette 1945).

The tests by Zaynoun, Johnson & Frain-Bell (1977 p. 232) also showed that using paraffin molle flavum (PMF) as the carrier resulted in increased speed of penetration through the horny layer and produced a shorter period in which phototoxicity persists than when using ethanol, and it is possible that the effects using a vegetable oil as a carrier more closely resemble those results using PMF than those using alcohol.

The IFRA Committee recommends a level of 5-MOP (bergapten, a naturally occurring analogue of psoralen) of 75 ppm in a (fragrance) compound, and assuming a 5-MOP content of 0.35% this equates to a level of expressed bergamot oil in the compound of 2% (Jouhar 1991) and this translates to 0.4% (about eight drops in 100 ml) in the aromatherapy preparation applied to the skin. The use of 5-MOP is forbidden in the EU except as a normal component of essential oils.

In our practical experience over two decades, there has been no reported problem for thousands of therapists who have followed our training and numerous clients who have followed our advice. On this basis, it is suggested that following application of bergamot oil using the normal aromatherapy dilution (usually less than 1%, as essential oils are usually used in synergistic blends, and not individually) it is reasonably safe to expose the skin of normal people to sunlight provided that more than 2 hours have elapsed since the application. This advice may be tempered by the holistic approach and any unusual sensitivity of the individual client.

On the other hand, it is interesting to note that some other simple coumarin derivatives, such as umbelliferon, herniarin and aesculetin have a sunlight filter effect because they absorb ultraviolet light of 280–315 nm (Schilcher 1985 p. 228).

Contact sensitization

There are some oils which do not produce any reaction on first contact with the skin, but may do so on a subsequent application. The body's reaction involves the immune system, via the cells in the basal layer of the epidermis. There are several oils which are sensitizing, and there seems to be no common denominator. Poor storage of oils containing a significant amount of monoterpenes can lead to the formation of sensitizing hydroperoxides: an infamous example is turpentine, which is responsible for skin allergies to workers in the paint industry. Oils to be wary of in this respect are shown in Appendix B.8.

Cross-sensitization

Once a person is sensitized to one substance, then that person is more likely to be susceptible to other similar substances, although the risk is low. This need not cause concern, but any aromatherapist who is sensitive to substances should be aware of the possibility. This is a complex topic, not well understood, but one example is when people become sensitive to benzoin after sensitization to Peru balsam or turpentine. There is a similar relationship between turpentine and peppermint (see Appendix B.8).

Other sensitivities and toxicities

Prolonged use

If any one oil is used for a very long period of time then there may be a risk of sensitization even though none exists for normal usage. It is relevant to note here that when eau de Cologne (which contains bergamot and other citrus essences) was much in vogue many people wore it daily over a period of years and developed raised erythematous rough skin where the eau de Cologne had been applied—usually on the neck (berloque dermatitis). This reaction can be semi-permanent, lasting for years after cessation of use of the fragrance before disappearing (Shirley Price's personal experience). Many perfumes have ingredients in common with eau de Cologne and may produce similar reactions.

Tea tree oil was identified as a possible cause of relapsing eczema in a 53-year-old woman who had prolonged exposure to the oil (Schaller & Korting 1995). She was also allergic to other essential oils including lavender, jasmin and rosewood, which may have resulted from prolonged exposure to the oils, but was in addition allergic to laurel and eucalyptus, to which she had not been previously exposed. This report emphasizes the importance of treating essential oils with respect, especially when using them for prolonged periods of time. To obviate toxicity as a result of overuse of any one oil, it is good aromatherapy practice to employ essential oils for short-term use and to change the oils used during a treatment of long duration.

A survey of 120 aromatherapists carried out by Wong (1995), in conjunction with Aromatherapy Quarterly, of the personal effects of essential oils on therapists using essential oils in treatments, revealed that they took place on many levels. A few suffered adverse effects but it was felt that these were due to reactions to clients rather than to the oils themselves. It is emphasized that this was a survey, not a properly constituted trial. Of the 120 therapists surveyed:

- most felt the effects were beneficial
- only two were men
- most had been in practice for less than 4 years
- most gave fewer than 10 treatments per week
- 40 different oils were mentioned.

Effects on particular systems included the following.
The skin:

- 105 therapists experienced insignificant or no effect.
- Several therapists experienced skin irritation, often between the fingers, and sweet almond oil and geranium were mentioned by two therapists as the offenders.
- Two therapists appeared to have developed eczema, and one previous dermatitis had disappeared.

Emotional and mental state:

- Only seven therapists surveyed felt that the oils had had no effect, with a majority feeling a moderate to great effect, usually beneficial, helping to calm, relieve headache and help sleep.
- Sleeplessness was mentioned in connection with geranium, bergamot, lemongrass, peppermint and rosemary.

Female reproductive system:

- About 28% of the women surveyed felt some effect on their reproductive system, but most did not know whether this was due to the essential oils or to other factors.

- Some said they felt no effects when using oils on clients but experienced considerable effects when using oils on themselves.
- Most experienced positive effects such as an improvement in PMS, period pains, and menopausal symptoms, and a more regular menstrual cycle.
- Clary sage was mentioned many times in this context.
- Six aromatherapists had been pregnant while practising; some found their sense of smell became more acute and they could not tolerate strong aromas.
- A few therapists felt adverse effects such as tender breasts, irregular or heavy menstruation, a change in menstrual cycle and fluctuating hormone levels, but these are common and may not be linked to essential oil use.

Digestive system:

- 109 found a slight or no effect.
- Some found that the calming effect of the essential oils helped digestive problems; a few reported flatulence; others had disturbed bowel movements.

Urinary system:

- 106 reported a slight or no effect, with 11 reporting moderate to great effect.

Lymphatic system:

- 96 felt no effects.
- Of the 22 who reported effects, about half were positive and half negative regarding fluid retention, congestion and swollen glands (some felt their symptoms were due to standing).

Immune system:

- 96 felt a positive effect on their immune system and three felt negative symptoms.

Respiratory system:

- Approximately half of those surveyed felt improved symptoms in catarrh, coughs, hay fever, asthma, breathing or chest infections.
- A few thought that their symptoms were made worse.

Circulation, muscles and joints:

- Any adverse effects were felt to be due to performing massage rather than to essential oils.
- Some felt their joint and muscle problems had improved.

(Note: the quality and purity of the oils used by those surveyed is unknown and it is well known that synthetics added to essential oils can have effects of their own. In a general survey such as this other circumstances may well have had an effect, e.g. diet, medication, general state of health, allergies, etc.; the performance of the massage itself may be responsible for some of the joint and circulation problems reported.)

Mutagenicity and teratogenicity

There is no available evidence that any natural essential oil has ever provoked mutagenicity or teratogenicity in an embryo or developing fetus. No tests have been carried out because the possibility of fragrant materials causing either genetic mutation or malformation is regarded as unlikely.

Carcinogenicity

A few oils have been tested for carcinogenicity on animals and the essential oil components safrole and dihydrosafrole have been implicated in the formation of hepatic tumours in rats; calamus oil containing β-asarone produced duodenal tumours (Taylor et al 1967). For this reason sassafras, which contains safrole as an important constituent, is not used in aromatherapy. Safrole is also significantly present in Brazilian sassafras oil, and in trace amounts in white camphor oil.

Beta asarone (found in calamus oil) is restricted in foods and drinks to 0.1–1 mg/kg. Despite the evidence from animal testing (where the doses used were large), it is thought that there is minimal risk in humans undergoing aromatherapy treatment.

Neurotoxicity

Special care must be taken with a few essential oils containing significant amounts of a ketone,

which can be aggressive to nerve tissue. Not all ketones are neurotoxic (Tisserand 1985 p. 61, Winter 1984 pp. 62–63), but as a class they must be regarded as hazardous in this respect. Particular care must be exercised when using oils containing apiole (e.g. *Petroselinum sativum* (fruct.)[PARSLEY SEED]) and ascaridole (e.g. *Peumus boldus*). (For risks of using neurotoxic oils in pregnancy see Ch. 10.) The molecules in essential oils are lipid soluble and as such can pass the blood–brain barrier and access the central nervous system. The degree of lipid solubility varies from one class of molecule to another; e.g. esters are more fat soluble than are alcohols. Once past this barrier there is a potential for toxicity; accidental overdose of *Syzygium aromaticum* [CLOVE] produced convulsions in a child. It is thought that the ketone thujone (found in *Thuja occidentalis*, *Salvia officinalis*, *Tanacetum vulgare*, *Artemisia vulgaris* and *A. absinthium*) is toxic to the central nervous system, as is the ketone asarone (found in *Acorus calamus*) (Wenzel & Ross 1957).

Hepatotoxicity

When using essential oils having appreciable quantities of aldehydes there is a risk of toxicity due to build-up in the liver. People taking fennel essential oil over a long period of time show a colour change in the liver tissue (Franchomme & Pénoël 1990). Thujone, thymol and turpentine oil may damage the liver following oral ingestion in high doses (Schilcher 1985 p 229). Liver toxicity seems to arise when innocuous essential oil components are metabolized to toxic chemicals, as with pulegone, found in many of the mint oils. Also to be treated with caution (based largely on animal testing using very high doses) are methyl chavicol (found in *Artemisia dracunculus* [TARRAGON]), safrole (in *Sassafras albidum*), myristicin and elemicin (in *Myristica fragrans* [NUTMEG]) and apiole (in *Petroselinum sativum* (fruct.)[PARSLEY SEED]).

Nephrotoxicity

Some essential oils have an effect on the kidneys which is regarded as stimulating and beneficial in low doses, but could be classed as toxic if the quantity of oil used is excessive or it is used for too long a time. *Juniperus sabina* [SAVIN] is mentioned by Schilcher (1985 p. 229) as causing damage to the kidneys, even when applied externally. Large quantities of the ester methyl salicylate, found in the oils of *Gaultheria procumbens* [WINTERGREEN] and *Betula lenta* [SWEET BIRCH], and of safrole (found in *S. albidum* [SASSAFRAS]) are nephrotoxic. Sandalwood and turpentine taken orally in excessive doses can also cause kidney damage (Tukioka 1927).

Respiratory sensitivity

See Chapter 5, Section on inhalation.

OCCUPATIONAL HEALTH AND SAFETY

Although used only in very small amounts by aromatherapists to utilize their healing properties, essential oils are complex chemical compounds. When used knowledgeably and with due caution, essential oils do not present a threat to health, but there are considered to be certain hazards associated with their use. This section considers the difference between 'hazard' and 'risk', and goes on to discuss the workplace regulatory requirements which must be observed when essential oils are being used.

Essential oil risk

Essential oils are complicated chemicals; although natural, they should nevertheless be a part of workplace risk assessment. Having said that, if they are used in correct amounts, with knowledge and all known precautions adhered to then they are relatively safe. However, until training in aromatherapy is of a consistent and high standard at every training school, there are several oils which may be hazardous and are therefore better used with caution in certain conditions, e.g. epilepsy and pregnancy. The latter is a moot point as any caution required is mainly in the first 4 months, becoming less necessary as the pregnancy progresses. This means that the most important time to be heedful could be before the

person concerned even knows she is pregnant. Nevertheless, it is important to be seen to be judicious especially as many people without qualifications use essential oils without considering any risk that may be involved.

The following was contained in the report from the research and scientific subcommittee at an Aromatherapy Organisations Council (AOC) meeting in November 1997: 'In a recent article in Complementary Therapies in Medicine it was said that since neither medicines nor cosmetics fall under COSHH and/or CHIP regulations but under the relevant Safety Sections of their respective regulations, the Health and Safety Executive (HSE) is uncertain as to whether they would actually apply to essential oils (AOC 1997)'. However, further enquiries show that regulations are needed—although these are mainly for bulk suppliers.

The molecular makeup of chemicals influences local or systemic toxicological effects and their elimination from the body. Some are known to be harmless and others harmful to varying degrees. For the vast majority there remains ambiguity over their effects and some are still a complete mystery.

(Fowler & Wall 1997)

Risk assessment

A hazard is anything that has the potential to cause harm. Essential oils have the potential to cause harm and could thus be labelled as hazardous, because they:

- are flammable
- should be kept away from the eyes
- may be irritants
- may be sensitizers
- should be avoided or used with caution in certain circumstances
- should not, in general, be taken internally without specific training.

However, many substances have the potential to cause harm if used incorrectly: oranges and potatoes are not named as hazardous, yet a surfeit of oranges or the ingestion of underripe or 'green' potatoes can cause health problems; too much alcohol can impair the liver; too many aspirins can damage the lining of the stomach. None of these products are labelled as hazardous—it is simply a question of correct, controlled and informed use; their overuse is almost always by personal choice.

Just because something is hazardous does not mean a problem exists, but rather that caution is necessary, especially for the uninformed. The likelihood that a hazard will lead to actual harm is the risk of it happening. So, in order to obtain a clear picture of what could go wrong and how serious an accident could be, an assessment of risk must be carried out. The Management of Health and Safety at Work regulations (HMSO 1992) require employers to carry out such assessments. In this way all workplace hazards can be identified, along with the associated risks and the actions necessary to eliminate or reduce risks of accidents and injuries.

Hazard assessment

If a material has the potential to harm a person it is considered to be a hazardous substance and the Control of Substances Hazardous to Health (COSHH) regulations of 1994 (Health and Safety Commission 1994) apply. These regulations do not set out specific requirements for specific circumstances; their aim is rather to assess, monitor and reduce the presence of possibly hazardous substances to the lowest possible level of risk, thereby preventing anyone who may come into contact with the materials from being harmed in any way. COSHH requires that:

- the current situation is identified
- a decision is made on what to do about it.

These demands are met by carrying out a specific risk assessment. The legal obligation is that the assessment be suitable and sufficient; simpler and lower risk situations will require less consideration than will more serious and complex risks. The aim is to reach reliable conclusions based on informed judgement.

For most essential oils their presentation, the amount used and the frequency of use together with the use of correct packaging (e.g. integral drop dispensers), means that any possible harmful effects are minimized. A simple assessment

for each essential oil in use, drawing attention to this, will meet the requirements of COSHH. The assessment must include not only the effects of essential oils on patients and clients but also on anyone else exposed to them, where cognitive function could be affected, thus altering the person's behaviour and reaction time, resulting in suppression of the cerebral inhibiting systems (Boyle 1993); the relaxation effects are now well established (Birchall 1990, Buchbauer et al 1991, Hardy 1991, Karamat et al 1992) so there may be the masking of warning signals, perhaps due to smell habituation or insensitivity to slow changes (Boyle 1987).

Assessment is not a one-off exercise; the regulations demand the situation is reviewed on a regular basis, the Approved Code of Practice (HSE 1997a) recommending an interval of no longer than 5 years. However, the assessment must be reviewed if anything changes—for example, if a new essential oil is in use.

Some essential oils, e.g. tea tree, have been classified in such a way (HSE 1997b) that the Chemical Hazard Information and Packaging for Supply (CHIP 2) regulations of 1994 apply. As with COSHH, the CHIP 2 regulations are designed to protect people from the ill effects of chemicals. Suppliers and manufacturers are required to provide safety data sheets, identify hazards associated with the chemicals and package them safely. The materials have to be classified, and assigned a formal category of danger together with an appropriate risk phrase.

CHIP 2 safety data sheets can be an important source of the information needed when completing COSHH risk assessments. However, the safety data sheet alone is not sufficient as a COSHH assessment, and not all essential oils have been categorized by CHIP 2. For example, essential oils are not included in Guidance Note EH40 (HSE 1995), which lists the maximum exposure limits and the occupational exposure standards for substances hazardous to health.

Safety data sheets

CHIP 2 applies only to the supply and storage of bulk quantities of material and retailers do not have to provide a safety data sheet for domestic use of essential oils. However, if a therapist intends to use the oils at work, a sheet can be requested. Furthermore, CHIP 2 does not specify exactly what should go into a safety data sheet; it gives headings under which information has to be provided and says that this information has to be sufficient. In this context 'sufficient' means adopting a commonsense approach and giving enough information to ensure that both people at work and the environment can be properly protected.

Accordingly, any data sheet supplied should address the following issues:

- name and location of the supplier
- product identification
- composition/ingredients
- first aid measures
- fire-fighting measures
- accidental release and disposal precautions
- handling and storage
- health hazards
- physical and chemical properties
- other appropriate information.

Suppliers are responsible for the accuracy of the safety data sheet, and any doubts or worries should be addressed to them. A particular concern with essential oils is the variability in quality, which cannot be guaranteed, as there are no regulations about this (Trevelyan 1993). Adulteration and mislabelling are not uncommon, and clearly this will influence the accuracy of any related data sheets. This is yet another reason for ensuring that only genuine essential oils are used therapeutically; in other words, as they come from the still, with nothing added and nothing taken away.

Summary

The need for a dispassionate and scientific attitude towards media charges of the dangers of essential oils has been demonstrated, as has the need for skill in their selection and prescription. Various types of potentially toxic situations have been identified. These should not occur if the guidelines for safe administration are followed. Despite this, essential oils must be treated as hazardous substances. In order to comply with the requirements of COSHH a thorough assessment of the potential risks associated with their use must be carried out in order to prevent anyone who may come into contact with them from being harmed.

REFERENCES

AOC 1997 Report from research and scientific sub-committee for Executive and Council meetings on 27 November 1997

Arora S K, Willis I 1976 Factors influencing methoxsalen phototoxicity in vitiliginous skin. Archives of Dermatology 112: 327

Bennett G 1990 Allergy and substance sensitivity. Course notes. Shirley Price Aromatherapy College, Hinckley

Birchall A 1990 A whiff of happiness. New Scientist 127(1731): 45–47

Blum H F 1964 Photodynamic action and diseases caused by light. Hafner, New York

Boyle A J 1987 Human reliability; risk assessment and control. Occupational Health and Safety Open Learning, pp 26/2–26/30

Boyle R J 1993 Human reliability; risk assessment and control. Version 2. Occupational Health and Safety Training Unit, Portsmouth University Enterprises Ltd, Section 9–13

Buchbauer G, Jirovetz L, Jäger W, Dietrich H, Plank C 1991 Aromatherapy: evidence for sedative effects of the essential oil of lavender after inhalation. Zeitschrift für Natürforschung 46(11–12): 1067–1072

Duraffourd P 1982 En forme tous les jours. La Vie Claire, Périgny

Fowler P, Wall M 1997 COSHH and CHIPS: ensuring the safety of aromatherapy. Complementary Therapies in Medicine 5: 112–115

Franchomme P, Pénoël D 1990 L'aromathérapie exactement. Jollois, Limoges

Gattefossé R-M 1937 Aromatherapy (trans 1993). Daniel, Saffron Walden, p 34

Griggs B 1977 New green pharmacy. Vermilion, London, p 305

Hall C 1904 cited in Valnet J 1980 The practice of aromatherapy. Daniel, Saffron Walden

Hardy M 1991 Sweet scented dreams. International Journal of Aromatherapy 3(2): 13

Health and Safety Commission 1994 The control of substances hazardous to health regulations. HMSO, London

HMSO 1992 Management of Health and Safety at Work regulations. HMSO, London

Hosokawa H, Ogwana T 1979 Study of skin irritations caused by perfumery materials. Perfumer and Flavorist 4(4): 7–8

Hotchkiss S 1994 How thin is your skin? New Scientist (29 January) 141(1910): 24–27

Howes A, Chan U, Caldwell J 1990 Structure specificity of the genotoxicity of some naturally occurring alkenylbenzenes determined by the unscheduled DNA synthesis assay in rat hepatocytes. Food and Chemical Toxicology 28(8): 537–542

HSE 1995 Occupational exposure limits—EH40. HSE Books, Sudbury

HSE 1997a General COSHH ACOP, carcinogens ACOP and biological agents ACOP (1996 edition): Control of Substances Hazardous to Health Regulations 1994. HSE Books, Sudbury

HSE 1997b Approved supply list: information approved for the classification and labelling of substances and preparations dangerous for supply, 3rd edn. HSE, Sudbury

IFRA (International Fragrance Association) 1992 Code of practice. IFRA, Geneva

Jenner P M, Hagan E C, Taylor J M, Cook E L, Fitzhugh O G 1964 Food flavourings and compounds of related structure. I. Acute oral toxicity. Food and Cosmetics Toxicology 2: 327

Johnson B E 1984 Light sensitivity associated with drugs and chemicals. In Jarrett A (ed) The physiology and pathophysiology of the skin. Academic Press, New York, pp 541–606

Jouhar A J (ed) 1991 Poucher's perfumes, cosmetics and soaps, vol 1, 9th edn. Blackie, Glasgow, p 40

Kaidbey K H, Kligman A M 1974 Photopigmentation with trioxsalen. Archives of Dermatology 109: 674

Kammerau B, Klebe U, Zesche A, Schaefer H 1976 Penetration, permeation and resorption of 8-methoxypsoralen. Comparative in vitro and in vivo studies after topical application of four standard preparations. Archives of Dermatological Research 255: 31

Karamat E, Ilmberger J, Buchbauer G, Rößlhuber K, Rupp C 1992 Excitatory and sedative effects of essential oils on human reaction time performance. Chemical Senses 17: 847

Kligman A M 1966 The identification of contact allergens by human assay. III. The maximization test, a procedure for screening and rating contact sensitizers. Journal of Investigative Dermatology 47: 393

Kligman A M, Epstein W 1975 Updating the maximization test for identifying contact allergens. Contact Dermatitis 1: 231

Kochevar I E 1987 Mechanisms of drug photosensitization. Photochemistry and Photobiology 45: 891–895

Lamola A A 1974 Fundamental aspects of spectroscopy and photochemistry of organic compounds; electronic energy transfer in biologic systems; and photosensitization. In: Fitzpatrick T B (ed) Sunlight and man. University of Tokyo Press, Tokyo, pp 17–55

Levenstein I 1976 Report to RIFM 18 August. Cited in Food and Cosmetics Toxicology 16: 673

Lovell R C 1993 Plants and the skin. Blackwell Scientific, London, p 65

Low D, Rawal B D, Griffin W J 1974 Antibacterial action of the essential oils of some Australian Myrtaceae with special references to the activity of chromatographic fractions of oil of Eucalyptus citriodora. Planta Medica 26: 184–189

Opdyke D L 1973 Bergamot oil expressed. Food and Cosmetics Toxicology 11: 1031–1033

Opdyke D L J 1976 Inhibition of sensitization reactions induced by certain aldehydes. Food and Cosmetics Toxicology 14(3): 197–198

Opdyke D L J 1979 Fragrance raw materials monographs. Food and Chemical Toxicology 17(3): 253–258

Pathak M A, Fitzpatrick T B 1959 Relationship of molecular configuration to the activity of furocoumarins which increase the cutaneous responses following long wave ultraviolet radiation. Journal of Investigative Dermatology 32: 255

Pénoël D 1992/93 Winter shield. International Journal of Aromatherapy 4(4): 11

Price L 1990 Clinical practitioners aromatherapy course notes. Shirley Price International College of Aromatherapy, Hinckley

Price S 1993 The aromatherapy workbook. Thorsons, London

Römelt H, Zuber A, Dirnagl K, Drexel H 1974 Münchner Medizinische Wochenschrift 116: 537 cited in Schilcher H 1985 Effects and side effects of essential oils. In: Baerheim Svendsen A, Scheffer J J C (eds) Essential oils and aromatic plants. Martinus Nijhof/Junk, Dordrecht, p 228

Schaller M S, Korting H C 1995 Allergic airborne contact dermatitis from essential oils used in aromatherapy. Clinical and Experimental Dermatology 20(2): 143–145

Schilcher H 1985 Effects and side-effects of essential oils. In: Baerheim Svendsen A, Scheffer J J C (eds) Essential oils and aromatic plants. Martinus Nijhof/Junk, Dordrecht p 229

Schröder J 1689 Pharmacopoea medico-chymica, thesaurus pharmacologus. (Ulm 1641, 1649, 1655, 1662, 1705) (Frankfurt 1640, 1669, 1677) (Lyons 1649, 1656, 1665, 1681) (Leyden 1672) (Geneva 1689) (Nürnberg 1746)

Spikes J D 1977 Photosensitization. In: Smith K C (ed) The science of photobiology. Plenum, New York, pp 87–110

Taylor J M et al 1967 Toxicity of oil of calamus (Jammu variety). Toxicology and Applied Pharmacology 10: 405

Tisserand R 1985 The essential oil safety data manual. Association of Tisserand Aromatherapists, Brighton

Tisserand R, Balacs T 1995 Essential oil safety. Churchill Livingstone, New York

Trevelyan J 1993 Aromatherapy. Nursing Times 89(25): 38–40

Tukioka M 1927 Proceedings. Imperial Academy Tokyo 3: 624

Tyman J H P 1990 Essential Oils Trade Association Symposium, Brunel University, June

Valette C 1945 Société de Biologie Comptes Rendus 13 October cited in: Katz A E 1947 Pénétration transcutanée des essences. Parfumerie Modern 39: 64–66

Valnet J 1980 The practice of aromatherapy. Daniel, Saffron Walden, p 11

Wenzel D G, Ross C R 1957 Journal of the American Pharmaceutical Association 46: 77

Winter R 1984 A consumer's dictionary of cosmetic ingredients. Crown, New York

Wong M 1995 The healing touch: survey results. Aromatherapy Quarterly 46: 26–29

Zaynoun S T, Johnson B E, Frain-Bell W 1977 A study of bergamot and its importance as a phototoxic agent. II. Factors which affect the phototoxic reaction induced by bergamot oil and psoralen derivatives. Contact Dermatitis 3: 225–239

Traditional use, modern research

Introduction

The use of essential oils as part of traditional plant-based medicine has led to the accumulation of a large body of empirical knowledge about their effectiveness in different conditions. This chapter looks systematically at their therapeutic properties, and shows where possible how modern science confirms traditional usage.

ORTHODOX MEDICINE AND PHYTOTHERAPY

There have always existed many different approaches to the healing of people. Today these approaches are generally viewed as being complementary and supplementary to each other rather than competitive and antagonistic. Two of the different medical approaches are contrasted here: orthodox medicine and phytotherapy.

The orthodox approach

The predominant contemporary approach is that adopted by orthodox allopathic medicine, where illness is regarded as being due to an outside agent. Throughout the ages this outside agent concept has been looked upon in various ways and illness attributed to 'evil spirits', 'ill will' or 'microbes' and, in more modern times, 'bacteria' and 'viruses'. In classical medicine the aim is to target and exterminate this outside agent, so freeing the body from further attack; the body is left to repair itself (Verdet 1989). It has, however, been estimated that 85% of all illness is self-limiting (see Ch. 8).

This selective focusing on the causative agent has brought about an enormous increase in the knowledge of the separate body systems and organs. However, the sheer volume of knowledge acquired has resulted in specialization and compartmentalization becoming the norm, and it is left to the general practitioner to preserve an overview of the whole person.

For many decades now medicine, and consequently pharmacy, has lived under the reign of analysis, of simplification. This philosophy shows itself in the production of medicines which are for the most part composed of a single well defined molecule, well-known regarding its structure and properties, particularly the pharmacodynamics or therapeutic action on the organism. This style of analysis and simplification is the heritage of Descartes, who said quite rightly that to know the body better it was necessary to divide it into its constituent parts.

(Duraffourd 1982 p. 14)

This excellent principle has, however, been pursued to such a degree that there now exists a detrimental imbalance in medical care as the large number of iatrogenic illnesses shows.

The phytotherapy approach

Phytotherapy (herbal medicine, but without the old-fashioned connotation of 'herbalism') deals exclusively in whole plants or isolated plant principles, and aromatherapy may be considered to be one of its branches (unlike homoeopathy, which uses plant, animal and mineral materials). It is essentially an empirical medicine, which recognizes the importance of the individual, and that each person lives his/her own ill health. This means that each person must receive individual treatment and care in his/her own environment, which may take longer than orthodox medicine but has a long-lasting effect. As well as treating illness, phytotherapy and aromatherapy are valuable for everyday prophylactic use, reinforcing weak points in the person to maintain good health. The following theoretical comparison illustrates the different approaches taken by orthodox and complementary practitioners in treating a person.

• **Allopathy.** Should an apparently healthy person suddenly develop a gastroenteric prob-lem, a gastroenterologist will investigate only the digestive system and not pay too much attention to neighbouring organs and systems. The offending bacteria will be identified in the laboratory and an antidote will be prescribed, most probably an antibiotic. After treatment the symptoms will disappear and the client is said to have regained health.

• **Aromatherapy.** The therapist will look at the patient and will say that the defence system has broken down, allowing the bacteria to enter and thrive, and that this is the cause of the illness. The weakness will be considered in relation to other systems—kidneys, liver, lungs, skin—and all this is then studied in the context of the living environment. The illness may be a problem relating to food, a stressful experience or climate, and a balance must be sought; the therapist using the properties of essential oils has the necessary weapons to effect this.

I had seen the miracles of modern medicine in Intensive Care; in daily practice it was not the same. Sick people fell ill again; sick people suffered side effects; new sicknesses appeared when I treated them with chemical medicines. But what struck me most of all was the complete absence of the human dimension.

(Dr Jean-Claude Lapraz, quoted in Griggs 1997)

Recent history of plant-based medicine

At the beginning of this century many medicines were based on plants and plant extracts. One reason for the former popular use of plants in healing was their easy availability in a still largely rural environment—people could gather plants and process their own medicines. Another reason for their use was the prevailing poverty at the time. In many areas of Europe money was scarce, there was little state assistance and private health insurance was practically unknown. Bonnelle (1993) quotes some older people's memories:

Before the social security, when people had to pay, they didn't call the doctor out … That's why people used to treat themselves with plants then. My mother had 50 plants which she used to dry … The doctor never came to our house. 20 franc pieces came in but never went out, except to buy a field.

However, after the Second World War, orthodox medicine took advantage of recent developments in science and technology. This resulted in an accelerating shift in emphasis from natural medicines to rapidly acting drugs. Dr Jean-Claude Lapraz made this observation:

When I was a boy my grandfather had a farm in the country, and I noticed that everybody used plants: they drank them in infusions, they made an oil to treat burns—oh yes, plants worked, I saw that clearly. But later, in all the years I spent in medical school, nobody ever mentioned plants. Not a single one.

(quoted in Griggs 1997)

Decline and fall of popular plant medicine

As part of the fresh start after the Second World War, state medicine was introduced in some Western European countries, including France and the UK. This was one of the greatest advances in civilization the world has seen, and we should all be very much the worse off, both as individuals and as a society, if it did not exist. Unwittingly though, this wonderful step forward struck a near-mortal blow at folk plant medication because, with the availability of free treatment and advice from doctors, the knowledge of centuries was discarded, or at best put to one side and little used. People were no longer content with the gentle use of plants which took rather a long time both to prepare and to bring about healing. They had great expectations of the new synthetic drugs, which genuinely appeared then to produce immediate and startling results without any real effort on the part of the sufferer.

Nowadays, speaking for myself, plants are not strong enough. I used nothing else before ... but now you have to get the doctors' medicines. When they discovered the new drugs, everyone forgot about the plants.

(Bonnelle 1993)

Both doctors and vets have used antibiotics extensively and liberally since 1945, and people's expectations of medical practice have changed, in that instant cures are asked for, without any effort or responsibility on the part of the sufferer. In a broad sense the relationship of people to their own health has changed and, as plant remedies have fallen into disuse and lost ground to high tech instant medicine, popular knowledge has disappeared inexorably. The older generation who used to practise self-healing with plants still talk about plants but no longer use them and do not pass on their knowledge to their successors.

In the flower-power and Beatles age of the 1960s and 1970s there was a resurgence of many ideas, including caring for the ecological balance of nature, the use of natural as opposed to synthetic products, and the idea of eating organically grown foods. This new vision also encompassed the field of medicine and as a result many alternative (as they were viewed then) approaches to healing took root and flourished. These are now known as energetic, parallel or complementary approaches and, in contradistinction to the idea of conquering the illness by destroying the disease, there is much attention paid to a holistic style of treatment, of strengthening the body's own natural defences to cope with attacks by pathogens, of helping a person to live in harmony with their own body, with other people and with the environment. When a person is successful in this, then good health is enjoyed, and illness strikes when the balance of the person within the environment is disturbed.

Today plant remedies are beginning to become more popular again, chiefly for small problems (such as headaches and twinges) which are too insignificant to warrant troubling the busy doctor and for chronic complaints (which by definition are not easily susceptible to orthodox treatment). Here, people are prepared to try, at their own expense, alternative procedures for the 'you must learn to live with it' conditions. It is significant that the most popular aromatherapy treatment and therefore one which might be regarded as successful is, in our experience, for chronic arthritis and rheumatism.

Modern research and traditional usage

Huge sums are spent on research, clinical trials and licensing for each orthodox medicine, pill or tablet which appears on the market. This is done with the best will in the world—to help alleviate suffering and disease—but medical science is now faced with the situation, despite all the care and time spent on research, that there are still many serious side-effects. Essential oils have not been clinically tested in this way because it would cost billions, not millions, of pounds to test each oil and synergistic mix for each therapeutic effect of which it is capable. In the absence of scientific proof, orthodoxy finds it difficult to accept a discipline such as aromatherapy, which is still more art than science. Nevertheless essential oils have been used traditionally for hundreds of years to good effect. Had they manifested serious side-effects their use would certainly not have survived to the present day; yet in the recent past clinical tests on animals (which have a different physiology from humans) have allowed the creation of drugs which have had disastrous effects on humans; Thalidomide and Opren passed such recognized tests. Apart from animal testing being abhorrent to the whole philosophy of natural holistic medicine, it has often proved impossible to extrapolate the results of animal testing to the human physiology. The enormous beneficial advances made in the field of orthodox medicine should not be underestimated, but appreciation and inclusion of the available natural ways are needed too—there is room for more than one approach in the healing arena.

Acceptance of aromatherapy

Litigation in all fields of medicine has increased dramatically over the last decade and it has now reached a significant level of cost. Where midwifery is concerned, the Congenital Disabilities (Civil Liabilities) Act 1976 provides for a child to be entitled to recover damages where he/she has suffered as a result of a breach in duty of care, and litigation can be instigated up to 21 years after the event. With this in mind it is understandable to a degree that 'unproven' complementary treatments and medicaments are viewed with a certain amount of caution. Nevertheless, the attitude of doctors to alternative and complementary therapies is changing, as is shown by the following surveys carried out in the UK, Canada, Israel and USA.

• **UK.** A survey of doctors revealed that 93% of all general practitioners (GPs) and 70% of hospital doctors had suggested a referral to alternative treatment at least once; 20% of GPs and 12% of house doctors practised an alternative therapy (Perkin, Pearcy & Fraser 1994). Researchers at the University of Exeter reviewed 12 surveys of doctors and found that, on average, 46% considered complementary therapies to be effective, but noted that young doctors were significantly more favourable to complementary therapies than were older doctors (Ernst, Resch & White 1995).
• **Canada.** 73% of doctors surveyed wanted to know more about the major alternative therapies; they believed that alternative therapies were most needed for chronic pain or illness and musculoskeletal disorders (Verhoef & Sutherland 1995).
• **Israel.** There were similar findings in a survey of Israeli doctors, where 60% of all physicians had made referrals to alternative health practitioners at least once (Borkan et al 1994).
• **USA.** Doctors are showing growing interest in alternative/complementary remedies, with over 70% in one survey indicating that they would like to learn more about the available therapies (Berman et al 1995).

The intrinsically safe practice of aromatherapy is finding acceptance in many hospital departments today. The following comparison may help to explain why.

• **Orthodox drugs.** These are predominantly synthetic but may include isolated natural components, and are mostly used in a symptomatic way. Side-effects (iatrogenic disease) are always present to some degree and may necessitate further medication. The newer antidepressants (e.g. fluoxetine) can cause side-effects including nausea, vomiting and diarrhoea, and this may be the reason for the continued use of tricyclic drugs (e.g. dothiepin hydrochloride) despite the risks shown by research. The drugs themselves are usually available only on prescription, but less powerful drugs and tablets are sometimes available over the counter. The clinical testing of drugs is rigorous but carried out over a comparatively short timescale compared with traditional plant usage.

The United States Patent Office is ready to grant patents for medicines, although it is an open question in professional ethics whether a physician should patent a remedy. Synthetic medicines, prepared by chemical processes, often coal tar products, are now invading the field of Nature's simples, and it is possible that there may yet be a number of patentable compounds invented, to replace quinine and other vegetable alkloids and extracts.

(Scientific American, 1886)

Side-effects come not only from the drug itself but also are due to additives, such as colouring. Pollock et al (1989) carried out a survey of 2204 orthodox drugs and found 419 different additives present in 930 formulations; these additives may cause a variety of reactions in some people, e.g. nettle rash, watery eyes and nose, blurred vision, oedema, bronchoconstriction (Bowker no date) and hypersensitivity reactions and photo-allergy (Lawrence 1987). Artificial colourings and preservatives are not added to essential oils.

- **Essential oils.** These are natural products extracted by steam distillation, those used in aromatherapy being obtained from a single, specified botanical source. Only whole, non-standardized, unadulterated oils should be used in aromatherapy.

Aromatherapy seeks to instil respect for the therapeutic powers inherent in natural aromas that have not been tampered with by humans. It also tries to show how the wider ecosystem which produces natural essential oils is of ultimate importance, for this wider ecosystem will have a profound effect on the intimate ecosystem of human health. The way we treat nature—either by polluting it or maintaining its integrity—will ultimately have a bearing on the natural products (such as the essential oils) that we use for our own well-being. And therein lies the importance of holism.

(Eccles 1997)

For aromatherapists to be able to carry out this aspect of holism, they have to depend on honest suppliers with a similar philosophy to their own—suppliers who can guarantee not only the exact source of their oils, but also that they are not the 'commercial' products used by the perfume and food industries. Pharmacists look for cost effectiveness; they do not always realize that any essential oil conforming to a BP formula will have been modified to fit a specification.

As a general rule the quantity of essential oils used is extremely small and unwanted side-effects are rare in practice; most side-effects are positive and wanted. It is usual for ample time to be devoted by the aromatherapy practitioner for discussion with the client and for the treatment. Individual treatment is necessary because clients are regarded as individuals. Germs do not necessarily produce the same reaction in different hosts, and it may be necessary to specify different oils to tackle the same infection in different people (Valnet 1980 p. 42). With one mix of essential oils it is possible to care for more than one health problem (the shotgun effect—see pp. 39, 50).

THE THERAPEUTIC PROPERTIES OF ESSENTIAL OILS

There are many reasons why essential oils need to be included in the armoury of weapons in the fight against disease. They have many positive properties and effects which are desirable—and few drawbacks. They are capable of being anti-inflammatory, antiseptic, appetite stimulating, carminative, choleretic, circulation stimulating, deodorizing, expectorant, granulation stimulating, hyperaemic, insecticidal, insect repelling and sedative (Schilcher 1985 p. 217). They are natural antimicrobial agents able to act on bacteria, viruses and fungi, and many trials have been performed in this field (see below). Tropical countries have traditionally used lots of spices in their cuisines, not only for the flavour, but also to kill the microbes which flourish in hot climates. It is thought that the antiseptic powers of essential oils are due to their lipid solubility (Malowan 1931) and their surface activity (Rideal, Rideal & Scriver 1928).

Essential oils are applied to the skin by various methods, ingested or inhaled (see Ch. 5), and all of these are harmless unless used incorrectly. A significant point in their favour is their pleasant aroma. They are much used in products for the home (examples are lemon and lavender) and are well accepted—they are much more pleasant and safer in use than bleach or carbolic acid. The aroma itself has effects on the person using them (see Ch. 8).

The healer should have precise control over, and full knowledge of, the substances being employed in the treatment. If this is the case, and the healer determines the therapeutic materials to be used, not some faraway laboratory, the medicine may be tailored precisely to the individual patient. Generally speaking there is an absence of unwanted side-effects arising from the use of essential oils in a healing situation (see Synergy in Ch. 3), and plant extracts are ecologically sound, causing no pollution, unlike antibiotics, which are flushed down the drain and pollute the land (Verdet 1989).

Case 4.1 Aromatologist: Dr D Pénoël, France

A's case is a 'princeps' one because it was the first time that a full medical aromatherapeutic treatment was undertaken in Australia, and it completely succeeded where all the other therapies, official or alternative, had failed.

One month after her premature birth, A began to suffer from recurrent ear, nose and throat (ENT) infections that were repeatedly treated by antibiotics. Her parents, very worried by this situation, which seemed to become worse every time, consulted a renowned homoeopath in Auckland. However, this treatment did not prevent the recurrence of the infections, together with very high fever, so the homoeopath reluctantly turned to antibiotics.

At 18 months, the condition was so bad that the parents decided to leave the wet climate of New Zealand and settle in 'the driest state of the driest continent of the world'—South Australia. This change did not help A's internal condition, and again she received lots of antibiotics, each time worsening her state of health. Tetracyclines had rotted her teeth and her knees hurt whenever the weather was wet. After repeated infections artificially suppressed, her immune system was beginning to turn against her own organism.

When A was 7 years old, the ENT children's specialist asked for an X-ray of the sinuses. The radiography showed a complete blockage of the left maxillary sinus, a thickening of the wall of the right maxillary sinus and an infectious condition of the enlarged adenoids. The specialist decided to perform a surgical operation, under general anaesthesia, in order to flush the pus out of the sinuses. Beforehand, A was to receive another course of antibiotics over 15 days and a fresh X-ray examination. A's parents refused this procedure and announced to the specialist that they had decided to try aromatherapy. The specialist said: 'Do it at your own risk and I will see you in a fortnight'.

A's condition was miserable. She had tubes in her ears and impaired hearing, frequent pains in her knees and her breathing was affected by her permanent chronic infection. She was skinny, pale, permanently tired and sad, and she was backward at school owing to absence from illness.

I had 2 weeks to prove the worth of medical aromatherapy, compared with 7 years of continuous disease and allopathic treatments. A complete programme of treatment was established, involving 2 hour sessions in the surgery each day and treatments at home. A's diet was corrected and nutritional advice was scrupulously followed by the family.

When dealing with a chronic and complex medical situation, it is of crucial importance to consider essential oils from an analytical perspective, i.e. knowing the molecules they contain and their percentages and linking this data with the different pathological aspects of the case and the capacity of the aromatic molecules to fight and correct these.

In A's case, the pathology included infection, mucus production and stagnation. The chronic inflammatory state of the mucous membrane was the result of the first two factors. The essential oils were carefully selected in relationship to how they could enter her body. Here, two errors had to be avoided: first, thinking only of the local treatment and forgetting the general one, and secondly believing that correcting the overall state of health would be sufficient to clear the local situation.

Local treatment. High tech aerosol equipment, using sonic vibrations, penetrated deeply into the sinuses (a drop of *Mentha* × *piperita* in some liquid honey, kept 30 seconds in the mouth as a pretreatment, helped to open the nostrils). The essential oil used in the aerosol was *Inula graveolens*, which contains a small percentage of sesquiterpenic lactones, endowed with a strong mucolytic power. Besides, it contains an antiinfectious and immunoregulator monoterpenic alcohol (borneol) plus an antiinflammatory and antispasmodic ester (bornyl acetate) which work in conjunction, making an excellent synergy within a single oil.

Cutaneous treatment. Here, essential oils were applied neat on different parts of the body—mainly on the back and thoracic area. The blend, 10 ml of which was used neat daily, included: *Rosmarinus officinalis* ct. cineole (respiratory), *R. officinalis* ct. verbenone (mucolytic and antiinflammatory), *Melaleuca alternifolia* (antiseptic) and *Thymus satureioides* (antiinfectious, antiinflammatory, immunobalancing).

Internal treatment. Orally, five to six drops of the following essential oils were blended in honey and taken four times a day with warm water, like a herbal tea: *M. alternifolia*, *M.* × *piperita*, *T. satureioides* and *Satureia montana*. Other complementary techniques used were: Swiss reflex massage on the feet, dynamic drainage of the face area by suction cups and magnetic field therapy on the face, liver, spleen and kidney areas.

After 2 weeks, A had received 11 sessions in my practice and it was clear that an overall and local improvement had taken place. When the new X-ray was taken it showed that the sinus and adenoid infections had totally cleared.

The ENT specialist, on seeing the X-ray, simply said 'cases of spontaneous healing are known among children'. Nevertheless, medical aromatherapy had won the first battle, in a case where everything else had failed.

Four months later, during winter, A had acute tonsillitis. Looking at the case holistically, we did not conclude that a 'bug' had jumped into A's throat, but that her whole organism had won enough strength, through the continued aromatherapeutic treatment,

to expel toxins and waste matters coming from all the medications and accumulated infections, that had been locked inside until then. Every morning for 4 days an enormous quantity of thick brown mucus had been found on A's pillow. To keep this acute elimination process under control (but not to counteract it!), essential oils were used in the same intensive way as before, and after a battle of 4 days, her throat was completely cleansed, the fever stopped, and A was feeling like a new child! Whenever the acute stages of a disease are dealt with successfully by implementing natural medicine treatments, it really marks a turning point in the evolution of the underlying illness.

A is now 15 years old and has taken no antibiotics since she was 7. She is strong, healthy, excels at school (especially in French!), in art and in sport and believes that the intervention of medical aromatherapy thoroughly changed her life.

Antiseptic and antibacterial

Essential oils have multiple actions and effects, e.g. when used for a respiratory infection an oil may be not only antiseptic, but also mucolytic, antiinflammatory and so on (Duraffourd 1987 p. 17). Another example is the use of oils on the digestive system, where the oils are antiseptic but do not act unfavourably on the flora and on the digestive secretions, in contrast to the unwelcome effects of antibiotics.

The molecules of essential oils occur naturally and are not inimical to the human body. They support the immune system and can be considered as pro- and eubiotic as opposed to the synthetic antibiotics. There is a natural variation in the chemical composition and physical characteristics of essential oils from year to year but this variation does not seem materially to affect their antiseptic properties, although it is always necessary to be aware of the analysis of the actual sample being tested. It is possible to have two factors for the one essential oil, depending on the method of use, e.g. the antiseptic use of liquid or vaporized oil.

Essential oils are especially valuable as antiseptics because their aggression towards microbial germs is matched by their total harmlessness to tissue—one of the chief defects of chemical antiseptics is that they are likely to be as harmful to the cells of the organism as to the cause of the disease ... It is very important

to remember that [chemical] antiseptics will destroy not only the micro-organisms but also the surrounding cells.

(Valnet 1980 p. 44)

A 45-year-old woman had a motor vehicle accident, resulting in a comminuted fracture of the ankle. It was operated on but the operation site became infected, and was open for 4 months. At this stage I was asked if I could try and treat the wound with essential oils. The orthopaedic surgeon gave his permission and before I started I took a wound swab for microscopy, culture and sensitivity. On the wound swab *S. aureus*, *Streptococcus pseudomonas* and *Escherichia coli* were isolated and from this I formulated my programme. The treatment consisted of a daily footbath with three drops each of *Thymus vulgaris* ct. alcohol, *Citrus limon* and *Melaleuca alternifolia* (the essential oils were put on a small spoon of salt as an emulgator and then put into the water). The wound was then cleaned with dry compresses, and a gauze (on which was put three drops of tea tree) put on. This acted as a compress and was covered with a mull bandage; this change was carried out once daily.

During this treatment the patient was given no antibiotics and only 20 drops of Tramal when it was needed for her pain. After 3 days she no longer needed any analgesics; 2 weeks later when a wound swab was tested none of the original bacteria were present. The wound closed after 3 weeks of using aromatherapy.

The use of essential oils is a sure way of avoiding the phenomenon of developed resistance in microbes as experienced with antibiotics, because the aromatic essences are able to destroy even the resistant strains selectively (Pellecuer, Allegrini & De Buochberg 1974). Germs resistant to synthetic antibiotics are susceptible in certain cases to some essences in dilutions as low as 1 in 16 000, e.g. *Satureia montana* (Belaiche 1979 p. 31) (see Table 4.1).

It is wise to avoid any possible resistance on the part of a germ by always prescribing the use of three or four essential oils in combination. This multimix approach will tend to minimize any risk of acquired resistance to any one oil, and it is unlikely that bacteria will be resistant at the same time to the other oils in the mix. This is one of the reasons why the authors strongly advise using a powerful synergistic mix of oils in any treatment. Moreover this risk is further reduced, even though the metabolism of the microbe changes continually, because essential oils are natural products and their composition varies with each fresh batch.

Testing for antiseptic and antibacterial activity

Tests have been carried out on the antiseptic and antibacterial properties of essential oils for more than a century. Two of the first were Chamberland's in 1887, concerning the activity of cinnamon oils, angelica and geranium (Valnet 1980 p. 33), and Koch's 1881 investigation of turpentine with respect to the anthrax bacillus. Since then the antiseptic and bactericidal powers of well-grown natural essential oils have been tested many times in laboratories across the world using the aromatogram technique (see below). This is a recognized standard test and the results obtained are repeatable (provided the essential oils themselves are repeatable) and are universally acceptable: it is virtually the same as the antibiogram test.

Tests proving the antiseptic effects of essential oils are numerous, and the following are cited as examples: Belaiche (1985a,b), Beylier (1979), Bonnaure (1919), Carson & Riley (1993), Carson et al (1995), Cavel (1918), Chamberland (1887),

Table 4.1 Antibacterial spectrum of *Satureia montana* on some species and strains resistant to antibiotics (after Pellecuer et al 1976).

Bacteria tested	Origin of bacteria	Type of resistance	Active dose in mg/ml
Staphylococcus aureus	IP 6454	penicillin	0.250
Staphylococcus aureus	IP 6455	penicillin streptomycin tetracycline	0.250
Staphylococcus aureus	IP 52149	penicillin streptomycin tetracycline	0.250
Staphylococcus aureus	IP 52150	streptomycin	0.250
Sarcina lutea	natural	100 γ of tetracycline	0.062
Bacillus subtilis	natural	streptomycin	0.250
Escherichia coli	natural	ampicillin colomycin	0.250
Staphylococcus pathogen	natural no. 1	⎫	0.062
Staphylococcus pathogen	natural no. 2	⎪	0.062
Staphylococcus pathogen	natural no. 3	Resistant	0.062
Staphylococcus pathogen	natural no. 5	to 500 γ of	0.125
Staphylococcus pathogen	natural no. 8	virginiamycin	0.250
Staphylococcus pathogen	natural no. 10	⎭	0.125

Courment, Morel & Bay (1938), Deans & Svoboda (1988), Deans & Svoboda (1990a,b), Gattefossé (1919, 1932), Gildemeister & Hoffmann (1956), Hinou, Harvala & Hinou (1989), Holland (1941), Jalsenjak, Pelinjak & Kustrak (1987), Jasper, Maruzella & Laurence Liguori (1958), Jasper et al (1958), Juven et al (1994), Kienholz (1959), Knobloch et al (1989), Low, Rowal & Griffin (1974), Martindale (1910), Moleyar & Narasimham (1992), Onawunmi (1988, 1989), Onawunmi & Ogunlana (1986), Onawunmi, Yisak & Ogunlana (1984), Pellecuer, Allegrini & De Buochberg (1974), Pellecuer et al (1975, 1976), Raharivelomanana et al (1989), Ramanoelina et al (1987), Ritzerfeld (1959), Shemesh & Mayo (1991), Tukioka (1927) and Yousef & Tawil (1980).

There is a wide variation in the antiseptic and bactericidal effects between different individual essential oils as shown by their phenol coefficients (Martindale 1910, Poucher 1936, Rideal, Sciver & Richardson 1930). This is illustrated in Table 4.2.

It is well known that essential oils provide a very pleasant and effective means of disinfecting the air in an enclosed area (Kelner & Kober 1954,

1955, 1956) and are therefore ideal for use in sick rooms, burns units, reception areas, waiting rooms, etc. A test describing the use of a blend of pine, thyme, peppermint, lavender, rosemary, clove and cinnamon essential oils for the bacteriological purification of the air concluded that 'the atmospheric dispersion of the prepared liquid brought about a very marked disinfection of the air, as demonstrated by the considerable reduction in the number of pre-existing microorganisms, some types being destroyed completely' (Valnet 1980 pp. 36–38).

Poucher (1936) quotes the results of an early investigation of the effect of 33 essential oils and phenol on beef tea which had been infected with water taken from a sewage tank. The trial referred to was originally carried out by Cavel (1918) and a selection from the results is shown in Table 4.3. The figures denote the dilution (per) 1000 at which the oils no longer showed effective antiseptic action, hence the lower the figure the

Table 4.2 The phenol coefficients of some essential oils and their isolated compounds (from Schilcher 1985 p. 221 reprinted by permission of Kluwer Academic Publishers). The phenol coefficient gives an indication of the antiseptic strength or weakness of a substance compared with that of phenol (which has a coefficient of 1.0)

Whole essential oil	Compound	Phenol coefficient
Aniseed		0.4
Peppermint		0.7
	menthol	0.9
Lavender		1.6
Lemon (Java)		2.2
	cinnamaldehyde	3.0
	citral	5.2
	camphor	6.2
Clove		8.0
	eugenol	8.6
Fennel		13.0
Thyme		13.2
	thymol	20.0
	synthetic chlorothymol	75.0

Table 4.3 Antiseptic effect of essential oils in sewage water (from Poucher 1936 vol. 2 p. 361 with permission)

Essential oil	Dilution
Thyme	0.70
Origanum	1.00
Orange (sweet)	1.20
Verbena	1.60
Cassia	1.70
Rose	1.80
Clove	2.00
Eucalyptus	2.50
Peppermint	2.70
Vetiver	2.25
Gaultheria	3.00
Palmarosa	3.10
Spikenard	3.50
Star anise	3.70
Cinnamon (Ceylon)	4.00
Anise	4.20
Rosemary	4.30
Cumin	4.50
Neroli	4.75
Lavender	5.00
Melissa	5.20
Ylang ylang	5.60
PHENOL	5.60
Fennel (sweet)	6.40
Lemon	7.00
Angelica	10.00
Patchouli	15.00

greater the antiseptic power. It is interesting to note that phenol (the standard for comparison) appears fairly low in the table.

Antibiogram and aromatogram

An antibiogram can test the validity of an antibiotic agent for the treatment of, say, a chest infection. A sample of sputum is taken and a culture grown in a dish. The antibiotic is introduced into the centre of the culture and its activity against the offending microorganism may be measured by the appearance of a clear 'killing zone'. The diameter of this clear area indicates the power of the antibiotic: the greater the diameter, the greater the effectiveness of the antibiotic agent. The aromatogram is carried out in exactly the same way as the antibiogram, except essential oil is used instead of an antibiotic. Both methods are subject to the proviso that in vitro activity is not always echoed in vivo, which is modified by absorption, metabolism, bioavailability, etc. Finding the most effective and appropriate essential oil to counteract any particular germ can be a lengthy undertaking: if there is no previous experience to go on it will be necessary to test all the oils in the therapist's repertory, perhaps 60 or more. It goes without saying that the essential oils used in the treatment should be from the same batch as the sample tested, because essential oils from different sources can vary in chemical composition. This testing procedure has confirmed the antiseptic powers of many oils but at the same time has revealed in some other oils antiseptic powers which were hitherto unsuspected, or at least underrated. At one time in aromatherapy, fennel (*Foeniculum vulgare* var. *dulce*) was known only for being an appetite stimulant, nutmeg (*Myristica fragrans*) as a stomachic and tarragon (*Artemisia dracunculus*) as an antispasmodic, but now the antiseptic qualities of these oils are also recognized. These tests allow essential oils to be used precisely and effectively, without the consequences which sometimes follow the use of antibiotics (such as tiredness, lowered immune system activity and destruction of intestinal flora). Because of the huge number of aromatogram results which

have now been published, it is possible to list the major essential oils by their antimicrobial properties (Roulier 1990 p. 55)—see Table 4.4.

Other properties

Analgesic

Many essential oils have analgesic properties to some degree and there seems to be no single reason why they do, just as pain itself is complicated. It is thought that the effect is partly due to the antiinflammatory, circulatory and detoxifying effects of some oils and to the anaesthetic effect of others. The phenol eugenol found in the oil of clove is well known for its use in calming dental pain, wintergreen oil (containing methyl salicylate, an ester) has traditionally been used in rubs for muscle pain, and menthol has been used specifically for headaches. On the skin, oils rich in terpenes have an analgesic effect, especially those containing *p*-cymene (Franchomme & Pénoël 1990 p. 86). Many aromatherapists report that the oil of *Melaleuca alternifolia* has this effect. Azulene and chamazulene (found in the chamomiles) can be used on the skin also. Some essential oils have a universal sedative or soporific action leading to an easing of pain, e.g. *Chamaemelum nobile*, *Cananga odorata*, *Citrus reticulata* (fol.) (Rossi et al 1988), *Citrus bergamia* (per. and fol.) (Franchomme & Pénoël 1990 p. 86). According to Roulier (1990), the analgesic and antalgic essential oils are: white birch, chamomile, frankincense, wintergreen, clove, lavender, mint (common names only given). A study into the use of complementary therapies to help treat patients suffering chronic pain was carried out at Monklands Hospital in Scotland. More than 75% of patients referred by local GPs suffering from a range of complaints (e.g. back or shoulder pain, long term problems, premenstrual tension, depression, anxiety or mood swings) found that such therapies helped to provide short term relief of their symptoms. The patients were treated with essential oils, reflexology or acupuncture during an 8 week trial (Anderson 1998). (See Appendix B.9 for a list of effective oils.)

Case 4.3   Aromatherapist: Jill Baxter SEN, UK

Jim's main problem area is on the sciatic nerve, left-hand side. He has had several operations and the deep creases, puckering and scar tissue on the site means that surgeons would be against further incisions—in fact they say there is little they can do, apart from giving morphia for the pain.

Jim told me that 4 years ago, when a wart first needed surgery, it was found to be benign. Following that, a severe injury against the angle of a piece of furniture was thought to trigger malignant growths. When I first saw him he moved very stiffly indeed and lay on the couch most awkwardly. I massaged his back, shoulders, legs and feet with lavender and rosemary in a blend of wheatgerm and grapeseed oil and afterwards applied lavender (neat) freely to the site of the wound.

Jim tells me he would never have believed the measure of relief he has found since having aromatherapy treatments. He says he gains immediate relief from constant aching, has a greater range of movement and a good night's sleep. He has noticed his skin is more supple and is looking forward to being able to sit more squarely in an easy chair, instead of sideways, one leg extended, as at present.

Case 4.4   Aromatherapist: R.A.H. RGN, RM, UK

Mr H had acute back pain in July after lifting heavy weights at work. He was treated with conventional drugs by his general practitioner and returned to work fairly quickly. However, the pain recurred and he was off sick from work in September, again not benefiting from conventional treatment, which consisted of analgesics, antiinflammatory drugs and physiotherapy. He developed an allergy to Ibuprofen, an antiinflammatory drug, but this was detected before any harm was done. Several of the doctors in the practice had been called out to administer analgesia, by tablet, injection or suppository. Obviously, this could not go on and he was admitted to hospital over Christmas with chronic back pain.

I was asked to see whether aromatherapy could bring him some relief. The essential oils selected were: three drops of *Chamaemelum nobile*, two drops of *Lavandula angustifolia* and one drop of *Origanum majorana* in 10 ml grapeseed oil. Having given him a full back massage, I gave special attention to his lower legs and feet, as I had observed how rigid his feet were, with virtually no flexibility in his ankles. I taught him foot exercises, massaging his lower extremities and counselling him. That night he slept very well without sedation.

26–29 December. Massaged as before. Now walking better during day and pain less. Being apprehensive as I was to be off duty for several nights, I prepared white lotion containing the same essential oils so that the other night nurses could stroke this on his back every night. He promised to continue his foot exercises.

7–11 January Massaged back and feet as before: Excellent effect. Mr H was confident and talking about the possibility of going on holiday. Had been to physiotherapy and had used the exercise bike, but disliked it (his legs were aching). He had continued with his leg and foot exercises, and on 29 January said he was pain free.

Antifungal

Many essential oils have been reported as having an antifungal effect (Table 4.5) and many investigations have taken place, some more than half a century ago (Schmidt 1936) showing the fungicidal and fungistatic effects of cinnamon, clove, fennel and thyme; these were active against *Candida albicans*, *Sporotrichon* and *Trichophyton* species (Gildemeister & Hoffmann 1956 p. 140). The fungicidal activity of the oil of *Chamomilla recutita* and its components, including chamazulene and (–)-α-bisabolol, has been well investigated and shown to be effective against *Trichophyton rubrum*, *T. mentagraphytes*, *T. tonsurans*, *T. quinckeanum* and *Microsporum canis* in concentrations of 200 mg/ml (Janssen et al 1984, 1986, Szalontai, Verzar-Petri & Florian 1976, 1977, Szalontai et al 1975a,b). *Satureia montana* also has been found to be active against candida (Pellecuer et al 1975). A general review of some essential oils with antifungal properties has been carried out (Pellecuer et al 1976) and in other trials a number of compounds found in essential

oils, especially the aldehydes and esters, are effective against various fungi, including candida infection (Larrondo & Calvo 1991, Maruzella 1961, Thompson & Cannon 1986). The oil of *Melaleuca alternifolia* has been investigated in vaginal infection with candida and has been found to be effective (Belaiche 1985c, Pena 1962, Shemesh & Mayo 1991). Rosemary, savory and thyme also have antifungal properties (Pellecuer, Roussel & Andary 1973) and *Ocimum basilicum* has both antifungal and insect-repelling properties (Dube, Upadhyay & Tripath 1989).

Table 4.4 Antibacterial properties of essential oils according to Belaiche P 1979, Franchomme & Penoël 1990, Valnet J 1980, Deans & Ritchie 1987, Deans & Svoboda 1988, 1989; Juven et al 1994, Beylier 1979. Not all the oils in this table have been tested for all the bacteria shown

The x's indicate effectiveness—xxx is the most effective

Essential oil	Bacillus subtilis	Candida albicans	Clostridium perfringens	Clostridium sporogenes	Corynebacterium diphtheriae	Diplococcus pneumoniae	Enterobacter aerogenes	Enterococci	Escherichia coli	beta-Hemolytic streptococci	Klebsiella	Mycobacterium tuberculosis	Neisseria gonorrhoeae	Neisseria meningitidis	Proteus	Pseudomonas aeruginosa	Salmonella pullorum	Salmonella typhi	Salmonella typhimurium	Sarcina	Staphylococcus albus	Staphylococcus aureus	Staphylococcus faecalis	Streptococcus faecalis	Vibrio cholerae	Yersinia enterocolitica
Artemisia dracunculus [TARRAGON]		×				×		×	×	×	×					×	×				×	×				×
Carum carvi [CARAWAY]							xx		×	×	×				xx		×					xx				×
Cedrus atlantica? (not specified) [CEDARWOOD]								×																		
Cinnamomum verum (cort.) [CINNAMON BARK]		xx				xxx		xxx	xxx	xxx	xxx				xxx	×	xxx				xxx	xxx				xx
Citrus aurantium var. amara (flos) [NEROLI]						×		×	×	×	×				×						×	xx				
Citrus aurantium var. amara (fol.) [PETITGRAIN]		xxx						×	×	×	×										×	xx				
Citrus bergamia (per.) [BERGAMOT]						×	×				×													×		
Citrus limon (per.) [LEMON]						×								×								×				
Coriandrum sativum (fruct.) [CORIANDER]						×		×	×	×	xx				×							×				xx
Cupressus sempervirens [CYPRESS]								×	×	×		×														
Eucalyptus citriodora [LEMON-SCENTED GUM]		xx				xx			xx													xx				
Eucalyptus dives [BROAD-LEAVED PEPPERMINT]		xx							xx													xx				
Eucalyptus globulus [TASMANIAN BLUE GUM]		xx				xxx		×	xx	?	xx	xx			xx	×					xx	xx				×
Eucalyptus radiata [GREY PEPPERMINT]		xx																				×				
Eucarya spicata [AUSTRALIAN SANDALWOOD]		xxx																				xxx				
Foeniculum vulgare var. dulce (fruct.) [FENNEL]						×																×				
Hyssopus officinalis [HYSSOP]						xx		xx			×				×						×	×	×			
Lavandula angustifolia [LAVENDER]		xx			×	xx		xx	xx	×	xx				×	xx	×				×	xx		xx		×
Melaleuca alternifolia [TEA TREE]		xx			xx			xx	xx		×		×		×	xx	xxx	xxx			×	xx				
Melaleuca leucadendron [CAJUPUT]		xx				xxx		xx	×		xxx				xx						xx	xx				

Table 4.4 Antibacterial properties of essential oils according to Belaiche P 1979, Franchomme & Pénoël 1990, Valnet J 1980, Deans & Ritchie 1987, Deans & Svoboda 1988, 1989; Juven et al 1994, Beylier 1979. Not all the oils in this table have been tested for all the bacteria shown (contd)

The x's indicate effectiveness—xxx is the most effective

Essential oil	Yersinia enterocolitica	Vibrio cholerae	Streptococcus faecalis	Staphylococcus faecalis	Staphylococcus aureus	Staphylococcus albus	Sarcina	Salmonella typhimurium	Salmonella typhi	Salmonella pullorum	Pseudomonas aeruginosa	Proteus	Neisseria meningitidis	Neisseria gonorrhoeae	Mycobacterium tuberculosis	Klebsiella	beta-Hemolytic streptococci	Escherichia coli	Enterococci	Enterobacter aerogenes	Diplococcus pneumoniae	Corynebacterium diphtheriae	Clostridium sporogenes	Clostridium perfringens	Candida albicans	Bacillus subtilis
Melaleuca viridiflora [NIAOULI]		x													x	x	x	x	x						x	xx
Mentha × piperita [PEPPERMINT]	xx		x	x	xx					xx	xx	xx			xx	xx	x	xx			x				xx	
Myristica fragrans (sem.) [NUTMEG]	x									x	x	x				xx	x	xx		x	x					
Ocimum basilicum var. album [BASIL]	x				x													x		x	x		xx			
Origanum majorana [MARJORAM]	xx		xx		x					xx		xx				xx	xx	xx		xx	x		xx			
Ormenis mixta [MOROCCAN CHAMOMILE]																		xx								
Pelargonium × asperum [GERANIUM]	xx				x	xx				xx		x				x	xx	x	x	xx	xx				x	
Pimpinella anisum [ANISEED]		x		x					x																	
Pinus sylvestris [PINE]						xx						xx									xx				xx	
Piper nigrum [BLACK PEPPER]	x				xx					x								x								
Rosa damascena [ROSE OTTO]	x				x																					
Rosmarinus officinalis [ROSEMARY]					x	x				x	x	x				xx	x	xx	x	xx	x				x	
Salvia officinalis [SAGE]			xx		xx					x	xx					xx	x	xx	x		xxx				x	
Satureia hortensis and S. montana [SAVORY]	xx		x		x	xxx				xx	xx	x			x	xx	xxx	xx	xxx	xx	xxx				xx	
Syzygium aromaticum (flos) [CLOVE BUD]	xx		x		xx	xxx				xx	xx	xx				xx	xx	x	xxx	xx	xxx			xx	xx	
Thymus capitatus [SPANISH OREGANO]					xxx	xxx						xxx				xxx	xxx	xxx	xxx		xxx				xxx	
Thymus serpyllum [WILD THYME]					x							x				x	xx	x	x		x				x	
Thymus mastichina [SPANISH MARJORAM]															xx											
Thymus vulgaris ct. thymol [THYME]	xxx		xxx		xxx	xxx	xxx	xx		xxx	xxx	xxx				xxx	xxx	xxx	xxx	xxx	xxx				xxx	

Case 4.5   Aromatologist: Alan Barker, UK

In July 1990 Mrs F (aged 40) was referred to a consultant, suffering from a continuous urinary tract infection (with inflammation, incontinence and pain), which antibiotics failed to control. She was given intermittent self-catheterization (ISC) and by April 1992 major surgery (removal of the bladder) was considered. She also developed a vaginal inflammation—thrush. By September 1992, Mrs F was unable to perform the ISC owing to thrush and inflammation and a cystectomy was again discussed.

In November, the sister suggested to the consultant that aromatherapy should be tried, and as Mrs F was interested the consultant gave his permission. I was asked if I was happy to start treatment and a meeting was finally arranged between myself, the continence adviser, Mrs F and her husband in March 1993.

Mrs F complained of constant pain and swelling of the abdomen (caused by having to have residual catheterization using microcatheters). She felt (and it was apparent on inspection) that her vagina was the consistency of 'raw liver' and she suffered frequent discharges. Intercourse was impossible. I had asked her husband to attend with her so that I could check him over, as this side of the partnership, although important, is often overlooked. Mrs F had had this recurrent form of candida for about 15 years with very few periods of respite—the relationship was beginning to suffer and credit was due to the couple for the level of understanding shared.

The couple's normal diet plan for an average week was looked at and changes arranged to help the body balance itself. These changes were to be gradual, over a period of time, so as not to add to the stress of the situation. Because of the latter, massage was to be part of Mrs F's treatment. A colonic massage was decided upon, with essential oils to benefit the swelling, pain and infection: *Citrus bergamia* (per.), *Eucalyptus globulus*, *Melaleuca alternifolia* and *M. viridiflora*. These were mixed together in equal quantities and a 15 minute massage given. At the first treatment a high concentration of 2.5 ml of the essential oils was put into 5 ml grapeseed oil—a 50% dilution.

I taught Mr F how to perform a simple abdominal massage in a clockwise direction consisting of very few strokes, to be carried out once daily to aid Mrs F's constipation. This was a good morale booster for him, as he had previously felt helpless—and he now became part of her recovery process. For this, he was given a 3% mix of: *Zingiber officinale* (antispasmodic and laxative), *Foeniculum vulgare* var. *dulce* (appetite stimulant, laxative and circulation stimulant) and *Mentha* × *piperita* (analgesic, antiinflammatory and stomachic).

Treatment with live yogurt and essential oils was discussed; this could not be carried out by using a tampon as the client was too swollen. It was decided to pour the yogurt mixture into the vagina, the client being propped up, legs raised, to allow the mix to penetrate. Mrs F found this was messy and difficult. However, after several days the swelling had reduced enough to insert a tampon soaked in the mixture, changing it morning and night.

Colonic massage treatment at the hospital involved using different strengths of essential oil; for 3 days a dilution of five drops in 5 ml was used. Several weekly treatments followed, using only one drop of the synergistic blend in 5 ml grapeseed oil.

Treatment at home involved the following: marigold flowers used for making tea (plus one drop *C. bergamia*) three times a day for 3 weeks, acidopholus tablets (six daily); a combination of essential oils to be used in the bath; abdomen massage oil—3% mix for Mrs F to use at home as above; yogurt treatment—five drops *M. alternifolia* was put with 10 ml yogurt—used as above.

By the end of the month Mrs F was already beginning to feel the benefits from the treatment. In June 1993, the abdominal swelling was going down; the yogurt treatment was changed to oral yogurt tablets as insertion was sometimes difficult. By the end of July the urinary tract was almost clear. Mrs F was on three acidopholus tablets (daily), marigold tea, occasional yogurt and *M. alternifolia* taken internally. Abdomen massage was still carried out by her husband once or twice a week with a reduced concentration of 1.5%. The couple's relationship is now close once more, partially due to Mr F's eagerness to help by giving his wife a daily massage.

Antiinflammatory

The oils of *Lavandula angustifolia* and *Chamomilla recutita* are widely used to soothe minor inflammations such as sunburn, small burns and insect bites, and plenty of people can testify to their effectiveness in this respect. Jakovlev, Isaac & Flaskamp (1983) showed the antiinflammatory effect of yarrow, chamomile containing chamazulene, arnica flower and turpentine. Azulenes are sesquiterpene derivatives and have the empirical formula $C_{15}H_{18}$. While chamazulene and (−)-α-bisabolol found in chamomile oils are antiinflammatory agents (Weiss 1988 p. 24), other azulenes which may be added to antiinflammatory preparations are not so effective, e.g. guaiazulene (manufactured from guaiol) and elemazulene (from elemol). Also (+)-α-bisabolol and synthetic (−)-α-bisabolol are not as effective as the natural form. There do appear to be differences in some cases between natural and synthesized molecules: synthetic myristicin does not

Table 4.5 Antifungal effects of essential oils

	General antifungal properties*	Aspergillus flavus	Aspergillus nidulans	Aspergillus niger	Aspergillus parasiticus	Candida albicans	Chaetomium	Cryptococcus neoformans	Fusarium oxysporum	Fusarium moniliforme	Microsporum audounii	Microsporum canis	Nigrospora oryzae	Penicillium chrysogenum	Sclerotium rolfsii	Sporotrichium species	Tinea pedis	Trichophyton species	Trichophyton mentagrophytes	Trichophyton quinckeanum	Trichophyton rubrum	Trychophyton tonsurans
Cinnamomum verum (cort) [CINNAMON BARK]					x	x		x								x		x				
Chamomilla recutita [GERMAN CHAMOMILE]												x							x	x	x	x
Coriandrum sativum [CORIANDER]						x																
Cuminum cyminum [CUMIN]						x																
Eucalyptus citriodora [LEMON-SCENTED EUCALYPTUS]				x							x								x			
Eucalyptus dives [BROAD-LEAVED PEPPERMINT]				x																		
Eucalyptus globulus [TASMANIAN BLUE GUM]						x																
Eucalyptus radiata [GREY PEPPERMINT]				x																		
Eucarya spicata [AUSTRALIAN SANDALWOOD]				x																		
Foeniculum vulgare var. *dulce* [FENNEL]						x										x	x					
Lavandula angustifolia [LAVENDER]						x										x						
Lavandula × intermedia 'Super' [LAVANDIN]																x						
Melaleuca alternifolia [TEA TREE]				xx		x																
Melaleuca leucadendron [CAJUPUT]						x																
Melaleuca viridiflora [NIAOULI]				x																		
Mentha × piperita [PEPPERMINT]																						x
Nardostachys jatamansi [SPIKENARD]		x	x	x					x	x				x	x							
Ocimum basilicum [BASIL]	x	x	x	x	x		x		x	x				x	x							
Pelargonium graveolens [GERANIUM]						?		x														
Pinus sylvestris [PINE]						x																
Rosmarinus officinalis [ROSEMARY]	x			x																		
Satureia montana [WINTER SAVORY]	x					x																
Syzygium aromaticum (flos) [CLOVE BUD]						x										x		x				
Tagetes glandulifera, T. patula [MARIGOLD]																	x					
Thymus mastichina [SPANISH MARJORAM]						x																
Thymus vulgaris (population) [THYME]	x					x										x		x				
Thymus vulgaris ct. linalool, geraniol [SWEET THYME]						x																
Thymus vulgaris ct. thymol, carvacrol [THYME]	x				x	x		x								x		x				

* Oils mentioned as having antifungal properties but without mention of a specific fungus produce hallucinations (D'Arcy 1993), unlike natural myristicin extracted from nutmeg oil (in which it is present at 4%). (See Appendix B.9 for a list of effective oils.)

Antitoxic

Chamomile oil has been found to be capable of inactivating toxins produced by bacteria. The amount of oil obtained by distilling 0.1 g of chamomile is sufficient to destroy, within 2 hours, three times that amount of staphylococcal toxins—the highest concentration of toxin so far found in the human organism. Streptococcal toxins proved even more sensitive (Weiss 1988 p. 26).

Antiviral

Most people practising aromatherapy have reported success in the control of herpes viruses causing herpes simplex type I, but there is no consistency in the choice of oils used (as can be seen from Table 4.6). Speaking from personal experience, we have always found the oils of *Melissa officinalis* and *Eucalyptus smithii* to be helpful for herpes simplex type I. The use of melissa agrees with tests showing this plant to be antiviral (Cohen, Kucera & Herrman 1964, Herrman & Kucera 1967, Kucera & Herman 1967). For herpes zoster (shingles) the oil of *Pelargonium graveolens* is specifically recommended, but it is best applied at the first sign of an attack to prevent the viruses from replicating. Used early it prevents blisters from forming and damps down the pain. Although attempts have been made to treat herpes simplex type II—the many oils suggested include *Melaleuca alternifolia* and *M. viridiflora* (Franchomme & Pénoël 1990)—little success has been reported. Despite the lack of scientific support, many aromatherapists still feel that herpes simplex type II and other viral infections such as glandular fever and influenza do respond to essential oil treatment. There is also some research to support the use in this area of black pepper oil (*Piper nigrum*) (Lembke & Deininger 1988). The oils of *Cymbopogon flexuosus*, *Mentha arvensis* and *Vetiveria zizanioides* (Pandey et al 1988) and *Eucalyptus viminalis*, *E.*

macarthurii and *E. dalrympleana* appear to be effective in vitro and in ovo on two strains of influenza virus (Vichkanova, Dzhanashiya & Goryunova 1973). There have been other papers published on this topic in India, Russia and China and a Swiss patent was filed in 1979 for an antiviral preparation using essential oils.

Table 4.6 shows the essential oils which have been recommended for antiviral use. The information has been culled from many sources, which often used only the common name for the plant volatile oil.

The following oils are also mentioned as having antiviral properties, but without specific indications (Franchomme & Pénoël 1990): *Aniba rosaeodora, Cinnamomum camphora* var. *glavescens Hayata, C. cassia, C. zeylanicum* and *C. zeylanicum* ct. eugenol, *Cistus ladaniferus* ct. pinene and *C. ladaniferus, Citrus limon* (per.), *Corydothymus capitatus, Cymbopogon martinii* var. *motia* and *C. martinii* var. *sofia, Eucalyptus polybractea* ct. cryptone and *E. radiata, Hyssopus officinalis* var. *decumbens* and *H. officinalis, Lantana camara* ct. davanone, *Lavandula × intermedia* 'Reydovan', *Ocimum gratissimum* ct. eugenol and *O. gratissimum* ct. thymol, *Origanum compactum* and *O. heracleoticum, Ravensara aromatica, Satureia hortensis, Thymus vulgaris* ct. geraniol, *T. vulgaris* ct. linalool and *T. vulgaris* ct. thujanol-4, *Trachyspermum ammi*.

Several constituents which are found naturally in a wide range of essential oils (anethole, β-caryophyllene, carvone, cinnamic aldehyde, citral, citronellol, eugenol, limonene, linalool, linalyl acetate, α-sabinene, γ-terpinene) were found to be active against herpes simplex (Lembke & Deininger 1985, 1988). Thus it can be seen that there is no one molecule or even one class of molecule involved. If the oils are effective it could well be because of some property common to all of them—perhaps lipid solubility.

Balancing

Aromatherapists are well aware of the remarkable balancing powers of essential oils. At times this can cause puzzlement because of the apparently contradictory effects of the oils, but

Table 4.6 Essential oils mentioned as having antiviral effects (from various authors)

	Adenovirus	Glandular fever	Herpes simplex	Influenza	Viral enteritis	Viral enterocolitis	Viral hepatitis	Viral neuritis	Zoster
Citrus aurantium var. *bergamia* (per.) [BERGAMOT]			x						
Citrus limon (per.) [LEMON]			x	x					
Commiphora molmol [MYRRH]			x				x		
Cupressus sempervirens [CYPRESS]			x						
Eucalyptus globulus [TASMANIAN BLUE GUM]			x						
Eucalyptus smithii [GULLY GUM]			x						
Lavandula latifolia, L. spica [SPIKE LAVENDER]						x			
Melaleuca alternifolia [TEA TREE]			x		x	x			
Melaleuca leucadendron [CAJUPUT]								x	
Melaleuca viridiflora [NIAOULI]			x	x			x		
Melissa officinalis [MELISSA]			x						x
Mentha × *piperita* [PEPPERMINT]							x	x	
Ocimum basilicum [BASIL]								x	
Pelargonium graveolens, P. × *asperum* [GERANIUM]			x						x
Piper nigrum [BLACK PEPPER]	x				x	x	x		
Ravensara aromatica [RAVENSARA]					x	x	x		
Rosa damascena [ROSE OTTO]			x						x
Rosmarinus officinalis [ROSEMARY]			x				x		
Satureia montana [WINTER SAVORY]						x			
Salvia officinalis [SAGE]		x			x	x		x	x
Syzygium aromaticum (flos) [CLOVE BUD]							x		
Thymus serpyllum [WILD THYME]					x				
Thymus vulgaris ct. phenol [THYME]		x			x				
Thymus vulgaris ct. alcohol [SWEET THYME]									x

essential oils are complex mixtures of many natural constituents, some of which are stimulating and others sedative, so a single oil may demonstrate an arousing effect on one occasion and a sedative effect on another. This is known as the adaptogenic effect.

Hyssop essential oil contains the ketone pinocamphone and is said to be toxic in high doses, causing epileptic attacks in those so predisposed (Valnet 1980). Yet this oil is used in Case study 4.6 (and has been used by the authors in an epilepsy case) with beneficial effects. *Lavandula angustifolia* is well known for its sedative effect but rather less known for its ability to prevent sleep at high doses (observed and experienced by many aromatherapists). Similarly hawthorn berries (used in herbal medicine) can lower blood pressure in some but raise it in others (Mabey 1988 p. 179). In aromatherapy this balancing of blood pressure is often ascribed to *Cananga odorata* but is not proven.

The skill of the aromatherapist lies in using such effects in skilful blends to the best advantage of the client.

Case 4.6 Aromatologist: Alan Barker, UK

M is 7 years old. He is hyperactive and epileptic: in a few seconds he went from daydreaming to petit mal convulsions. He is on a high dose of Epanutin, which his mother is not very happy about.

I used essential oils in high concentration as recommended in Valnet (1980). The essential oils used were: *Hyssopus officinalis, Salvia officinalis* and *Ocimum basilicum*, altogether 60 drops in 30 ml of carrier oil (10% dilution). The mix was used only on the kidney area on the back, therefore the quantity of essential oils being applied was in reality quite small.

The convulsions ceased within a week. M is now on a minimum dose of Epanutin, the massage oil concentration reduced to 1.5% and treatments to one a month. M's mother is now looking at withdrawing conventional drug therapy.

Deodorant

Bad smells sometimes arise from the disease process, and the sweet-smelling oils act to prevent degradation, replace the odours and tackle the bacteria causing these effects. The use of sweet-smelling and familiar essential oils is more acceptable to the client (who may be in a weakened state) than is the imposition of harsh synthetics. This attribute is also helpful in a healing situation where bad smells are generated, for example in some severe burn injuries. Essential oils do not merely disguise these unpleasant odours which clients and nurses have to suffer, but actually cancel them out. 'The odour of essential oils does not cover up the bad smells of infected gangrenous or cancerous wounds; it suppresses them by physicochemical action' (Valnet 1980 p. 44).

We have supplied a mixture of essential oils designed for this purpose for a number of years to a burns unit at the request of the consultant surgeon. The nurses find it particularly useful when bathing patients with burns. Essential oils find a similar use in incontinence cases, making life a great deal more pleasant for all concerned. Bad-smelling wounds can be deodorized by the use of hypericum oil (see p. 106), thyme and citrus oils (Schilcher 1985 p. 222). Chamomile preparations are also known for their deodorizing effect.

Because of the deodorizing effect of some fragrant materials they are useful in underarm and foot deodorants. Compounds and oils recommended as effective against body odour are eugenol, linalool and the essential oil *Pogostemon patchouli* (Decazes 1993). Elsewhere *Salvia sclarea*, *Cymbopogon flexuosus*, *Zingiber officinale* and *Myristica fragrans* are also mentioned in this respect.

Digestive

Essential oils have strong effects on the digestive system (Table 4.7) and are used in appetite-stimulating and digestive drinks as carminatives and stimulants for the stomach, liver and gall bladder. The carminative effect of many essential oils is strong, and there are other benefits, such as increased secretory activity of the stomach and gall bladder, antiseptic and spasmolytic effects. The essential oils concerned are mainly from the Umbellifer botanical family—*Carum carvi*, *Coriandrum sativum*, *Foeniculum vulgare* var. *dulce*, *Pimpinella anisum* and also *Mentha × piperita*, *Ocimum basilicum* and the chamomiles (Schilcher 1985 p. 224). Wild thyme (*Thymus serpyllum*) has been shown to stimulate bile production (Chabrol et al 1932), and essential oils containing the alcohols menthol and thujanol-4 seem to be beneficial to liver function (Gershbein 1977, Zara 1966).

The citrus oils generally have a favourable effect on the digestive system, being mildly appetite stimulating and digestive. *Citrus aurantium* var. *amara* (per.) is given as a treatment for constipation as it encourages intestinal peristalsis and also acts as a cholagogue (Duraffourd 1982 p. 95); this oil is also mentioned for dyspepsia, flatulence and gastric spasm (Franchomme & Pénoël 1990 p. 337). *Rosmarinus officinalis* has always been associated with improving the liver function. In animals an intravenous infusion of rosemary doubled the volume of bile secreted (Valnet 1980 p. 177); it is given as a carminative and cholagogue (Lautié & Passebecq 1984 p. 74) and to stimulate hepatobiliary secretions (Duraffourd 1982 p. 107).

Diuretic

Just as rosemary oil is traditionally associated with the liver, so juniper berry oil—*Juniperus communis* (fruct.)—is associated with the kidneys. At normal dosage it is a beneficial stimulant, although it has a toxic effect on inflamed kidneys. There is a diuretic effect (Duraffourd 1982, p. 67, Franchomme & Pénoël 1990 p. 361, Lautié & Passebecq 1984 p. 51, Viaud 1983) although this is denied by Schilcher (1985 p. 226) and omitted by Roulier (1990). However, one authority (Gattefossé 1937 p. 71) states that nearly all essences are diuretic and endorses juniper oil. It is also claimed that terpene-free oil containing mainly terpinen-4-ol has marked diuretic effects

Table 4.7 Essentials oils and the digestive system. Sources same as for Appendix A

	Properties									Indications									
	Antispasmodic	Aperitive	Astringent	Carminative	Choleretic	Hepatic stimulant	Litholytic (g=gall, k=kidney, u=urinary)	Pancreatic stimulant	Colic	Colitis, gastroenteritis	Constipation	Diarrhoea	Digestion painful	Digestive stimulant	Diverticulitis	Enteritis, gastritis	Indigestion	Nausea	Ulcers (duodenal, gastric)
Achillea millefolium [YARROW]				x			k							x					
Carum carvi [CARAWAY]	x			x	x			x									x		
Chamaemelum nobile (flos) [ROMAN CHAMOMILE]		x		x						x		x					x		
Chamomilla recutita (flos) [GERMAN CHAMOMILE]	?													x	x			x	x
Citrus aurantium var. *amara* (flos) [NEROLI BIGARADE]						x		x											
Citrus aurantium var. *amara* (fol.) [PETITGRAIN BIGARADE]																	x		
Citrus aurantium var. *amara* (per.) [ORANGE BIGARADE]						x			x	x						x	x		
Citrus bergamia (per.) [BERGAMOT]	x	x		x					x							x	x		
Citrus limon (per.) [LEMON]	x	x	x	x			g,u	x	x			x	x	x				x	x
Citrus reticulata (per.) [MANDARIN]				x	x						x						x		
Commiphora myrrha [MYRRH]														x					
Coriandrum sativum [CORIANDER]	x			x						x				x					
Cupressus sempervirens [CYPRESS]	x		x									x							
Eucalyptus smithii [GULLY GUM]														x					
Foeniculum vulgare var. *dulce* [FENNEL]				x	x		u			x				x			x		
Hyssopus officinalis [HYSSOP]							u	x						x			x		
Juniperus communis (fruct.) [JUNIPER BERRY]		x	x	x		x	u,k	x	x	x				x					
Melaleuca alternifolia [TEA TREE]												x							
Melaleuca leucadendron [CAJUPUT]	x																		
Melaleuca viridiflora [NIAOULI]				x		x	g			x		x			x	x			x
Melissa officinalis [MELISSA]	x			x	x				x					x			x	x	
Mentha × piperita [PEPPERMINT]	x		x	x	x				x	x		x	x	x	x		x	x	
Myristica fragrans (sem.) [NUTMEG]	x			x										x					
Nepeta cataria [CATNEP]							g												
Ocimum basilicum var. *album* [BASIL]	x			x	x				x	x				x			x		
Origanum majorana [MARJORAM]	x			x					x	x	?	x		x			x	x	x
Pelargonium graveolens [GERANIUM]			x		x			x		x				x	x				
Pimpinella anisum [ANISEED]	x	x		x					x					x			x	x	
Pinus sylvestris [SCOTS PINE]							g												
Piper nigrum [PEPPER]						x					x			x					
Rosmarinus officinalis [ROSEMARY]				x	x	x	g		x	x	x	x		x			x	x	
Salvia officinalis [SAGE]		x	?	x					x					x			x		
Santalum album [SANDALWOOD]			x							x									
Satureia montana, S. hortensis [WINTER AND SUMMER SAVORY]	x			x	x				x	x	x	x	x						
Syzygium aromaticum (flos) [CLOVE BUD]	x																		
Thymus serpyllum [WILD THYME]									x										
Thymus vulgaris (population) [THYME]				x										x					
Zingiber officinale [GINGER]				x					?	x	x	x		x				x	

(Schneider 1975), although juniper oils consist of more than 90% hydrocarbon monoterpenes and the level of this alcohol may be only 2–5%.

Energizing

Plants capture electromagnetic energy from the sun and some of this is stored in the essential oil. The biosynthesis of the terpenes has as a starting point acetyl coenzyme A (Hay & Waterman 1993 p. 52) and in certain plants this process of synthesis goes beyond terpenes to the production of steroids with hormonal properties. Plant metabolic mechanisms have much in common with those of humans, and this starting point of acetyl coenzyme A is analogous to the process in the human body by which steroids are synthesized—cortisone, vitamin D and cholesterol. The phenylpropanoids are another building block of essential oils and provide another example. They are in effect the precursors of some of the amino acids, the basic elements for the synthesis of proteins. Proteins are the building blocks of the human body, the agents for transformation and energy transfer which maintain the fabric of the body and all the physiological activity (Duraffourd 1987 p. 26). This may help us in understanding the special nature of essential oils; because of their molecular energy and because they have elements in common with human physiology, they can help to correct either deficits or blockages (Duraffourd 1987 p. 27).

Granulation promoting

This effect helps in healing where there has been damage or removal of tissue. Probably the best-known use is that of lavender oil for minor burns, which yields positive and rapid results (Gattefossé 1937). Hypericum oil and chamomile oils have been used traditionally for wound healing, and the validity of this has been borne out in the case of chamomile by studies (Glowania, Raulin & Swoboda 1987, Thiemer, Stadler & Isaac 1973). Red oil of hypericum is available: it is a fixed oil—usually with a base of olive oil or sunflower oil—in which the flowers of St John's wort (*Hypericum perforatum*) have been macerated.

This oil contains as active constituents not only the essential oil but also hypericin and was much used in the past for the external treatment of wounds and burns (Weiss 1988 p. 296).

Hormonal

Some essential oils have a tendency to normalize hormonal secretions, and it is thought that this action may be direct or effected via the hypophysis (Franchomme & Pénoël 1990). No work has so far been done to establish precisely how the oil molecules could do this, and there is little likelihood of this being carried out in the foreseeable future. For the present, treatment is easy and pleasant for the client and, so far as is known, without any side-effects. The hormone-like action of some plant extracts has been widely noted. Extracts of fennel seed have a slight oestrogenic effect in animal experimental models (Foster 1993). Bernadet (1983) and others advise the use of essential oils for such disorders as dysmenorrhoea and amenorrhoea. The essences

---

Case 4.7   Aromatherapist: Lynne Reed, UK

A community colleague of mine was called out one evening to see a client (a medical practitioner) with extremely sore nipples. On arrival, the nipples were cracked, bleeding and extremely painful—made worse by the application of a nipple cream which the client said had caused stinging. The baby was unable to be latched on. My colleague hand-expressed the mother and the baby was fed. She then left her with a small bottle of the nipple oil which is used in the hospital and arranged to call back the following morning.

When she revisited, the baby was back feeding on the breast and both client and colleague were surprised by the amount of healing that had taken place. The mother said that she had felt instant relief as soon as she applied the nipple oil.

Nipple oil. *Chamaemelum nobile, Lavandula angustifolia* and *Rosa damascena*, one drop each in 30 ml carrier oil made up of 20% calendula and 80% sweet almond. The blend is divided into 10 ml bottles for use in hospital. Apply to sore nipples after feeding the baby, remembering to wash the breasts with warm water just before the next feed.

The oils used are analgesic, antiseptic, bactericidal, antiinflammatory, granulation stimulating, haemostatic and antidepressant (rose). The analgesic effect has had a response of 7+ on a scale of 0–10 from patients using this oil in a small study.

of pine (needles), borneol, geranium, basil, sage, savory and rosemary stimulate the cortex of the suprarenal gland, while anise excites the anterior pituitary body, as does mint (Valnet 1980).

Valnet also writes that the essence of cypress seems to be a homologue of the ovarian hormone. There are compounds in some volatile oils which have structures similar to natural human hormones, and these promote efficient endocrine gland activity by natural means. Sclareol, viridiflorol and *trans*-anethole are examples of compounds which have structures similar to folliculin or analogous to oestrogen. Other compounds found in *Pinus sylvestris* are similar to cortisone (Franchomme & Pénoël 1990) (Table 4.8).

Hyperaemic

Essential oils promote local peripheral circulation owing to a primary irritation of the skin, and the effects of this are twofold:

- the freeing of mediators (e.g. bradykinin) which cause vasodilatation
- humoral reactions resulting in the antiinflammatory effect.

On the skin there is a sensation of warmth, comfort and pain relief following the use of rubefacients such as *Eucalyptus globulus, Rosmarinus officinalis* and *Juniperus communis*, which cause increased local blood circulation. Local skin irritation may also have some effect on internal organs (e.g. cardiac ointment used in angina). Some essential oils are vesicants, e.g. *Brassica nigra* [MUSTARD] and *Armoracia lapathifolia* [HORSERADISH] due to the principal constituent allylisothiocyanate. Croton oil is also a vesicant, and its use is proscribed by the Medicines Act 1968.

Immunostimulant

Melaleuca viridiflora has been reported to have an immunostimulant effect by increasing the level of immunoglobulins (Pénoël 1981), and many other oils have been mentioned by various writers as strengthening the immune system. There is a wide variety and no common agreement, and this may be so because many oils possess a range of properties (antifungal, antiseptic, antiviral, etc.) that are beneficial to the immune system (see Ch. 15). (See Appendix B. 9 for a list of effective oils.)

Insecticidal and repellent

Plant volatile oils may be used over a long period of time without promoting resistance. Some plants use essential oils to repel attacking insects, and they are still effective after millions of years. In the south of France, citronella is universally used as an insect repellent, and tests show other oils to have this property too, e.g. *Ocimum basilicum* (Dube, Upadhyay & Tripath 1989). Of a number of essential oils and some of their components investigated for insecticidal activity, only a few demonstrated this attribute—*Cinnamomum camphora, C. verum, Cymbopogon nardus, Syzygium aromaticum* and *Eucalyptus* oils, plus two aldehydes and a ketone (cinnamic aldehyde, citral and carvone) (Gildemeister & Hoffmann 1956). Our past experience indicates that *Thymus vulgaris* ct. thymol and *Melaleuca alternifolia* are effective parasiticides (head and pubic lice), and tests in which we were involved tend to confirm this.

Mucolytic and expectorant

Accumulated secretions in the mucous linings can hold germs and it is necessary to break down the mucus in order to kill them. Many oils are mucolytic thanks to their content of powerful ketones (carvone, menthone, thujone, pinocamphone, etc.) and in some cases lactones. The expectorant effect is due to the breaking down of secretions and to cilial activity, and several oils have in the past been tested to determine expectorant properties (Boyd & Pearson 1946, Gordonoff 1938, Schilcher 1985 p. 223). Besides *Eucalyptus globulus* and other essential oils containing the oxide 1,8-cineole, *Pimpinella anisum, Foeniculum vulgare* var. *dulce, Pinus sylvestris* and *P. mugo* var. *pumilio, Thymus vulgaris* ct. phenol and *T. serpyllum* are also expectorants. These oils, whether used by

Table 4.8 The influence of essential oils on the hormonal system (from various authors)

Species [common name]	Adrenal (cortex)	Adrenal (medulla)	Anaphrodisiac	Emmenagogic	Frigidity, impotence	Hypophysis gonads	Hypophysis ovarian	Hypophysis pancreas	Hypophysis suprarenal cortex	Hypophysis	Hypothalamus	Lactogenic	Oestrogen like	Pancreas (diabetes)	Pituitary (anterior)	Pituitary (posterior)	Reproduction (ovaries)	Sex hormones (testes)	Thymus	Thyroid	Thyroxine production	Uterotonic (facilitates delivery)
Chamomilla recutita [GERMAN CHAMOMILE]				?																		
Citrus aurantium var. *amara* (per.) [ORANGE BITTER]										X	X				X							
Citrus limon (per.) [LEMON]			X							X	X					X						
Commiphora myrrha [MYRRH]				?															X		X	
Cymbopogon citratus, C. flexuosus [LEMONGRASS]																						
Foeniculum vulgare var. *dulce* (fruct.) [FENNEL]				X								X	X									X
Juniperus communis (fruct) [JUNIPER BERRY]				?																		
Melaleuca leucadendron [CAJUPUT]				?																		
Melaleuca viridiflora [NIAOULI]				X		X	X						X				X					
Mentha × piperita [PEPPERMINT]				?																		X
Myristica fragrans (sem) [NUTMEG]				X																		X
Ocimum basilicum [BASIL]				?																		
Origanum majorana [SWEET MARJORAM]			X	?																		
Pelargonium graveolens, P. × asperum [GERANIUM]														X								
Pimpinella anisum [ANISEED]				X		X						X										X
Pinus sylvestris [PINE]								X	X											X		
Rosa centifolia, R. damascena [ROSE OTTO]				?	X																	
Rosmarinus officinalis [ROSEMARY]	X			?																		
Salvia officinalis [SAGE]		X		X									X									
Salvia sclarea [CLARY]				?									X									
Santalum album [SANDALWOOD]																		X				
Syzygium aromaticum (flos) [CLOVE BUD]																						X
Thymus vulgaris ct. geraniol [SWEET THYME]																						X
Thymus vulgaris ct. thymol [THYME]	X																					
Vetiveria zizanioides [VETIVER]				?													X					

external application or by inhalation, reach the bronchi and are eliminated from the lungs in the exhaled air. Russian research endorsed this property of some essential oils when inhaled (Eremenko et al 1987); all 96 patients suffering from chronic bronchitis showed a significant increase in the permeability of the respiratory tracts and clearing of the airway as well as a decrease in immunoglobulin E, indicating reduced infection levels. The study shows that the vapour of some essential oils (camphor, eucalyptus, peppermint and menthol) can improve the function of the lungs and bronchials, and so relieve mucous congestion, chest infections, colds and influenza.

Sedative

In the past there has been little apart from anecdotal evidence for the sedative properties of essential oils, but now several oils have been investigated and found to be effective. They include *Melissa officinalis*, which is calming to the central nervous system because of its citronellal and other monoterpene content (Becker & Förster 1984, Mills 1991), and the valerian oils, which contain small amounts of valepotriates (Becker & Reichling 1981, Becker 1983, Boeters 1969, Schmiedeberg 1913). *Valeriana officinalis* contains only about 1.5% of these but this figure can rise to 12% in other species. Recently other tests have been carried out which prove for the first time the sedative, calming effects of other oils, such as *Citrus aurantium* var. *amara* (flos) [NEROLI] and *Passiflora incarnata* [PASSION FLOWER] (Buchbauer 1993, Buchbauer, Jirovetz & Jäger 1992, Buchbauer et al 1993) (Table 4.9). The aromatic water collected during the distillation of orange flowers (orange flower water) also has sedative properties, and more effective still is the essential oil of petitgrain *C. aurantium* var. *amara* (fol.) (Duraffourd 1982 p. 97). Lavender is recognized as a calming oil (Guillemain, Rousseau & Delaveau 1989) (Table 4.9) and is now used in many hospital wards to aid sleep (see Ch. 14). It is thought that the sedative effect of *Lavandula angustifolia* is due in part to the presence of coumarins in the oil, even though the content is low at 0.25% (Franchomme & Pénoël 1990 p. 364).

Table 4.9 Effects of fragrance compounds and essential oils on the motility of mice after a 1 hour inhalation period (from Buchbauer et al 1993 p. 661)

Compound	Effect on motility %[a]	Effect on motility after caffeine %[b]
Anethole	−10.81	−1.26
Anthranilic acid methyl ester	+17.70	+38.22
Balm leaves oil (Austria)	−5.21	+16.29
Benzaldehyde	−43.69	−34.28
Benzyl alcohol	−11.21	−23.68
Borneol	−3.05	−1.88
Bornyl acetate	−7.79	+2.27
Bornyl salicylate	−17.29	−2.99
Carvone	−2.46	−47.51
Citral	−1.43	+17.24
Citronellal	−49.82	−37.40
Citronellol	−3.56	−13.71
Coumarin	−15.00	−13.75
Dimethyl vinyl carbinol	+5.36	−2.11
Ethylmaltol	+9.73	+2.09
Eugenol	+2.10	−38.73
Farnesol	+5.76	+36.34
Farnesyl acetate	+4.62	−30.71
Furfural	+3.04	−4.51
Geraniol	+20.56	+1.20
Geranyl acetate	−29.18	−7.46
Isoborneol	+46.90	−11.23
Isobornyl acetate	+3.16	−22.35
Isoeugenol	+30.05	−74.34
β-ionone	+14.20	−27.97
Lavender oil (Mont Blanc)	−78.40	−91.67
Lime blossom oil (France)	−34.34	+30.41
Linalool	−73.00	−56.67
Linalyl acetate	−69.10	−46.67
Maltol	+13.74	−50.04
Methyl salicylate	+16.64	−49.88
Nerol	+12.93	+29.31
Neroli oil	−65.27	+1.87
Orange flower oil (Spain)	−4.64	−14.62
Orange terpenes	+35.25	−33.19
Passion flower oil (USA)	+8.15	−27.93
2-phenyl ethanol	+2.67	−30.61
2-phenylethyl acetate	−45.04	+12.42
α-pinene	+13.77	+4.73
Rose oil (Bulgaria)	−9.50	+4.31
Sandalwood oil (East India)	−40.00	−20.70
α-terpineol	−45.00	−12.50
Thymol	+33.02	+19.05
Valerian root oil (China)	−2.70	−12.01

[a] motility of untreated control animals = 100%
[b] motility of control animals after pretreatment with 0.1% caffeine solution (0.5 mL, ip) = 100%

Spasmolytic

Essential oils have been found to relieve smooth muscle spasm (Debelmas & Rochat 1964, 1967a,b, Taddei et al 1988), hence their usefulness for some problems of the digestive tract. The oils with this property are chamomile oils containing (–)-α-bisabolol (Achterrath-Tuckerman et al 1980, Melegari et al 1988), *Carum carvi, Cinnamomum zeylanicum* (cort.), *Citrus aurantium* var. *amara* (per.), *Foeniculum vulgare* var. *dulce, Melissa officinalis* and *Mentha × piperita* (Schilcher 1985 p. 225).

There is value in successful practical experience, and essential oils have been used to ease spasm in skeletal muscle also, despite the lack of clinical trials. We have used *Ocimum basilicum* and *Origanum majorana* successfully over the years, and a fuller list has been published (Price 1993 p. 278). *Cupressus sempervirens* is also credited with this property (Franchomme & Pénoël 1990 p. 346).

Case 4.8 Aromatherapist: Rosalind Mere BA, RN, Australia

In March 1990 I was asked by the Deputy Director of Nursing of Jindalee Nursing Home in Canberra ACT, Australia if I would give weekly aromatherapy massages to one of their residents, the purpose being to reduce muscle spasm and help prevent the onset of joint confracture. A further purpose was to induce relaxation in this client who had been hospitalized since the age of 19 with multiple injuries from a horrific motor accident. Both her doctor and the occupational therapist had recommended massage for Amanda.

My work with her commenced 2 years before she died under anaesthetic at the age of 30. Over the months that I worked weekly with Amanda, I used various essential oils which included mental stimulants (e.g. lemon, peppermint, basil and rosemary), antispasmodics (e.g. neroli, bergamot, lavender, chamomile and clary) and relaxing oils (e.g. melissa, marjoram, sandalwood and vetiver).

On my first visit to Amanda I tried a smell preference test with her but as she was relatively uncommunicative in those early days I was not sure of the precision of her reactions. Although she appeared to resist rosemary at first, I did use this oil on her at times when she seemed withdrawn and depressed—with good result. Senior staff felt that the treatments made her more socially receptive and commented that Amanda's mental attitude had improved since the commencement of massage.

Other considerations

Essential oil interaction with drugs

Essential oils are composed of chemicals which are known to be active, gain access to cells by virtue of being fat soluble, and are metabolized by the body. It has been found by experience that some oils are relaxing, some sedative, some sharpen the memory, some promote the circulation and so on. Therefore it may be assumed that as active agents they may react with other drugs present in the body, although there has been no evidence so far which would imply any adverse significant reaction between essential oils and allopathic drugs, and they have been used together successfully in hospitals (Barker 1994 personal communication). In a study on rats, eucalyptol administered subcutaneously or by aerosol was found to increase the in vitro liver metabolism of aminopyrine, *p*-nitro-anisol and aniline, and in vivo the metabolism of pentobarbital (Jori, Bianchetti & Prestini 1969). Animal studies have shown enhanced skin penetration for some drugs with eucalyptus oil, camphor and limonene, and, in laboratory tests on excised human skin, penetration of 5-fluorouracil was increased with aniseed oil (2.8 times), ylang oil (7.8 times) and eucalyptus oil (34 times) (Williams & Barry 1989). Drug interaction with essential oils is discussed in Tisserand & Balacs (1995).

Nevertheless this is a cloudy area and, until laboratory investigations into possible reactions between essential oils and other drugs have been carried out and results made known, it is possible only to surmise what may happen. If sedative pills to help sleep are being prescribed then it may be unwise with our present level of knowledge to use an essential oil such as rosemary, which keeps the mind alert. It would be better to choose oils like lavender, vetiver and valerian, which are known to aid relaxation and sleep. It has been suggested that when a person is on medication the drugs involved could possibly affect metabolization of essential oil molecules. In some cases metabolism may be increased, e.g. with clofibrate (a blood lipid level reducer), steroids and phenobarbitones (antiepileptics). In other cases the drugs involved may reduce the metabolism of essential oil molecules, e.g. imidazole (antifungal), plant drugs, caffeic acid, myristicin or tannic acid. The study by Buchbauer et al (1993) indicates an area of possible future study in that some essential oils or their components may interact with caffeine, e.g. neroli, methyl salicylate, isoeugenol.

Some essences have been found to complement the action of antibiotics. Laboratory tests have shown that the essence of niaouli will increase the activity of streptomycin, cocaine and, more especially, of penicillin (Quevauviller & Panousse-Perrin 1952a,b). Reporting the results obtained when using turpentine derivatives in conjunction with antibiotics, Mignon has shown, from tests in vitro and on mice, the action of the antibiotics to be considerably augmented by being administered in a solution of oxygenated turpentine derivatives. There are, however, some constituents of some essential oils (aldehydes, ketones and some alcohols) which inactivate antibiotics and so limit their use in ointment form.

(Valnet 1980 p. 39)

Homoeopathy. For many years now we have been questioning practitioners of homoeopathy as to whether homoeopathic treatment is affected in any way by the concurrent use of essential oils, and the answers have varied from the total prohibition of all essential oils to the unrestricted use of any. However, the chief common ground is that peppermint should be avoided and probably eucalyptus and camphor as well, and this is what is advised in the absence of a definitive answer.

Molecular structure

A possible relationship between the molecular structure of the essential oil components and their therapeutic effect has been studied and published (Franchomme & Pénoël 1990). This is an interesting piece of work and although not proven rigorously is nevertheless very useful to therapists when studying and choosing oils; the principles involved are to be found in Price (1993 pp. 49–55). 'It is based on the presence of key chemical groups in the oil molecules. If this approach is valid, then it may well be that essential oil molecules are interacting with the same

receptors on nerve cells and in other tissues which respond to drugs' (Balacs 1991).

British Pharmacopoeia

Mabey (1988 p. 190) points out that no less than 80% of the medicines in the BP were plant based at one time (e.g. aspirin)—and even today 30% are still plant based (e.g. digitalis). Current pharmaceutical formulae demonstrate that essential oils and oleoresins derived from spices and herbs are valued not only as flavouring agents but also for other properties they possess, for instance, they:

• stimulate the appetite by increasing salivation
• act as carminatives to relieve gastric discomfort and flatulence
• counteract the griping action of purgatives
• contribute as mild expectorants in cough mixtures and pastilles
• check profuse secretion and relieve congestion of the bronchioles when used in inhalants
• act as counterirritants and rubefacients, for the chest in bronchitis and pleurisy, and for the relief of rheumatic pain, when formulated as ointments, creams and liniments.

As flavouring agents, essential oils are acceptable for repeated dosage, e.g. in tablets to be chewed and for repeated usage in such products as toothpaste. As perfumes they are present in a variety of cosmetics which are used daily over long periods of time.

The essential oils as specified in the BP are not suitable for use in aromatology or aromatherapy because the specification is too broad or does not reflect the materials currently available; 'the analytical figures for the present English lavender oil do not correspond with the existing BP standards' (Trease & Evans 1983). There are many different varieties of eucalyptus used in aromatherapy, each with its own characteristics, but many are lumped together in the BP where eucalyptus essential oil is given as *E. globulus* Labill., *E. fruticetorum* F von Muell, *E. polybractea* R T Baker, or *E. smithii* R T Baker. Each of these indeed has 1,8-cineole as its major component but the other constitutents modify the effects of the whole oil. The BP gives the results of thin layer chromatography on some of the oils listed, but for some there is not even this specification; a critical commentary on the BP monograph for peppermint oil can be found in Hay & Waterman (1993).

Lemon is listed as *Citrus limon* (L.) Burm, f. with not less than 2.2% w/w and not more than 4.5% w/w of carbonyl components (calculated as citral) $C_{10}H_{16}O$. Also listed as *C. limon* is terpeneless lemon oil containing not less than 40% w/w of aldehydes (calculated as citral) $C_{10}H_{16}O$. However, the deterpenated essence is not used in aromatherapy or aromatology as defined today because only unadulterated and unrectified oils may be used. Some of the oils mentioned in the BP lack any complete specification: anise, caraway, cardamom, cedarwood, cinnamon, clove, coriander, dill, eucalyptus, lemon, nutmeg, orange, peppermint, spearmint and turpentine.

A survey of the European pharmacopoeia (Bischof et al 1992) shows that only a few oils are common to the major pharmacopoeia—caraway, eucalyptus, lemon, peppermint. Surprisingly, lavender is not one of them, but the Pharmacopoeia Helvetica does allow synthetic lavender. The Formulaire national de France has three monographs on lavender.

Summary

The numerous therapeutic properties of essential oils have been examined in some detail, and scientific confirmation of traditional wisdom given where possible. It is to be hoped that more controlled trials will take place, and the importance of the totality of effects of any essential oil will be given precedence over the activity of its components. There is also an urgent need for official sources such as the BP to be revised to take into account modern botanical and therapeutic knowledge of essential oils.

REFERENCES

Achterrath-Tuckerman U, Kunde R, Flaskamp O, Theimer I, Theimer K 1980 Pharmacological investigations with compounds of chamomile. V. Investigations on the spasmolytic effect of compounds of chamomile. Planta Medica, Stuttgart 39: 38–50

Anderson M 1998 Sweet smell of success for Monklands hospital. Scottish Nurse 1998 2(8): 7

Balacs T 1991 Essential issues. International Journal of Aromatherapy 3(4): 24

Becker H 1983 Deutsche Apotheker Zeitung 123: 2470

Becker H, Förster W 1984 Biologie, Chemie und Pharmakologie pflanzlicher Sedativa. Zeitschrift Phytotherapie Stuttgart 5: 817–823

Becker H, Reichling J 1981 Deutsche Apotheker Zeitung 121: 1185

Belaiche P 1979 Traité de phytothérapie et d'aromathérapie, 3 vols. Maloine, Paris

Belaiche P 1985a L'huile essentielle de *Melaleuca alternifolia* (Cheel) dans les infections cutanées. Phytothérapie 15 September: 15–18

Belaiche P 1985b L'huile essentielle de *Melaleuca alternifolia* (Cheel) dans les infections urinaires colibacillaires chroniques idiopathiques. Phytothérapie 15 September: 9–12

Belaiche P 1985c L'huile essentielle de *Melaleuca alternifolia* (Cheel) dans les infections vaginales à *Candida albicans*. Phytothérapie 15 September: 13–14

Berman B M, Singh B K, Lao L, Singh B B, Ferentz K S, Hartnol S M 1995 Physicians' attitudes towards complementary or alternative medicine: a regional survey. Journal of the American Board of Family Practitioners 8(5): 361–366

Bernadet M 1983 La phyto-aromathérapie pratique. Dangles, St-Jean-de-Braye

Beylier M F 1979 Bacteriostatic activity of some Australian essential oils. Perfumer & Flavorist 4(23) (April/May): 23–25

Bischof C, Holthuijzen J, Löwenstein C, Stengele M, Stahl-Biskup E, Wilhelm E 1992 Essential oil analysis in the European pharmacopoeia. 23rd International Symposium on Essential Oils, West of Scotland College, Ayr, Scotland. Copies available from Lehrstuhl für Pharmakognosie der Universität Hamburg, Bundesstraße 43, D-2000 Hamburg 13

Boeters M 1969 Behandlung vegetativer Regulationsstörungen mit Valepotriaten (Valmane). Münchner Medizin Wochenschrift 11: 1873–1876

Bonnaure F 1919 Essais sur les propriétés bactericides de quelques huiles essentielles. Parfumerie Moderne 12: 151

Bonnelle C 1993 Des hommes et des plantes. Editions du Parc Naturel Régional du Vercors, Lans-en-Vercors, p 32

Borkan J, Neher J O, Anson O, Smoker B 1994 Referrals for alternative therapies. Journal of Family Practitioners 39(6): 545–550

Bowker (no date) Food additives and the patients they affect. CBA and Associates Ltd, London (leaflet)

Boyd E M, Pearson G L 1946 The expectorant action of volatile oils. American Journal of Medical Science 211: 602–610

Buchbauer G 1993 Biological effects of fragrances and essential oils. Perfumer & Flavorist 18 (January/February): 19–24

Buchbauer G, Jirovetz L, Jäger W 1992 Passiflora and lime blossoms: motility effects after inhalation of the essential oil and of some of the main constituents in animal experiment. Archiva Pharmaceutica (Weinheim) 325: 247–248

Buchbauer G, Jirovetz L, Jäger W, Plank C, Dietrich H 1993 Fragrance compounds and essential oils with sedative effects upon inhalation. Journal of Pharmaceutical Sciences 82(6) (June): 660–664

Carson C F, Riley T V 1993 Antimicrobial activity of the essential oil of Melaleuca alternifolia. Applied Microbiology 16(2): 49–55

Carson C F, Cookson B D, Farrelly H D, Riley T V 1995 Susceptibility of methicillin-resistant Staphylococcus aureus to the essential oil of Melaleuca alternifolia. Journal of Antimicrobial Chemotherapy 35: 421–424

Cavel L 1918 Sur la valeur antiseptique de quelques huiles essentielles. Comptes Rendus Académie des Sciences, p 827

Chabrol E, Charonnat R, Maximum M, Busson A 1932 Le serpolet: cholagogue. Comptes Rendus Société Biologie 109: 275–276

Chamberland M 1887 Les essences au point de vue de leurs propriétés antiseptiques. Annales Institut Pasteur 1: 153–154

Cohen R A, Kucera L S, Herrman E C 1964 Antiviral activity of Melissa officinalis extract. Proceedings of the Society of Experimental Biology and Medicine 117: 431–434

Courmont P, Morel P, Bay I 1938 The antiseptic action of essential oils. Parfumerie Moderne 21: 161

D'Arcy P F 1993 Drug reactions and interactions. International Pharmacy Journal 7(4) (July/August): 140–142

Deans S G, Ritchie G A 1987 Antibacterial properties of plant essential oils. International Journal of Food Microbiology 5: 165–180

Deans S G, Svoboda K P 1988 Antibacterial activity of French tarragon (Artemisia dracunculus L.) essential oil and its constituents during ontogeny. Journal of Horticultural Science 63: 135–140

Deans S G, Svoboda K P 1989 Antibacterial activity of summer savory [Satureia hortensis L.] essential oil and its constituents. Journal of Horticultural Science 64: 205–211

Deans S G, Svoboda K P 1990a Essential oil profiles of several temperate and tropical aromatic plants: their antimicrobial and antioxidative properties. Proceedings 75th International Symposium of Research Institute for Medicinal Plants, Budakalasz, Hungary, pp 25–27. (Copies obtainable from authors at Scottish Agricultural College, Ayr)

Deans S G, Svoboda K P 1990b The antimicrobial properties of marjoram (Origanum majorana L.) volatile oil. Flavor & Fragrance Journal 5(3): 187–190

Debelmas A M, Rochat J 1964 Etude comparée sur la fibre lisse des solutions aqueuses saturées d'essence de thym, de thymol et de carvacrol. Bulletin des Travaux. Société de Pharmacie de Lyon 4: 163–172

Debelmas A M, Rochat J 1967a Action des eaux saturées d'huiles essentielles sur la musculature lisse. 25th International Congress of Pharmaceutical Science. Butterworth, London, pp 601–607

Debelmas A M, Rochat J 1967b Activité antispasmodique étudiée sur une cinquantaine d'échantillons différents. Plantes Médicinales et Phytothérapie 1: 23–27

Decazes J-M 1993 The masking effect of perfume ingredients. Symposium at Stoke-on-Trent: Fragrance—more than just a pleasant smell? Society of Cosmetic Chemists

Dube S, Upadhyay P D, Tripath S C 1989 Antifungal, physiochemical, and insect-repelling activity of the essential oil of Ocimum basilicum. Canadian Journal of Botany 67(7): 2085–2087

Duraffourd P 1982 En forme tous les jours. La Vie Claire, Périgny, p 107

Duraffourd P 1987 Les huiles essentielles et la santé. La Maison du Bien-Etre, Montreuil-sous-Bois

Eccles S 1997 Editorial. Aromatherapy Quarterly 55: 5

Eremenko A E, Nikolaevskii V V, Kostin N F, Meshkov V V 1987 Letuchie fraktsii fitontsidov na osnove efirnykh masel v sostav lechebno-reabilitatsionnykh kompleksov pri khronicheskikh bronkhitakh. Volatile fractions of essential oil based phytoncides as a component of therapeutic–rehabilitative complexes in chronic bronchitis (in Russian). Tikhomirov AA Ter. Arkh. 59(3): 126–130

Ernst E, Resch K L, White A R 1995 Complementary medicine. What physicians think of it: a meta analysis. Archives of Intern Medicine 155(22): 2405–2408

Foster S 1993 Herbal renaissance. Gibbs Smith, Layton, Utah p 93

Franchomme P, Pénoël D 1990 L'aromathérapie exactement. Jollois, Limoges

Gattefossé R M 1919 Propriétés bactéricides de quelques huiles essentielles. Parfumerie Moderne 13: 152

Gattefossé R M 1932 Rôle antiseptique de la lavande. Parfumerie Moderne 26: 543–553

Gattefossé R M 1937 Aromatherapy (transl 1993). Daniel, Saffron Walden, p 87

Gershbein L E 1977 Regeneration of rat liver in the presence of essential oils and their components. Food and Cosmetics Toxicology 15: 173–181

Gildemeister E, Hoffmann F 1956 Die ätherischen Öle, vol 1. Akadamie Verlag, Berlin, p 119

Glowania H J, Raulin C, Swoboda M 1987 Effect of chamomile on wound healing—a clinical double-blind study. Zeitschrift für Hautkrankheiten (Berlin) 62(17): 1262, 1267–1271

Gordonoff T 1938 Ergebnisse der Physiologie, biologischen Chemie und experimentallen. Pharmakologie 40: 53

Griggs B 1997 New green pharmacy. Vermilion, London, p 293

Guillemain J, Rousseau A, Delaveau P 1989 Neurodepressive effects of the essential oil of Lavandula angustifolia Mill. Annales Pharmaceutiques Françaises 47(6): 337–343

Hay R K M, Waterman P G 1993 Volatile oil crops. Longman, Harlow, p 52

Herrman E C Jr, Kucera L S 1967 Antiviral substances in plants of the mint family (Labiatae). II. Nontannin polyphenol of *Melissa officinalis*. Proceedings of the Society for Experimental and Biological Medicine 117: 369–374

Hinou J B, Harvala C E, Hinou E B 1989 Antimicrobial activity screening of 32 common constituents of essential oils. Pharmazie 44(4) (April): 302–303

Holland E H 1941 Results of a series of investigations carried out on the germicidal, disinfectant and bacteriostatic action of Melasol (*Melaleuca alternifolia*). Unpublished paper, Sydney University

Jakovlev V, Isaac O, Flaskamp E 1983 Pharmacological investigations with compounds of chamomile. VI. Investigations on the antiphlogistic effects of chamazulene and matricin. Planta Medica 49: 67–73

Jalsenjak V, Peljnjak S, Kustrak D 1987 Microcapsules of sage oil: essential oils content and antimicrobial activity. Pharmazie 42(6) (June): 419–420

Janssen A M, Scheffer J J C, Baerheim Svendsen A, Aynehchi Y 1984 Pharmazeutisch Weekblad (scientific edn) 6: 157

Janssen A M, Chin N L J, Scheffer J J C, Baerheim Svendsen A 1986 Screening for antimicrobial activity of some essential oils by the agar overlay techniques. Pharmazeutisch Weekblad (scientific edn) 8: 289–292

Jasper C, Maruzella J C, Laurence Liguori L 1958 The in vitro antifungal activity of essential oils. Journal of the American Pharmaceutical Association 47(4): 294–296

Jasper C, Maruzella J C, Percival A, Henry P A 1958 The antimicrobial activity of perfume oils. Journal of the American Pharmaceutical Association 47(7): 471

Jori A, Bianchetti A, Prestini P E 1969 Effect of essential oils on drug metabolism. Biochemical Pharmacology 18: 2081–2085

Juven B J, Kanner J, Schved F, Weisslowicz H 1994 Factors that interact with the antibacterial action of thyme essential oil and its active constituents. Journal of Applied Bacteriology 76: 626–631

Kellner W, Kober W 1954 Möglichkeiten der Wewendung ätherischer öle zur Raumdesinfektion. I. Mitteilung: Die Wirkung gebräuchlicher ätherischer öle auf Testkeime. Arzneimittel-Forschung [Drug Research] 4(5): 319

Kellner W, Kober W 1955 Möglichkeiten der Werwendung ätherischer öle zur Raumdesinfektion. II. Arzneimittel-Forschung [Drug Research] 5(4): 224

Kellner W, Kober W 1956 Möglichkeiten der Werwendung ätherischer öle zur Raumdesinfektion. III. Arzneimittel-Forschung [Drug Research] 6(12): 768

Kienholz M 1959 Action antibactérienne des huiles essentielles. Arzneimittel-Forschung [Drug Research] 9(8): 518–519

Knobloch K, Pauli A, Iberl B, Weigand H, Weis N 1989 Antibacterial and antifungal properties of essential oil components. Journal of Essential Oil Research 1: 119–128

Kucera L S, Herman J C Jr 1967 Antiviral substances in plants in the mint family (Labiatae). 1. Tannin of *Melissa officinalis*. Proceedings of the Society for Experimental and Biological Medicine 124: 865

Larrondo J V, Calvo M A 1991 Effect of essential oils on *Candida albicans*: a scanning electron microscope study. Biomed Letters 46(184): 269–272

Lautié R, Passebecq A 1984 Aromatherapy. Thorsons, Wellingborough, p 74

Lawrence F (ed) 1987 Additives—your complete survival guide. Century, London

Lembke A, Deininger R 1985 Preparation and method for stimulating the immune system. German Patent 3508875 A 1 21 November 1985

Lembke A, Deininger R 1988 Virus inactivating pharmaceutical containing formates and black pepper oil. European Patent (EP) 259617 A 2 16 March 1988

Low D, Rowal B D, Griffin W J 1974 Antibacterial action of the essential oils of some Australian Myrtaceae. Planta Medica 26: 184

Mabey R 1988 The complete new herbal. Elm Tree, London

Malowan S L 1931 Zeitschrift für Hygiene 1(1): 93

Martindale W H 1910 Antiseptic powers of essential oils. Perfumery & Essential Oil Record 1: 266, 274

Maruzella J C 1961 Antifungal properties of perfume oils. Journal of the American Pharmaceutical Association 50: 655

Medicines Act 1968 HMSO, London

Melegari M, Albasini A, Pecorari P, Vampa G, Rinaldi M, Rossi T, Bianchi A 1988 Chemical characteristics and pharmacological properties of the essential oil of *Anthemis nobilis*. Fitoterapia 59(6): 449–455

Mills S Y 1991 Essential book of herbal medicine. Penguin, London, p 452

Moleyar V, Narasimham P 1992 Antibacterial activity of essential oil components. International Journal of Food Microbiology 16: 337–342

Onawunmi G O 1988 In vitro studies on the antibacterial activity of phenoxyethanol in combination with lemongrass oil. Pharmazie 43(1) (January): 42–43

Onawunmi G O 1989 Antifungal activity of lemongrass oil. International Journal of Crude Drug Research 27(2): 121–126

Onawunmi G O, Ogunlana E O 1986 A study of the antibacterial activity of the essential oil of lemongrass *Cymbopogon citratus* (DC) Stapf. International Journal of Crude Drug Research 24(2): 64–68

Onawunmi G O, Yisak W A, Ogunlana E O 1984 Anti-bacterial constituents in the essential oil of *Cymbopogon citratus* (DC) Stapf. Journal of Ethnopharmacology 12(3): 279–286

Pandey M P, Prasad J, Awasthi L P, Kaushik P 1988 Antiviral effect of the essential oils from lemongrass (*Cymbopogon flexuosus*), mint (*Mentha arvensis*) and vetiver (*Vetiveria zizanioides*). Indigenous medicinal plants including microbes and fungi. National seminar on conservation and ethnobotanical aspects. Today and Tomorrows Printers and Publishers, New Delhi, pp 47–49

Pellecuer J, Roussel J L, Andary C 1973 Propriétés antifongiques comparatives des essences des trois Labiées méditerranéennes: romarin, sarriette et thym. Travaux de la Société de Pharmacie de Montpelier 33(4): 587

Pellecuer J, Allegrini J, De Buochberg S 1974 Etude in vitro de l'activité anti-bactérienne et antifongique de l'essence de *Satureia montana* L. Labiées. Journal de Pharmacie de Belgique 29(2): 137–144

Pellecuer J, Allegrini J, De Buochberg S, Passat J 1975 Place de l'essence de *Satureia montana* L. Labiées dans l'arsenal thérapeutique. Plantes Médicinales et Phytothérapie 9(2): 99–106

Pellecuer J, Allegrini J, Seimeon M, De Buochberg S 1976 Huiles essentielles bactéricides et fongicides. Revue de l'Institut de Lyon 1(2): 135–159

Pena E F 1962 *Melaleuca alternifolia* oil—its use for trichomonal vaginitis and other vaginal infections. Obstetrics and Gynecology June: 793–795

Pénoël D 1981 Phytomédecine. CIMP, La Courtête 1/2: 63

Perkin M R, Pearay R M, Fraser J S 1994 A comparison of the attitudes shown by general practitioners, hospital doctors and medical students towards alternative medicine. Journal of the Royal Society of Medicine 87(9): 523–525

Pollock I, Young E, Stoneham M, Slater N, Wilkinson J, Warner J 1989 Surveys of colourings and preservatives in drugs. British Medical Journal 299: 649–651

Poucher W A 1936 Perfumes, cosmetics and soaps, 3 vols. Chapman & Hall, London

Price S 1993 The aromatherapy workbook. Thorsons, London, pp 49–55

Quevauviller A, Panousse-Perrin J 1952a Exaltation du pouvoir anesthétique local de la cocaïne par l'essence de Niaouli purifiée. Anesthésie 9: 421

Quevauviller A, Panousse-Perrin J 1952b Influence du Gomenol sur l'activité in vitro de certains antibiotiques. Revue de Pathologie Comparée et Hygiene Générale 637: 296

Raharivelomanana P J, Terrom G P, Bianchini J P, Coulanges P 1989 Study of the antimicrobial action of various essential oils extracted from Malagasy plants. II: Lauraceae. Archives Institut Pasteur de l'Afrique (Madagascar) 56(1): 261–271

Ramanoelina A R, Terrom G P, Bianchini J P, Coulanges P 1987 Antibacterial action of essential oils extracted from Madagascar plants. Archives Institut Pasteur de l'Afrique (Madagascar) 53(1): 217–226

Rideal S, Rideal E K, Sciver A 1928 An investigation into the germicidal powers and capillary activities of certain essential oils. Perfumery & Essential Oil Record 19: 285

Rideal E K, Sciver A, Richardson N E G 1930 Perfumery & Essential Oil Record 21: 341

Ritzerfeld W 1959 Arzneimittel-Forschung 9: 521

Rossi T, Melegari M, Bianchi A, Albasini A, Vampa G 1988 Sedative, antiinflammatory and antidiuretic effects induced in rats by essential oils of varieties of *Anthemis nobilis*: a comparative study. Pharmacology Research Communications 5 (December 20): 71–74

Roulier G 1990 Les huiles essentielles pour votre santé. Dangles, St-Jean-de-Braye

Schilcher H 1985 Effects and side effects of essential oils. In: Baerheim Svendsen A, Scheffer J J C (eds) Essential oils and aromatic plants. Martinus Nijhof/Junk, Dordrecht

Schmidt P W 1936 Zentralblad für Bakteriologie, Parasitenkunde und Infektionskrankheiten 138: 104

Schmiedeberg O 1913 Grundriss der Pharmakologie, 7th edn. Pharmakologie, Leipzig

Schnaubelt K 1994 Aromatherapy and chronic viral infections. In: Aroma 93 Conference Proceedings. Aromatherapy Publications, Brighton, pp 34–41

Schneider G 1975 Pharmazeutische Biologie. Wissenschaftsverlag, Mannheim, p 128

Scientific American 1886 [quoted in Scientific American 1996 50, 100 and 150 years ago.] September: 14

Shemesh A U, Mayo W L 1991 Tea tree oil—natural antiseptic and fungicide. Journal of Alternative and Complementary Medicine 9 (12 December): 11–12

Szalontai M, Verzar-Petri G, Florian E, Gimpel F 1975a Pharmazeutische Zeitung 120: 982

Szalontai M, Verzar-Petri G, Florian E, Gimpel F 1975b Deutsche Apotheker Zeitung 115: 912

Szalontai M, Verzar-Petri G, Florian E 1976 Acta Pharmaceutica [Hungary] 46: 232

Szalontai M, Verzar-Petri G, Florian E 1977 Contribution to the study of antimycotic effect of biologically active components of *Matricaria chamomilla* L. Parfümerie und Kosmetik [Hungary] 58: 121

Taddei I, Giachetti D, Taddei E, Mantovani P, Bianchi E 1988 Spasmolytic activity of peppermint, sage and rosemary essences and their major constituents. Fitoterapia 59: 463–468

Thiemer K, Stadler R, Isaac O 1973 Arzneimittel-Forschung 23: 756

Thompson D P, Cannon C 1986 Toxicity of essential oils on toxigenic and nontoxigenic fungi. Bulletin of Environmental Contamination and Toxicology 36(4) April: 527–532

Tisserand R, Balacs T 1995 Essential oil safety. Churchill Livingstone, New York, pp 41–43

Trease G E, Evans W C 1983 Pharmacognosy, 12th edn. Baillière Tindall, London, p 424

Tukioka M 1927 Proceedings, vol 3. Imperial Academy, Tokyo, p 624

Valnet J 1980 The practice of aromatherapy. Daniel, Saffron Walden

Verdet 1989 Why phytotherapy? Aromatherapy Study Trip Lecture notes. Price Publishing, Hinckley, p 10

Verhoef M J, Sutherland L R 1995 General practitioners assessment of and interest in alternative medicine in Canada. Society Scientific Medicine 41(4): 511–515

Viaud H 1983 Huiles essentielles. Présence, Sisteron

Vichkanova S A, Dzhanashiya N M, Goryunova L V 1973 Antiviral activity displayed by the essential oil of *Eucalyptus viminalis* and of some frost-hardy eucalypti. Farmakologiia Toksikologiia 36(3): 339–341

Weiss R F 1988 Herbal medicine. Arcanum, Göteborg, p 296

Williams A C, Barry B W 1989 Essential oils as novel human skin penetration enhancers. International Journal of Pharmaceutics 57: R7–R9

Yousef R T, Tawil G G 1980 Antimicrobial activity of volatile oils. Pharmazie 35(11): 698–701

Zara M 1966 Association atoxique de dérivées terpéniques d'huiles essentielles possédant une triple action en hépatologie (cholérétique, antispasmodique, lipotrope). Vie Méd 47(10): 1549–1553

The foundations of practice

SECTION CONTENTS

5

How essential oils enter the body

Introduction

Essential oils follow three main pathways to gain entry to the body: ingestion, inhalation and absorption through the skin (Fig. 5.1). Ingestion is little used in the UK. Of the two remaining pathways, inhalation is a very effective method and indeed is regarded by some (e.g. Buchbauer 1988) as the only method truly deserving the name aromatherapy. However, topical application via the skin has also been found to be effective—the route selected depends on the problem being helped.

INGESTION

Ingestion is the main route employed by aromatologists and doctors in France, but is not widely used by aromatherapists in other countries. This is because in the UK and elsewhere there are wide variations in training standards, ranging from those designed for simple beauty therapy to that enabling a therapist to practise clinical aromatherapy/aromatology. Therapists who have successfully completed an advanced aromatology training course accredited by the IAM (see p. 376) are in a position to advise the use of essential oils per os.

Most of the research carried out by medical aromatologists in France has involved internal use of essential oils. In this case every drop of oil used reaches the body systems, unlike inhalation, when only a tiny amount of essential oil vapour enters the body, and external application, where some of the essential oils are lost by evaporation.

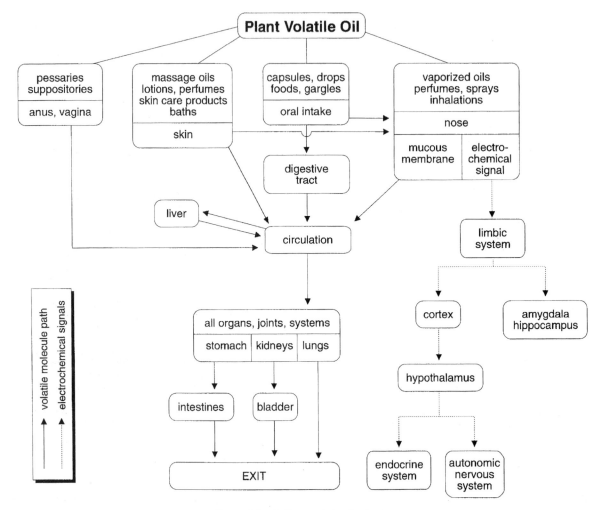

Figure 5.1   Pathways into the body.

Methods of ingestion

Per os (See also Ch. 14)

When essential oils are taken by mouth, knowledge of the constituents of the oils is of paramount importance. This is not to say that an oil containing a potentially hazardous component cannot be ingested—these components are sometimes effective for certain disorders. It simply means that it is essential to know the strength of concentration, the nature of any diluent used and the length of time for which it is to be taken. Alcohol and honey water are the most usual diluents (Valnet 1980) though vegetable oils (such as hazelnut and olive oils) are excellent for this pur-

pose and are preferred by many doctors and naturopaths practising in France (Collin 1994 personal communication), who have studied phytotherapy and are experienced in prescribing essential oils for internal use. Special dispersants are available for use to ensure essential oils dissolve thoroughly in an excipient, including water. Although higher doses can be found in aromatherapy books (particularly those written by French authors) a rough guide to the maximum safe dose is three drops, three times a day, for 3 weeks (see Ch. 3), although the individual and the particular oils used must be taken into consideration. As mentioned above, all the oil is taken into the body via ingestion. Although this

Case 5.1 Aromatologist: Jane Fletcher, UK

Approximately 2 years ago I began experiencing symptoms associated with myalgic encephalomyelitis (ME). The symptoms of mental and physical fatigue developed to the point where I had to spend the greater proportion of the day in bed. My condition then became chronic for about 7 months, when I was unable to read or watch television.

I consulted two general practitioners, one Chinese doctor, had numerous blood tests, plus a separate brain scan in Bristol to confirm I had ME, because having spent so much time in bed I had wanted to try my aromatology skills to effect a recovery if possible.

With the help of my partner I made a combination of essential oils with aloe vera and other herbal ingredients to create a synergistic formula. The essential oils were in a suitably diluted condition for internal use and the formula was taken over a 20 day period at 50 ml per day.

Day 1: took my first 50 ml of the formula.

Day 2: felt brighter and was able to read the Sunday papers.

Day 3: felt tired, though not desperate for sleep; by 5:00 p.m. I suddenly felt much better.

Day 4: felt much less like a zombie today; and was able to rewrite my whole address book.

Days 5/6: was able to work on a court case with my partner; I had not been able to concentrate like this for a whole year and did 2 full days' work. I was very tired but not exhausted.

Day 7: feeling more like my old self; went out with a friend for lunch. In the afternoon I read my book and took notes on the herbs I needed for other formulae. Cooked dinner for the first time in 6 months. My eyes were not itching and dry any more.

Day 8: a whole week is gone by and I feel much brighter; tired but able to make myself do things. Did quite a bit of housework and drove to the market (haven't driven in months). Stripped all the beds and did the washing—felt exhausted then; slept for 1 ½ hours and felt refreshed.

Day 9: had slept for 11 hours. Made some curtains for my clinic, spring-cleaned the bedroom and cooked the evening meal. Worried I may have a relapse.

Days 10/11: active both days, cleaning the silver, making cushions for my clinic.

Days 12/13: had a good day. Went for a special seafood dinner with a friend (Brian).

Day 14: woke up with a sore throat, cough, streaming cold and aching all over—must have caught a flu virus. Took some different essential oils to cope with this and felt fine after 2 hours.

Day 15: had booked a Chinese meal months ago for Brian but he had come down with a tummy bug and I was bit queasy.

Days 16/17: ill in bed with nausea and tummy bug. Thought I may have relapsed, but the symptoms were completely different from ME and, in any case, Brian felt the same.

Day 18: felt much better. Concluded it must have been food poisoning. Did 3 hours of ironing, went out for a drink and then I cooked an evening meal for everyone.

Days 19/20: felt certain I did not have ME anymore and came to terms with the fact that I am no longer ill. My whole life had then to be readjusted to working, and not to being an invalid for months at a time.

I am now working a full 8 hours a day and walking, swimming, dancing and going out frequently—and loving every minute of my life.

A year later the story is the same; I am leading a happy, busy and eventful life!

is not harmful when used correctly, continual ingestion for too long a period of time can eventually lead to toxic build-up in the liver. This is particularly true of the powerful oils. It is for this reason that, after 3 weeks, several days' rest from the oils is indicated, to allow the liver the opportunity to eliminate any accumulated toxic matter.

Because they are usually tasteless and do not cause irritation, many conventional drugs are given by mouth. However, essential oils often taste quite bitter and may irritate the mucous lining; for this reason essential oils to be taken by mouth are frequently put into capsules. Most aromatherapists are cautious about using ingestion, particularly as there is much greater danger of an excessive dose reaching the liver than by external application. Further, there is the possibility of change in the essential oil molecules by digestive enzymes, strong acids and metabolization. Nevertheless, the authors have used essential oils in this way for nearly two decades for sore throats, stomach upsets, etc., with no reported adverse effects. After specialized training in this field (i.e. aromatology), therapists should be confident in using this method. Aromatherapists often advocate tisanes (herbal teas) and while these can be helpful they are not the same as essential oils in composition and do not have exactly the same action.

Per rectum or vagina

Another method of internal use is by means of suppositories and pessaries, which can be useful in cases of irritable bowel syndrome, haemorrhoids, vaginal infections and candida.

Suppositories, though not much favoured in the UK, allow the essential oils direct access to the bloodstream with little chance of metabolization. The maximum dose for suppositories and pessaries is six drops (Collin 1994 personal communication). Toxic or irritant essential oils should not be used.

INHALATION

Access via the nasal passages is indisputably the quickest effective route in the treatment of emotional problems such as stress and depression (and also some types of headache). This is because the nose has direct contact with the brain, which is responsible for triggering the effects of essential oils regardless of the route they use to gain access to it. The nose itself is not the organ of smell, but simply modifies the temperature and humidity of the inhaled air and collects any foreign matter which may be breathed in. The first cranial (olfactory) nerve is responsible for the sense of smell and serves the receptor cells, of which there are two groups of about 25 million, each occupying a small area (of about 4 cm^2) at the top of the nostrils (van Toller 1993).

Inhalation and the mucous membranes

When inhaling any vapour, some molecules from it inevitably travel down the pathway to the lungs where, if they are appropriate essential oils, they can have an immediate and beneficial impact on many breathing difficulties. In the nose the endothelium is thin and the site is close to the brain, therefore it must be assumed that essential oil molecules reach the local circulation and the brain fairly easily and quickly. On their journey to the lungs some molecules are undoubtedly absorbed by the mucous linings of the respiratory pathways, the bronchi and multitudinous bronchioles, where access is very easy. Arriving at the point of gaseous exchange in the alveoli, the tiny molecules are transferred to the blood circulating the lungs. It can be seen that deep breathing will increase the quantity of essences taken into the body by this route. Ill

effects from inhalation of the essential oils normally used in aromatherapy are rare.

Methods of inhalation

Inhalation is an unobtrusive way of using essential oils in a healthcare setting. They may be given via a tissue, the hands (in an emergency), a vaporizer, etc., and all are effective in the appropriate situation. To choose oils for particular conditions, see the tables in Chapter 4 and Appendix B.9.

Tissues

Inhalation from a tissue with five to six drops of essential oil (three drops for children, the elderly and pregnant women) is most effective for immediate results, requiring two or three deep breaths to ensure good contact with the cilia. To give further benefit, and easier with children and the elderly, the tissue can be placed inside the shirt, blouse or nightwear so that the effects may continue as the heat of the body causes the oil molecules to evaporate and float upwards to the nose. Firm tissues such as kitchen towels hold the aroma longer than do paper handkerchiefs.

Q-tips

This method uses less essential oil than does a tissue, because it is concentrated in a small area. The Q-tip is held against the dropper and one drop allowed to wet it. Unlike a crumpled tissue, it cannot be placed next to the skin, but has the advantage of slower evaporation, so the person can use it for longer.

Hands

This is an excellent method, but should be confined to emergencies only and is not suitable for children. A solitary drop of essential oil (single, or from a mix) should be put into one of the patient's palms, which is then rubbed briefly against the other palm to disperse and warm the oil. With eyes closed, the patient should place the cupped hands over the nose, avoiding the eye area, and should then take a deep nasal breath. It is usually respiratory or stress conditions which require this sort of help.

Steamers

Allowing a patient to hold a basin of hot water is not acceptable in many hospital situations, on account of the Health and Safety Act (1994). Even if the nurse holds it there is always the possibility that some people, especially those with learning difficulties, may strike out (involuntarily or otherwise) and knock the scalding water over themselves or the nurse. Home-visiting health professionals may find in certain circumstances, and with people whose movements are stable, that the method can be used safely, but it is our opinion that dry inhalation is safer for those not enjoying full health and living alone, unless a proprietary brand diffuser is used—which can be expensive.

Nebulizers are safer but unfortunately the essential oils can attack some kinds of plastic, so care must be taken not to damage the equipment. A precautionary test is advisable for any plastic which may come into contact with essential oils. This applies also to facial steamers. These methods are normally used for respiratory problems and the common cold, though any problem which can benefit from inhalation may obtain speedier relief when steam is used. The heat of the water evaporates the oil molecules more quickly, increasing the strength of the vapour and for this reason only half the number of drops (i.e. three) are needed compared with inhalation from a tissue (or one to two drops for a child, elderly person or pregnant woman). The following cautions may be helpful:

• Ensure the patient's eyes are kept closed and watch carefully for any adverse reaction such as choking or coughing, which can happen if too many drops have been used or too deep a breath is taken.
• One drop only—with water of not too high a temperature—is adequate for asthmatics because the overpowering effect of the vapour (stronger because of the speedy evaporation referred to above) may have an adverse effect.

Baths

Treatment by putting oils into the bath is effective because not only do they come into gentle contact with the skin, but also they are inhaled at the same time; thus a double benefit is derived. For details, see Methods of percutaneous absorption on page 99.

Spray bottle

A quick way of freshening the air when dressings are being changed for patients with bed sores, gangrene, etc. is using 10–12 drops of essential oil in 250 ml of water, shaking the bottle well before spraying the room. The essential oils to use in this case are *Pinus sylvestris* [SCOTS PINE], *Thymus vulgaris* [THYME] (all chemotypes, though phenolic thymes are the most powerful antiseptics), *Syzygium aromaticum* [CLOVE], *Eucalyptus smithii* [GULLY ASH], *Mentha × piperita* [PEPPERMINT].

Vaporizers and diffusers

Possibly the most favoured way of using inhalation in a healthcare setting at the moment is from a vaporizer. This liberates the lightest molecules from the oil first, releasing the heavier ones progressively. Although there are many different types of vaporizers available, only electric ones are considered safe where patients are concerned (the British Safety Standard mark should be looked for on the model to be used). Electric vaporizers should be thermostatically controlled at a low temperature, preventing the essential oils from becoming too hot. If this occurs, not only are they used up too quickly to be economical but the heaviest molecules burning off last may produce an unpleasant acrid smell.

Diffusers (units with a small blown-glass container for the essential oils) are more efficient in that they push out all the differently sized molecules at the same time. Unlike vaporizers using heat, there is no burning of residue when the essential oil is used up. Their only disadvantage is cost: both of the oils (which are used up fairly rapidly) and the price, which can be up to three times greater than that of an electric vaporizer. A recent development on the market uses a new technique to deliver evenly and economically all sizes of molecules contained in the essential oils into the atmosphere. The essential oils are released in a regulated manner so that the air does not become overloaded; there are time switches for selecting both operating and rest times, making this method suitable for clinical use.

Ethical considerations. A few hospitals use vaporizers and diffusers in single-occupancy rooms only—not in general ward areas, as it is felt by some therapists to be unethical to impose aromas (which may be disliked or unwanted by some) on other occupants. Nevertheless, when the effects required for a whole ward are the same for each occupant, e.g. when conducting a trial or keeping a ward free from infection, the method is viable and effective; it can also be useful in the reduction of stress and insomnia as well as in the destruction of germs. It seems strange that there is not equal ethical consideration regarding piped music, the wearing of perfume, the use of perfumed spray cleaners or the pollution of air through cigarette fumes, the last three of which can adversely affect the health of those in the vicinity. Unfortunately, large vaporizer units used in hotels and offices are often run on commercial-grade essential oils and aromas to keep costs down, without taking into account what effect long term exposure may have on people's health. It is already known that artificial perfumes and adulterated essential oils cause sensitivities in asthmatics and skin reactions in those susceptible to such effects. 'Environmental fragrancing', as this practice is termed, is most advanced in the USA, where there is growing concern at the use of synthetic aromas (see Ch. 17). The liberty of the individual is an important consideration and, unlike shoppers irritated by 'muzak' or 'fragrancing' designed to alter their mood, hospital patients are not free to walk away from an environmental influence which they may not like.

ABSORPTION VIA THE SKIN

Until the second half of the 20th century the skin was thought to be almost impermeable (Maibach & Marzulli 1977, Stoughton 1959). This old idea still persists, even though the skin is now known to be a poor barrier to lipophilic substances (Brun 1952) and essential oils in a base oil applied to the skin are absorbed into the bloodstream (Jäger et al 1992). Most chemicals are absorbed to some degree and this is made use of in patch therapy, e.g. glyceryl trinitrate must penetrate the skin to reach the blood vessels and heart to treat angina, and many other substances—including oestradiol, scopalamine and nicotine—are administered in this way, while others are being tested—e.g. beta blockers, testosterone and antihistamines (Cleary 1993). Water comprises 90% of any cell and therefore the skin has developed as a barrier specifically to resist water, nevertheless it is slightly permeable to water soluble substances, to water itself and to lipids (Riviere 1993).

The absorption of drugs and poisons through the skin was studied by Macht (1938) and there has been a considerable amount of research on pesticides and the skin. Pesticides, which dissolve in essential oils, are lipid-like and can therefore get through the skin—every farmer is aware of this health hazard, and thousands of people are killed each year by pesticides, mostly in third world countries. The amount absorbed through human skin varies enormously; for example less than 1% of cypermethrin pesticide is absorbed whereas up to 65% of of the antifungal agent benzoic acid may penetrate the skin (Hotchkiss 1994).

The skin's success as a barrier is due in the main to the stratum corneum, the tough and durable, self-repairing keratinized layer, which is only about 10 μm thick. Once a chemical gets past the epidermis—the only great obstacle—the rest of the journey into the body is easy, because the presence of lipids in all cell membranes negates the dermis's effectiveness as a barrier. For example, the antibacterial substance hexachlorophene is absorbed through the skin, and was shown in 1969 to cause microscopically visible brain damage in rats (Winter 1984 p. 138), and chloasma in humans; in the 1970s hexachlorophene was used as an antiseptic in baby soaps and talcum powders, causing brain damage and even death in some babies after it had penetrated the skin (Jackson 1993). The lipid solubility of essential oil components allows these compounds to cross the blood–brain barrier (where certain substances are held back by the endothelium of cerebral capillaries) and make contact with the fluids around the brain (Anthony & Thibodeau 1983).

There are many factors which dictate the rate and quantity at which any given substance penetrates the skin, but it is now generally recognized that the skin is a semipermeable membrane susceptible of penetration by substances to a greater or lesser degree (Lexicon Vevy 1993a). Obviously the physicochemical properties of the molecules, such as the molecular weight, spatial arrangement, polarity, optical activity, liposolubility, coefficients of diffusion and dissociation, are fundamental to skin penetration. Mills (1993) states that an advantage of the percutaneous route for remedies is the avoidance of the 'first-pass liver' effect, i.e. they are not subject to immediate metabolization by the liver as they are in oral administration.

The skin as a barrier

On account of their solubility in the lipids found in the stratum corneum, lipophilic substances (such as essential oils) are considered to be easily absorbed. The absorption of organic compounds with anionic or cationic groups (weak acids and alkalis) takes place when they are found in undissociated form—then they are more lipophilic than when dissociated; it also depends on their dissociation constant and on the pH of the substance and of the skin. Most essential oils used in aromatherapy pass through the skin and the organism and can be detected in exhaled air within 20–60 minutes (Katz 1947).

Once the essential oil constituents have passed the epidermis and entered the complex of lymph and blood vessels, nerves, sweat and oil glands, follicles, collagen, fibroblasts, mast cells, elastin and so on (known as the dermis), they are then carried away in the circulation to pervade every cell in the body. There is no research at the moment comparing percutaneous absorption with the gastrointestinal route (Torii et al 1991).

The main factors affecting the penetration of the skin by essential oils are detailed below.

Intrinsic factors

Area of skin. The very large area of the skin—in the region of $2\,m^2$—makes it possible for a significant quantity of essential oils to be applied to the skin and so taken into the body. If a set quantity of essential oil in a carrier is applied to a small area of skin, then less will enter than if the same quantity were to be applied to a greater area.

Thickness and permeability of the epidermis. On palmar and plantar skin, because the epidermis is quite thick and there are no oil glands, the time taken to cross the skin is longer, especially for any lipid soluble components. There is less resistance to water soluble components, however, and garlic placed on the feet is soon detected on the exhaled breath, for instance. Easy penetration may occur on parts of the body where the skin is thinner, e.g. behind the ears, eyelids and inside wrist. The skin regions of the legs, buttocks, trunk and the abdomen area are less permeable than are those of the soles, palms, forehead, scalp and armpits (Balacs 1993).

Gland openings and follicles. Hydrophilic molecules can find a path through the skin using the sweat glands; lipophilic molecules may use the sebaceous glands as a pathway, also travelling between the cells through the fatty cement and through the cells themselves, all of which contain lipids (Lexicon Vevy 1993b). The skin of the forehead and scalp contains numerous oil glands, and here the epidermis is thinner. This again makes for easy penetration of lipophilic substances, although the water layer on the skin must present a partial barrier for the lipophilic molecules. The number of follicles and sweat glands is another factor; generally speaking, the more openings the speedier the access. When sweating, because of a fever or after a sauna for example, the body is exuding and ingress of essential oils is slower.

Reservoirs. Essential oils are lipid soluble and gain access to lipid rich areas of the body (Buchbauer 1993), therefore it is possible that essential oils may be sequestered (stored apart) in the body, as happens in the plants that produce them. If so, there would be reservoirs of essential oils (or at least of some of their constituent molecules) in the outer layers of the epidermis and subcutaneous fat, and these may persist for some time. It might be considered that lipophilic components can, at least temporarily, be retained in this layer and consequently will not be available for rapid diffusion to other adjacent levels (Lexicon Vevy 1993b). Subcutaneous fat has a poor blood supply and although essential oils are slow to enter they probably tend to stay there for a long time.

A Dutch Government Commission report in 1983 showed that many MAC (maximum acceptable concentrations) for toxic chemicals failed to take into account the significant physiological differences between the sexes. Women's skin is more permeable to toxic chemicals than that of men and because they carry more fat their body levels of fat soluble chemicals are generally higher and take longer to disperse (Eisberg 1983).

Enzymes. Enzymes in the skin can activate and inactivate many drugs and foreign compounds. They can also activate and inactivate the body's own natural chemicals such as hormones, steroids and inflammatory mediators. The activities of these skin enzymes may vary greatly between individuals and with age (Hotchkiss 1994).

The skin contains many enzymes and therefore provides a 'laboratory' where metabolism can take place. Certainly some enzymes will effect a change in some essential oil molecules and even a slight change of shape in an essential oil molecule will mean a change in the effect on the body. In the case of some phthalic esters, enzymatic action effects complete metabolization during skin absorption; enzymes in the skin can either activate or inactivate drugs and other alien compounds and there is great variation between individuals and with age. Bacterial action breaks down the triglycerides in sebum to organic free fatty acids and incompletely esterified glycerol derivatives, and it is reasonable to suppose that similar sorts of processes may happen with the essential oils.

Damaged skin. Broken, inflamed and diseased skin is not a great barrier and ingress is rapid through cuts, abrasions, ulcers, psoriasis, burns, etc. Aged skin and skin dehydrated through exposure to sunlight does not accept substances easily: some dermatological problems (e.g. ichthyosis) may also have this same effect.

Other physiological factors

Rate of circulation. Where there is an increase in the rate of blood flow, perhaps due to rubbing (massage) or inflammation, there is an increased rate of absorption. Massage not only increases the speed of blood flow (causing hyperaemia) but also raises the local skin temperature slightly, hence we can expect an increased rate and degree of absorption of essential oils owing to the lowering of the viscosity and dilation of the blood vessels (Pratt & Mason 1981). Proof that essential oils in a base oil applied to the skin are absorbed into the bloodstream has been provided by Jäger et al (1992) by the detection of linalyl acetate and linalool in a blood sample taken 5 min after the oil was applied.

Rate of distribution. As far as distribution is concerned, the speed of the lymph and blood circulation is a limiting factor because the circulation is slower in the capillary loops than in the veins. The speed may be increased, for example, by massage or by warmth (e.g. infrared). Both these methods may be used to increase the rate of distribution of essential oils. It has been proved that the blood vessels constantly resorb and expel terpenes so that a balance of flow results (Römmelt et al 1974, Schilcher 1985).

External factors

Hydration. Hydrated skin is very permeable, hence the effectiveness of what the authors term aromabalneotherapy (the use of essential oils in a bath). It has been shown that in a bath the essential oils penetrate the skin 100 times faster than does water and 10 000 times more quickly than do the ions of sodium and chloride (Römmelt et al 1974). Conversely, if the stratum corneum is dehydrated its permeability is decreased.

Degreased skin. Although detergents, degreasants, soaps, etc. increase the permeability of the skin to essential oils, they are not necessarily recommended.

Warmth. A warm room, warm oils, warm hands and body all help to speed up absorption. Care must be taken that the body is not made too warm (e.g. after exercise) as it is then exuding and eliminating, making ingress of oils difficult.

Occlusion. Occlusion due to a covering, e.g. a compress, has a sealing-in effect—it decreases the ability of the essential oils to volatilize, and it also aids warming. Oils applied under occlusion, as with all other substances, have an enhanced effect because of the increase in the quantity absorbed, due probably to local warming, and reduced loss of molecules from the site of application through evaporation: as evaporation is reduced, absorption may be increased (Bronaugh et al 1990). Clothing may be regarded as being partially occlusive.

Oil-related factors

Viscosity. All essential oils have a low viscosity, but some oils with a relatively high viscosity, e.g. sandalwood, which comprises 90% alcohols, will still cross the skin at a rate similar to other oils. Viscosity plays a more important part with regard to the carrier oils because some, such as hazelnut, are quite viscous and others, such as grapeseed and sunflower, are less so.

Molecular size. If the molecular weight exceeds 500 then it is unlikely to pass the skin. Essential oils, being products of distillation, are limited to a maximum molecular weight of 225 (rarely reaching 250). In some cases it may be worth considering the use of a carrier that is partially hydrophilic (e.g. wheatgerm oil, walnut oil) even if to only a small extent.

The size and shape of the individual essential oil molecules also has a bearing on the speed at which they penetrate the skin. Small molecules pass easily down the follicular and sebaceous ducts, and the smaller the molecule the faster it penetrates. Dissociation may also be relevant. When dissolved in a carrier the essential oil molecules may split into ions, thus becoming even more tiny. The bigger molecules, being less volatile, are less likely to be lost to the atmosphere, stay on the skin longer and therefore have a greater opportunity for penetration. Even though essential oils are quite volatile and evaporate from the warm surface of the skin, absorption may be 20–40% of the oil applied, and up to double that, depending on the extent of occlusion.

Frequency of use. There is some evidence that repeated use of the same oil makes the skin more permeable (see Ch. 3).

Carriers. The carrier medium can have a significant effect on absorption of essential oils (see discussion on phototoxicity in Ch. 3, p. 51). In a laboratory test using rat skin, absorption of phenol was enhanced when a barrier cream was used; in humans, penetration of fragrance chemicals was increased when mixed with ethanol (Hotchkiss 1994). Saturated oil carriers such as lard, wool-fat and mineral oil (e.g. baby oil) all prevent or seriously delay absorption: the higher the degree of unsaturation of a fat the easier the absorption process becomes. Zatz (1993) found that when phenol was applied to the skin in a saturated fat the antiseptic effect was inhibited.

Methods of percutaneous absorption

Many of the techniques used on the skin entail the use of water, vegetable oil or a bland lotion to dilute and spread the essential oils over an area of skin.

Compresses

Compresses are sometimes required on open wounds such as leg ulcers, bedsores, boils, etc., and on bruising or areas of severe localized pain such as arthritis, stomach pain, fractures, etc. A non-adherent silicon dressing such as Mepitel should be used on ulcers, and a low adherent absorbent dressing such as Melolin on open wounds. The size of compress, number of drops of essential oils and amount of water used are dependent upon the size of the area to be treated. A septic finger requires only a minuscule square of the dressing material chosen, and an eggcupful of water to which two drops of essential oil have been added, whereas a swollen rheumatic knee would require a piece of cloth large enough to cover the swelling, and a small basinful of water (about 200 ml) containing five to six drops of essential oils. As always, the quantities of essential oil should be halved for children and the elderly.

The chosen material should be immersed in the mixture of water and essential oil, squeezed gently and placed over the required area. It should be covered in the normal manner, and a piece of Clingfilm can be ideal as a first layer to prevent evaporation of the essential oils. The compress should be left on for about 2 hours, or overnight if practicable. Some therapists apply essential oils diluted in a vegetable oil to the site, if the skin is unbroken, then cover it. During the 1914–1918 war, other media used for wet dressings for large wounds with considerable tissue loss were ether and ointment bases, into which the essential oils were mixed (Valnet 1980 p. 67). If a cream or lotion base is used for open wounds

(see Useful addresses, p. 375), this can be applied directly on to the dressing.

Gargles and mouthwashes

After the removal of tonsils or complicated dental surgery, gargling with essential oils helps to relieve any pain or inflammation, stem blood flow and aid healing; at the same time the oils are antiseptic to the mucous surfaces. Two to three drops in quarter of a tumbler of water is all that is needed—the most important rule to follow being that the water should be stirred before each mouthful to disperse the essential oils each time. For children, blend only one drop of essential oil in a teaspoonful of honey before adding the water. *Syzygium aromaticum* (flos) [CLOVE BUD] is the most used for pain in this context (but see Appendices also).

Case 5.2   Aromatologist: Penny Price MISPA MIAM, UK

Basic details: K was a widower of 91 years, retired and living alone.

Aetiology: a keen gardener, he lived in a small street in the middle of a market town; the residents of this street formed a close-knit community.

Lifestyle: K had few hobbies except cleaning his house and working in his garden. He took very little exercise outside of these activities. His diet was simple yet sufficient.

Medical history
Medication: K's ulcer was being treated with compression bandages by a community nurse once a week. He also had help with bathing, dressing, etc. at other times in the week. The nurse was reluctant to give information on the dressing used.

Emotional balance: K was a happy, contented soul whose only regret was that he was unable to spend more time in his garden because of his immobility.

Presenting symptoms: the ulcer was 3 inches in diameter, situated on the outside calf of the left leg. K had been told that he could not expect any improvement because everything possible was being done for him and the condition had remained static for some considerable time.

Proposed treatment plan
For the first week of treatment essential oils were to be used in distilled water in a spray. The four oils chosen were: *Melaleuca alternifolia, Lavandula angustifolia, Citrus bergamia* and *Commiphora myrrha*. These oils were selected very carefully for their constituent properties, which collectively addressed the pain, the malodour, the healing and the infection.

General advice: K was to spray the wound directly (and was thereby involved in his own care) when his bandage was removed by the nurse; he was to do this six times a day. After consultation with the doctor it was agreed that the bandage could remain off for 3 days during the daytime, being replaced at night.

Treatment
First visit (morning): K's wound was sprayed when the nurse removed his bandage, K himself spraying the leg at intervals during the day until the nurse replaced the bandage at night. This was repeated each day.

Second visit (evening, 3 days later): after these 3 days the healing was evident. Wearing protective gloves, I applied the same synergy of essential oils directly to the wound (this time in a 3% mix using *Calendula* as a carrier) before the nurse applied the compression bandage. This was to be left for a week until the next bandage. During this week I massaged Joe's feet every day with the same blend and noticed improvement in the circulation.

Third evening visit: the above procedure was repeated.

Conclusion
After 3 months the ulcer was closed. The only evidence of it having been there was that there was a small area of discoloured skin. This was later to improve. K was consistent in the use of his oil blend for the rest of his life and the ulcer did not recur. The quality of K's life was greatly improved as a result of the treatment—not least because his improved mobility meant he could work longer in his beloved garden.

Sprays

The spray method mentioned above (see Methods of inhalation, p. 95) can also be used as a method of application when the client is unable to be touched, e.g. in the case of severe burns, zoster or wounds. A higher concentration is needed when treating burns this way, e.g. 15–20 drops in 50 ml of distilled or sterilized water. Appropriate essential oils in this case are *Citrus limon* [LEMON], *Lavandula angustifolia* [LAVENDER], *L. × intermedia* 'Super' [LAVANDIN], *Chamomilla recutita* [GERMAN CHAMOMILE], *Melaleuca viridiflora* [NIAOULI] and *Pelargonium graveolens* [GERANIUM].

Baths

A valuable method of use involving water and inhalation is the addition of six to eight drops of essential oils to the bath water after running it to the correct temperature. This amount of essential oil in a bathful of water can appear to be too little, but it must be borne in mind, as mentioned above, that skin penetration is increased 100 times in this method and also that inhalation plays a significant part. There are those who advise adding the essential oils to another medium first, such as vegetable oil, dried milk, high proof vodka, bubble bath mix, etc. While useful for certain skin conditions, vegetable oil is not necessary in most circumstances (and it can leave an oily ring on the bath which is difficult to remove). Although the essential oils are not completely soluble in water, it is a simple matter to disperse them by vigorously agitating the water (efficiently, so no globules can get into the eyes). For water births the essential oils are best dissolved first in a small amount of powdered milk (adding enough water to make a thin paste). Blend three to four drops in honey or dried milk for children and the elderly. For maximum benefit, the patient should remain in the bath for 10 minutes if possible.

Foot, hand and sitz baths

It is sometimes easier to use a washing-up bowl for bathing individual areas—the sitz bath, for example, is ideal for haemorrhoids and stitches after childbirth. Three to four drops of essential oils are needed, and a kettle should be available to keep the bath warm during the 10 minutes. This method may not be found to be necessary for children but, should the occasion arise, remember to follow the recommendation above for baths.

Topical application

Application means the 'putting on' of oils—either for self-use or via a third party. Treatment by massage employs an organized routine using specific movements to achieve specific aims, e.g. lymph drainage, relaxation, etc. Professional aromatherapists mostly employ essential oils with massage, and this subject is covered in detail in Chapter 7 together with massage techniques suitable for nurses to administer without having qualified in whole-body massage.

Unless aromatherapists are paid by the health authority or the patient concerned, or they are offering their services voluntarily, there is not usually time in a busy nursing schedule for a nurse to spend an hour or more with a patient requiring an aromatherapy treatment. However, nurses do have time to apply a ready-diluted oil or lotion on the relevant area daily as an embrocation. It takes no longer than giving more usual forms of medication and adds the magic of touch and care to the prescription.

The normal dilution is 15–20 drops in 50 ml of suitable carrier oil or lotion, but for the very young, elderly, heavily medicated or those with learning difficulties half this amount is advised. When essential oils are to be applied daily, it is less messy to dilute them in a non-greasy lotion base of emulsified oil and water (garments and bed linen can become permanently soiled by vegetable oil). A number of rheumatology wards, including the Royal Devonshire Hospital, Buxton, apply an aromatherapy lotion as part of the daily treatment, resulting in a reduction in the use of painkillers (see Ch. 14). For effectiveness in certain conditions, e.g. lowered immune system activity or toxic build-up, an essential oil lotion should be applied liberally to the lymph node areas such as the armpits and groin.

The significance of macerated carrier oils

It is well worth taking care to select a carrier which is of holistic and/or symptomatic use, i.e. one of the macerated oils such as calendula. Lime blossom carrier oil can help to induce sleep or soothe rheumatic pain, carrot or hypericum carrier oils will help to reduce skin inflammation or accelerate the healing of burns, calendula or hypericum carrier oils will help to soothe and heal bruising, and calendula, hypericum or rosehip carrier oils will relieve skin rashes, etc. (Price 1993). The quantity of essential oil added should be the same as if using a basic carrier oil.

Carrier oils

Carrier oils constitute the bulk of the material used in an aromatherapy massage. Their function is to 'carry' or act as a vehicle for administering the essential oils to the body. They also function as lubricants, making it possible to carry out massage movements. This section discusses the nature of carrier oils, and details the properties and applications of those more frequently used in aromatherapy.

Fixed oils

The oils used as carriers in aromatherapy are known as fixed oils, because they do not evaporate, in contrast to the plant essential oils, which are volatile and therefore do evaporate. Fixed oils constitute a different chemical family from essential oils, which is why their properties are so different. Fixed oils leave a permanent oily mark on paper because of their lubricating quality and non-volatile nature; essential oils do not leave an oily mark, although any colour present will leave a stain. All essential oils dissolve easily and completely in fixed oils in all proportions.

Chemical nature

Chemically speaking, carrier oils are classed as lipids, which are a diverse family of compounds found naturally in plants and animals. Oils and fats have similar structures, but at room temperature (15°C) fats are solid and oils are liquid.

Lipids are formed when an alcohol (glycerol) reacts with a type of organic compound known as a fatty acid; this results in a type of ester (a triacylglycerol), and carrier oils are made up of these. As glycerol is common to almost all vegetable oils, the differences that exist between carrier oils can be attributed to the nature of the fatty acids. Fatty acids all have a long hydrocarbon chain (typically containing 16–18 carbon atoms) with an organic acid group, often written as -COOH, attached to one end. The number of carbon atoms they contain can be used to refer to these long chain fatty acids. This is octadecanoic acid, also known as stearic acid, an 18-carbon fatty acid:

$$CH_3CH_2CH_2CH_2CH_2CH_2CH_2CH_2CH_2CH_2CH_2CH_2CH_2CH_2CH_2CH_2CH_2COOH$$

Reference is often made to the fatty acid content of vegetable oils, but the acids are present only in a combined state and are not 'free' to take part in reactions. They have already reacted with the glycerol to form a triacylglycerol, and so are present only as 'bonded' components.

Fatty acids can be further classified as *saturated* or *unsaturated* depending on the type of covalent bonds that exist between the carbon atoms. This is because carbon atoms can form double bonds as well as single bonds with each other:

C–C	C=C
single bond	double bond

Compounds that contain only single bonds are said to be saturated whereas those with one or more double bonds are unsaturated. With this in mind, the 18-carbon fatty acids can be described as:

C18:0	saturated	no double bond	stearic acid
C18:1	mono-unsaturated	one double bond	oleic acid
C18:2	poly-unsaturated	two double bonds	linoleic acid
C18:3	poly-unsaturated	three double bonds	linolenic acid

This indicates that stearic acid is a fatty acid which has 18 carbon atoms in the chain and does not contain any double bonds whereas oleic acid, which also has 18 carbon atoms in the chain, contains one double bond, and so on.

The so-called 'hard' fats are mostly made up of triacylglycerols containing saturated carbon chains such as those based on stearic acids. The most saturated of all the vegetable-based products is coconut oil, which contains triacylglycerols based on caproic acid (also found in butter). Oils, which are liquid at room temperature, are based on triacylglycerols containing high proportions of unsaturated fatty acid units such as those found in palmitoleic and oleic acids.

Vegetable oils contain a high level of unsaturated fatty acid units (>80%), which is why they are important for our health. The double bonds are less strong than single bonds and introduce an element of weakness into a compound. Once opened up they can absorb other molecules for transportation elsewhere in the body, and can also facilitate the natural digestive breakdown of the triacylglycerols. However, oils with a high degree of unsaturation are less stable than those that are highly saturated, owing to the weakness of the double bonds; thus they are open to attack by oxygen and moisture, which can lead to breakdown and rancidity.

Cold-pressed oils

Carrier oils used in aromatherapy should, wherever possible, be cold pressed, although this term is a slight misnomer, as the extraction process generates a certain amount of heat and cooling is normally required. Temperatures are usually maintained below 60°C, however, and in this way changes to the natural characteristics of the oil are kept to a minimum.

Vegetable oils may also be refined to meet the particular requirements of large scale users such as the pharmaceutical industry, cooking oil manufacturers, food processors and the cosmetics companies. Processing here frequently involves the use of high temperatures and chemicals. Many of the natural properties of the oil are lost, the character is altered, and its use in

aromatherapy is not desirable. This is the type of oil usually found on supermarket shelves.

Mineral oils are high molecular weight hydrocarbons, and a different class of compound from the triacylglycerols. They are oily and greasy, with a tendency to clog the pores, and are less able to be absorbed by the skin; they are not normally used in aromatherapy.

Types of carrier oil

There are three broad categories:

1. **Basic oils.** These can be used with or without essential oils for body massage; they are generally pale in colour, not too viscous and have very little smell. They include sweet almond, apricot kernel, peach kernel, grapeseed and sunflower.

2. **Special oils.** These tend to be more viscous, heavier and more expensive. They include avocado, sesame, rose hip and wheatgerm. The really rich oils such as avocado and wheatgerm are seldom, if ever, used on their own. It is more normal to use them as 10–25% of carrier oil blend.

3. **Macerated oils.** These have certain additional properties because of the way they are produced. Chopped plant material is added to a selected fixed oil (often sunflower or olive oil) and the mix is agitated gently for some time. All of the oil soluble compounds present (including the chemicals that make up the essential oil) are transferred to the carrier oil, which consequently has extra therapeutic effects.

Fixed oils and skin penetration

It has generally been considered that triacylglycerol molecules are too large to penetrate the skin but this observation has perhaps been brought into question. Tests on rat skin suggested that the oils of linseed, safflower and avocado were of interest in carrying active substances into the skin (Valette & Sobrin 1963).

Essential fatty acid deficiency is recognized as a complication of long term fat-free parenteral nutrition, and consideration has been given to the use of cutaneously applied vegetable oils as a way of avoiding this problem. Sunflower seed oil was used on three patients who had developed essential fatty acid deficiency after major intestinal resections (Press, Hartop & Prottey 1974, Prottey, Hartop & Press 1975). The deficiency was corrected by the application of 2–3 mg of the oil per kg of body weight per day for 12 weeks. Friedman et al (1976) reported the correction of essential fatty acid deficiency in two infants given 1400 mg/kg per day of topically applied sunflower oil. In order for the essential fatty acid to be made available the molecules of triacylglycerol have to undergo hydrolysis. This implies that the topically applied oil has been metabolized and so skin penetration has taken place. In a report assessing the safety of sweet almond oil it is stated that pharmacological studies reveal that sweet almond oil is slowly absorbed through intact skin (Expert Panel 1983). Sweet almond oil has been used as a solvent for parenterally administered drugs (Hizon & Huyck 1956).

However, other investigators have reported that essential fatty acid deficiency cannot be influenced by cutaneously applied vegetable oils (Hunt et al 1978, McCarthy et al 1983, O'Neill, Caldwell & Meng 1976). Miller et al (1987) examined the use of safflower oil on five patients, and deduced that topical application may improve plasma fatty acid profiles but adequacy of tissue stores remained unanswered.

Clearly, uncertainty remains. However, there is evidence that oils rich in bonded essential fatty acids do benefit the skin. A deficiency in essential fatty acids increases transepidermal water loss resulting in dryness; this may be corrected by the topical application of borage and evening primrose oils for 14 days with a resulting 2% increase in the level of γ-linolenic acid in the stratum corneum (Hoffmann-La Roche 1989).

Carrier oils used in aromatherapy

There are more than 20 suitable carrier oils available (Price, Smith & Price 1999); detailed below is a small selection. Table 5.1 gives a more complete list including particular properties and indications for each.

Almond sweet (Prunus amygdalis var. dulcis). Sweet almond oil is one of the most used carrier oils; it is pale yellow in colour, slightly viscous and very oily. Apricot kernel (*P. armenaica*) and peach kernel (*P. persica*) oils are very similar, and it can be very difficult to discriminate between them. An advantage which these oils have over some others is that they have less of a tendency to become rancid. The unrefined oil has a delicate, sweet smell and a flavour with a hint of marzipan. It has a high proportion of bonded mono- and polyunsaturated fatty acid units. Sweet almond oil is used in laxative preparations and is said to be effective in reducing blood cholesterol levels (Leung & Foster 1996). It is an excellent emollient and nourishes dry skin; it also helps to soothe inflammation (Stier 1990). Almond oil is beneficial in relieving the itching caused by eczema, psoriasis, dermatitis and all cases of dry scaly skin, and is absorbed slowly through the intact skin (Expert Panel 1983 p. 97). It is said to be non-irritating, non-sensitizing and considered safe for cosmetic use (Leung & Foster 1996) but a few people are allergic to cosmetics containing almond oil, suffering a stuffy nose and skin rash (Winter 1984 p. 49).

Grapeseed (Vitis vinifera). First produced in France, grapeseed oil is now produced mainly in Spain, Italy and California. Grape seeds cannot be cold pressed. The oil is tasteless, almost odourless and is very fine (it is used to lubricate watches). It contains a high proportion of bonded units based on linoleic acid (an essential fatty acid), it is easily digested and is one of the few oils not to contain cholesterol. Grapeseed oil is a gentle emollient and leaves the skin with a smooth satin finish without feeling greasy.

Rose hip (Rosa mosquette, R. rubiginosa). The bush grows wild in the Andes, principally in Chile and and Peru, and bears white and pink flowers that ultimately form hips. Seeds make up 70% by weight of the fruit and these are the source of the oil. Rose hip oil is a golden-red colour and contains high levels of reacted linoleic and linolenic acids along with significant amounts of vitamin C. It also contains small quantities of *trans*-retinoic acid, which contribute to its therapeutic properties. Studies in Chile

Table 5.1 Properties and indications of carrier oils

Fixed oils ('indicates macerated)

Common name	Scientific name	Analgesic (light)	Antiinflammatory	Antipruritic	Astringent	Arthritis	Circulatory	Haemorrhoids	Laxative	Lowers blood cholesterol	PMT	Rheumatism	Sprains/bruises	Varicose veins	Wounds	Acne	Broken veins	Burns	Eczema	Emollient, dry skin	Psoriasis	Scars	Shingles zoster	Sunburnt skin	Sun protection	Wrinkles, mature skin
ALMOND SWEET	*Prunus amygdalis* var. *dulcis*	X	X	X		X			X	X									X	X	X					
APRICOT KERNEL	*Prunus armeniaca*			X					X	X									X	X	X					X
AVOCADO	*Persea gratissima*								X				X	X	X		X		X	X						X
CALENDULA*	*Calendula officinalis*		X	X	X										X		X	X	X							
CARROT*	*Daucus carota*		X	X														X	X			X				
EVENING PRIMROSE	*Oenethera biennis*					X				X	X				X				X	X	X					
GRAPESEED	*Vitis vinifera*																			X						
HAZELNUT	*Corylus avellana*		X	X	X	X	X									X									X	
JOJOBA	*Simmondsia chinensis*		X									X				X			X		X					X
LEMON BALM*	*Melissa officinalis*																							X		X
LIME BLOSSOM, LINDEN*	*Tilia europoea*							X				X														X
MACADAMIA	*Macadamia ternifolia*																								X	
OLIVE	*Olea europoea*			X	X				X	X			X					X		X						
PASSIONFLOWER	*Passiflora incarnata*	X																		X						
PEACH	*Prunus persica*			X					X	X										X						X
ROSE HIP	*Rosa canina, R. mosquetta*	X	X									X	X		X			X	X			X				X
ST JOHN'S WORT*	*Hypericum perforatum*	X										X	X		X			X	X					X		
SUNFLOWER	*Helianthus annuus*									X															X	
TAMANU	*Calophyllum inophyllum*	X	X																X		X	X	X			
WALNUT	*Juglans regia*						X		X										X		X		?			
WHEATGERM	*Triticum vulgare*						X			X				X					X							X

have identified that the oil is a tissue regenerator and has an effect on the skin to minimize premature ageing and wrinkles, also to reduce scar tissue. It is helpful on wounds, burns and eczema.

Sunflower *(Helianthus annuus)*. The Aztecs worshipped the flower as a representation of the sun; it originated in South America and was brought to Europe in the 16th century. Each flower head yields on average about 250 g of seeds that contain a light and slightly scented oil. Much of the oil available commercially has been obtained by solvent extraction so care must be taken to ensure that only cold-pressed material is used. Sunflower oil has slight diuretic properties; it is said to aid cholesterol metabolism and may be used to counteract arteriosclerosis (Stier 1990). It is expectorant and, as it contains inulin, it may be useful in the treatment of asthma. The oil is beneficial for skin complaints and bruises, and is effective on leg ulcers. It has been reported as being efficacious in the treatment of multiple sclerosis (Anon 1990, Millar et al 1973, Swank & Dugan 1990).

Wheatgerm *(Triticum vulgare)*. Wheatgerm is a rich orange-brown colour and very viscous. It is seldom used on its own, being commonly employed as 10–25% of the carrier oil mix. Because of its high content of vitamin E, a natural antioxidant, it is added to less stable oils to increase their useful life. The oil is rich in lipid soluble vitamins, and so is good for revitalizing dry skin. It is also said to be useful on ageing skin where its natural antioxidants are an effective weapon against free radicals. The oil is beneficial for tired muscles and should be included in the mix for after-sports massage.

Macerated oils

Calendula *(Calendula officinalis)*. Calendula oil is typically obtained by macerating the plant material in sunflower oil, and clearly its chemical and physical characteristics will depend partly on the type and quality of the fixed oil used. The normal orange-yellow colour of the calendula flowers is reflected in the colour of the oil. The oil has a favourable effect on the skin and can be used on its own for broken veins, varicose veins, bruises, etc., although it is preferable also to add one or two drops of appropriate essential oils to help with these and other conditions. Calendula extracts have been used to promote healing and to reduce inflammation (Fleischner 1985), and calendula is specifically indicated for enlarged or inflamed lymph nodes, sebaceous cysts and acute or chronic skin lesions (Casley-Smith & Casley-Smith 1983).

It should be noted that although calendula is sometimes referred to as 'marigold' it is a very different plant from *Tagetes patula* and *Tagetes minuta* [TAGETES, FRENCH MARIGOLD], which are also known as marigold.

St John's wort *(Hypericum perforatum)*. Again, the chemical and physical characteristics of the finished product will depend partly on the fixed oil (traditionally olive oil) used in the mac-eration process and the resulting macerated oil is a deep red colour, owing to the presence of hypericin. An antiinflammatory oil, hypericum is useful on wounds where there is nerve tissue damage and it is also useful for inflamed nerve conditions, hence it is used in cases of neuralgia, sciatica and fibrositis. A 20% hypericum tincture has been used in the treatment of suppurative otitis, and extracts are stated to have been used clinically in Russia to treat infection (Shaparenko et al 1979). The use of hypericum in the treatment of vitiligo (Newall, Anderson & Phillipson 1996) has also been reported, as has its use as an astringent and diuretic (Martindale 1993). Hypericin, the red pigment, is being studied as a possible antiviral agent in the management of acquired immune deficiency syndrome (AIDS) (Abrams 1990, Anon 1991).

Summary

This chapter has identified the principal routes by which essential oils can enter the body—and the principal hindrances. Detailed information has been given so that the aromatherapist can select the optimum pathway to achieve the desired therapeutic effect. Carrier oils comprise the major part of the blend used in an aromatherapy massage and should be selected with care; vegetable based oils with their inherent high degree of unsaturation provide the most suitable medium.

REFERENCES

Abrams D I 1990 Alternative therapies in HIV infection. AIDS 4: 1179–1187

Anon 1990 Lipids and multiple sclerosis. Lancet 336: 25–26

Anon 1991 Treating AIDS with worts. Science 254: 522

Anthony C P, Thibodeau G A 1983 Nervous system cells in anatomy and physiology. Mosby, St Louis

Balacs T 1993 Essential oils in the body. In: Aroma '93 Conference Proceedings. Aromatherapy Publications, Brighton, pp 12–13

Bronaugh R L, Webster R C, Bucks D, Maibach H I, Sarason R 1990 In vivo percutaneous absorption of fragrance ingredients in rhesus monkeys and humans. Food and Chemical Toxicology 28(5): 369–373

Brun K 1952 Les essences végétales en tant qu'agent de pénétration tissulaire. Thèse Pharmacie, Strasbourg

Buchbauer G 1988 Aromatherapy: do essential oils have therapeutic properties? In: International Conference on Essential Oils, Flavours, Fragrances and Cosmetics, Beijing. International Federation of Essential Oils and Aroma Trades, London, pp 351–352

Buchbauer G 1993 Molecular interaction. International Journal of Aromatherapy 5: 11–14

Casley-Smith J R, Casley-Smith J R 1983 The effect of Unguentum lymphaticum on acute experimental lymphedema and other high-protein edemas. Lymphology 16: 150–156

Cleary G 1993 Transdermal drug delivery. In: Zatz J L (ed) Skin permeation: fundamentals and applications. Allured, Wheaton, pp 207–237

Eisberg N 1983 Male chauvinism in toxicity testing? Manufacturing Chemist 3 (July): 3

Expert Panel 1983 Cosmetic ingredient review: 4: Final report on the safety of sweet almond oil and almond meal. Journal of the American College of Toxicology 2(5): 85–99

Fleischner A M 1985 Plant extracts: to accelerate healing and reduce inflammation. Cosmetics and Toiletries 100: 45

Friedman Z, Shochat S, Maisels M, Marks K, Lamberth E 1976 Correction of essential fatty acid deficiency in newborn infants by cutaneous application of sunflower seed oil. Pediatrics 58: 650–654

Health and Safety Commission 1994 The health and safety at work act. HMSO, London

Hizon R P, Huyck C L 1956 The stability of almond and corn oils for use in parenteral solutions. Journal of the American Pharmaceutical Association 45: 145–150

Hoffmann-La Roche 1989 Information leaflet HHN-5379A/589

Hotchkiss S 1994 How thin is your skin? New Scientist 141(1910): 24–27

Hunt C E, Engel R R, Modler S, Hamilton W, Bissen S, Holman R T 1978 Essential fatty acid deficiency in neonates: inability to reverse deficiency by topical application of EFA-rich oil. Journal of Pediatrics 92(4): 603–607

Jackson E 1993 Toxicological aspects of percutaneous absorption. In: Zatz J L (ed) Skin permeation: fundamentals and applications. Allured, Wheaton, pp 177–193

Jäger W, Buchbauer G, Jirovetz L, Fritzer M 1992 Percutaneous absorption of lavender oil from a massage oil. Journal of the Society of Cosmetic Chemists 43(1) (January-February): 49–54

Katz A E 1947 Parfüm Mod 39: 64

Leung A Y, Foster S 1996 Encyclopedia of common natural ingredients used in food, drugs and cosmetics. John Wiley, New York

Lexicon Vevy 1993a La peau: siège d'absorption et organ cible. In: Skin Care Instant Reports (Vevy Europe, Genova) 10(4): 35–41

Lexicon Vevy 1993b La peau: siège d'absorption et organ cible. In: Skin Care Instant Reports (Vevy Europe, Genova) 10(6): 68

McCarthy M C, Turner W, Whatley K, Cottam G 1983 Topical corn oil in the management of essential fatty acid deficiency. Critical Care in Medicine 5: 373–375

Macht D 1938 The absorption of drugs and poisons through the skin and mucous membranes. Journal of the American Medical Association 110: 409–414

Maibach H I, Marzulli F N 1977 Toxicologic perspectives of chemicals commonly applied to skin. In: Drill V A, Lazar P (eds) Cutaneous toxicity. Academic Press, New York

Martindale 1993 The extra pharmacopoeia, 30th edn. Pharmaceutical Press, London, p 1378.3

Millar J H D, Zilkha K J, Langman M J S, Payling Wright H, Smith A D, Belin J, Thompson R H S 1973 Double blind trial of linoleate supplementation of the diet in multiple sclerosis. British Medical Journal 31 March 1(5856): 765–768

Miller D G, Williams S K, Palombo J D, Griffin R E, Bistrian B R, Blackburn G L 1987 Cutaneous application of safflower oil in preventing essential fatty acid deficiency in patients on home parenteral nutrition. American Journal of Clinical Nutrition 46: 419–423

Mills S 1993 The essential book of herbal medicine. Penguin, London, pp 333, 334

Newall C A, Anderson L A, Phillipson J D 1996 Herbal medicines. The Pharmaceutical Press, London, p 251

O'Neill J A, Caldwell M D, Meng H C 1976 Essential fatty acid deficiency in surgical patients. Annals of Surgery 185(5): 535–541

Pratt J, Mason A 1981 The caring touch. Heyden, London

Press M, Hartop P J, Prottey C 1974 Correction of essential fatty acid deficiency in man by the cutaneous application of sunflower-seed oil. The Lancet 6 April: 597–599

Price L, Smith I, Price S 1999 Carrier oils for aromatherapy and massage. Riverhead, Stratford upon Avon

Price S 1993 The aromatherapy workbook. Thorsons, London, pp 162, 166

Prottey C, Hartop P J, Press M 1975 Correction of the cutaneous manifestations of fatty acid deficiency in man by application of sunflower seed oil to the skin. Journal of Investigative Dermatology 64(4): 228–234

Riviere J E 1993 Biological factors in absorption and permeation. In: Zatz J L (ed) Skin permeation: fundamentals and applications. Allured, Wheaton, pp 113–125

Römmelt H, Zuber A, Dirnagl K, Drexel H 1974 Münchner Medezin Wochenschrift 116: 537

Römmelt H, Drexel H, Dirnagl K 1978 Heilkunst 91(5): 21

Schilcher H 1985 Effects and side effects of essential oils. In: Baerheim Svendsen A, Scheffer J J C (eds) Essential oils and aromatic plants. Kluwer Academic, Dordrecht, p 218

Shaparenko B A, Slivko B A, Bazarova O V, Vishnevetskaya E N, Selesneva G T, Berezhnala L P 1979 On the use of medicinal plants for treatment of patients with chronic suppurative otitis. Zhurnal Ushnykh I Gorlovykh Boleznei 39(3): 48–51

Stier B 1990 Secrets des huiles de première pression à froid. (Publisher not given), Quebec

Stoughton R B 1959 Relation of the anatomy of normal and abnormal skin to its protective function. In: Rothman S (ed) The human integument, normal and abnormal. American Association for the Advancement of Science: 3–24

Swank R L, Dugan B B 1990 Effect of low saturated fat diet in early and late cases of multiple sclerosis. Lancet 336: 37–39

Torii S, Fukada H, Kanemoto H, Miyanchi R, Hamauzu Y, Kawasaki M 1991 Contingent negative variation (CNV) and the psychological effects of odour. In: Van Toller S, Dodd G (eds) Perfumery: the psychology and biology of fragrance. Chapman & Hall, London, pp 107–118

Valette G, Sobrin E 1963 Percutaneous absorption of various animal and vegetable oils. Pharmica Acta Helvetica 38(10): 710–716

Valnet J 1980 The practice of aromatherapy. Daniel, Saffron Walden

Van Toller S 1993 The sensory evaluation of odours. Paper on clinical practitioners course, Shirley Price International College of Aromatherapy, Hinckley

Winter R 1984 A consumer's dictionary of cosmetic ingredients. Crown, New York

Zatz J L 1993 Modification of skin permeation by solvents. In: Zatz J L (ed) Skin permeation: fundamentals and applications. Allured, Wheaton, pp 127–148

Essential waters

Introduction

The subject of aromatic waters is intriguing, yet not one on which very much has been written. It has been necessary to search many books on herbalism and aromatherapy to glean snippets of information. Even then the quality of information is not always very good, and none of it would stand up to rigorous examination (save for the information on kekkik water (Aydin, Baser & Öztürk 1996)). Most has been found in French literature, the country that most uses aromatic waters, although even there not to a great extent today.

Water has the remarkable capability of picking up information relating to the vibrational energy found in a living plant, of storing this information and, under certain circumstances, of transferring this to the human body. This means that distilled aromatic waters pick up and store not only physical plant particles (Roulier 1990) but possibly also subtle energetic information; consequently such products have an almost homoeopathic aspect.

There are several kinds of water-based aromatic products used in therapies, including infusions, teas (it has been estimated that over 1 000 000 cups of chamomile tea are taken every day worldwide (Foster 1996)), tisanes, wines, vinegars, as well as aromatic waters, which may be distilled or prepared. Distilled aromatic waters contain the water soluble compounds of the plant, but not the tannic acid and bitter substances, and make an excellent complement to that other product of distillation, the powerful essential oils. They are, however, very different in nature from the volatile essential oils, even though obtained from the same plant, in as much as they are without aggression and are active on a different level; these 'gentle giants' are subtle, safe and effective, although any treatment must be carried out over a longer period of time than when using essential oils.

Some plants, whether containing essential oils or not, are distilled specifically for the aromatic water and not for the essential oil; when plants are distilled specifically for the aromatic water the quality of the water used is of great importance. Although there may be no volatile or aromatic molecules in these plants, and hence no aromatic oil, all water soluble molecules (large and small) within the plant are taken up by the steam; thus the aromatic waters stand intermediate between, and represent to some extent a fusion of, aromatherapy and herbalism, containing as they do some of the useful plant molecules from both worlds. Aromatic waters are used in conjunction with both essential oil treatments and herbalism, as well as on their own.

As these valuable products of the distillation process are so safe in use, they deserve to be much better known and far more widely used, especially by aromatherapists already familiar with that other product of the distillation process, the essential oils. Aromatic waters last featured in the French Codex in 1965.

TERMINOLOGY

In France the term *hydrolat* is used to describe the condensed steam which has passed through the plant material; the translation of hydrolat is given as 'aromatic, medicated water' (Mansion 1971), but many names are in use, some more accurate than others.

Terms used for these products are:

- aromatic water—this is adequate and reasonably accurate (even though some do not smell very pleasant)
- floral waters—this is inaccurate as by no means all distilled waters are from flowers.

- hydrosol—this is inappropriate, as this is a generic term applied to a wide range of products and is not specific: a hydrosol may be defined as a colloidal solution (i.e. a dispersion of material in a liquid, characterized by particles of very small size, of between 0.2 and 0.002 micrometres) where water is the dispersant medium
- essential water—this is an ancient name and aptly describes the aromatic distilled water from the still
- prepared water—this is an assembly of products to simulate a natural product.

Prepared aromatic waters

These are not produced by the distillation process but are put together in a laboratory. They consist of distilled water with the addition of one or more essential oils; these oils may be genuine plant extracts (volatile oil, absolute or concrete) or they may be partly or wholly artificial or synthetic. Essential oils are not generally soluble in water—probably on average only about 20% of any given oil is water soluble—but many of the oils can be 'knocked' into solution by shaking to produce a saturated solution. For each litre of distilled water 2–3 grams (40–60 drops) of essential oil can be added; this must be shaken frequently and vigorously for 2 or 3 days and then stored in a cool place; it can be stored successfully at 10–15°C for several months. Essential oils suitable for use by this method are anise, basil, borneo camphor, chamomile, caraway, cinnamon, citron, coriander, cypress, eucalyptus, fennel, garlic, geranium, hyssop, juniper, lavender, lemon, marjoram, melissa, niaouli, nutmeg, orange, origanum, peppermint, rosemary, sage, savory, tangerine, tarragon, verbena and ylang ylang (Lautié & Passebecq 1979 p. 91).

They may be used for gargles, mouthwashes, bathing wounds and for ingestion, where 20 ml of the made water contains one drop of essential oil and therefore one teaspoonful contains about a quarter of a drop (about 0.25% concentration). Many essential oils exhibit significant bactericidal power at a concentration of 0.25%, as found in prepared waters, e.g. in a concentration of 0.18% clove essential oil kills the tubercular bacillus in a few minutes without causing any tissue damage or risk of toxicity, in contrast to some other preparations and antibiotics (Lautié & Passebecq 1979 p. 92).

Prepared waters do not have the same make-up as essential (distilled) waters, and therefore cannot have the same therapeutic properties. Some prepared waters are made with the use of alcohol, and these are not recommended for use alongside aromatherapy. The main volume of sales of prepared waters is to skin care manufacturers for use in 'natural' skin toners, refreshers and washes. Water which has had essential oil(s), synthetics or alcohol added to it is not an essential water and the two should not be confused. To achieve a genuine plant water, distillation alone is the true method.

WHAT ARE ESSENTIAL WATERS?

Essential waters are a product of distillation and can be considered as true partial extracts of the plant material from which they are derived. They may be by-products of the distillation of volatile oils, e.g. chamomile water and lavender water, or of the distillation of plant material which has no volatile oil, e.g. elderflower, cornflower, plantain. Their method of preparation, by definition, necessitates that they be totally natural products with no added synthetic fragrance components. Essential (distilled) waters are obtained from aromatic and other plants by steam distillation, and during this process a proportion of the water soluble compounds of the essential oil contained in the plant matter is absorbed and retained by the water. As some essential oils have a relatively high proportion of water soluble compounds, much of the essential oil can be lost to the water during the distillation process, e.g. *Melissa officinalis* [LEMON BALM]; in such cases it is imperative to use cohobation. This is a system whereby the water/steam in contact with the biomass during distillation is continuously recirculated, giving maximal opportunity for the water soluble elements of the essential oil and the plant to pass into the water. Eventually this water reaches saturation point, when no more of the essential oil components can pass into solution (it is at this stage that the complete essential oil is gained); thus a water is produced that is rich not only in some essential oil molecules but also in other hydrophyllic molecules found in the plant which are not usually part of the essential oil. When distilling for essential waters, it is important that the water used in the distillation process should be of good quality, preferably from a non-polluted spring, and free of any chemical cleansers that may have been used to clean the still.

Aromatic waters contain about 0.2% to 0.5% (or perhaps more, according to the plant) of the water soluble parts of the essential oil freely dispersed in an ionized form. They may have similar properties to the parent oils but not to the same degree, and often their properties are different.

Which plants yield an essential water?

Many aromatherapists think that only plants containing an essential oil are distilled but this is not so. Many plants containing very little or no essential oil at all are processed primarily to gain the essential water. The essential water from each plant, like the essential oil, is unique and reacts according to its constituents. *Hypericum perforatum*, often macerated in olive oil to gain its therapeutic properties (see carrier oils in Ch. 5, p. 102) is an example of a plant that contains an essential oil but which is rarely distilled for this on account of the minute yield, which would cause the price to be prohibitive; it is therefore distilled for its essential water. *Plantago lanceolata* (plantain) is an example of a non-aromatic plant which is distilled only for its essential water. This illustrates that water soluble molecules other than volatile essential oil molecules can be taken into the steam, yielding a therapeutic water at the end of the process.

Yield

It is not possible to gain an almost unlimited or even a large quantity of water from a small amount of plant material. The quantity of essential water is proportionately limited to the plant weight and therefore aromatic waters of excellent quality are obtained when cohobation is an integral part of the distilling process. This method is used to produce a number of essential waters, e.g. rose, and yields a saturated essential water; melissa is another case where a whole essential oil cannot be achieved until the steam water is saturated with the water soluble molecules of the essential oil, thus preventing the loss of these from the essential oil.

Yields of distilled waters usually lie between the limits of 1 to 1.5 and 2 to 5 litres per kilogram of plant matter, and vary according to the particular plant. The waters of thyme, savory and rosemary require a less quantity of plant than do lettuce, hawthorn, yarrow or hemp agrimony. Some waters are known as 'weight for weight' products since the quantities of plant matter and water product are equal, e.g. 100 lb of roses are distilled with sufficient water to yield 100 lb of fragrant rose water (Poucher 1936).

Appearance and aroma

Distilled waters are not strongly coloured and are clear, with the exception of cinnamon water, which is always opalescent; for the most part they have only slight, delicate colouration (Viaud 1983 p. 23). Their smell may be generally reminiscent of the original plant material, but this is not always the case; an example is distilled lavender water, which often disappoints.

Keeping qualities and storage

Waters need to be stored at a temperature of less than 14°C, and in the shade. At higher temperatures certain waters tend to show flocculation. The maximum storage period under the conditions given must not, in general, exceed 1 year as some essential waters are fragile and break down after a relatively short time. They are best purchased in small quantities, although Rouvière & Meyer (1989) say that the plant waters resulting from the distillation process of essential oils have a life of 2 to 3 years, owing to the presence of soluble compounds from the

essential oils, which inhibit bacterial growth. Those hydrolats which have a good content of antiseptic phenols keep well; the distilled waters of *Satureia hortensis* and *Origanum vulgare* can be kept for more than 2 years with no discernible change.

Composition

It is known that, besides certain volatile compounds (isovalerianic, cyanhydric, benzoic and cinnamic acids), distilled aromatic waters can contain many other volatile principles, although these are rarely properly identified. Analysis of three essential waters (*Lavandula angustifolia*, *Salvia officinalis*, *Matricaria recutita*) showed that they contain substances present in the plant (Montesinos 1991 p. 24). The pH of an essential water is closely linked to the concentration of alcohols and phenols present and to the degree of dissociation; they are usually neutral, and sometimes have a weak acid reaction.

Quality

The basic criteria for obtaining a good quality hydrolat is the same as those for the procurement of a genuine essential oil, i.e. using a known botanical species, grown organically or wild, with a known chemical make-up; a distillation of sufficient duration and at low pressure, and a hydrolat that itself has had nothing added and nothing extracted. It is imperative that only products obtained during steam distillation and without colouring matter, stabilizers and preservatives be used. Products procured from a high street chemist shop do not usually conform to this high standard, often containing synthetic materials; alternatively, they may be entirely artificial.

As with an essential oil, it is difficult to judge the quality of a distilled water from the smell; a true distilled water does not necessarily smell the same as the oil from the same plant because it has a different chemical make-up; when freshly distilled it may have an odour and taste of the still, although this is not long lasting.

Unfortunately, most essential waters from plants distilled for their essential oils are discarded and are saved only if ordered beforehand. It is generally thought that because hydrolats are often thrown away, they should be inexpensive; unhappily this is not the case, as the cost of transporting the bulk (volume and weight) of the product is reflected in the final cost.

USES OF ESSENTIAL WATERS

A nice attention, however, is certainly necessary in the use of them.

(John Farley (1783), principal cook at the London Tavern, Dublin, referring to the water and infusions of bay)

Waters are ultra mild in action compared with essential oils and are useful for the treatment of the young, the elderly and those in a state of delicate health. The less volatile odorous molecules are integrally dispersed in the water in ionized form, therefore irritation of the skin and mucous surfaces is avoided. Essential waters have a higher concentration of volatile elements than do teas and so are more efficacious and quicker acting, with a very easy method of use, i.e. drinking small quantities.

Essential waters work synergistically with essential oils and so they can be prescribed as a complement to either phytotherapy (Streicher 1996) or aromatherapy. Herbalists in France do not use these waters on their own to any great extent, but they are used as a complement to other phytotherapeutic treatments both internally and externally; they are used both singly and as ready-prepared mixes.

General

Being non-aggressive, waters can be used safely for disinfection of open wounds and on mucous surfaces; they have been mentioned for use in cases of eczema, ulcers, bronchitis, tracheitis, colitis, burns and pain, whether local or generalized (e.g. *Chamaemelum nobile* [ROMAN CHAMOMILE] is said to ease post-zoster pain).

They are used in gargles, nasal sprays, skin sprays and vaginal douches.

Skin care

Aromatic waters are nearly free of irritating components, and their mild action and lack of toxicity make them ideal for use as skin care products; they have long been used in this way in the form of cleansers, toners (all skin types especially sensitive skin), conditioning creams and lotions. They are also used in baby care, bath preparations, hair rinses, aftershave preparations and facial sprays.

Children

Essential waters do not contain alcohol, and so are suitable for children, especially as they may be sweetened with sugar if necessary. They are recommended for young children for external and internal use because they do not irritate the skin or mucous surfaces.

Eye care

Some essential waters are used in preparations for eyewashes; e.g. *Myrtus communis* [MYRTLE] and *Chamaemelum nobile* [ROMAN CHAMOMILE] soothe pains resulting from inflammatory states of the eyes.

Traditional medicine

Essential waters are often prescribed by some complementary practitioners to adjust the 'energy balance' and the 'environment' (both internal and external) of the person, for instance according to Chinese medicine. The conditions treated include disorders of the digestive system such as constipation, rheumatism, migraine (from liver irritation), parasites, and ear, nose and throat problems.

Routes of absorption

First there is the oral route through the walls of the digestive tract. The culinary aspect is

Case 6.1   Aromatologist: Dr D Pénoël, France

At the beginning of August 1994, I received a phone call from a mother who was extremely worried by the disease diagnosed by the GP for her young son. Clément was suffering from *Molluscum contagiosum*, a dreadful viral infection, which had developed while the family were on holiday in Corsica. For several days, his whole body (including his genitals) had been covered with boils; he was feverish and screaming with pain day and night.

The parents firmly believed in natural medicine and, for them, sending Clément to the hospital did not represent the adequate answer, in particular for a viral disease for which no real allopathic cure existed. As the boy was also prone to eczema and allergic reactions, they decided to refuse the antibiotics and to seek an alternative in medical aromatherapy, which proved successful very swiftly.

Clément was indeed in an appalling situation and his suffering was so intense that a proper examination was not even possible (I took two slides before beginning the aromatic care). I not only assessed the medical condition of the child, but also took into account the capacity of the family to understand and undertake the therapeutic intensive programme that I would establish with them. This holistic feasibility diagnosis is much more important in our alternative medical approach than in current medicine and the parents had to be prepared to follow each step with continuity and perseverance over several days.

In such severe cases, aromatologists will know that we apply the concept of the relationship between the external interfaces and their capacity to receive and distribute the relevant aromatic extracts.

For a viral condition with such extreme external cutaneous manifestation, the first choice is *Melissa officinalis*—not the essential oil, but the aromatic water. Genuine essential oil of melissa is extremely rare (and more expensive than rose otto) and the main producer of this essential oil (and therefore the cohobated aromatic water) is in the Drôme valley in France.

A fine spraying technique (using a compressor) of the neat aromatic water was used and, a few seconds after I began to spray the fine melissa mist around the little boy, relief was felt for the very first time—after so many days of intense suffering! That was already a great result in order to gain his confidence and to prepare the further steps of the treatment.

To continue the treatment, the following essential oils were chosen:

- *Chamaemelum nobile* (ROMAN CHAMOMILE), for its antiinflammatory calming and vulnerary properties
- *Matricaria recutita* (GERMAN CHAMOMILE) with antiviral, antiallergic and antiinflammatory properties

- *Melaleuca alternifolia* (TEA TREE) with analgesic, antiinfectious, antiinflammatory, antiviral and immunostimulant properties
- *Thymus vulgaris* ct. linalol with antiinfectious, antiinflammatory, antiseptic, antiviral, soothing and immunostimulant properties
- *Juniperus communis* fruct. with analgesic, antiseptic, antiviral and depurative properties.

These were made up in a 5% concentration in a 95% blend of vegetable carrier oils, also active in the healing process: macerated oils of calendula (60%), St John's wort (25%) and oil of *Calophyllum inophyllum* (5%). The parents were advised to apply the blend upon each boil, using a fine paint brush.

The essential oils above were also given to the parents to be used internally—one drop blended in honey six times per day orally and three drops three times per day diluted in vegetable oil and used in capsule form as a suppository.

A second blend of essential oil was made with: *Melaleuca cajuputi* (CAJUPUT), *M. alternifolia* and *Myrtus communis* (RED MYRTLE) to be applied without dilution mainly under the sole of each foot six times a day.

These products were given to the parents together with the spraying equipment, lent for this period of intensive aromatic care, which they had to implement by themselves 200 kilometres further south at their home, from where they would keep us informed of the progress day by day.

After 3 days the problem had enormously improved. The parents then had to continue the treatment with decreasing intensity. During all that time, a toxin-free diet had been established for Clément by my wife in order to help the detoxification process, which accompanies any infectious disease.

Nine days later the family returned to see me. Clément was in wonderful shape (another slide was taken); the skin was almost perfect and he had regained his vitality. This remarkable success, in particular its unbelievable swiftness, had been made possible only by the synergistic conjunction of several factors:

- the strong will and full determination of the parents
- the experience, competence and confidence of the therapist
- the availability of high quality aromatic and vegetal products (extremely important)
- the choice of method for the application of the aromatic water
- the willingness of the parents to continue the treatment at home.

Table 6.1 Properties and indications: essential waters

Essential water	General	Skin	Emotion
Achillea millefolium [YARROW]	circulatory problems (women)	eczema, skin drainer, pyodermatitis	
Calendula officinalis [MARIGOLD]	emmenagogue, hypertension, staphylococcus; skin problems of intestinal origin		
Centaurea cyanus [CORNFLOWER]			
Chamaemelum nobile [ROMAN CHAMOMILE]	cardiac calmative? healing, ophthalmic	antiinflammatory, infections	calming
Citrus sinensis [ORANGE FLOWER]	cardiac calmative, anticollibacillus		seasonal nervous depression, uplifting
Cupressus sempervirens [CYPRESS]	haemorrhoids, broken veins		
Eucalyptus globulus [TASMANIAN BLUE GUM]	bronchi, kidneys, pancreas, antidiabetic	acne	
Foeniculum vulgare [FENNEL]	galactogen, antiseptic		nervous depression, sedative
Helichrysum angustifolium [EVERLASTING]	diabetes, aerophagy, pulmonary depurative	bruises, abscesses, couperose skin, cicatrizant	
Hypericum perforatum [ST JOHN'S WORT]	low dose—clears the lungs; high dose—antiepileptic	soothing	
Hyssopus officinalis [HYSSOP]	diuretic, kidney deflocculant, rheumatoid arthritis	skin astringent, oily skin, refreshing	
Juniperus communis [JUNIPER]	intestinal antibiotic, rheumatism	soothing, pimples, burns, insect bites	
Lavandula angustifolia [LAVENDER]		acneic skin, herpes	
Lavandula × intermedia [LAVANDIN]			
Melissa officinalis [LEMON BALM]	blepharitis, conjunctivitis, digestive, headaches	irritated skin, insect bites, herpes	sedative, relaxing, uplifting, depression
Mentha × piperita [PEPPERMINT]	eupeptic, antiseptic	itching, inflammation, cooling	refreshing
Myrtus communis [MYRTLE]	soothing antiseptic		
Ocimum basilicum [BASIL]	carminative, digestive		
Origanum majorana [MARJORAM]	clears the liver, gall bladder		
Origanum onites [KEKIK]	cardiovascular stimulant		
Pinus sylvestris [SCOTS PINE]	balsamic, diuretic		
Rosa damascena [ROSE]	mouth ulcers	toning all skin types, dermatitis, wrinkles, couperose	mental strain, calming, sedative
Rosmarinus officinalis [ROSEMARY]	emmenagogue, rheumatism, circulation stimulant	toning oily and mixed skins	stimulating, alertness
Salvia officinalis [SAGE]	emmenagogue, pelvic congestion, diuretic, rheumatism, ulcers	astringent, oily skin, acne, eczema	
Salvia sclarea [CLARY]	sore throat, period pain	astringent, oily skin, acne, inflamed, mature skin	depression, anxiety
Satureia montana [SAVORY]	revitalizing		
Thymus serpyllum [WILD THYME]	intestinal antiseptic, Gram −ve		
Thymus vulgaris (population) [THYME]	intestinal antiseptic, Gram +ve	acne, dermatitis, insect bites, eczema	stimulating, revitalizing
Thymus vulgaris ct. alcohol [SWEET THYME]	eye problems		

attractive here as essential waters are easily added to foods and are palatable.

The rectal route using an enema is also used, and the active substance is here absorbed across the mucous surfaces of the large intestine.

Finally there is the skin; here the substance is absorbed from the whole surface of the body.

Methods of use and dosage

- Put 50 ml of essential water into a bath to aid relaxation and promote a soothing effect.
- Use it on a cotton wool pad as a skin tonic after cleansing.
- Use it as a mouthwash or gargle.
- Put a teaspoonful (5 ml) into tea (without milk), fruit juice or fruit salads, coffee (petit-grain or orange flower water is delicious in coffee and fruit salads) or in a morning glass of water.
- Oral (internal) use may safely be recommended where appropriate; up to three teaspoonfuls (15 ml) per day may be ingested.

Duration of treatment is dependent on the particular organ and person being treated:

- For treatment of the liver, two teaspoonfuls should be taken before supper or before going to bed.
- For treatment of the kidneys and bladder, three teaspoonfuls should be taken between 3 p.m. and 7 p.m.
- For treatment of the lungs, six teaspoonfuls should be spread throughout the day in acute cases or three teaspoonfuls for chronic cases.
- For gargles essential waters may be used neat, but in general use they should be diluted, up to 1 in 10 depending on the water.

Table 6.1 lists the properties and indications for use of essential waters for general conditions, skin conditions and emotional states: it is based, almost wholly, on anecdotal evidence in the absence of any other kind of proof. There is a general table giving the properties of these waters in Appendix B (p. 357). Waters have certainly been in continual use for three and a half centuries, and perhaps longer, in cooking, for medicine and for personal cleanliness (Genders 1977).

Cautions

It should be noted that preservative is often added to shop-bought natural essential waters to improve the shelf life and these should be avoided for culinary or therapeutic purposes. When purchasing waters it may also be necessary to obtain a certificate from the supplier to ensure that the proper conditions of harvesting, processing and stocking have been observed.

Essential waters, as with other partial plant extracts, will possess the claimed activity of the plant only if its constituents giving this activity are contained within that fraction of the plant forming the partial plant extract. Many partial plant extracts, particularly distillates, have the advantage of being virtually colourless, making them easy to incorporate into a range of products. Unfortunately, this has led over the years to the production of distillates from a wide range of plant materials which are not suitable for this form of processing, and therefore little credence can be given to any claimed activity of the plant material or to its extract (Helliwell 1989).

Summary

Continued use of essential waters over centuries indicates that these substances have a potential for therapeutic use and are worthy of investigation. Physically they contain some water soluble molecules known to be therapeutic, in common with essential oils and some compounds found in other types of herbal preparations, and it may be that they also carry information and energy in a manner somewhat analogous to homoeopathic remedies. They are gentle in use and may safely be used in some cases where the use of the more powerful essential oils would be inadvisable, and may also be used to complement other forms of treatment; they have the advantage of being relatively inexpensive.

REFERENCES

Aydin S, Başer K H C, Öztürk Y 1996 The chemistry and pharmacology of origanum (kekik) water. 27th International Symposium on Essential Oils, September, Wien

Farley J 1783 The handbook on art of cookery and housekeepers complete assistant, p 307

Foster S 1996 Chamomile: *Matricaria recutita* & *Chamaemelum nobile*. Botanical series 307. American Botanical Council, Austin, p 6

Genders R 1977 A book of aromatics. Darton, Longman and Todd, London, p 13

Helliwell K 1989 Manufacture and use of plant extracts. In: Grievson M, Barber J, Hunting A L L (eds) Natural ingredients in cosmetics. Micelle, Weymouth, pp 26–27

Lautié R, Passebecq A 1979 Aromatherapy; the use of plant essences in healing. Thorsons, Wellingborough

Mansion J E 1971 Harrap's new standard French and English dictionary.

Montesinos C 1991 Eléments de réflexion sur quelques hydrolats. Study written for Ecole Lyonnaise de Plantes Médicinales, Lyons

Poucher W A 1936 Perfumes, cosmetics and soaps, vol II. Chapman & Hall, London, pp 34–35

Roulier G 1990 Les huiles essentielles pour votre santé. Dangles, St-Jean-de-Braye, p 115

Rouvière A, Meyer M-C 1989 La santé par les huiles essentielles. M A Editions, Paris, pp 82–83

Streicher C 1996 Hydrosols—the subtle complement to essential oils. plexus 1: 22

Viaud H 1983 Huiles essentielles—hydrolats. Présence, Sisteron

SOURCES

Claeys G 1992 Précis d'aromathérapie familiale. Equilibres, Flers, p 74

Grace U-M 1996 Aromatherapy for practitioners. Daniel, Saffron Walden, pp 84–85

de Bonneval P 1992 Votre santé par les plantes. Equilibres, Flers

Price S 1997 Aromatic water. The Aromatherapist 3(2): 44–47

Price L, Price S 1999 Essential waters. Riverhead, Stratford upon Avon

Rose J 1994 Hydrosols: the other product of distillation. Aromatherapy correspondence course notes, California

Touch and massage

7

Introduction

Many studies exist to show the importance of touch in the development of healthy human beings. This chapter considers the reintroduction of touch to healthcare settings, and gives a practical grounding in simple massage.

TOUCH

Touch is a basic human behavioural need (Sanderson, Harnison & Price 1991), and its importance for both mental and physical health has been well researched (Montagu 1986). Animals and humans alike thrive and remain in better health when stroked or touched caringly. 'Take it away from the baby and the baby will not thrive' (Anckett 1979). Even the carer derives benefit—stroking a pet regularly can effectively reduce a person's blood pressure. 'We all have great technical skills, but forget how much good we can do with just 10 minutes of holding someone's hand' said one nurse in an interview (Wilkinson 1991). Executed with love, the effect of this simple action on the recipient is a feeling of pleasure and eventual relaxation of body and mind (Worrell 1997). This is especially so during the experience of sudden stressful situations. 'We need to touch each other in ways besides aggression or sex' (Rouse 1993).

Nurse/patient contact

As research and scientific developments in the efficacy of drugs forged ahead, so close patient contact diminished until, in the 1960s, massage more or less lost its therapeutic status in medical care. A senior nurse at Battle Hospital in Reading summed up the feeling among many nurses when she said: 'I felt more of a super-technician than anything else; my caring role was just not being fulfilled' (Wilkinson 1991).

This unfortunate situation is now changing. In recent years nurses have shown a renewed interest in the value of touch where patients are concerned and massage has been introduced to several hospitals for general relaxation, relief of side-effects and to encourage recovery. 'Massage may be the only therapy which is instinctive: we hold and caress those we wish to comfort; when we hurt ourselves, our first reaction is to touch and rub the painful part' (Vickers 1996 p. 6).

At a nursing conference at St Catherine's College, Oxford (1991), the subject was essential oils and massage. Sister Helen Passant spoke of their use on the elderly, and how massage provided nursing staff with a new way of communicating with their patients. Senior Nurse Chrissie Dunn outlined the study carried out at Battle Hospital, Reading in the intensive therapy unit, where blood pressure and heart rate had both been reduced by the use of essential oils and massage. Sheena Hildebrand described how they were used on oncology patients at the Royal Marsden Hospital, London (Sutton branch), where essential oils and massage brought about relief of tension, promoting peace and tranquillity. (Chs 13, 14 and 15 discuss these in detail.)

The Churchill Hospital, Oxford, was possibly the first hospital (well before 1987) to introduce massage for the care of the elderly, and Sister Helen Passant used aromatherapy there many years (Wise 1993). Others followed closely, including the Royal Marsden Hospital, Sutton and Battle Hospital, Reading. All the nurses involved have been extremely encouraged by the results, and, on the strength of patient satisfaction, up to 60% of the costs at the Marylebone Health Centre are now met by the local health authority (Wilkinson 1991).

Massage has been further enhanced in many hospitals by the addition of essential oils, transforming the treatment into one of aromatherapy (Buckle 1997). The benefits not only can be enhanced by the choice of oil used—increased energy levels, side-effects of drugs lessened, symptoms not being treated by the hospital relieved and emotional problems eased—but the effects themselves can last longer owing to the therapeutic action of the essential oil components (see Chs 12–15).

Benefits

The physiological benefits of massage may be easily assessed—it increases the circulation of both blood and lymph (helping in the elimination of toxins from the body), slows the pulse rate, lowers blood pressure, releases muscle tension, tones underworked or weak muscles and relieves cramp. The psychological benefits, though perhaps not so easy to evaluate, are also notable and play their part in the holistic healing effect: relaxing an apprehensive mind, uplifting depression and despair, relieving panic or anger and, importantly, giving a person the feeling that someone cares enough to spend time giving the specialized contact brought by touch and massage. Many aromatherapy schools, including the authors' own, teach a specialized massage, now termed an aromatherapy massage. However, patients can also benefit greatly from:

- professional massage given by a physical therapist without essential oils
- professional massage given by a physical therapist using essentials oils ready mixed by an aromatherapist or aromatologist
- a caring nurse with no professional training in massage, but with sound theoretical knowledge of essential oils (or under the direction of an aromatherapist or aromatologist), using them with touch and gentle, non-manipulative massage movements.

Sharon MacNish, who practised aromatherapy once a week at a London hospice, said:

The techniques I was in the habit of using were totally inappropriate in a hospice setting, so I had to revise completely the way I work with an individual. It became a case of re-learning what I knew, so that instead of using textbook massage, I was free to work with the gentlest touch and the most loving attitude.

(MacNish 1991)

MASSAGE—A THERAPY IN ITS OWN RIGHT

The relationship of massage to aromatherapy

It would be preferable, and would prevent misunderstanding of the word aromatherapy, if qualifications in professional massage were totally separate from qualifications in essential oil knowledge. 'Massage and aromatherapy should be judged on their own merits' (Vickers 1996 p. 15). Those people who have studied aromatherapy are at the moment called aromatherapists, though their massage training is not usually as thorough as that of a physical therapist. Aromatology training (that is, training in aromatic medicine) involves full theoretical knowledge of essential oils, their chemistry and all their holistic possibilities and methods of use as in aromatherapy (to at least the standard required by the Aromatherapy Organisations Council)—plus intensive external undiluted use of neat essential oils and internal use by os, rectum or vagina; the massage taught involves simple techniques for hand, foot, scalp, back, abdomen and shoulder massage and is practised by health practitioners who do not have the time either to learn—or to give in the course of their work—a 90 minute full-body massage. We agree with Caroline Stevensen who believes that it is not necessary to spend an hour massaging patients in order to be effective: 'Patients can benefit from a very short period of high-quality time' (quoted in Tattam 1992). There is already some acceptance that aromatology (i.e. aromatic medicine) will be the path in the UK for health professionals wishing to use essential oils at a professional level, but who do not wish, or are unable, to use full-body massage in their work. The aromatology approach not only modifies the idea that treatment with essential oils necessarily implies a specialized aromatherapy massage, but also eradicates the unfortunate popular association of aromatherapy with bath bubbles, shampoos, soap and even tobacco and washing-up liquid.

Massage training

Massage therapists have a slightly different problem with the status of their therapy, which in the past has had other, unsavoury, connotations.

Case 7.1   Therapist: Rosemary Holder LIAM, UK

Mrs X is a middle-aged teacher, divorced and 'putting' her second son through university with the usual accompanying financial strain. She attended regularly every 2 months for an aromatherapy massage, mainly for stress-related muscular aches. During one of these sessions, she casually mentioned that she had chronic bronchitis every winter, exacerbating her usually well-controlled asthma. She had omitted to mention these problems during a comprehensive initial assessment because she felt if she ignored them they would lose some of their power over her! We discussed aromatic medicine and she was keen to try a prophylactic aromatic mixture in the period before the approaching winter. I subsequently made and gave her the following mixture:

Eucalyptus smithii—3 ml	analgesic, anti-catarrhal, decongestant
Melaleuca leucadendron—3 ml	analgesic, antiinfectious, expectorant
Abies balsamea—1 ml	muscle relaxant, respiratory action
Melaleuca alternifolia—12 drops	analgesic, antiinfectious, immunostimulant
Eucalyptus dives—4 drops	anticatarrhal, mucolytic
Rosmarinus officinalis ct. camphor—4 drops	analgesic, muscle relaxant
Myrtus communis—4 drops	anticatarrhal, expectorant
Cinnamomum zeylanicum (fol.)—2 drops	immunostimulant, neurotonic

This was made up to 30 ml in total with *Echinacea purpurea* (macerated in sunflower oil), which helps raise tissue permeability and stimulates phagocytosis.

Six drops of this mixture were to be applied to warmed soles of both feet night and morning. (Preferably, this should have been applied three times a day but I was aware this would not be possible for her.)

One week before the end of last Christmas term, she telephoned me and excitedly reported that it was the first time she had ever managed to work through that particular term without being off sick with bronchitis and subsequent further problems.

She was quite convinced it was because of the aromatic mixture I had prepared for her. She is currently using a similar mixture this year, and of course I am hoping for an equally favourable feedback from her!

Numerous books have been written for the general public on the subject, and several colleges teach short courses which are not sufficiently comprehensive to confer a recognized full massage qualification. Only bona fide massage schools can do this. Beard & Wood (1964) considered that, to be recognized as a physical therapist, one must be trained in an accredited educational programme which is adequate to meet both the medical and the physical therapy professions' definition of professional standards:

A physical therapist who gives massage must know human anatomy and physiology. He must understand the relationship between the structure and function of the tissues being treated and the total function of the patient. He must know pathology, so that he can understand how to use massage to obtain the effects that are desired to alleviate the pathological condition being treated. He must be skilled in the proper manipulation of tissues, so that he can accomplish this aim and at the same time not cause further damage to the tissues or harm to the patient.

(Beard & Wood 1964 p. 1)

The main object of an aromatologist using simple massage with essential oils is to enable oils to penetrate the skin. For the lay person, or the busy nurse, knowledge of a few of the simpler techniques is an extremely valuable asset which can only bring benefit to those needing care. Aromatologists (and many aromatherapists) are not qualified to give remedial massage and further training would be required in order to incorporate this into their work.

Beneficial effects of massage

Massage is widely recognized as providing the following benefits:

- it induces deep relaxation, relieving both mental and physical fatigue
- it releases chronic neck and shoulder tension and backache
- it improves circulation to the muscles, reducing inflammation and pain
- it relieves neuralgic, arthritic and rheumatic conditions
- it helps sprains, fractures; breaks and dislocations heal more readily
- it promotes correct posture and helps improve mobility
- it improves, directly or indirectly, the function of every internal organ

- it improves digestion, assimilation and elimination
- it increases the ability of the kidneys to function efficiently
- it flushes the lymphatic system by the mechanical elimination of harmful substances (especially toxins due to bacteria) and waste matter
- it helps to disperse many types of headache (or migraine) originating from the gall bladder, liver, stomach and large intestine, and also those of emotional origin (including premenstrual syndrome or PMS)
- it stimulates both body and mind without negative side-effects
- it helps to release suppressed feelings, which can be shared in a safe, confidential setting
- it is a form of passive exercise, partially compensating for lack of active exercise.

These combined benefits not only result in increased body awareness, but also produce better overall health. Furthermore, studies carried out in hospitals and private practice have shown that massage with essential oils greatly enhances and prolongs the health-giving effects.

Touch and the emotions

Before forging ahead with enthusiasm, it should be remembered that close contact with patients can become 'a psychologically daunting commitment. Staff may need training to deal with the emotions massage may bring up for the patient' (quoted in Tattam 1992). In order not to take on board the patient's anxieties, the therapist (in this case, the nurse) should endeavour to be empathetic, rather than sympathetic (a course in counselling could be of benefit here).

It must be said that not everyone enjoys the thought of being touched (or even of touching others)—perhaps lack of love in childhood or a bad experience is responsible for this. As Burnside said (1973): 'Adults find it difficult to be asked to be touched'. However, with the right approach, once a small non-intrusive movement is made, both the giver and the receiver can come to love the care they are sharing and open up, becoming not only more relaxed in body, but also happier in mind (Worrell 1997).

SIMPLE MASSAGE SKILLS

The most easily acquired skills of massage are:

- Stroking, which comes under the heading of effleurage movements (perhaps the most important for hospital use), for which the whole of both hands from fingertips to wrist are usually used. Stroking is simply an extension of touch and, as well as being one of the simplest, is one of the most important movements in massage.
- Frictions, which come under the heading of petrissage (a deeper and more energetic series of movements than effleurage), and in which either the thumb or one or more fingers are employed. 'Rubbing it better' is nothing other than a simple friction movement. The Hippocratic writings (from the Hippocratic collection 460–357 BC, quoted in Beard & Wood 1964 p. 3) contain the remark that 'the physician must be experienced in many things, but assuredly also in rubbing … for rubbing can bind a joint that is too loose and loosen a joint that is too hard'.

All of us have an innate ability to perform these two movements correctly and safely without the necessity of long training; both are taught thoroughly on aromatherapy and aromatology/ aromatic medicine courses. Two further techniques, requiring greater skill and best learned on an accredited massage course, may be mentioned:

- Kneading (a form of petrissage), involving use of the palm, palmar surface of the fingers, the thumb, or thumb and fingers working together, is a squeezing movement.
- Percussion, including all movements in which the hands and fingers continually make and break contact with the body in a definite rhythm—like the percussion group in an orchestra or band. Vibratory and shaking movements are sometimes included in percussion movements.

These last two movements are usually used on healthy individuals and have little place in the treatment of pathological conditions (Beard & Wood 1964 p. 45). They are not normally employed by aromatherapists, though they are occasionally used by massage therapists, together with essential oils, to good effect—another reason for keeping in mind the distinction between the two therapies. Lymph drainage is also a specialized form of massage, only briefly covered in an aromatherapy training programme.

Effleurage

Effleurage is the basis of all good massage, used not only on its own, and to begin and end massage on a given area, but also in between other types of movements. It consists of two types of stroking movement and normally uses the whole hand or hands, which should mould themselves to the shape of the part of the body being massaged. The strokes are either deep (i.e. with pressure) or superficial (without pressure). Sometimes only part of the hand is used— perhaps only two fingers on a small area.

Deep stroking with both hands is accomplished by moving up the body with pressure, usually towards the heart (see below) and its purpose is to assist the venous and lymphatic circulation by its mechanical effects on the tissues.

Superficial stroking is effected without pressure of any kind, and in any direction (the pressure is so light that the circulation is not directly affected). The perfection of this technique can require skill and long practice. However, in simple massage, superficial effleurage is mostly used as the return movement of deep effleurage, moving away from the heart back to the starting position.

Effleurage is used mainly to relax the recipient both mentally and physically and to improve the vascular and lymphatic circulation. Many different types of strokes come under this heading, but all should follow the basic principles above.

Frictions

Frictions are another form of compression massage, or kneading. They may be performed with the whole or proximal part of the palm of the hand, or with the palmar surface of the distal phalanx of the thumb or of the fingers, which carry out circular movements over a restricted area. There are two types of frictions:

- Fixed frictions move the superficial tissues over the underlying structures—i.e. the part of the hand used is 'stuck' firmly to the client's skin, which is moved over the tissues beneath by the act of making circles.
- Gliding frictions move part of the hand over a small area of the skin surface and may also progress along a specific path.

Frictions are primarily used to break down fibrous knots, loosen adherent skin, loosen scar tissue, relieve tension nodules in the muscles and increase the circulation in a specific area.

Other considerations

Learning the different types of movements is only part of massage training. Equally important is the way in which these movements are performed. Essential factors to consider are the direction of movement, the amount of pressure, the rate and rhythm of the movements, the medium used, the position of both patient and therapist and the duration and frequency of the treatment (Beard & Wood 1964 pp. 37–40). Further factors include the need for full contact with the patient and complete relaxation of the masseur's own hands and arms because hard, tense hands transfer tension (and possibly pain) to the recipient. The mind should also be cleared of any intruding, disruptive thoughts.

The following principles need to be absorbed at the same time as the actual movements are learned.

Contact

No part of the human body is flat; nevertheless, when using effleurage (stroking movements) there should be full hand contact with every part of any large area to be massaged. Hands and fingers when fully relaxed can maintain this contact by following the body's contours closely, draping themselves over the body like silk. The hands should remain in contact with the body for both outward and return journeys of all movements made in sequence. Neither should the hands be lifted off between changes in

movements, because this disrupts the flow of the massage as a whole (Price 1993 pp. 202–203).

Pressure

In effleurage, when using the whole hand on a large area, pressure should always be concentrated on the palm of the hand (Price 1993 p. 202). The fingers should be kept completely relaxed because pressure from them at this time does not provide the relaxation required from effleurage, and finger pressure should be kept for friction movements only. Normally, palm pressure should be applied only when moving towards the heart, with none on the return journey. One of the aims of massage is to stimulate the circulation, and the return of the venous blood is not as easily accomplished by the pumping action of the heart as is the movement of the arterial blood—therefore pressure towards the heart increases the rate of circulation. The lymphatic flow is also increased, ridding the body more quickly of any harmful substances.

Pressure in frictions, using the thumb or finger pads as described above, needs to be firm, but care must be taken to use the whole finger pad and not to dig in with the tip.

In Japanese shiatsu massage, pressure usually follows the acupuncture meridian lines and can therefore sometimes be applied moving away from the heart. This kind of massage works on body energy—not necessarily the circulation of blood and lymph—and the technique should be learned independently from Western techniques.

Speed

This depends to a certain extent on the effects to be achieved. Generally speaking, massage is given to relax the recipient, and a rate of approximately 15 strokes a minute for a long stroke (e.g. hand to shoulder) is considered correct (Mennell 1945) or 18 cm (7") per second (Beard & Wood 1964 p. 38). Anything faster than this can induce a state of agitation, and is used only if the massage is intended to be stimulating.

Rhythm

Uneven or jerky movements are not conducive to relaxation and care should be taken to maintain a smooth, unbroken rhythm (Price 1993). While practising, relaxing music with a regular gentle beat can be of great help in sustaining continuous, fluent and flowing effleurage movements. Frictions should also be performed rhythmically (Beard & Wood 1964 pp. 10–11).

Continuity

Nothing breaks the relaxing effect of massage more than the repeated lifting off and replacing of the hand or hands. Because most massage is carried out to relax both mind and body, the movements themselves (and the changeover from one movement to another) should be smooth and unnoticeable to the recipient. The whole area receiving massage should be covered without a break in continuity, contact or rhythm. Nevertheless, should a stimulating effect be required then staccato-type massage can be effective.

Duration

The duration of a massage session depends on how much of the body is to be massaged, the age of the individual, the size of the body and by no means least, the enjoyment level of the recipient. The massage sequences suggested in this book each last between 5 and 15 minutes, taking into consideration only the size of the area to be massaged. Ten minutes of massage should provide sufficient relaxation to induce a good night's sleep (Breakey 1982).

Frequency

The frequency of massage treatment depends to a great extent on the pathological condition of the patient, as does the type of massage given. 'It is generally believed that massage is most effective daily, although some investigators have suggested that it is more beneficial when administered more frequently and for a shorter duration' (Beard & Wood 1964 p. 39).

CONTRAINDICATIONS FOR MASSAGE

Contraindications for massage depend very much on the type of condition suffered. The lists below should be consulted to determine whether massage of any kind is appropriate or not.

Illness

Whole-body massage is not taught in this book and is contraindicated in the situations described below. Although whole-body massage should not be given, specific area massage (e.g. shoulders, hands and arms, feet and lower legs, face and scalp) is acceptable in most instances.

Infection. The advice of the microbiologist or the infection control nurse should be sought if considering any type of massage for the infectious or contagious patient.

Pyrexia. If the client feels well enough an appropriate specific area could be massaged gently, using oils to give a cooling effect (e.g. include 0.5–1% peppermint in the blend).

Severe heart conditions. Permission from the doctor or specialist must be obtained for whole-body massage.

Medication. If on strong (and/or many types of) medication, specific-area massage only should be used.

Cancer. There is some controversy over massage where this condition is present, and reports from aromatherapists show that consultants can give conflicting advice. Some consultants say that it is not advisable to encourage movement of the lymph, because this may promote migration of the cancer to another area of the body: others say that to move the lymph and therefore encourage the elimination of toxins, and possibly some of the cancer cells also, could be beneficial (see Ch. 15). Horrigan (1991) offers the opinion that, although surface massage will not cure cancer by natural means, equally it will:

- not make the cancer grow owing to an increased blood supply
- not make the cancer spread
- not interfere with chemotherapy and radiotherapy.

Localized damage

In the following situations, the site of any trauma should be avoided, although other areas can be massaged.

Inoculations. The site of an inoculation given within the previous 24 hours should not be massaged.

Recent fractures and recent scar tissue. The healing of scar tissue can be hastened by the gentle application of essential oils in a carrier oil or lotion, or spraying them in a water carrier on to the site if touch cannot be tolerated.

Bruises, broken skin, boils and cuts. If small, they can be covered with thin transparent tape and treated as normal.

Normal physiology

In the following situations, whole-body massage is contraindicated, although specific-area massage is allowed.

Hunger. If 6 hours or more have passed since any food intake, or if the patient feels hungry, fainting may occur with whole-body massage.

Digestion. Immediately following a heavy meal, the digestive system is working full time and whole-body massage could cause either nausea or fainting.

Alcohol. After recent alcohol intake, massage and certain essential oils can intensify the effects of alcohol, possibly causing dizziness, or a floating feeling. Specific-area massage does not have this effect, and the amount of any essential oil used (in the recommended dilution) would be too small to make their use contraindicated.

Perspiring. Immediately after exertion, sport, a long hot bath or sauna, the body absorbs essential oils with difficulty. It is advisable to wait 20–30 minutes before whole-body massage, although a wait of 10–15 minutes is adequate for specific-area massage.

Menstruation. During the first 2 days of menstruation, bleeding could be increased by whole-body massage. However, specific-area massage can help to relieve congestion and soothe any pain or discomfort.

Varicose veins and oedema

These two conditions are often believed to be unsuitable for massage. In fact, they can both be alleviated by essential oils used in light massage. Special care is needed in the execution of the massage, and only gentle, almost superficial, *upward* effleurage strokes should be used.

Varices. The area above the damaged valve should be cleared first with deep, firm, upward effleurage strokes.

Oedema. This condition must be treated by a precise technique. When it is present in an extremity, then the massage should begin with the proximal portion, because it is important to clear and improve the circulation in this area first before attempting to relieve the oedema. Treatment of the distal part should then be carried out, returning to the proximal part at intervals during the massage and to finish with. The affected part must be elevated while giving the massage (Beard & Wood 1964 pp. 38, 60, 104).

MASSAGE SEQUENCES

The following are simple techniques, easily carried out after attending an introductory course.

Introducing massage

The hand is a good place to begin a massage, because few people have a hang-up about shaking hands—we all do it as a matter of course when the occasion arises. At the same time, the 'handshake' technique described below can also be used to introduce the aromas of essential oils. To prepare to give such a handshake, add to a carrier oil a blend of two or three relaxing essential oils which have an aroma you feel would be acceptable to your client or patient. Place a little of this oil in your hands, rubbing them briefly together to distribute the oils evenly, then follow steps 1–3 below.

1. Take your patient's right hand in yours as if about to give a firm handshake (palm to palm—see Fig. 7.1a) and place your left hand

Case 7.2   Therapist: Sue Naylor (aromatherapist and aromatologist), UK

a   Mr P was aged 67 years and was referred to me in October 1996. He had had prostate cancer and had developed bone secondaries. He had not had any lymph nodes removed but had developed severe lymphoedema in both legs, the right leg being significantly worse than the left.

Mr P was on a significant number of medications, which included diuretics. As well as the swelling in his legs, the skin around his heels was becoming very sore and cracked. I discussed with Mr P the need for elevation, good skin hygiene, etc. and taught his wife how to do simple drainage massage and how to apply the two lotions which I dispensed: one to try and alleviate the problem with his feet, the other to apply after the drainage massage. The latter lotion contained six drops each of *Juniperus communis* (JUNIPER), *Citrus limon* (LEMON) and *Cupressus sempervirens* (CYPRESS) in 50 ml of white lotion.

I saw Mr and Mrs P 2 weeks later. There was a significant improvement to the legs and the skin on his feet was beginning to heal. The improvement was so marked that in retrospect I wished I had taken a photograph to compare the 'before' and 'after'. Mr and Mrs P were so pleased with the improvement that they were quite happy to continue with the massage and application of lotion without any further appointments—so long as he could contact me for further lotion.

b   Mrs M was referred to me at the beginning of May 1996 as 'a joke/test'. She had had treatment for a lump in her right breast and shortly after that had developed a very localized oedema in the breast. The consultant in palliative care and the MacMillan nurse did not know what to suggest as an intervention because they did not think medication was appropriate. The referral was given to me to 'see what you can do'.

I dispensed 30 ml lotion with eight drops *J. communis*, four drops *C. limon* and three drops *C. sempervirens*. Because the oedema was so localized I did not think a drainage massage was appropriate. I suggested she just apply the lotion three times a day using gentle circular movements. The client rang me 2 weeks later and said that the lumps were going and the breast was smoother and softer to the touch. She agreed to continue applying the lotion. Contact continued by telephone. At the end of June, Mrs M said the problem was resolved and was quite excited about seeing the consultant to tell him. She decided to stop applying the lotion, but agreed to restart it if the need arose.

c   Mrs B was referred to me in June 1996 to see if I could 'make her feel better'. She was quite poorly and in hospital. She had an unknown primary to the chest causing blockage in the superior vena cava. She also had lung cancer and was suffering from generalized lymphoedema. She was having chemotherapy, and was taking painkillers and diuretics. Emotionally Mrs B seemed quite well. She was most concerned about the discomfort in her back from prolonged immobility, and a developing bed sore on her bottom that she was too embarrassed to mention to the nursing staff. She was also not sleeping very well. Since her priority was her aching back, I gave her a very gentle back massage, and dispensed neat *Lavandula angustifolia* (LAVENDER) for her to apply to the bedsore. I also dispensed 30 ml lotion containing six drops each of *C. sempervirens, C. limon* and *J. communis*, for her to apply to her legs and arms. I opted for equal amounts of the essential oils because there did not seem to be one indicated over another. I did not instruct her in drainage massage as she did not feel physically able to do it but, more importantly, because vena cava obstruction is a contraindication for manual lymph drainage (MLD), and even though I was not doing MLD it seemed prudent to be cautious. She was quite happy simply to apply the lotion twice a day and to elevate her legs as much as possible. I saw Mrs B the next day. She had slept well and the skin to her legs appeared slightly less taut. On this occasion Mrs B wanted her legs and arms massaging so I did a simple drainage massage and then applied the lotion. Mrs B agreed to continue applying the lotion in between visits. I saw Mrs B in hospital again 3 days later. She said the bed sore felt better and when I looked at it, it was beginning to dry and form a scab. She had continued to sleep well and generally felt much better. Regarding the lymphoedema, the skin to her arms and legs was definitely less taut. She was discharged 2 days later and the consultant did not feel it appropriate for me to continue seeing her at home although Mrs B had felt much better as a result of the treatments.

over the dorsum of the hand, relaxing your fingers to 'cradle' your patient's hand (Fig. 7.1b). While you are holding her hand, ask your usual questions such as 'Did you have a good night?' or 'How is your back this morning?' Your patient is bound to notice the aroma and comment on it. As you explain, you can say essential oils are used for massage too, and if the interest is there, you can demonstrate by continuing as follows.

2. Gently raise the patient's forearm slightly, leaving the upper arm resting on the bed. Keeping your fingers in complete contact with the arm, begin to move your left hand firmly up the outer side of the lower arm (Fig. 7.1c); turn at the elbow towards the lateral

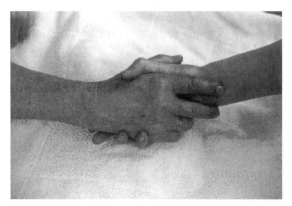

Figure 7.1a

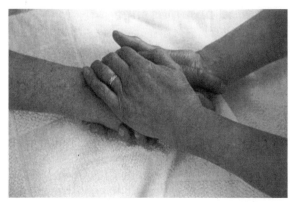

Figure 7.1b

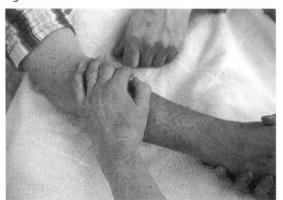

Figure 7.1c

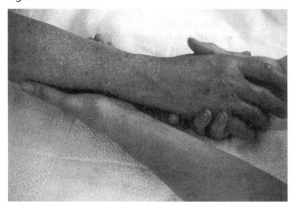

Figure 7.1d

Figure 7.1 The 'handshake' technique.

epicondyle, moving your palm underneath the arm and return gently to the wrist down the inner side of the arm (Fig. 7.1d). Turn your hand, bringing it back to the starting point.

3. Repeat the movement a few times, then suggest to your patient that you do the other hand to keep the body in balance.

Once you are confident and the patient is happy about being touched (and for those who already know about the benefits of massage), the following sequences can then be carried out, allowing the essential oils to enter the bloodstream and give the desired benefits.

Hand and arm massage

1. Start with movements 1, 2. and 3 above, repeating three or four times. Where possible, take this stroke right up to and around the deltoid

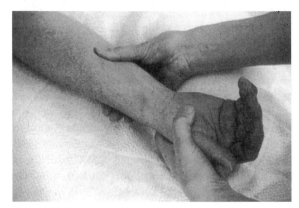

Figure 7.2a

muscle and 'cradle' the whole shoulder, returning via the inner side of the arm, to finish at the wrist.

2. Still holding the patient's hand as in Fig. 7.1a, make large friction circles with the left thumb from wrist to elbow on the upper side of

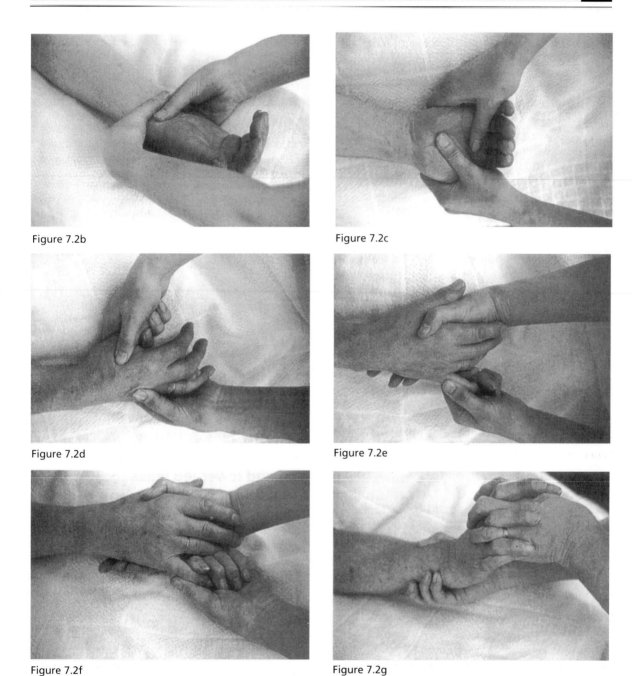

Figure 7.2b

Figure 7.2c

Figure 7.2d

Figure 7.2e

Figure 7.2f

Figure 7.2g

Figure 7.2 Hand and arm massage.

the arm, returning with a single superficial stroke as in step 1. Repeat three or four times.

3. Turn the arm over, leaving the left hand holding the medial side of the patient's hand and placing the fingers of the right hand on the lateral side of the forearm, make friction circles with the right thumb between the radius and ulna as far as the medial epicondyle, returning gently via the lateral side of the forearm to the wrist, with fingers underneath (Fig. 7.2a). Repeat three or four times.

4. Leaving the fingers of both hands over the extensor retinaculum, push the thumbs across the inside wrist firmly in a zig-zag movement, back and forth several times with one thumb in front of the other (Fig. 7.2b).

5. Slide the fingers down until they cover the back of the hand and stroke up the palmar interosseous muscles firmly, using the whole length of each thumb alternately, from finger level to wrist, several times (Fig. 7.2c).

6. Turn the hand over and repeat wrist zig-zags as in step 4, on the dorsal side of arm.

7. Move your fingers down until they cover the patient's palm and stroke firmly between the metacarpals along their full length, right thumb between patient's thumb and first finger (returning via the radial side of the hand) and left thumb between third and fourth fingers (returning via the ulnar border of the hand). Repeat these strokes, this time with your right thumb between the patient's first and second fingers, and the left between the fourth and fifth fingers (Fig. 7.2d).

8. With the fingers of your right hand still supporting the patient's palm make friction circles with your left thumb up the little finger; at the base, turn your own palm uppermost and, using your first finger and thumb, slide down the sides of the finger to the tip (Figs 7.2e and 7.2f). Move to the ring finger and repeat the frictions and return movement. Repeat on the other two fingers, using your right thumb to massage the patient's thumb.

9. Push the fingers of your left hand through your patient's fingers (Fig. 7.2g) and, holding the patient's forearm with your right hand, rotate the wrist slowly and firmly anticlockwise, then clockwise.

10. Smoothly change to the handshake hold and repeat step 1 several times.

To treat the patient's left hand, reverse the directions for 'right' and 'left' in the above text.

Foot and lower leg massage

When learning to massage the feet, one very important factor has to be borne in mind. The foot must be touched or held *firmly*. Many people have a dread of someone touching their feet and in the majority of cases it can be attributed to having had their feet held so lightly that it was tickled or felt insecure and therefore unpleasant.

1. Place your hands across the dorsum of the patient's right foot at toe level (Fig. 7.3a) and move them firmly up the lower leg to the patella. Separate them towards the lateral and medial sides of the leg, returning gently via these to the ankle (Fig. 7.3b), turning the hands again as you reach the toes, ready to repeat the movement three or four times.

2. When you have mastered this, incorporate the following 'sandwich' into the last part of the movement. As you approach the foot on the return journey, let the fingers of your right hand slide across the instep onto the sole of the foot,

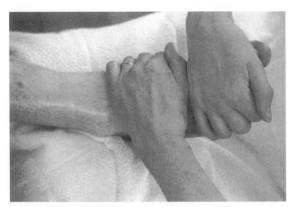

Figure 7.3a

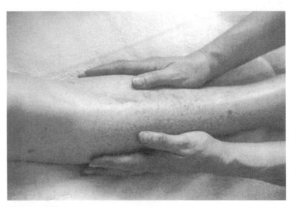

Figure 7.3b

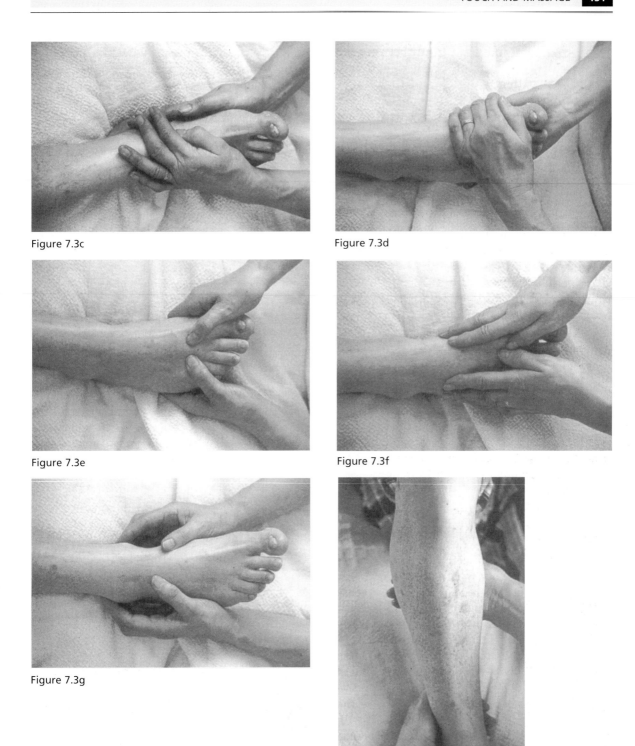

Figure 7.3c

Figure 7.3d

Figure 7.3e

Figure 7.3f

Figure 7.3g

Figure 7.3h

Figure 7.3   Foot and lower leg massage.

meanwhile turning the fingers of the left hand across the dorsum of the foot towards the wrist of your right hand (Figs 7.3c, 7.3d), squeezing both hands together as they move towards the toes. Lift off your right hand only, replacing it in front of or behind the left hand, ready to repeat the whole of movement 1 (with the sandwich) several times.

3. On the last journey hold the foot firmly in the sandwich for a moment or two, before progressing to the next movement.

4. Turn your hands so that your fingers are underneath the foot and with your thumbs carry out gentle frictions on the metatarsals—as in the hand massage (Fig. 7.3e). The frictions need to be gentle because this reflex area of the foot is often tender, owing to poor lymphatic circulation or bronchial conditions (which the movement can help if done regularly).

5. Bring your fingers back to the anterior surface of the foot and move them towards each malleolus (Fig. 7.3f). Take the first and second fingers, pressing firmly, in a circle behind each malleolus (Fig. 7.3g), relaxing the pressure as you come to the front of the foot. Repeat these circles several times. This movement covers the foot reflex point for the groin lymph and is ideal for relieving lymphatic congestion in the groin and increasing circulation in the legs generally.

6. Turn your hands into the position for movement 1 and repeat this movement (together with the sandwich, as in movement 2) several times, finishing by continuing the squeezing movement until you are no longer in contact with the foot.

For the left foot, reverse directions for 'right' and 'left' in the text.

Should you wish to increase leg circulation further, ask the patient to bend her knee, placing the foot flat on the bed. Sit on the toes (place a towel over them to protect your clothes from the oil if necessary) and continue as follows:

7. Carry out movement 1 several times, but only from and to the ankle.

8. Slide one hand on to the tendo calcaneus and move it with pressure up the gastrocnemius muscle, following with the other hand, then the

first hand again, etc.—about 10 alternate strokes in all (Fig. 7.3h).

9. Repeat movement 5 around the ankle bones.

10. Finish with movement 1.

Swiss reflex massage

This technique was devised by Shirley Price when in Switzerland in 1987, and is based on reflexology, while differing from it. Reflexology is 'an ancient technique which makes use of somewhat mysterious connecting pathways or energy flow lines in the body' (Price 1994 p. 59). These culminate in various areas of the body and occur mainly in the feet, hands, ears and tongue, where reflexes representing every part of the body can be found. These reflexes are valuable as a diagnostic aid and the body can also be treated effectively using these points. As in professional aromatherapy, it is necessary to undertake an accredited training in order to be able to understand thoroughly the position, significance and interpretation of each bodily system and each reflex point.

In a Swiss reflex treatment, these same reflexes are massaged, together with a specific dialogue between therapist and client. A bland cream base is used to which are added essential oils selected by the same method as for an aromatherapy massage treatment. The ratio of oil to cream is 30 drops to 30 ml. The treatment is simpler to learn than the techniques involved in reflexology, but knowledge of the location of the representative reflexes is of primary importance before the treatment can be carried out successfully. As with all practical subjects, attending a practical course is the best way to learn. However, the basic principles are described below.

Swiss reflex treatment involves special client participation, including daily practice by the client at home. Without daily participation by the client, the results are approximately the same as they are using reflexology or normal massage; with daily participation, positive results are gained much more quickly than by reflexology alone. Therapists trained in this method at the Shirley Price International College of Aromatherapy have had some extraordinarily positive results (see Cases 7.3, 7.4, 7.5).

NB. Always begin with the solar plexus reflex area (Fig. 7.4a) and finish on the kidney–bladder area (Fig. 7.4b).

1. Apply a very small amount of cream all over the dorsum and sole of the right foot.
2. Carry out foot movement 1 (as on p. 130—but up to the ankle only) and 2, several times to warm the foot, then wrap in a towel.
3. Repeat the two movements on the left foot and wrap in a towel.
4. Holding the right foot by placing the palm of the left hand over the phalanges and metatarsal of the big toe, begin by massaging the whole of the solar plexus reflex area with the whole of the length of your right thumb (Fig. 7.4a) in a circular motion as firmly as the tolerance of the individual patient will allow (if the patient is highly stressed even a gentle stroking will seem painful). Maintain just enough pressure to give the patient slight discomfort until the client is able to tell you that discomfort is no longer evident. If the discomfort is still present after 1 minute, the original pressure was too strong and the movement should be repeated with just enough pressure to take the patient to her lowest pain threshold.

5. Massage (as described above) any reflex areas whose representative organs are presenting

---

Case 7.3   Aromatherapist: Lynn Cartwright, UK

Medical condition
The patient had plantar fascitis—movement-related pain under sole of foot at the anterior margin of calcaneum. Pain can manifest from the lower back down the legs, and can be caused by the overstretching of the plantar fascia due to poor posture or prolonged standing.

Aetiology/presenting symptoms
In R's case the symptoms occurred during lambing time when he had been standing for long hours in cold and damp conditions. The pain was not relieved by painkillers, and unfortunately it was a time when he could not stop work.
    R was normally very fit, was the ex-captain of a rugby team, had four young children and also ran a sheep farm. He leads an active lifestyle.

Proposed treatment plan
I decided to give R a Swiss reflex treatment and a leg massage using the following essential oils:

* *Syzygium aromaticum* [CLOVE BUD] for its pain-relieving properties and warmth
* *Juniperus communis* [JUNIPER BERRY] for pain relief and detox
* *Origanum majorana* [SWEET MARJORAM] for pain and swollen joints and warmth
* *Rosmarinus officinalis* [ROSEMARY] for pain relief in muscles
* *Zingiber officinale* [GINGER] for sprains and relieving cramp.

These were mixed with Swiss reflex cream base for use on the feet (six drops of each in 30 ml) and into hypericum carrier oil (15 drops in 50 ml) for his wife to massage on to his legs.

First visit: Swiss reflex treatment was followed by a leg massage. The heels on both feet were very painful to touch. R found it easier to get off the couch at the end of treatment than it had been to get on.
    His wife was asked to continue massaging his legs and feet on a daily basis. I suggested he rest with his legs up as much as possible and that he visit his GP to confirm his condition. His GP diagnosed lower back pain or plantar fascitis. X-ray and physiotherapy appointments were made. On his way home from the GP he called in at his rugby club and saw the coach, an osteopath, who confirmed the diagnosis of plantar fascitis—and advised R to rest. After 2 days the pain was much easier and continued to abate.
    Second visit (1 week later): Swiss reflex treatment. Although his heels were still slightly tender, they were much less sensitive, and he had been back about his work for 4 days. R's wife continued daily treatments at home and the response was such that he found he did not need a third treatment.

Conclusion
R was very pleased with the outcome. I was surprised how quickly he responded to the oils and Swiss reflex treatment, as two professional treatments and those carried out by his wife were sufficient to cure the problem. The condition has never recurred, and he did not experience any problems during lambing time the following year.
    Six weeks after treatment ceased he received notice of an appointment from the physiotherapy department of the local hospital. He took great delight in ringing them up to say that it would no longer be required.

Case 7.4 Therapist: Shirley Price

Mrs A, who had just recovered from a second attempt on a hip replacement (the healing of the second was helped considerably by aromatherapy), was to undergo an operation in 6 months' time to fuse her cervical vertebrae on account of the severe arthritic pain there. She was reluctant to undergo this, as due to the death of her husband she needed to be able to drive. She wore a surgical collar, which she hated.

On the first visit, Mrs A received Swiss reflex treatment on her feet and was shown how she could carry it out herself at home. The following essential oils were added to a 30 ml pot of bland, non-greasy Swiss reflex cream base:

- 10 drops *Rosmarinus officinalis* [ROSEMARY] for its antiinflammatory action
- 4 drops *Origanum majorana* [SWEET MARJORAM] for its antiinflammatory and analgesic properties
- 8 drops *Juniperus communis* [JUNIPER BERRY], properties as above
- 8 drops *Lavandula angustifolia* [LAVENDER], properties as above.

The client was given the pot of cream to take home for her daily use.

At the second visit 2 weeks later, I was disappointed that no improvement had been made. However, I discovered my 58-year-old client had faithfully been massaging the wrong reflex! This experience indicated the importance of giving the client a marked chart, illustrating exactly not only the sequence of the treatment but also the reflex points to be massaged.

Two weeks later, Mrs A was experiencing somewhat less pain and a slight improvement in neck mobility. The improvement continued over the next 2 weeks and at the fourth appointment Mrs A arrived smiling and wearing a collar homemade from firm foam sponge wrapped in a pretty scarf.

Six weeks after this, with no further clinic treatments, but a visit every 2 weeks to confirm all was progressing well, she had her appointment with the consultant prior to the operation. He was amazed at the change in her mobility and the lack of pain. He asked her what she had been doing, and unfortunately Mrs A was too embarrassed to say she had been rubbing her big toe—as it was early in the history of complementary therapies in the UK, her reluctance was probably understandable.

Case 7.5 Therapists: Shirley Price and Debbie Moore

The case concerns a gentleman who had been in a mining accident 19 years previously. One of the beams had fallen on his shoulder, which was damaged; a rib was broken, which had pierced his lung, so apart from being unable to move his arm away from his side, and walking by moving his feet only 6 or 7 inches (15–17 cm) at a time, he was having breathing difficulties.

He had been under a consultant for the whole 19 years and was becoming progressively worse, rather than better. His wife had heard me speaking on the radio about aromatherapy and decided to try this treatment for Frank. When they arrived, it was obvious that administering essential oils by a body massage would not be the best for Frank. The answer was the Swiss reflex treatment, which was given to him twice a week for the first 2 weeks, once a week for 2 further weeks, once a fortnight for the next month, then once a month and eventually once every 2 or 3 months. The oils selected for Frank, in 30 ml of the bland reflex cream base, were:

- *Piper nigrum* [BLACK PEPPER] for its expectorant, antispasmodic and analgesic properties
- *Juniperus communis* [JUNIPER BERRY], properties as above
- *Boswellia carteri* [FRANKINCENSE] for its immunostimulant and expectorant properties
- *Lavandula officinalis* [LAVENDER] for its antispasmodic, analgesic and general tonic properties.

Frank's wife was taught how to do the daily treatment and it was obvious she never missed a day; after 6 weeks Frank could raise his right arm about 10 cm; after another 2 months this was increased to 30 cm, his shoulders and head were halfway to being erect and his feet were able to take steps as long as his foot.

Six months later, not having seen him for 3 months, I saw him leaving our centre with his head erect and an almost normal, albeit slow, step. When I went up to him, he proudly showed me how he could lift his arm almost up to his shoulder and was looking forward to the day he could comb his own hair.

---

a problem to the patient—e.g. lung area for bronchial problems, digestive system area for constipation (concentrating on the large intestine reflex area, in a clockwise direction), spinal areas for rheumatism or arthritis. Change your hand positions when necessary.

6. Placing your right hand across your body and placing it over the patient's toes, massage in

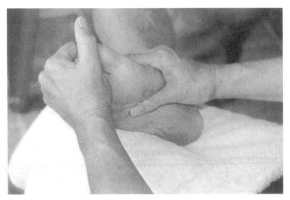

Figure 7.4a

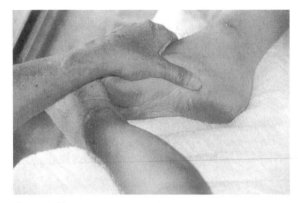

Figure 7.4b

Figure 7.4 Swedish reflex massage.

a firm circle, following the kidney–ureter–bladder line (Fig. 7.4b) and relaxing the pressure on the return half of the circle.

7. Repeat movements 2 and 3 and rewrap in the towel.

8. Repeat movements 2–7 on the left foot, reversing 'right' and 'left' in the text.

Shoulder massage

As a general rule the tensions and anxieties we feel manifest themselves first of all as tension nodules in the trapezius muscle. It is not always apparent as continual pain, but can be felt immediately when someone presses firmly on the precise area of taut muscular fibres we call nodules.

The best time to give a shoulder massage (unless needed at any time to dissipate a headache) is just before retiring; this not only hastens sleep itself, but ensures a more relaxed body during slumber, which in turn puts the body into a healing mode (see Ch. 8).

If a special back and shoulder massage stool is not available, the best position for the patient to receive a shoulder massage is sitting straddled on a chair with a low back. There should be a pillow over the chairback, on which the arms and head can rest. This position is not always possible, and depends on the age and health of the patient. If it is impractical, the patient may sit normally on a stool or low-backed chair. Then proceed as follows:

1. One foot should be in front of the other, the front foot pointing towards the chair, with the rear foot at right angles to it and about 30 cm behind it. Shake your own hands to ensure that they are completely relaxed, before placing them gently over each clavicle of the patient (Fig. 7.5a).

2. Take your relaxed hands (you should see spaces between each finger) across the clavicles, cradling each deltoid muscle and across the latissimus dorsi to the base of each scapula—when your wrists will be pointing towards the spine; turn your hands until the fingers almost face one another (Fig. 7.5b) and move firmly with pressure up the back—one hand on either side of the spinal column—until you reach the clavicles again, with your fingers curving (draped) over the shoulders as at the start. Repeat this three or four times.

3. Keeping your fingers on each clavicle, make friction movements with your thumbs across the upper trapezius from the neck to the acromion process (Fig. 7.5c) and repeat this several times.

4. Still keeping fingers in same position, stretch the thumbs down the spine as far as they will go without undue effort. Place them in the spinal channels and make friction circles up the channels as far as you can go without exertion (Fig. 7.5d). Repeat this several times, circling several times on any spot where you feel there is tension before continuing.

5. Move round to the left side of the chair (keeping your hands in contact with the patient), so that the patient's shoulder is directly facing

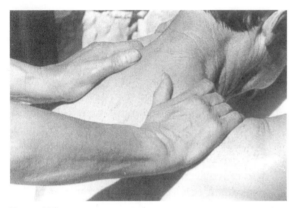

Figure 7.5a

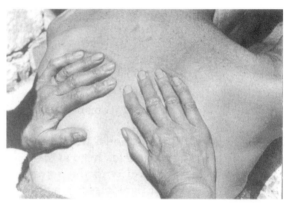

Figure 7.5b

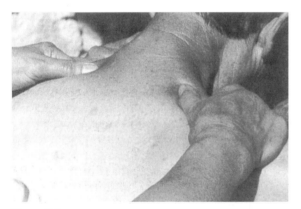

Figure 7.5c

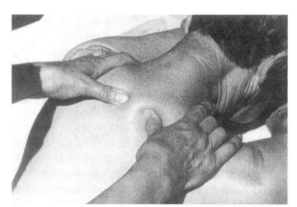

Figure 7.5d

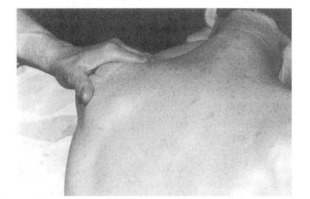

Figure 7.5e

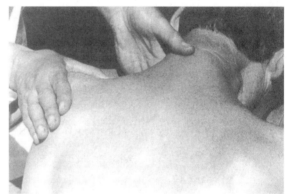

Figure 7.5f

the centre of your body. For this movement your feet should be about 45 cm apart, so that you can bend your knees in order to carry out the movement effectively, without strain.

Open your hands as shown in Fig. 7.5e and, as you place the 'V' of the left hand at the head of

the humerus (level with the acromion process), bend your right knee (swinging the body to the right) and stroke up the deltoid to the hair line—your fingers will be in front of the shoulder and your thumb behind. As you reach the hair line, swing your body over to the left, bending

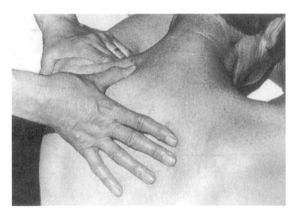

Figure 7.5g

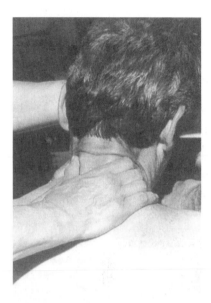

Figure 7.5h

Figure 7.5 Shoulder massage.

your left knee, and stroke up the same area with your right hand as your left hand slides off the back of the neck (Fig. 7.5f). This time your thumb is in front of the shoulder and your fingers behind. Continue this alternate effleurage for a moment or two.

6. With your thumb, feel for painful tension nodules in the deltoid muscle. Firmly make friction circles over the knotty tissue with your thumb cushion (Fig. 7.5g). Use the full length of both thumbs in single alternate strokes if the thumb tires too quickly.

7. Repeat the shoulder effleurage described in movement 5.

8. Leaving your right hand on the shoulder, place your left hand on the patient's forehead and, keeping the fingers of your right hand apart from your thumb (as in movement 5), place it at the base of the neck (Fig. 7.5h); squeeze your thumb and fingers together as you move firmly up the rotator muscles of the neck (sternocleidomastoid and upper trapezius) to the hair line. Without lifting your hand from the patient, relax down to the base of the neck and repeat several times.

9. Keeping your hands on the patient, walk round to the back of the chair and repeat movement 2.

10. Without lifting your hands, walk round to the right-hand side of the chair and repeat movements 4, 5, 6 and 7 on the other shoulder.

11. Keeping contact with the patient, walk round to the back of the chair and repeat movement 2, finishing at the base of the scapula with wrists together, and gradually and gently bring your fingertips to the centre and lift off.

Forehead massage

Starting with the fingertips of the left hand on the right temporalis muscle (the length of the hand lying along the frontalis as in Fig. 7.6a), move the hand slowly and gently across to the left temporalis (Fig. 7.6b), keeping contact as long as possible until the fingertips are almost on the hair; before lifting off, place the fingertips of the right hand on to the left temporalis, laying the length of the hand across the frontalis and moving across to the right temporalis (Fig. 7.6c); keeping the continuity and rhythm, repeat the two strokes with alternate hands for a few minutes. This stroke can also be done in an upward direction, but teaching may be needed to master this (Figs 7.6d–f).

Scalp massage

If you have been giving a forehead massage, scalp massage follows naturally. No further oil is needed because your hands will still be lubricated from stroking the forehead. When executed gently and firmly, massage of the scalp is exceedingly relaxing. If the patient wishes to receive a scalp massage only, gently place on to the face a small amount of the diluted oil you would have selected had you been massaging part of the body. Then proceed as follows:

1. Place the hands on the scalp as shown in Fig. 7.7a and, without moving the fingers through the hair, move the scalp firmly and slowly over the bone beneath.
2. Place the hands as shown in Fig. 7.7b and, once again, firmly and slowly move the scalp over the bone beneath.
3. Move the hands to another position and repeat.
4. Repeat movements 1, 2 and 3 several times.

5. Place the hands as shown in Fig. 7.7c and bring the thumbs and fingers (stroking the scalp all the way) to meet each other at the centre of the scalp (Fig. 7.7d), then gently draw the fingers and thumbs through the hair to the ends.
6. Repeat this movement several times.

Simple back massage

In a hospital situation this should be kept reasonably brief unless it can be carried out on a massage bed of the right height, to ensure the correct posture of the therapist, and prevent backache. Where possible, the feet should be approximately 45 cm apart, the rear foot facing in towards the bed, the front foot pointing towards the patient's head. Your hip should be level with the patient's gluteus maximus, enabling you to reach the shoulders without strain. To follow the directions given here, it is necessary to stand on the patient's right side.

1. Check your hands are relaxed and use the whole hand, starting with hands on either side of the patient's spine at sacrum level, fingers pointing towards the opposite shoulder (Fig. 7.8a). Use effleurage up the latissimus dorsi muscle (covering as much of the back as possible with your relaxed hands), pushing both hands up

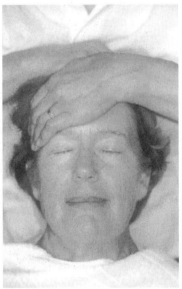

Figure 7.6a

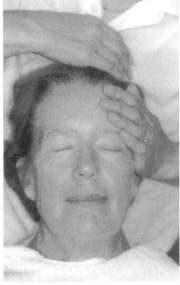

Figure 7.6b

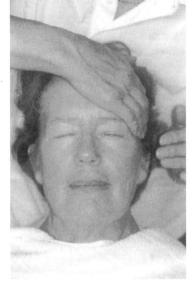

Figure 7.6c

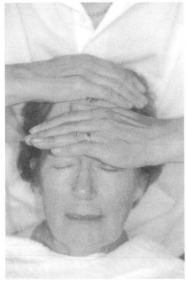

Figure 7.6d

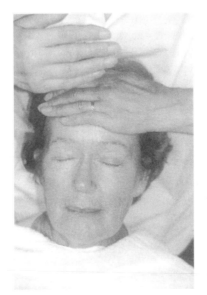

Figure 7.6e

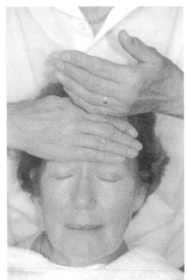

Figure 7.6f

Figure 7.6 Forehead massage.

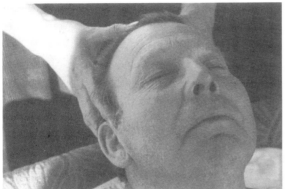

Figure 7.7a

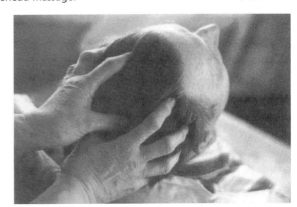

Figure 7.7b

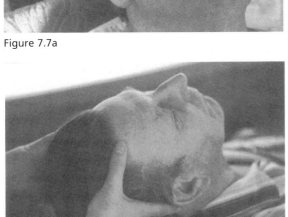

Figure 7.7c

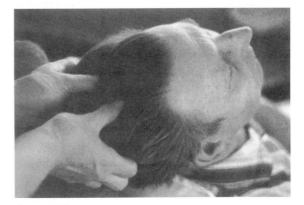

Figure 7.7d

Figure 7.7 Scalp massage.

either side of the back and around the deltoid (Fig. 7.8b). Return with a superficial stroke right down the lateral sides of the body before bringing the hands back to the starting point. Turn the hands and repeat the movement several times.

2. Repeat the same movement, but only around the scapula, several times, finishing with your fingers over the shoulders.

3. Lift up your palms only, leaving your fingers anchored at the clavicle and, using your thumbs, make friction circles on the deltoid across the shoulders (Fig. 7.8c).

4. Place your thumbs into the hollow channels on either side of the spine at the hair line, and make small circles with the pressure on the upward half of each circle. The return journey should be extended downwards so that the circular movement will be accomplished a little lower down the back each time, until the thumbs are just above the coccyx. Repeat movement 1 several times, then turn to face the patient, with your feet 45 cm apart and the centre of your body opposite the patient's waist line.

5. Place both your hands on the gluteus maximus muscle farthest from you (Fig. 7.8d). Move your left hand towards you, to the right gluteus maximus, with pressure (Fig. 7.8e) on the initial lift. As your left hand returns to the left side of the body, your right hand moves towards you to the right side of the body (Figs 7.8f and 7.8g). As your right hand returns to the left side of the body, your left hand moves towards you

again—to the right side. At every move, each hand is directed slightly higher up the body. Continue this two-way movement up to the top of the latissimus dorsi, sliding both hands in a superficial movement down the lateral sides of the back, ready to repeat the whole movement several times.

6. Return to the position required for movement 1 and repeat that movement several times.

7. Using the whole of the length of the thumb and thenar muscle (Fig. 7.8h) push up firmly

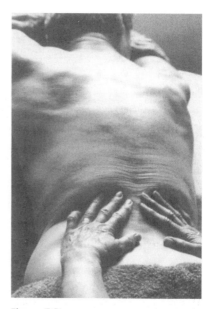

Figure 7.8a

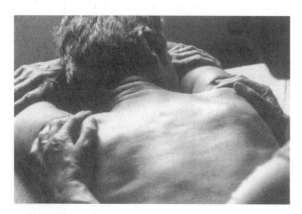

Figure 7.8b

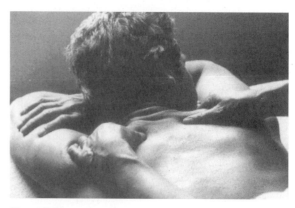

Figure 7.8c

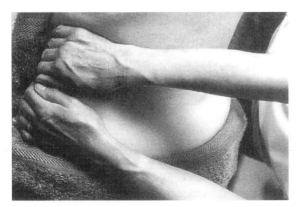

Figure 7.8d

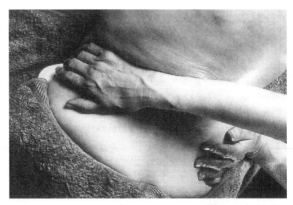

Figure 7.8e

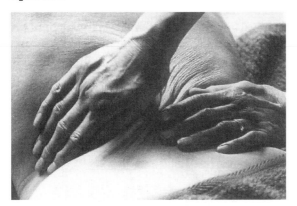

Figure 7.8f

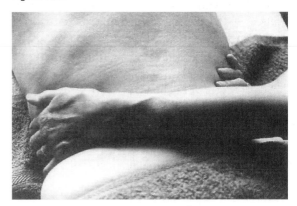

Figure 7.8g

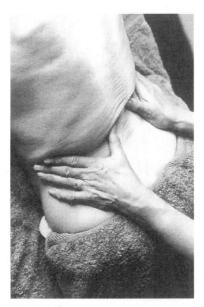

Figure 7.8h

Figure 7.8   Back massage.

from the sacrum past the waist level until the thenar muscle is lying in the waist itself. Take your thumb over to the fingers, then turn your hands towards the sides of the body until your fingertips touch the bed. Do not take your fingers around the body, but when your fingertips make contact with the bed allow them to bend as the thenar muscle comes to meet them, making a fist on the bed.

8. Repeat movement 1 several times.

Abdominal massage

Abdominal massage has been well documented since the beginning of the 20th century as a natural method of relieving constipation (Hertz 1909). It is also used on people hospitalized for differing reasons such as the elderly, those with cerebral palsy, Parkinson's disease and those who are HIV positive etc. (Emly 1993). Movements which follow the peristaltic action of the colon are particularly important. Stand at the side of the bed and place one hand on top of the other at the top of the patient's diaphragmatic arch (Fig. 7.9a). Check your hands are relaxed and think about your palm when directing the movement. Then proceed as follows:

1. Bring the hands gently down the centre of the body until you can see the patient's navel at the tips of your fingers (Fig. 7.9b). Turn your fingers outwards (Fig. 7.9c) and take them to just under the waist. Lift both hands, keeping full contact and bringing them towards each other downwards (keeping palms down) to the pelvic bone. With your fingers in the original overlapped position, gently slide up the centre of the

body to the sternum. Repeat the whole movement several times.

2. Taking both hands (overlapped) to the right iliac fossa (Fig. 7.9d), move them slowly and gently in a clockwise circle up the ascending colon, across the transverse colon and down the descending colon several times, finishing where you began.

3. Keeping your hands reinforced and fingers relaxed, make small clockwise circles, in one big circle, with your palms, following the colon as in movement 2 (Fig. 7.9e).

4. Place both hands on the far, lateral side of the abdomen (Fig. 7.9f) and do movement 5 from the back massage above, but gently, with less pressure.

5. Repeat movement 3. For severe constipation, the fingers of the underneath hand may be

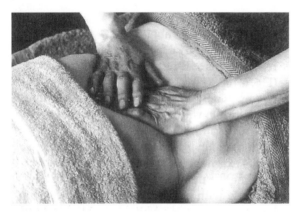

Figure 7.9a

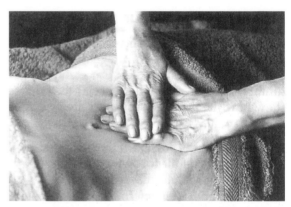

Figure 7.9b

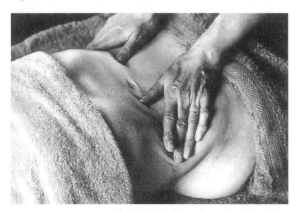

Figure 7.9c

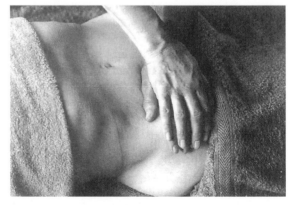

Figure 7.9d

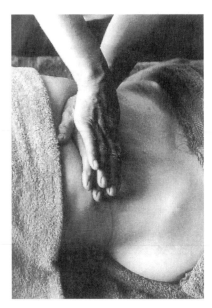

Figure 7.9e

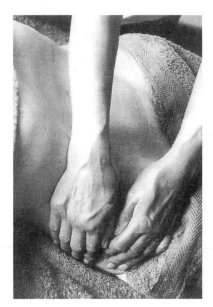

Figure 7.9f

Figure 7.9 Abdominal massage.

made into a fist in order to give a slow, more determined stimulus to the colon.

6. Repeat movement 2.

Pregnancy and labour

During pregnancy normal massage is encouraged up to the 5th month. As the pregnancy develops, the mother-to-be cannot lie comfortably on her tummy, and the following special techniques show how the massage sequences above can be adapted at this stage:

- Back massage is possible if the mother-to-be can be in any of the following positions—whichever she finds most comfortable:
  - semiprone, often referred to as Sims's position; on the left (or right) side and chest, the opposite knee and thigh drawn up so that it can rest on the bed, the trailing arm along the back (Fig. 7.10a)
  - sitting on the bed with legs in a squatting position, resting the top half of the body on the backrest plus pillows (Fig. 7.10b)
  - sitting straddled on a chair as suggested for

shoulder massage above
  - sitting on a stool facing the side of the bed, resting arms and head on a pillow on the bed (Fig. 7.10c).
- Leg massage can take place with the patient in a sitting position on the bed, supported by a backrest and pillows.
- Abdominal massage should be very gentle and is excellent for calming the baby and relaxing the mother. Raise the upper half of the body with pillows. Movement 1 has been found to be very effective during a contraction (Fern 1992).

Summary

Massage has profound benefits, not only for the recipient, and its recent neglect in official healthcare is slowly beginning to be remedied. This chapter has identified the main benefits, as well as the most important contraindications. It has also provided a basic grounding in simple massage techniques, and suggested some of the more useful massage sequences.

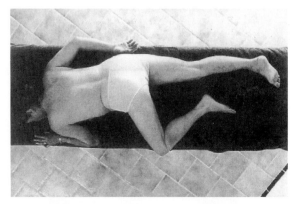

Figure 7.10a

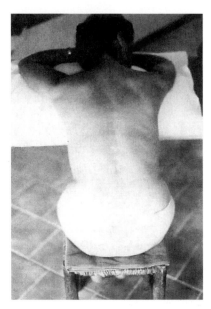

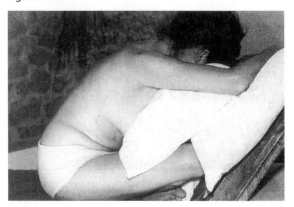

Figure 7.10b   Figure 7.10c

Figure 7.10   Massage during pregnancy.

REFERENCES

Anckett A 1979 Baby massage alternative to drugs.
  Australian Nursing Journal 9(5): 24–27
Beard G, Wood E C 1964 Massage—principles and
  techniques. Saunders, London
Breakey B 1982 An overlooked therapy you can use ad lib.
  Registered Nurse July: 50–54
Buckle J 1997 Clinical aromatherapy in nursing. Arnold, London
Burnside I 1973 Touching in talking. American Journal of
  Nursing 73(12): 2060–2063
Emly M 1993 Abdominal massage. Nursing Times 89(3): 34–36
Fern E 1992 Directorate of Maternity and Gynaecology.
  Practice Group (Midwifery, Gynaecology and Neonatal
  Care) Aromatherapy. Midwifery Procedure no 23. Ipswich
  Hospital
Hertz A F 1909 Constipation and internal disorders. Oxford
  University Press, Oxford
Horrigan C 1991 Complementing cancer care. International
  Journal of Aromatherapy 3(4): 15–17
MacNish S 1991 The soothing touch. International Journal of
  Aromatherapy 3(1): 17–19
Mennell J B 1945 Physical treatment, 5th edn. Blakiston,
  Philadelphia

Montagu A 1986 Touching—the human significance of the
  skin. Harper & Row, New York
Price S 1991 The aromatherapy workbook. Thorsons,
  London
Price S 1994 Practical aromatherapy. How to use essential
  oils to restore health and vitality, 3rd edn. Thorsons,
  London, p 59
Rouse J 1993 Touch for health. Spirit of the Age Spring:
  18–20
Sanderson H, Harrison J, Price S 1991 Aromatherapy and
  massage for people with learning difficulties. Hands On,
  Birmingham
Tattam A 1992 The gentle touch. Nursing Times 88(32):
  16–17
Vickers A 1996 Aromatherapy and massage. A guide
  for health professionals. Chapman & Hall, London
Wilkinson M 1991 The healing touch in an age of
  technology. Massage can soon become widely available on
  the NHS. The Independent October 15: 17
Wise R 1993 Flower power. Nursing Times 85(22): 45–47
Worrell J 1997 Touch: attitudes and practice. Nursing Forum
  18(1): 1–17

8

Aromas, mind and body

Introduction

This chapter explores the connections between a person's thoughts, feelings and immune status, and suggests that the ability of essential oils to affect all these makes aromatherapy worth considering as a truly holistic therapy.

THE IMPACT OF THE MIND AND EMOTIONS ON THE BODY

Throughout the ages, whatever their culture, tradition and background, whether surgeon–barber or medicine worker, people concerned with healing have always been aware that there is a connection between thoughts, emotions and the state of health of the physical body. The following quotation, from an article in the British Medical Journal of 1884, shows accurate observation of the connection between the state of the emotions and physical well-being: 'the depression of the spirits at these melancholy occasions (funerals) … disposes them to some of the worst effects of the chills' (Wood 1990a). In modern times this has been recognized not only by psychotherapists and those in psychosomatic medicine, but also in general medicine.

Can a pessimistic outlook influence our immune system directly? The answer must be yes. The way that we assess situations determines our emotional responses to them. Emotions release hormones and hormones can influence immunity. But it is important to realise that this process does not happen (or need not happen) automatically, without our knowing about it. In the last analysis it is the way we think and feel that triggers the immune change.

(Wood 1990b)

145

These effects can be real, and changes in blood chemistry have been recorded even when the emotions are conjured up artificially, as in the case of superstition. There is a superstition in the theatre, for example, that playing the part of Macbeth will bring bad luck of some sort, such as ill health. Three thousand years ago the impact and influence of the intangible human mind on the material body had been observed and recorded in the Bible: 'A merry heart doeth good like a medicine; but a broken spirit drieth the bones' (Proverbs 17: 22, King James version).

Psychoneuroimmunology

Since the mid 1980s there has been a significant advance in the study and understanding of the connections between mind and body. Previously, the psyche, the nervous system and the immune system were studied more or less as independent systems functioning alongside each other but without direct connections. However, a new scientific discipline, known as psychoneuro-immunology (PNI), has appeared, and a partial understanding of how the brain and the immune system communicate with each other is developing. They are being looked at now in terms of their intercommunicating system of chemical messengers, their interconnections via nerve tissue and their effects and interactions with one another.

The immune system

Neuropeptide messengers produced by the immune system and nerve cells, including those of the brain, provide two-way communication between the emotional brain and bodily systems via hormonal feedback loops. The limbic system (hypothalamus and pituitary), the spleen, the adrenal and thymus glands all have nerve interconnections. Thus emotions are capable not only of directing the body but also of receiving and being modified by information feedback from cells in the body.

Adrenalin and cortisol are two of the many chemical messengers whose release can be triggered by negative emotion associated with sudden or long term stress: these two hormones influence the immune system directly to switch it off (Borysenko 1988 p. 14). Adrenocorticotrophic hormone (ACTH) suppresses pituitary action by stimulation of the adrenal gland to produce adrenalin, which is a stimulator of the autonomic nervous system (ANS). In the wake of research like this, the idea has gradually gained ground that emotional states can translate into altered responses in the immune system: negative thoughts and sad emotions, perhaps resulting from such occasions as bereavement or because of other types of stress, can sometimes lessen the effectiveness of the immune system temporarily. Hence the body puts into physical effect non-material thoughts and emotions—to produce a beneficial healing effect or to inflict self-damage. This idea is echoed by many writers.

The effect of the emotions on health

It has not been possible up to the present for anyone to show a link between a particular emotion and any specific physical disease—'Pessimism is not linked to any particular disease' (Wood 1990b)—although pessimism or depression amplifies symptoms of pain. It can probably be said, though, that the course and eventual conclusion of nearly all disease is affected by non-physical thoughts, feelings, emotions and attitudes, which are in turn influenced by personality.

Studies have confirmed the power of the mind to bring about dramatic changes in the physiology of the body as evidenced in the fight-or-flight response.

Fight-or-flight response

Many thousands of years ago people developed a response to dangerous situations designed to protect the body. This is known as the automatic primary stress response and the arousal system is located in the brain stem. When a person is presented with a threatening set of circumstances, the median hemisphere of the hypothalamus instantly puts into the bloodstream chemical messengers (catecholamines). These, in conjunction with the sympathetic nervous system, trigger a whole array of interconnected reactions—release of steroids, glycogen and adrenalin, faster breathing, increased heart rate, raised blood pressure, dilated pupils and so on—all designed to prepare the body for instant action resulting from the awareness of danger. Today, in modern society, this ancient inbuilt fight-or-flight response is evoked many times, not only in response to short term acute physical risk (e.g. war, traffic, mugging, etc.) but also to threats such as job security, divorce and money problems. Long term stress conditions like these make the traditional response inappropriate: not only does it not do any good, it can actually be harmful to the body it is supposed to protect. The high tech, high pressure lifestyle lived by so many people is responsible for many threatening situations, both chronic and acute, and it is now generally recognized that some, if not most, physical problems in our society have a non-physical component in their aetiology. Helen Flanders Dunbar, one of the first researchers in this area, wrote: 'It is not a question of whether an illness is physical or emotional, but how much of each' (Dunbar 1954).

Anticipation stress

Some life events cast a shadow before them. It is known that students are prone to catch colds at examination times and it has also been shown that such times of stress for candidates reduce the efficiency of the immune system. This is due to lowered production of interferon leading to decreased function of natural killer cells. The effects of stress of this kind are popularly recognized in the case of brides-to-be who may catch a 'bride's cold'. Why stress should have the effect of decreasing the body's defences is not clear, and as yet, unexplained. It is noteworthy that some of the more ambitious students suffer a greater reduction in the immune system defences, perhaps because the examination represents a bigger threat to them (Borysenko 1988 pp. 12–16).

Grief

The effect of emotions on health is recognized by the insurance industry. Statistics exist for various stressful situations which make people more prone to accidents and poor health, e.g. divorce, marriage, holidays, death, etc. They show for instance that there are 50% more deaths than would normally be expected in widowers during the first year after the loss of a wife (even though the suicide rate amongst single men is very high to begin with). Depression following the death of a wife is likely to have an adverse effect on the protective immune system and so on the health of the survivor.

Voluntary stress

While repeated stressful situations may produce ill effects and people may suffer chronic illness as a result, many people joyfully expose themselves to repeated stress with no apparent ill effect, e.g. in sports such as mountaineering, car racing and skiing. This can be explained in the following way: on the one hand, if repeated stress is unwanted and creates unhappiness, then it will have unwanted effects; on the other hand, if the repeated stressful situations are sought and enjoyed, the resultant happiness will bring beneficial effects to the person as a whole. In sporting contexts the euphoria resulting from release of endorphins is recognized, for instance, as 'runner's high'.

Thinking and healing

Using the mind to control pulse rate and breathing, and to bring about general relaxation of the body has long been practised in many different cultures. A few people have mastered the technique to such a degree that they have almost reached a state of suspended animation. This has been documented in people practising transcendental meditation (Benson 1979). In the meditative state the brain waves drop from the β-rhythm to the slower α-rhythm, when the blood circulation is diverted more to the brain and vital organs, with less going to the muscles, the heart rate is slower, blood pressure is lower and little oxygen is used.

All this is initiated by thought alone, effected via the hypothalamus. Hesse, experimenting on cats in the 1950s, found that when the hypothalamus was stimulated, increased activity or relaxation was produced (Hesse & Akerl 1955). Sometimes, as in the case of people suffering a terminal illness, this mind-to-body effect means that healing is possible even though a cure is not.

Today there is a realization that for optimum healing the sufferer must be fully involved in all stages of the treatment from diagnosis to final cure, and it is generally recognized that all true healing comes from within (as demonstrated by the effectiveness of the placebo). Healing is accomplished by mental and physical routes, with primary roles played by the patient, doctor and nurse, while family and friends take secondary supportive parts. As Plato wrote in the 3rd century BC:

The curing of the part should not be attempted without treatment of the whole. No attempt should be made to cure the body without the soul, and, if the head and the body are to be healthy, you must begin by curing the mind. ... For this is the great error of our day in the treatment of the human body, that physicians first separate the soul from the body.

Trust and placebo

Another well-known example of the effect of thought on the physical body is the placebo effect. This happens when the cure or amelioration of an illness is due to the patient's trust and belief in either a prescribed substance (whether or not the substance in question is passive), or faith in the healer, or frequently a combination of both. For instance, it has been shown that dummy pain killers are 56% as effective as morphine in the treatment of severe chronic pain (Chaitow 1991). This remarkable and much-used placebo effect is important in all healing. When people are made to feel better, positive healing thoughts, which encourage the healing process, are generated. If an aromatherapy treatment does no more than make people feel better in themselves, it is at least a move in the right direction, for such feelings put the whole person into a healing mode. Positive healing thoughts in the mind can induce healing reactions in the bodily healing processes.

Similarly the efficiency of the immune system is reduced by negative belief and thought. It is not unreasonable to draw the conclusion that we are, in some measure, potentially masters of our own fate so far as our health is concerned, in the sense that immunity from disease appears to be enhanced or diminished by beliefs, and by the environment in so far as it affects our emotions. 'Immunity is to some degree under mental control' (Wood 1990a). Fortunately the human race is intrinsically optimistic, with a will to survive.

Relaxation response

When we are safe, in a calm atmosphere, we have the opposite of the stress response—in that tension, blood pressure, oxygen use and so on are all reduced. This highly desirable and very important state has been termed the 'relaxation response' (Benson 1975). It can be brought about by many means, including reading, listening to favourite music, contemplating nature and, indeed, aromatherapy.

WHERE DOES AROMATHERAPY FIT IN?

We must now consider how aromatherapy can play an effective and worthwhile part in the mental–physical sphere of healing. It is established beyond doubt that essential oils can have physical impact in that they are bactericidal, anti-inflammatory, antifungal, appetite stimulating, hyperaemic, expectorant, etc. (see Ch. 4 and Table 8.1) and that at the same time they possess properties which can affect the mind and emotions to sedate, calm and uplift.

Table 8.1 Effects of essential oils used internally and externally (from Schilcher 1984)	
External application	Internal application
hyperaemic antiinflammatory antiseptic/disinfectant granulation stimulating deodorizing insecticide/insect repellent	expectorant appetite stimulating choleric, cholekinetic carminative antiseptic/disinfectant sedative circulation stimulating

Case 8.1   Midwife/aromatherapist: Elizabeth Kell SRN, SCN, FP, UK

J came to the antenatal clinic at the Southern General Hospital in the early weeks of pregnancy and was extremely anxious and agitated. She was suffering from phobias, unable to enter a lift at any time and preferred rooms which were light and had windows with very open aspects. It became extremely difficult for J to attend for care because of her anxiety state due to her phobias.

I was asked by her consultant to use aromatherapy with her and the first consultation took place in the antenatal clinic in a quiet bright room. After an initial chat J relaxed slightly, when she felt she could relate to me and trust me. I offered her a hand massage, which I thought would be less threatening for her at the outset and would allow her to feel more confident with me. She relaxed very well, enjoying the hand massage (using neroli and lavender in a base oil of sweet almond). We then progressed to shoulder and back massage with J sitting astride a chair, relaxing her arms on a pillow placed on the back of the chair. The oils used were lavender and Moroccan chamomile in a base oil of peach kernel.

After this she felt much more able to discuss her fears and worries and counselling was able to take place. I was then more able to decide what J's problem was and we discussed how her partner K could help her to cope with her fears. I gave her a tape of simple relaxation techniques, such as breathing and visualization, which J used daily until her next visit. One of her main fears was coming into the labour suite in labour. We decided it would be beneficial to try and use aromatherapy with J in a suitable labour room, which we would hopefully use when she did eventually arrive in labour. This enabled her to become very familiar with her surroundings and with the midwives.

In the early stages J often cancelled visits to the clinic because of her anxiety state. I therefore visited her at home and occasionally when necessary would accompany her to the antenatal clinic. J was referred to a psychiatrist at one point during her pregnancy, but she did not wish to take the medication prescribed at that point. It was decided to continue with aromatherapy treatments and her pregnancy progressed well, although her anxiety state fluctuated considerably. Aromatherapy was used to calm and reassure her.

When she was admitted to the labour suite, I administered back and leg massage (using jasmine, lavender and Moroccan chamomile in a base oil of peach kernel) and inhalation of jasmine oil. She progressed well and surprised everyone, including herself, by remaining very calm throughout. Unfortunately, she did need to have a forceps delivery, but coped extremely well with this. J's feelings were that aromatherapy had a great deal to offer her during her pregnancy and labour. She was delivered of a beautiful baby boy and both mother and baby did extremely well.

They are therefore ideal tools for tackling not only physical problems but at the same time mental and emotional states, especially if the essential oils are carefully selected on a holistic basis.

Olfactory physiology

Speaking at the 12ième Journées Internationales Huiles Essentielles (1993), Professor André Holley of Lyons reported that changes in thinking have occurred about odour reception, following identification of a very large family of genes responsible for coding olfactory receptors (Buck & Axel 1991). Like receptors are grouped together, some specialized for one type of molecule, others more general but with weaker reactions. Considerable advances have also been made in the description of the transduction steps leading from receptor activation by odour molecules to ionic currents generating the peripheral message. Behind this peripheral activity there is a mass of intensely active neurons, involved in such things as memory of odours. Memory is distributed all over the brain, not just in one area, but studies on olfactory memory have revealed new properties of the olfactory bulb in the process of memory storage and it is thought that odour memories probably reside in the olfactory bulb and are modified by other information. Olfactive sensitivity could be dependent on environment.

The nose has two distinct functions, one to condition the air inhaled in preparation for its journey into the lungs, and another to act as the organ of the sense of smell. An average human breathes about 8 litres of air each minute; this probably means that more than a million molecules are taken in with each breath; a very few molecules of some odours mixed in the air intake can be detected by humans (Engen 1987). People have a very sensitive sense of smell, but have poor perception and have difficulty in describing the quality of a smell because olfactory input is widely distributed in the amygdala and phylogenetically primitive cortex, without direct projections to the neocortex (Klemm et al 1992).

When essential oils are inhaled, the volatile molecules in the oils are carried by eddy currents to the roof of the nose, where delicate cilia protrude from the receptor cells into the nose itself. When the molecules lock on to these 'hairs' an electrochemical message is transmitted via the olfactory bulb and olfactory tract to the limbic system (amygdala and hippocampus). This may trigger memory and emotional responses, which can cause messages to be sent via the hypothalamus, acting as relay and regulator, to other parts of the brain and the rest of the body. The received messages are converted into action, resulting in the release of euphoric, relaxing, sedative or stimulating neurochemicals as appropriate. Some researchers believe that subcortical processing yields behavioural responses without conscious awareness of stimuli (Weiskrantz et al 1974). It is worth remembering that the limbic system developed 70 million years ago and that it used to be called the rhinencephalon (from the Greek words *rhis* = nose, *enkephalon* = brain).

The limbic system is heavily implicated in the expression of emotion, although whether it generates emotion or merely integrates it is not clear (Stoddart 1990). The body can replace olfactory nerve cells, an unusual feature of human nerve tissue, which serves to underline their importance.

Michael Shipley, a neurophysiologist at Cincinnati University, has demonstrated that fibres from the olfactory nerve carry impulses to two small but significant parts of the brain, the locus ceruleus and the raphe nucleus. Noradrenalin is concentrated in the locus ceruleus and serotonin in the raphe nucleus (Godfrey-Hardinge 1993 personal communication). It is suggested that sedative aromas such as *Origanum majorana* [SWEET MARJORAM], *Lavandula angustifolia* [LAVENDER], *Chamaemelum nobile* [ROMAN CHAMOMILE], *Chamomilla recutita* [GERMAN CHAMOMILE] and *Citrus aurantium* (flos) [NEROLI] cause stimulation of the raphe nucleus, which then releases the neurochemical serotonin; stimulating aromas such as *Rosmarinus officinalis* [ROSEMARY], *Citrus limon* (per.) [LEMON], *Ocimum basilicum* [BASIL] and *Mentha* × *piperita* [PEPPER-

MINT] will affect the locus ceruleus, which then releases noradrenalin.

The use of essential oil aromas in aromatherapy treatments is not too far removed from intranasal drug delivery in common use today, e.g. steroid inhalers for allergies, peptides and anaesthetics (Chen, Su & Chang 1989). Lavender has been used in the treatment of insomnia (Hardy, Kirk-Smith & Stretch 1995) (see Ch. 14) and lavender consists largely of oxygenated terpenes, which interact with cell membranes to suppress cell action potentials (Teuscher et al 1990), which might account for a sedative effect. Animal tests using 42 essential oils and their components showed linalyl acetate and linalool from lavender oil to have the most sedative consequence (Buchbauer et al 1993), (see Ch. 4); a serum level in line with intravenous injection was produced, possibly owing to ready absorption by nasal and lung mucosa (Buchbauer et al 1991). The use of an essential oil for such a purpose has advantages, as lavender oil:

- does not have unwanted side-effects
- can be used to vary long term treatment, giving relief from powerful drugs and their side-effects
- masks malodours usually present in psychogeriatric wards.

Warren et al (1987) patented the use of a fragrance that included nutmeg oil to reduce stress in humans. Subjects were stressed with and without nutmeg oil in a fragrance: with the nutmeg oil the systolic blood pressure was reduced and subjects rated themselves as being calmer with decreased anxiety. Nutmeg oil contains the phenolic ethers myristicin and elemicin, which convert to the hallucinogens TMA (trimethoxyamphetamine) and MMDA (methoxy-methylenedioxyamphetamine); a higher than normal ambient concentration of the aroma was used. In their paper on the use of fragrances and essential oils as medicaments, Buchbauer & Jirovetz (1994) draw the conclusion that interaction between fragrance molecules and receptors in the central nervous system (in combination with reflectoric effects) is responsible for the sedation caused by the inhalation of fragrances or essential oils.

Aromas affect emotions

Odours are important in everyday life, though notoriously difficult to describe. We are surrounded—sometimes almost suffocated—by aromas, some natural but many synthetic. There are many natural aromatic messages; e.g. babies are able to recognize their own mothers by the individual odours of the latter, also synchronous menstruation occurs in groups of females. Some messages are imposed; e.g. fragrances are added to almost everything from floor polishes to foods in order to improve sales, buildings may be fragranced to manipulate the working environment, or shops and hotels to invoke a 'feel-good' factor in customers, in airports to reduce apprehension and in cars to reduce traffic stress. These aromas are inflicted on us regardless of our wishes and feelings—like background music—and the short and long term effects on people are not always known, since the emotions produced can be strong and unforgettable. The psychosomatic effect of smell is experienced by most people: the unfamiliar mixture of odours encountered in hospitals, for example, can produce a feeling of dread accompanied by physical manifestations such as sweating, nausea and fainting (in visitors as well as patients), and the memory of the smell of school cabbage can affect the appetite throughout life.

The chain of events involving aroma, emotion and physical change, for so long a mystery, is now beginning to be explained scientifically by PNI, as are the special benefits to be derived from the use of aromatherapy (Table 8.2). Essential oils consist of natural molecules and are to be welcomed, at the very least, as a means of introducing a little bit of nature into the mainly synthetic hospital environment. The use of carefully selected essential oils makes good sense therapeutically and financially, for they are simple and inexpensive to use and no costly equipment is required.

Conditioning, stimulus substitution

Pavlov (1849–1936) showed by experiments with dogs how the secretion of saliva could be stimulated not only by food but also by the sound of a bell which had been paired repeatedly with the presentation of food, and came to elicit saliva when presented alone. Here the sound of the bell was the *neutral stimulus*, which was paired, i.e. associated with, a natural *unconditioned stimulus* (namely the food), and the *response* was salivation; after repeated pairings the sound of the bell, previously a neutral stimulus, became a *conditioned stimulus*.

Classical conditioning, using a visual or an auditory (as above) stimulus, requires many pairings but in the case of olfaction sometimes only one pairing is needed, e.g. conditioning body production of natural killer cells (NKC), fever and cytotoxic T lymphocytes (CTL) to camphor (see below). This demonstrates the connection between the olfactory and immune systems; this communication is important for species survival (Hiramoto et al 1993). Taste and odour pair easily with illness (therapists should note this); this is useful in some cases but an odour may become associated with an unwanted state or illness. Aversive conditioning using an odour has been used to control overeating and this resulted in a significant loss of weight compared with a control group (Foreyt & Kennedy 1971).

Examples of pairing are:

- Hiramoto et al (1991) paired camphor with fever induction and found that a fever response could be elicited by camphor afterwards.
- Betts (1994) used olfaction to control arousal symptoms in epileptic seizures, not only in those who experience olfactory auras, but in any patient who has an aura sufficiently long enough to give them time to apply a countermeasure before the major seizure starts. Essential oils employed for this purpose include lavender, chamomile, ylang ylang and lemongrass; rosemary oil is avoided. Betts says that using the autohypnotic technique it is possible to train the patient to associate intense relaxation just with the smell of the oil, so that the remembered aroma is sufficient to act as a countermeasure.
- Ghanta, Hiramoto & Solvason (1987) implanted myeloma cells in mice and 2 days later injected them with PolyIC followed by 4 hours' exposure to camphor. Every 3rd day afterwards

Table 8.2   Mental and nervous system effects of essential oils mentioned by various authors. The figures indicate the number of mentions

	Anguish	Breathlessness (nervous)	Calming, relaxing	Depression (nervous)	Fatigue (nervous)	Hypochondria	Hysteria	Insomnia	Irritability	Melancholy	Memory loss	Migraine
Aniba rosaeodora (lig.) [ROSEWOOD]	1			2								
Boswellia carteri [FRANKINCENSE]	1		1	4					1	1	1	
Cananga odorata (flos) [YLANG YLANG]	2		1	1				1	1	1	1	
Carum carvi (fruct.) [CARAWAY]												
Cedrus atlantica (lig.) [ATLAS CEDARWOOD]	1		1						1	1	1	
Chamaemelum nobile (flos) [ROMAN CHAMOMILE]	2		1	2			1	1	1			1
Chamomilla recutita (flos) [GERMAN CHAMOMILE]												1
Cinnamomum zeylanicum (cort.) [CINNAMON BARK]			2	3								
Citrus aurantium var. *amara* (flos) [NEROLI BIGARADE]	1		1	2				1	1		1	
Citrus aurantium var. *amara* (fol.) [PETITGRAIN BIGARADE]	2		2	1				1	1			
Citrus aurantium var. *amara* (per.) [ORANGE BIGARADE]	2			2				2	1			
Citrus aurantium var. *sinensis* (per.) [ORANGE SWEET]	2		2					1				
Citrus bergamia (per.) [BERGAMOT]	1		1	1				2	1			
Citrus limon (per.) [LEMON]	2		2					2	1	1		2
Citrus reticulata (per.) [MANDARIN]	3		2	1				2	1	1	1	
Commiphora myrrha [MYRRH]	1			1					1			
Coriandrum sativum (fruct.) [CORIANDER]	1			1				1				
Cupressus sempervirens [CYPRESS]			2	2				1	3			
Eucalyptus globulus (fol.) [TASMANIAN BLUE GUM]	1	1										2
Foeniculum vulgare var. *dulce* [FENNEL]												
Hyssopus officinalis [HYSSOP]	1			1								
Juniperus communis (fruct.) [JUNIPER BERRY]				2				1	1		1	
Lavandula angustifolia [LAVENDER]	4	1	2	3		1	2	2	2			2
Lavandula × intermedia 'Super' [LAVANDIN]	1							1				1
Lippia citriodora [VERBENA]	2		1	1								
Melaleuca alternifolia (fol.) [TEA TREE]												
Melaleuca leucadendron (fol.) [CAJUPUT]				1			1					
Melaleuca viridiflora (fol.) [NAIOULI]	1			3					1		1	
Melissa officinalis [MELISSA]	2		1	1		1	2	2	1	2		2
Mentha × piperita [PEPPERMINT]	1	1		1					2	1		4
Myristica fragrans (sem.) [NUTMEG]												
Ocimum basilicum [BASIL]	4			2				1		1	1	3
Origanum majorana [MARJORAM]	5		1	2			1	3	2	1	1	4
Pelargonium graveolens [GERANIUM]	2		1	1				1	1	1	1	
Pimpinella anisum (fruct.) [ANISEED]												2
Pinus sylvestris (fol.) [PINE]				2								
Ravensara aromatica [RAVENSARA]				1				1				
Rosa damascena, Rosa centifolia [ROSE OTTO]	1			1				1	1		1	
Rosmarinus officinalis [ROSEMARY]				2			2			1	2	3
Salvia officinalis [SAGE]			1	1		1						
Salvia sclarea [CLARY]	1		1	1	1				1	1		
Santalum album (lig.) [SANDALWOOD]	1		1	1				1	1	1	1	
Satureia hortensis, S. montana [SUMMER AND WINTER SAVORY]	1			3	1							
Syzygium aromaticum (flos) [CLOVE BUD]											1	
Thymus serpyllum [WILD THYME]				2	1							
Thymus vulgaris ct. alcohol [SWEET THYME]	2			1	1				1	1	1	
Thymus vulgaris ct. phenol [THYME]	1			3								
Valeriana officinalis [VALERIAN]	1		1				1	2				
Vetiveria zizanioides [VETIVER]	1			1								
Zingiber officinale [GINGER]				1					1		1	

Table 8.2 Mental and nervous system effects of essential oils mentioned by various authors. The figures indicate the number of mentions (*contd*)

	Nervous breakdown	Nervous system balancer	Nervous debility	Nervousness (excitability)	Nightmares	Sedative	Sleep problems	Sorrow, sadness	Stress	Tinnitus	Vertigo	
Aniba rosaeodora (lig.) [ROSEWOOD]				1	1			1				
Boswellia carteri [FRANKINCENSE]				1	1			1				
Cananga odorata (flos) [YLANG YLANG]				2	1							
Carum carvi (fruct.) [CARAWAY]											1	
Cedrus atlantica (lig.) [ATLAS CEDARWOOD]				1	1							
Chamaemelum nobile (flos) [ROMAN CHAMOMILE]	1					1		1			1	
Chamomilla recutita (flos) [GERMAN CHAMOMILE]												
Cinnamomum zeylanicum (cort.) [CINNAMON BARK]												
Citrus aurantium var. *amara* (flos) [NEROLI BIGARADE]				2	1		1					
Citrus aurantium var. *amara* (fol.) [PETITGRAIN BIGARADE]					1			1				
Citrus aurantium var. *amara* (per.) [ORANGE BIGARADE]				2	1	1	1	1			1	
Citrus aurantium var. *sinensis* (per.) [ORANGE SWEET]				1								
Citrus bergamia (per.) [BERGAMOT]				2	1	1						
Citrus limon (per.) [LEMON]					2	1					1	
Citrus reticulata (per.) [MANDARIN]				2		1	1	1	2			
Commiphora myrrha [MYRRH]				1	1							
Coriandrum sativum (fruct.) [CORIANDER]	1		1		1				2		1	
Cupressus sempervirens [CYPRESS]		1		2					1			
Eucalyptus globulus (fol.) [TASMANIAN BLUE GUM]								1				
Foeniculum vulgare var. *dulce* [FENNEL]											1	
Hyssopus officinalis [HYSSOP]												
Juniperus communis (fruct.) [JUNIPER BERRY]	1			1								
Lavandula angustifolia [LAVENDER]	1	1	1	4		2	2				2	
Lavandula × intermedia 'Super' [LAVANDIN]	1			1			1					
Lippia citriodora [VERBENA]				1		2	1		1			
Melaleuca alternifolia (fol.) [TEA TREE]	1											
Melaleuca leucadendron (fol.) [CAJUPUT]												
Melaleuca viridiflora (fol.) [NIAOULI]							1	1				
Melissa officinalis [MELISSA]	1			2	1	2	1	1			1	
Mentha × piperita [PEPPERMINT]											1	
Myristica fragrans (sem.) [NUTMEG]						1						
Ocimum basilicum [BASIL]	1		1	1						1	1	
Origanum majorana [MARJORAM]			1	4	1	2	1		1		2	
Pelargonium graveolens [GERANIUM]	1			3	1		1					
Pimpinella anisum (fruct.) [ANISEED]											1	
Pinus sylvestris (fol.) [PINE]								1				
Ravensara aromatica [RAVENSARA]				1			1					
Rosa damascena, Rosa centifolia [ROSE OTTO]				1				1				
Rosmarinus officinalis [ROSEMARY]		1			1						1	
Salvia officinalis [SAGE]		1	1								1	
Salvia sclarea [CLARY]	1			1	1			1				
Santalum album (lig.) [SANDALWOOD]				1	1							
Satureia hortensis, S. montana [SUMMER AND WINTER SAVORY]	1											
Syzygium aromaticum (flos) [CLOVE BUD]	1											
Thymus serpyllum [WILD THYME]												
Thymus vulgaris ct. alcohol [SWEET THYME]	1			1				1				
Thymus vulgaris ct. phenol [THYME]	1		1			1					1	
Valeriana officinalis [VALERIAN]				2	1	3						
Vetiveria zizanioides [VETIVER]												
Zingiber officinale [GINGER]				1								

they were exposed to camphor again, and these mice had a better survival time than control groups.

• Hiramoto et al (1993) found that injected spleen cells provoke specific CTL. Camphor odour was paired with their injection for 1 hour, and this odour was able to elicit the CTL 1 week later.

A neutral odour can be easily paired with an emotional state, in a single session, so that it will evoke the same emotional state in another circumstance at a later time. This effect appears to be quite strong, and it is not even necessary for the odour to be perceived either during the pairing or when evoking the state; this is likely to be due to olfaction's relative lack of representation in the neocortex (Kirk-Smith, Van Toller & Dodd 1983). In a clinical application, Schiffman & Siebert (1991) found that an apricot fragrance paired with a relaxed state after progressive relaxation later 'triggers' the relaxed state. They claim that this conditioning was particularly useful in the treatment of lower back pain. King (1988) has similarly paired a 'sea fragrance' with relaxation training, measuring the effects of fragrance alone with forehead EMG (electromyogram). Neither of these reports appear to be controlled trials, however, so clinical evaluation remains to be carried out (Kirk-Smith 1995).

Rose & Behm (1994) found that inhalation of the vapour from an extract of black pepper serves to reduce the withdrawal symptoms experienced on cessation of tobacco smoking.

Inducing the relaxation response

When, during a massage, the touch of the therapist is combined with the mental and physical effects of the essential oils, the client is helped to achieve a temporary separation from worldly worries, somewhat akin to a meditative state. The massage itself induces the relaxation response, which activates the body's healing mode and this, in conjunction with the essential oils, is outstanding for the relief of tension and anxiety, both physical and mental.

Whatever the method of application, it is our feeling that most of the healing effect of true essential oils takes place primarily through inhalation (see Ch. 5) via the mind and emotional pathways, and that a lesser part of the healing effect takes place via the physical body. There is no doubt that smelling plant volatile oils can affect the mood and general feeling of well-being in the individual. This is especially true when the essential oils are applied with whole-body massage; the physical and mental relaxation achieved over a period of 90 minutes has to be experienced to be fully appreciated. In order to select essential oils to address the mental, emotional and physical needs of the client it is necessary to take the time to identify the cause(s) of the health problem. It is probable that all essential oils have an effect on the mind as well as the body, although much research needs to be done in this respect—natural unadulterated essential oils have undeniably powerful effects which need to be properly researched and directed.

The influence of aromas on the mind

Consider that aromatics, such as incense, were used first as calming agents to induce a state of contentment. This sounds like one of our modern day tranquilizers, however the aromatic—unlike the pills—is completely safe. As far back as ancient Greece, the physician Galen recommended the use of aromatic herbs against hysterical convulsions. Burning bay leaves were inhaled by the Oracle at Delphi to induce a trance-like state enabling communication with the gods. Aromatic woods were later burned to drive out 'evil spirits'. Even then, aroma was known to have an effect on the psyche.

(Lee & Lee 1992)

Over 70 years ago a series of experiments on rats provided confirmation of the anecdotal sedative effects of some oils: when the oils were dispersed in the air the rats took longer to perform tasks (Macht & Ting 1921). The oils used included lavender, rose and valerian. This method is effective (Jirovetz et al 1992) because of the huge area in the lungs available for absorption of airborne oils into the bloodstream.

In the 1920s three papers were published by Gatti & Cayola which looked at the action of essences on the nervous system (1923a), the therapeutic effects of essential oils (1923b) and the use of valerian oil as a cure for nervous complaints (1929) (see also Ch. 4). They noted that the physical effects of the sedative/stimulant action of the oils were achieved more quickly by inhalation than by ingestion, and that opposite reactions could be obtained depending on whether the dose was small or large. The authors' experience confirms this, having found, for instance, that a low dose of lavender is calming and helpful for sleep, but a high dose makes sleep difficult, even impossible.

Since the 1920s further experiments have been carried out and knowledge of the psychotherapeutic effects of essential oils has grown, but nevertheless much more research is needed; aromatherapy works but it is necessary to find out how. Some interesting studies which have been published, illustrating calming, stimulating and other effects, are given below.

Many patients undergoing magnetic resonance imaging (MRI), or body scans, find it to be a distressing and claustrophobic situation; this expensive procedure can be aborted by a stressed patient pressing the panic button, wasting a lot of time and money. At the Memorial Sloan-Kettering Hospital in New York, 'applespice' fragrance (constituents unknown) is used to calm patients receiving whole-body scans. Redd et al (1994) administered bursts of heliotropine (a vanilla-like scent) to patients undergoing this procedure and this reduced recalled anxiety by 63% in those who liked the smell. The calming brought about was thought to be attributable to the pleasing effect of the aroma, as pleasant conditions make stress more bearable.

Work by Professor Ammen at Tübingen University has shown that rosemary containing 39% 1,8-cineole was refreshing and improved locomotor activity in mice (Buchbauer 1988). According to Dember & Warm of the University of Cincinnati (New Scientist 1991), people do much better in a task that requires sustained attention if they receive regular puffs of an aroma. The test of concentration involved staring for 40 minutes at a pattern on a computer screen and hitting a key whenever the pattern changed very slightly. People generally did well to begin with, but performance eventually fell off and the fragrance effect was likened to a mild dose of caffeine. Peppermint was found to be stimulating, and lily of the valley relaxing.

The effects of peppermint have also been investigated at the Catholic University of America in Washington DC, where changes found in brainwave patterns were associated with alertness. It was also shown that the peppermint aroma enhanced the sensory pathway for visual detection, which allowed the subjects more control over their allocation of attention (Parasuraman 1991). This confirms the traditional use of peppermint oil in aromatherapy.

Schab (1990) found that presence of an ambient aroma during the process of learning words and at the later testing gave a 50% better recall than when an aroma was not present: Smith, Standing & Deman (1992) had a similar result. Another study showing that aromas can influence the way people think and behave was carried out by Baron (1990) where subjects were put in a room that was intermittently fragranced with air-freshener; under these conditions these people set themselves higher goals, were more inclined to negotiate in a friendly manner and were able to resolve conflicts more successfully.

In the early 1990s some patients at the Middlesex Hospital intensive therapy unit (ITU) were assessed for the effects of aromatherapy and massage on post-cardiac surgery patients (see Ch. 13). Foot massage for 20 minutes with and without the use of neroli essential oil on day 1 (postoperative) showed that significant physiological benefit was limited to respiratory rate as an immediate effect of massage. A further follow-up questionnaire on day 5 (postoperative) showed a marked reduction in anxiety compared with a control group using a bland vegetable oil, and indicated a trend towards greater and more lasting psychological benefit (Stevenson 1994).

Physiological effect of aroma

Klemm et al (1992) studied the physiological responses of 16 young women to aromas from seven essential oils (birch tar, galbanum, heliotropine, jasmine, lavender, lemon and peppermint); their responses were assessed by

EEG (electroencephalogram) recordings from 19 locations on their scalps. Topographic maps were plotted from the amplitude spectra in four frequency bands: delta (1–4 Hz), theta (4–8 Hz), alpha (8–13 Hz) and beta (13–30 Hz). Subjective responses to the odours differed, but the most consistently arousing and strong odours included galbanum, lavender, lemon and peppermint, with heliotropine being classed as weak. The most pleasant odours were lemon and peppermint, while birch tar, galbanum and lavender were consistently unpleasant. EEG map changes occurred in one or more frequency bands in each subject in response to one or more of the odours, and sometimes even occurred with weak odours and when the subject seemed unaware of the odour's presence. The most consistent responses to odours were in the theta frequency band, the odours causing the greatest increase being jasmine, lavender and lemon. All odours used affected the EEG in at least some subjects, and all subjects responded to at least some odours.

NB. The essential oils used in these tests were not identified; for example, the term lavender may cover oils from several quite different plants; it is hard to imagine that true lavender oil (*Lavandula angustifolia*) could consistently be rated as unpleasant, whereas it is possible that *L. latifolia* or *L. stoechas* could merit this description. That said, subjective reactions to odours do vary according to personal preference as well as the concentration and aroma make-up; lavender was found to be not pleasant in some tests (Klemm et al 1992, Lorig & Roberts 1990) but to be pleasant in others (Torii et al 1988); there are similar findings with jasmine; this should be taken into consideration when intending to put essential oils into the air for therapeutic purposes.

Children

The sense of smell becomes important to children with severe learning difficulties who may have diminished hearing and sight, and essential oils can be used to make their life easier and more friendly. Fragrances have been used on wrist bands to identify carers, each with their own aroma, to identify the child's possessions and to locate areas, rooms and facilities (Sanderson, Harrison & Price 1991).

The elderly

Aromas are well accepted in homes for the elderly, where they can create a pleasant atmosphere, either stimulating or relaxing, and some aromas may create an ambience which will bring old memories to the fore, possibly sparking off nostalgic conversation between the residents, with obvious benefits.

Anosmia

Not every person can smell every aroma. Unlike vision (where differences between people can be as obvious as the need for spectacles or a white stick), there is no easy means of recognizing differences in the ability to smell. Aromas are made up of individual chemicals and each cilium is equipped with uniquely contoured depressions into which a single aroma molecule can fit, somewhat like a jigsaw puzzle. However, if the appropriate 'docking' depression for the molecule being inhaled is absent, that smell will not be registered. Only when the molecule is keyed in is a specific signal generated.

Total, specific and temporary anosmia

Anosmia, the absence of sense of smell, can be total (where nothing is smelt at all), specific (an inability to register certain smells) or temporary. Almost everyone suffers from some form of the latter, and probably each of us has about five of these specific anosmias. It is interesting that about 5% of people are insensitive to the sweaty smell notes and, while about 50% of people are anosmic to androstenone, musk is almost universally noticed. Some aromas have exceptionally low detection thresholds (e.g. those of grapefruit and green pepper). It is a fact that there are differences between individuals in the perception of odours, even in young adults, who constitute the most consistent age group (Doty 1991), but these differences are due to more than genetic anosmias, as shown by experiments revealing that repeated exposures can alter detection thresholds (Wysocki, Dorries & Beauchamp 1989).

Temporary anosmia may be caused by colds, rhinitis and sinusitis, and results in a loss of taste. There are four types of taste cells (salt, bitter, sour and sweet) although appreciation of food flavour does not depend solely on these but also on food texture, acidity/alkalinity, hot/cold and the trigeminal nerve, and also chiefly on smell. The author remembers a case of chronic sinusitis (suffered for 17 years), when even after an operation the client was unable to smell his wife's cooking—his main cause for concern! After three treatments he was able to detect *Mentha × piperita*, one of the essential oils in the mix used (which also included *Eucalyptus globulus* and *Ocimum basilicum*). After 6 months he had recovered his sense of smell sufficiently to recognize some of the gastronomic aromas greeting him on his return from work.

Effect of aroma during sleep

The aromas of essential oils have measurable physiological effects on humans while asleep. Ten participants were monitored every 3 minutes to see whether any physiological changes occurred when they were subjected to 3 minute periods either of air alone or of peppermint odour during stage two sleep. The results revealed conclusively that humans do react behaviorally, autonomically and centrally to the aroma of essential oil of peppermint administered while sleeping. Significant differences in responsivity to odour periods versus non-odour periods were found for EEG, EMG, and heart rate as well as behavioural changes (Badia et al 1990).

Does anosmia, sleep or unawareness negate aromatherapy?

If a person is incapable of smelling an aroma, does this mean that aromatherapy will not be effective? There is no definitive answer to this question, but many aromatherapists believe that prolonged use of essential oils will restore the

sense of smell in some cases. This is in line with some surprising recent findings which indicate that in both humans and animals possessing specific anosmia, the sensitivity to some odours can be restored by repeated exposure to these odours (Holley 1993, Van Toller & Dodd 1992).

Nasel et al (1994) in a study noted an increase of cerebral blood flow in humans following inhalation of 1,8-cineole (found in eucalyptus and rosemary essential oils), and a similar result was obtained with an anosmic person. Although not concerned with anosmia, tests by Kirk-Smith & Booth (1990) are interesting to aromatherapists in that they used a fragrance at such a low level as to be imperceptible to the subjects, and found specific mood changes in both men and women rating their own mood compared with a non-perfume situation.

The results obtained in these tests point to the result that inhaled fragrances do have effects on humans:

- when the aroma is at an imperceptible level, and not noticeable
- whether the subject is anosmic or not
- when the aroma is not being consciously registered
- whether asleep or awake.

Therefore it can be concluded that everyone, anosmic or not, conscious of the aroma or not, awake or not, is likely to benefit from aromatherapeutic treatment.

Smell adaptation

It is a common assumption that the sense of smell, more than other modalities, is readily affected by adaptation as a result of continued exposure to a stimulus. For example, a room one has just entered may have a noticeable odour, but this is no longer apparent after a short while; presumably the odour quickly disappears because receptors fatigue and decrease their rate of firing in the continuing presence of odorous molecules in the mucus (Engen 1982). If the receptors do indeed stop firing, then the question arises of whether aromas can bring about changes in the client in these circumstances.

Engen goes on to say that, although olfactory adaptation is apparently commonly experienced, its effect has been exaggerated. He points out that animals using olfactory cues to find a mate would be frustrated if the cue should disappear halfway there. Broad experience in the field of aromatherapy massage says that the aromas are indeed effective throughout the treatment, even though the quality of perception at the end of the treatment may well be different from that at the beginning.

Trials

When the olfactory sense and odours are used therapeutically in clinical contexts they may be working in different ways at the same time. For example, lavender oil may act pharmacologically as a light sedative; it may also be alerting, simply by being there as a stimulus; it may be creating positive feelings because it is pleasant; it may aid recall of past personal situations, positive or negative; and it may have connotations due to social expectations, e.g. connoting health or cleanliness (Kirk-Smith 1995). The placebo effect has to be taken into account when conducting trials using aromas, because the memory, attitude and expectations of the subject may modify the outcome, in addition to any effects of the aroma employed. Although there are difficulties in carrying out trials using aromas, and it can be difficult to assess any results obtained because so many factors other than the aroma may impinge on the situation, aromatherapists should not be deterred from embarking on clinical trials. The use of olfaction in therapy—aromatherapy—is bound to increase and it is imperative that aromatherapy is put on a surer footing than at present; this can best be done by the thousands of therapists currently in practice. With a little expert help in setting up a simple trial, much useful information could be gained in a relatively short time. Kirk-Smith (1995) in his review of therapeutic processes involving olfaction agrees that further clinical evaluation of olfaction in therapy is needed, but trials involve many skills (therapeutic and scientific), and expectations or perceptions about the odour, as well as pleasantness, must be taken into account when predicting effects. It is not a simple matter to ascribe any reported benefits from the use of an aroma directly to that aroma.

Summary

Great advances have been made in our knowledge of the interactions of the mind, emotions, nervous system and immune system, and there is growing recognition of their combined impact on general health. Essential oils have an effect on everyone and have an important role to play in bringing about a state of relaxation, which can favour healing, and they are effective even during sleep or unawareness of their presence; everyone is capable of deriving benefit from aromatherapy.

REFERENCES

Badia P, Wesensten N, Lammers W, Culpepper J, Harsh J 1990 Responsiveness to olfactory stimuli presented in sleep. Physiology and Behaviour 48(1) (Jul): 87–90

Baron R A 1990 Environmentally induced positive affect: its impact on self efficacy, task performance, negotiation and conflict. Journal of Applied Social Psychology 20: 368–384

Benson H 1975 The relaxation response. Morrow, New York

Benson H 1979 The mind/body effect. Simon & Schuster, New York

Betts T 1994 Sniffing the breeze. Aromatherapy Quarterly 40 (Spring): 19–22

Borysenko J 1988 Mending the mind, mending the body. Bantam, Toronto

Buchbauer G 1988 Aromatherapy: do essential oils have therapeutic properties? In: Proceedings of the Beijing International Conference on Essential Oils, Flavours, Fragrances and Cosmetics. International Federation of Essential Oils and Aroma Trades, London

Buchbauer G, Jirovetz L 1994 Aromatherapy—use of fragrances and essential oils as medicaments. Flavour & Fragrance Journal 9: 217–222

Buchbauer G, Jirovetz L, Jäger W, Dietrich H, Plank C, Karamat E 1991 Aromatherapy: evidence for sedative effects of the essential oil of lavender after inhalation. Zeitschrift für Naturforschung 46c: 1067–1072

Buchbauer G, Jirovetz L, Jäger W, Plank C, Dietrich H 1993 Fragrance compounds and essential oils with sedative effects upon inhalation. Journal of Pharmaceutical Sciences 82(6): 660–664

Buck L, Axel R 1991 A novel multigene family may encode odorant receptors: a molecular basis for odor recognition. Cell 65: 175–187

Chaitow L 1991 Mind your immunity. Here's Health October: 19–20

Chen Y W, Su K S E, Chang S 1989 Nasal systemic drug delivery. Dekker, New York

Doty X 1991 Olfactory system. In: Gerchell T V et al (eds) Smell and taste in health and disease. Raven Press, New York, pp 175–203

Dunbar H F 1954 Emotions and bodily changes, 4th edn. Columbia University Press, New York

Engen T 1982 The perception of odours. Academic Press, New York

Engen T 1987 Remembering odors and their names. American Scientist 75: 497–502

Foreyt J P, Kennedy W A 1971 Treatment of overweight by aversion therapy. Behaviour Research and Therapy 9: 29–34

Gatti G, Cayola R 1923a L'azione delle essenze sul sistema nervoso. Rivista Italiana delle Essenze e Profumi 5(12): 133–135

Gatti G, Cayola R 1923b Azione terapeutica degli olii essenziali. Rivista Italiana delle Essenze e Profumi 5: 30–33

Gatti G, Cayola R 1929 L'essenza di valeriana nella cura delle malattie nervose. Rivista Italiana delle Essenze e Profumi 2: 260–262

Ghanta V K, Hiramoto R N, Solvason H B 1987 Influence of conditioned natural immunity on tumour growth. Annals of the N Y Academy of Science 496: 637–646

Hardy M, Kirk-Smith M, Stretch D 1995 Replacement of chronic drug treatment of insomnia in psychogeriatric patients by ambient odour. Lancet 346: 701

Hesse W R, Akerl K 1955 Experimental data on the role of the hypothalamus in mechanisms of emotional behaviour. American Medical Association Archives of Neurology and Psychiatry 73: 127–129

Hiramoto R N, Ghanta V K, Rogers C, Hiramoto N 1991 Conditioning fever: a host defence reflex response. Life Science 49: 93–99

Hiramoto R N, Hsueh C M, Rogers C F, Demissie S, Hiramoto N S, Soong S J, Ghanta V K 1993 Conditioning of the allogenic cytotoxic lymphocyte-response. Pharmacology Biochemistry and Behaviour 44(2): 275–280

Holley A 1993 Actualité du mécanisme de l'olfaction. In: 12èmes Journées Internationales Huiles Essentielles. Istituto Tetrahedron, Milano, pp 21–27

Jirovetz L, Buchbauer G, Jäger W, Woidich A, Nikiforov A 1992 Analysis of fragrance compounds in blood samples of mice by gas chromatography, mass spectrometry, GC/FTIR and GC/AES after inhalation of sandalwood oil. Biomedical Chromatography 6(3) (May/June): 133–134

King J R 1988 Anxiety reduction using fragrances. In: Van Toller S, Dodd G H (eds) Perfumery: the psychology and biology of fragrance. Chapman & Hall, London, pp 147–165

Kirk-Smith M D 1995 Possible psychological and physiological processes in aromatherapy. In: Aroma 95 One body–one mind conference proceedings, Aromatherapy Publications, Brighton, pp 92–103

Kirk-Smith M D, Booth D A 1990 The effect of five odorants on mood and the judgement of others. In: MacDonald D W, Muller-Schwartz D, Natynzcuk S (eds) Chemical signals in vertebrates. Oxford University Press, Oxford, pp 48–54

Kirk-Smith M D, Van Toller C, Dodd G H 1983 Unconscious odour conditioning in human subjects. Biological Psychology 17: 221–231

Klemm W R, Lutes S D, Hendrix D V, Warrenburg S 1992 Topographical EEG maps of human responses to odors. Chemical Senses 17(3): 347–361

Lee W H, Lee L 1992 The book of practical aromatherapy. Keats, New Canaan CT, p 125

Lorig T S, Roberts M 1990 Odor and cognitive alteration of the contingent negative variation. Chemical Senses 15: 537–545

Macht D I, Ting G C 1921 Experimental inquiry into the sedative properties of some aromatic drugs and fumes. Journal of Pharmacology and Experimental Therapy 18: 361–372

Nasel B, Nasel Ch, Samec P, Schindler E, Buchbauer G 1994 Functional imaging of effects of fragrances on the human brain after prolonged inhalation. Chemical Senses 19(4): 359–364

New Scientist 1991 On the scent of a better day at work. 2 March: 18

Parasuraman R 1991 Effects of fragrances on behavior, mood and physiology. Paper presented at the annual meeting of the American Association for the Advancement of Science, Washington DC

Plato (3rd century BC) The Republic. (transl Lee D) Penguin, Harmondsworth

Redd W H, Manne S L, Peters B, Jacobsen P B, Schmidt H 1994 Fragrance administration to reduce patient anxiety in MRI. Journal of Magnetic Resonance Imaging 4(4): 623–626

Rose J E, Behm F M 1994 Inhalation of vapor from black pepper reduces smoking withdrawal symptoms. Drug and Alcohol Dependence 34: 225–229

Rovesti P 1973 Aromatherapy and aerosols. Soap, Perfumery and Cosmetics 46: 475–477

Sanderson H, Harrison J, Price S 1991 Massage and aromatherapy for people with learning difficulties. Hands On Publications, Birmingham

Schab F R 1990 Odors and remembrance of things past. Journal of Experimental Psychology: Learning, Memory and Cognition 16: 648–655

Schiffman S S, Siebert J M 1991 New frontiers in fragrance use. Cosmetics and Toiletries 106(6): 39–45

Schilcher H 1984 Ätherische Öle—Wirkungen und Nebenwirkungen. Deutsche Apotheker Zeitung 124: 1433

Smith D G, Standing L, Deman A 1992 Verbal memory elicited by ambient odour. Perceptual and Motor Skills 74(2): 339–343

Stevenson C J 1994 The psychophysiological effects of aromatherapy massage following cardiac surgery. Complementary Therapies in Medicine 2: 27–35

Stoddart D M 1990 The scented ape. Cambridge University Press, Cambridge, p 132

Teuscher E, Melzig M, Villmann E, Moritz K U 1990 Untersuchungen zum Wirkungsmechanismus Ätherischer Öle. Zeitschrift für Phytotherapie 11: 87–92

Torii S, Fukuda H, Kanemoto H, Miyauchi R, Hamauzu Y, Kawasaki M 1988 Contingent negative variation and the psychological effects of odour. In: Van Toller S, Dodd G H (eds) 1988 Perfumery. The psychology and biology of fragrance. Chapman & Hall, London, pp 107–120

Van Toller S, Dodd G 1992 Fragrance: the psychology and biology of perfume. Elsevier, Barking, pp 99–101

Warren C B, Munteanu M A, Schwartz G E, Benaim C, Walter H G, Leight R S, Withycombe D A, Mookerjee B D, Trenkle R W 1987 Method of causing the reduction of physiological and/or subjective reactivity to stress in humans being subjected to stress conditions. US Patent No. 4671959

Weiskrantz L, Warrington E K, Sanders M D, Marshall J 1974 Visual capacity in the hemianopic field following a restricted occipital ablation. Brain 97: 709–728

Wood C 1990a Sad cells. Journal of Alternative and Complementary Medicine October: 15

Wood C 1990b Say yes to life. Dent, London, p 60

Wysocki C J, Dorries K, Beauchamp G K 1989 Ability to perceive androstenone can be acquired by ostensibly anosmic people. Proceedings of the National Academy of Science USA 86: 7976–7978

Aromatherapy in context

9

Primary healthcare

Introduction

Primary healthcare is the first level of contact which individuals and families in the community have with the National Health system, bringing healthcare as close as possible to where people live and work; it constitutes the first element of a continuing healthcare process (WHO 1978). Among its aims are the care, treatment and rehabilitation of those who are acutely or critically ill. This chapter shows how some of the conditions coming under the category of primary healthcare can benefit from aromatherapy.

PRIMARY HEALTHCARE TEAM (PHCT)

Nine out of every ten contacts between service users and health carers take place in primary care settings. For most people, a stay in hospital is a rare experience. Therefore, a health service for all must have its roots in the community—monitoring and promoting health amongst the well, and providing treatment and care for those who are ill (Primary Care Nursing 1997).

Primary healthcare consists of a team, beginning with the general practitioner (GP), who usually has first contact with the patient and can refer the patient to another member of the PHCT, secondary care or tertiary care (specialist, e.g. a cancer care centre, etc.) or, since 1994, to a complementary therapy (aromatherapy is one of the most popular), should this be found to be the best course of action—and should resources be available.

Aromatherapy as a form of treatment is initiated or approved by the GP or the management to whom nurses or midwives are responsible before they introduce it to their patients in the community. Aromatherapists working on a PHCT and wishing to take aromatherapy officially to their patients should present the team with a sound policy and guidelines for the use of aromatherapy in their particular field (see Ch. 16).

Primary healthcare includes practice nurses, those working within a health centre or GP premises, midwives and community nurses. Community-based nurses include district nursing teams, health visitors, those who visit schools, nurses at clinics, family planning nurses, paediatric nurses and nurses dealing with learning difficulties. Mental health nurses, e.g. community psychiatric nurses, also work in the community and may be based within a health centre or GP premises and may use essential oils. All of these people make an important contribution to community-based healthcare, and when the need arises for a specialist in a particular field the healthcare extends to physiotherapists, psychiatric nurses, occupational therapists, etc.

There is a great potential in the community for aromatherapists/nurses to help patients and many are already adding this skill to their caring; 'A significant number of nurses within the health authority are now using essential oils and/or massage in their practice' (Ersser 1990). Several GP practices now have a room where complementary practitioners can treat patients referred to them by one of the GPs and aromatherapy is one of the treatments most in demand. This agrees with the survey of nurses in relation to complementary therapies carried out by the Nursing Times (Trevelyan 1996).

A White paper from the Department of Health (December 1997) sets out three areas for action. One of these areas includes a local drive for quality through teams of local GPs and community nurses working together in new primary care groups and NHS trusts; another includes national standards and guidelines through a new national institute for clinical excellence to give a strong lead on the clinical and cost effectiveness of complementary medicine generally, drawing up new guidelines from the latest scientific evidence.

Perhaps one outcome on the cost-effective aspect will be that the use of essential oils will figure more prominently in community care as well as within a hospital setting.

CARE IN THE COMMUNITY

The elderly

Although community nurses are concerned with patients who have widely differing nursing needs and are of all ages, 'most of their patients, even as early as 1985, were 65 years and over' (Baly, Robottom & Clark 1987 p. 227). Work with these patients can take them into residential homes and day centres for the elderly, although a large number of elderly people still prefer to live in their own homes until necessity places them into a nursing home, hospital or hospice.

Around 25% of all drugs prescribed are for the elderly, many to treat the side-effects of a main drug. If more resources were made available, community nurse/aromatherapists could use their skills to alleviate any secondary effects being suffered, such as constipation, sleeplessness and anxiety (see Ch. 14).

Midwifery and health visiting

Another area where aromatherapy can be of benefit is in midwifery, in the care of mothers during their pregnancy, during labour and immediately after the birth of their babies. In secondary care, the midwife meets her patient only when labour is established, unless any complications have brought the mother-to-be in early. Within the White paper it is expected that there will be integration in midwifery; this is intended to remove the division between hospital and community care by basing midwifery in the community and utilizing the hospital facility only as and when needed. It is also intended to provide continuity of care throughout a woman's pregnancy as she will come into contact only with professional members of her particular team; this is already happening with shared GP care, GP units, etc. As pregnancy in the majority of cases is a normal physiological function it is also more appropriate to care for women in their

Case 9.1 Therapist: Sue Naylor MISPA MIAM

Mrs H (88 years old) was referred to me in March 1997 to see if I could alleviate the backache she was experiencing. She had a number of medical problems including angina and osteoporosis and had been diagnosed as having breast cancer the year before. The tumours had been removed by surgery about 18 months before I saw her; she had not had any radio- or chemotherapy, but was put on tamoxifen.

A few months previous to my seeing her, her legs had become swollen, especially the left leg. Although she was referred to me about her backache, Mrs H asked if there was anything I could do to help her legs as there was no specific intervention being done. She was quite distressed about this because she said her leg ached and often hurt. It was also leaking fluid, making movement and walking very difficult. I asked her if she would like me to show her a simple drainage technique she could do for herself. Mrs H was keen to try anything.

As with other clients, I instructed her on the need for elevation, good skin care, etc. I also taught her a simple drainage technique. After a week, Mrs H said there was no noticeable difference to her legs, but she was quite happy to continue with the massage. At this stage I dispensed 60 ml lotion containing 10 drops each of *Juniperus communis* (juniper), *Cupressus semperivens* (cypress), *Citrus limon* (lemon) and *Pelargonium graveolens* (geranium). I decided to increase the concentration slightly from that which I usually use because the condition was so bad. I instructed her on how to apply the lotion.

I saw her again 2 weeks later. There was a very slight improvement to the area just above her left ankle, but otherwise still a lot of swelling. However, she commented that her legs were no longer leaking, and when she thought about it she said it had stopped weeping some time after she started the drainage massage. She also said that often in an evening her ankles ached, but after she had done the massage and applied the lotion the ache went away.

As we discussed her legs she told me that she did the drainage massage regularly and at the same time went through the motions of what she did. I realized then that she needed correction on her technique as she had slipped into more of an effleurage type massage which was also deeper than a drainage one. We spent some time ensuring she was doing it properly. Because her legs were so swollen and it was difficult to tell what improvement there was, we decided to measure her leg at different points. This was done really out of curiosity so that we could see

if there was any difference the next time I saw her.

Her left foot at its narrowest measured 28.5 cm, just above the ankle 28.5 cm and just below the knee 32.5 cm. I saw her a week and a half later, during which time she applied the lotion three times a day after the massage. When I saw her, the change in her leg was dramatic. She was thrilled and remarked on how much better they were. Whilst her leg was still swollen, there was indeed a dramatic change in both size and contour. The change was borne out by the measurements, which were 24 cm at the narrowest part of the foot, 27 cm above the ankle and 30.5 cm just below the knee.

Mrs H said her legs no longer ached, and that she was finding it noticeably easier to walk. She also had more mobility in her ankle. She rotated her ankle, which was something she had been unable to do previously. She was also able to wear shoes that she had not worn for some time because they had not fitted her. She also said she no longer needed to put a pillow under her knees at night, which she had been doing to try and make them comfortable. All her visitors had commented on the improvement in her legs.

Mrs H asked if it would be all right to stop doing the massage because, whilst she did not mind doing it, she did find it difficult. I advised her that stopping was probably not a good idea as the massage would be needed to maintain improvement. However, she felt she wanted to stop 'just for a few days'. Whilst reluctant for her to do this, I was curious as to what would happen. Mrs H decided she would stop the massage but would continue to apply the lotion for a few days. I saw her a week later. She was quite upset because, whilst not back to its original dimensions, the leg had definitely swollen again. I felt this was probably due to the discontinuation of the massage, although Mrs H said that because of her new-found mobility she had been doing a lot of standing and walking. She agreed to restart doing the massage.

I saw Mrs H after another week. There was a slight improvement in her leg. I saw her after another week but she had fallen during the week and had broken bones in both feet. She had plaster up to her knee and was having to use a Zimmer frame. She was walking in a very lop-sided manner, and her left leg looked quite swollen again. Her GP told her that her accident would be causing increased swelling and would continue until she was back to normal. At the time of writing, Mrs H is still in plaster but continuing to use the lotion and massage.

'natural' home setting than in the medicalized environment of a hospital.

Aromatherapy can be used widely during labour and after the birth, but it is the primary health carer and aromatherapist who have the greatest opportunity to help with problems encountered during pregnancy (see Ch. 10), such as backache, fluid retention, emotional upsets, constipation, etc. Chapter 10 includes all the probable common symptoms of mothers-to-be, with the oils which were used, some by nurses in the community.

Health visitors are the team's experts in preventative healthcare within the family (Baly et al 1982 p. 90); they have a distinct role within the primary healthcare team, working across all age groups. For them, children and parents are a priority group (Primary Care Nursing 1997); it is their responsibility to visit every baby born in their area within 10 days and to monitor the child's health and development until he or she starts school.

Paediatrics

When a health visitor calls to see a patient, there may be occasions when that child, or another member of the family, may have a cold, a bruise, cut or wound, or perhaps a lowered immune response because of overfrequent use of antibiotics (Soulisbury Report 1998). Essential oils can be selected to assist healing in all these areas and more.

When selecting essential oils for children it is best to keep within a small range, excluding any

---

Case 9.2   Aromatologist: Penny Price MISPA MIAM, UK

Philip, aged 14, came to see me with tonsillitis. He had suffered on and off with this for several years, and each time he was given antibiotics, which eventually did not seem to have much effect, his attacks even becoming more frequent. In desperation his mother brought him to me. I decided to use *Eucalyptus smithii* [GULLY GUM], *Citrus limon* [LEMON] and *Melaleuca alternifolia* [TEA TREE] for use in the bath and in a carrier lotion for his throat, the latter to be used three times a day.

After 4 days Philip's mother reported that her son's symptoms had almost disappeared. I advised her to make sure he kept using the oils in the bath until he had recovered totally—and as a preventive against further attacks.

Two years later, Philip's mother was delighted to say that Philip had had no further attacks, which was apparently very unusual for him; it confirmed my belief that if we help the body (by the use of nature's products) to overcome a disorder, then in effect we make it stronger, fitter and better equipped for our environment. By helping the body to heal itself Philip was healthier after the illness than he was previously, because his immune system had been stimulated to deal with further infections that might come his way. Philip is now aged 29 and has had no further problems with tonsillitis.

Case 9.3   Aromatherapist: Michael Vanhove, Belgium

An osteopath colleague had to treat a child 5 years of age, attacked by juvenile polyarthritis. The young girl suffered various inflammations in different parts of her body, and was no longer growing. Her knees were already deformed and she could not walk normally. She was on heavy medication when the aromatherapy started. Besides diet changes suggested by the osteopath, they started on my advice to give massage with: *Pinus sylvestris* [SCOTS PINE], *Laurus nobilis* [BAY] and *Eucalyptus citriodora* [LEMON-SCENTED GUM] in a 4–5% dilution in jojoba oil.

The osteopath visited the girl three times a week to massage her; on the other days it was the mother who gave the massage, having been shown what to do.

Result: 2 months later the girl had grown by 2 cm and the medication was able to be reduced by 50%. She has not had much pain since, and her behaviour is more positive.

---

oils with a significant percentage of possibly hazardous components such as ketones, phenols, phenolic ethers and aldehydes (see Appendix A and Ch. 2). Aromatherapy for babies and children (Price & Price-Parr 1996) gives a list of 20 safe oils to use. The only eucalyptus oil which should be used on children is *Eucalyptus smithii* [GULLY GUM]; although it contains a high percentage of 1,8-cineole, the synergy between components renders it gentle, though effective, according to Pénoël (1992/3).

Aromatherapy for babies and young children is usually effected in the following ways:

- inhalation (tissues, vaporizers, cotton tips or balls concealed in the pillowcase or on night clothes)
- baths, using only one drop (for babies under 9 months, in a baby bath) and two drops (for babies over this age, who are in the 'big bath'), dispersed into a paste of dried milk and water or a base carrier lotion. As the number of drops used is so small, it is a good idea to add eight drops of the selected essential oil(s) to 50 ml of white lotion and use a dessertspoonful of this for each bath, swishing the water thoroughly (Price & Price-Parr 1996)
- massage: the health visitor can show the new mother how to do a simple massage, which is

of immense benefit to the mother as well as the baby—and later the child.

Other areas of care within the community

Many of the common and chronic ailments suffered by people of all ages will be cared for in the primary health sector (apart from any necessary visit to hospital); multiple sclerosis (MS), strokes not requiring hospitalization, myalgic encephalomyelitis (ME), Parkinson's disease (PD), burns and wound care are only a few of the areas to have been treated by aromatherapists or community nurses in the home. A trial study and a few case studies are given in this chapter; others appear in other chapters of this book, (e.g. Ch. 14).

Multiple sclerosis

Sometimes referred to as disseminated sclerosis, MS is a chronic disorder of the central nervous system, in which scattered areas of the brain and spinal cord degenerate while the nerve fibres lose their insulating myelin sheaths and their ability to conduct impulses (Wingate & Wingate 1996). It is thought that an infection of some kind may be the cause, but no specific virus has been implicated. Some recent research and thinking have identified allergy and food intolerance as playing a significant part in the process of the condition; the major culprits appear to include animal fats and gluten products (Swank & Dugan 1990, Swank 1991) and a few of the trials carried out have indicated that a diet rich in linoleic acid can considerably reduce the severity of the disease (Bricklin 1983 p. 340). MS is progressive but not continuous; symptoms may start with numbness in a part of the body or muscle weakness in a limb, and after weeks or months (sometimes it could be as long as 2 years) of the person being free from other symptoms, they may begin to experience shooting pains in the back and spasm in the limbs. Sight and speech can be affected, but the main long term problems are lack of control of the bladder, leading to urinary infections, and difficulty with walking, often resulting in the

patient being confined to a wheelchair (Ball 1990 pp. 201–2).

No allopathic treatment has yet proved to be of value; aromatherapy is not a cure either, but its holistic approach (i.e. consideration of the whole body and state of mind of the patient) has been found to be beneficial. For example, one aromatherapist was able to improve quality of sleep, strengthen muscles and relieve muscle tension or spasm (Mutch 1997). Another was able to help a patient in a nursing home who had reached the final stages of the disease and was suffering with persistent pain in both forearms, which 'subsided within two months' (Hulmston 1995). A person suffering from MS was helped by using aromatherapy to boost the immune system, alleviate muscle fatigue, and to stimulate both the circulation and the memory (Donald 1996); the oil chosen to address the latter three conditions was *Rosmarinus officinalis* [ROSEMARY]; other oils common to all three cases mentioned above were *Santalum album* [SANDALWOOD] and *Pelargonium graveolens* [GERANIUM]; *Cymbopogon citratus* [LEMONGRASS] was used in two of the cases. Lunny (1997) suggests using essential oils containing large proportions of esters and aldehydes in their composition, suitably diluted for massage.

Strokes

Strokes appear to occur more in women than in men and particularly in those with hypertension or diabetes—or in fact any condition leading to atherosclerosis, including smoking and familial hypercholesterolaemia (Ball 1990 p. 189). Usually, about a third of people who have a stroke will recover with time, though any further strokes considerably weaken the body. As far as the authors are aware, there have been no studies on strokes carried out in a healthcare setting. Nevertheless, it is possible to help those who have suffered even a severe stroke to regain movement in the limbs affected. The author's mother, who had high blood pressure, is one such case. On return from hospital, Mrs Price was unable to talk clearly or to move her left arm and leg sufficiently to walk. Essential oils to

---

Case 9.4 Aromatherapist: Josie Browne, UK

Aetiology/medical history
J was a 46-year-old married lady with three grown-up children and an 8-year-old daughter. She cared for her mother who had terminal cancer. She tried hard not to cry as she told me her mother was undergoing chemotherapy, her brother-in-law had just been diagnosed with lung cancer and her daughter had had a miscarriage 4 days ago. She herself had been diagnosed with MS 16 years previously. Her first relapse left her unable to walk for 2 years but, during a visit to Lourdes in France, she said 'a miracle happened' and she was able to walk again.

Presenting symptoms
She had spasm in her legs, poor memory, regular headaches, pain in her neck and shoulders and her sleep pattern was poor.

Proposed treatment plan
My aim was to improve her sleep, headache and lowered immune response and to help relaxation. Appointments were made fortnightly.
 First visit: the following essential oils were massaged into her back and head, noting that there was a lot of tension in her neck and thoracic region.

Chamaemelum nobile [ROMAN CHAMOMILE] two drops
Lavandula angustifolia one drop
Origanum majorana [SWEET MARJORAM] five drops.

 Home treatment: a blend of the oils used was supplied for her husband to massage her back before going to bed.
 Second visit (2 weeks later): J was sleeping a lot better. I massaged her back and legs with the previous essential oil mix with the addition of *Boswellia carteri* [FRANKINCENSE] as she was grieving.
 Home treatment: a blend of the essential oils in white lotion was supplied for her to apply to her chest and neck morning and evening. I also showed her how to meditate and suggested that she try to do so for 5 minutes five times a day if possible.
 Third visit (2 weeks later): J was sleeping well, but she was still uptight. I spent a long time counselling her as she needed to talk; since she was a devout Christian, I suggested that she visit a Church minister.
 I massaged her back and legs with the same oils as before and supplied a mixture of the neat oils, instructing her to put nine drops in the vaporizer and to massage one drop into her temples a few times each day.

 Fourth visit (2 weeks later): J was feeling much better in herself. Her muscle spasm was lessening and she was learning to relax more. I massaged her legs and back with:

Rosmarinus officinalis (two drops)
Chamaemelum nobile (two drops)
Lavandula angustifolia (two drops)
Cedrus atlantica (CEDARWOOD)

and supplied a blend of the oils to massage her legs morning and evening.
 Fifth visit (3 weeks later): J's sister, who lived alone and suffered from osteoarthritis, was looking to her for support; I pointed out to Jean the importance of having time and energy for herself. On this occasion I massaged her back and legs with two drops each of *C. nobile*, *O. majorana*, *Citrus bergamia* and *L. angustifolia*.
 Home treatment: we discussed a form of gentle exercise for her and chose swimming as it was something she could do with her daughter.
 Sixth visit (2 weeks later): J had been swimming twice a week. Her memory was better, her headaches were infrequent and she was more relaxed. I massaged her back and legs with two drops each of *O. majorana*, *C. nobile*, *L. angustifolia* and *C. atlantica*.

Outcome
J now had her own supply of oils which she used regularly at home. An aromatherapy appointment was made for 3 months' time. She thanked me for being there at that particular time with so many things happening. She felt she would have been unable to cope and might have had a relapse.
 During the 3 months of treatments a chart had been filled in and from that it was found that over the 3 months J had achieved:

85% relief from anxiety and depression
85% relief from aches and pains
86% relief from stiffness
73% improvement in sleep
78% improvement in mobility
75% improvement in skin condition
90% improvement in relaxation during and after treatment
80% improvement in relaxation for a few days following treatment.

---

stimulate the circulation were massaged daily in an upward movement only on her arms and legs (on both sides of the body to maintain balance) and Swiss reflex was carried out on the corresponding reflexes of her feet (plus the throat reflex). The doctor commented on her unusually rapid recovery.

Myalgic encephalomyelitis

Myalgic encephalomyelitis (ME) appeared as a medical problem during the 1970s but has only in recent years been accepted by the medical profession as a debilitating and distressing condition. Ball (1990 p. 194) says it is thought to be 'a variety of viral encephalitis, occurring both sporadically and in epidemics'. ME is known also as chronic fatigue syndrome (CFS) or postviral fatigue syndrome, the latter name being favoured by Wingate & Wingate (1996), who regard the name myalgic encephalomyelitis to be: 'a massive overstatement. Encephalomyelitis means inflammation of the brain and spinal cord, a serious and sometimes fatal result of infection. ME is an ill-defined collection of symptoms that include aching muscles, lassitude and depression'. It is usually accompanied also by mild fever, sore throat, tender lymph nodes, headache, sleep disorders, confusion, memory loss and visual disturbances (Encyclopaedia Britannica 1996). According to Bennett (1992 p. 157), although opinions differ as to its cause, it is believed to be possibly due to a viral infection compounded by a compromised immune system. He goes on to say: 'Experience suggests that nearly all the sufferers have been regular medical drug takers (particularly antibiotics and/or the oral contraceptive pill, which are known to undermine the immune system) and that most also appear to have developed *Candida albicans* as a consequence of their drug therapy, aggravated by a diet high in refined carbohydrates'.

There is very little that orthodox medicine can do for a person with ME, but it is included here because aromatherapy has had success in boosting the immune system with both ME and AIDS (see Ch. 15 for oils and studies on AIDS). Symptoms can also be helped by careful selection of the essential oils.

Aromatherapy is not contraindicated, although the ME Association booklet, 'Alternative approaches to ME', states that it is unlikely to produce anything more than symptomatic relief. This point of view is not supported by everyone, including two therapists known to the author and the chairperson of the Kirklees ME Support Group.

(Smith 1995)

Parkinson's disease

Parkinson's disease (PD), named after James Parkinson (1755–1824) was described in a paper he wrote in 1817 as 'the shaking palsy'. The disease is due to a lack of dopamine, a chemical substance which is needed in the brain to transmit messages to the distal muscles (Parry 1997). It is a slow, progressive disorder usually affecting people in later life, though it can occur earlier. It affects the parts of the brain which control movement; the symptoms include trembling and/or stiffness of the limbs, a shuffling walk and difficulty in speaking (Collin 1994). As the disorder progresses, the amount of medication needed increases; this means that more side-effects are evident—and so the vicious circle continues.

The community nurse can play an important part in the life of the patient with PD, providing research-based knowledge of the condition and education on how best to cope with manifestations before they arise. He can also obtain specialist advice and treatment for the patient when appropriate and provide continuity of care, coordinating the various aspects of treatment given by the multidisciplinary team (Livesy 1992).

Many people with PD are turning to aromatherapy to try to lessen the side-effects from their medication: at worst they find their condition remains unchanged; at best they find their mobility is increased, their pain is decreased and, due to the relaxing properties of the oils selected, they are less tense and anxious and sleeping much better.

PARKINSON'S DISEASE PROJECT

A project was carried out by the authors in 1992 (Price 1993) on three groups of people with PD. It was set up to determine whether or not essential oils can play a part in improving movement in a PD sufferer and perhaps in increasing the time span before stronger drugs need to be administered. It was intended only as a preliminary exercise for possible future research.

Objective of the trial

The objective of the trial was to discover whether daily application of essential oils, without massage, was as effective as using essential oils with regular full-body massage, thus making it possible for people to benefit

Case 9.5 Aromatherapist: Ian Smith, UK

Andrew, who was 25 years old, contracted ME 2½ years before coming for aromatherapy treatment and was forced to stop working 6 months later. He visits his doctor regularly but treatment consists only of tablets to combat nausea and depression. He has tried other forms of complementary medicine, such as acupuncture, in an attempt to get himself well, but with no success. Andrew also has candida infection of the bowel and attends a specialist clinic for colonic irrigation. At the time of consultation with me he was recovering from a stomach virus, which had kept him in bed for 4 weeks. He does not generally suffer from abnormal headaches or migraines. He is subject to stress-related pain across the shoulders, due to whiplash injuries done 3 years previously. He has become prone to depression, partly owing to a cartilage operation on his left knee, which meant he was no longer able to play cricket or football. He also has psoriasis on his right calf and sometimes on his scalp.

The reason for his visit was to seek relief from the symptoms and hopefully to gain overall improvement in health. It was pointed out to Andrew that although aromatherapy would not effect a cure it would help stimulate the body's own ability to self-heal, restoring and promoting the balance between mind and body.

His GP was aware that he was seeing an aromatherapist.

Treatment
Week 1: this focused on stimulating the depressed immune system, reducing the candida and treating his psoriasis. Essential oils can support and strengthen the immune system in two ways: by directly opposing the hostile microorganisms, or by stimulating and increasing the activity of the organs and cells involved. Those selected (and used in 20 ml carrier oil for full-body massage) were:

- *Lavandula angustifolia* (2 drops)
  — combines both actions on the immune system above
  — antifungal, therefore effective on the candida
  — beneficial to psoriasis
  — a balancing oil, of great value when emotions are unsteady
- *Melaleuca alternifolia* (2 drops)
  — powerful immunostimulant
  — antifungal, therefore effective in treating the candida
- *Chamaemelum nobile* (2 drops)
  — calming and soothing
  — antiinflammatory
  — antidepressant
  — digestive

- *Vetiveria zizanioides* (1 drop)
  — relaxing (works well on deep-seated anxiety).

After treatment Andrew felt there was some relief in his lower back pain.
Week 2: Andrew's shoulders had ached less and he felt good both emotionally and physically. He was experiencing pain in his lower back and stomach. His consultant had said that he had a gastrointestinal problem for which nothing could be done. Oils and treatment as above.
Week 3: Andrew's shoulders and back had been free of pain although he had had pain in his lower legs; the psoriasis had improved slightly. Oils and treatment as above.
Week 4: There was no pain in his shoulders or lower legs. Andrew said he felt much better emotionally and when he did have a 'down' day his spirits recovered much more quickly than usual. Others had commented on his improvement and his self-confidence seemed to be increasing. Oils and treatment as above.
Week 5: Andrew's general feeling of well-being was much improved and he had taken two short bike rides. The psoriasis on his scalp had improved, as had the large patch on his legs. His attitude was much more positive and although his stomach was not right it was getting better. Oils and treatment as above.
Week 6: Andrew continued to show an improvement but an infection in his gum (for which he had visited his dentist) had returned and the dentist had provided antibiotics; Andrew was reluctant to take these as apparently they can cause problems for ME sufferers. Oils and treatment as above.

A further two treatments using the same blend were given at weekly intervals and continuing progress was made. He was going out socially instead of refusing invitations, was feeling much less lethargic and, importantly, was adhering to his diet.

Evaluation:
Physically Andrew was much stronger. Candida was still present but the stomach pain was markedly reduced and the psoriasis was responding to treatment. The big change was in his state of mind; he was recovering his self-confidence and self-belief.

Conclusion
Although Andrew has made good progress there is still a long way to go and it may be hard to curb his impatience. Clearly aromatherapy is a treatment with which Andrew has a rapport, so benefit should continue to accrue.
(This report first appeared in Aromatherapy World Harvesting (autumn) 1995)

from essential oils at a reasonable cost, without full-body massage (which not everyone wants, because of

time and cost considerations). Because the blend of essential oils had to be identical for everyone in order to have a meaningful comparison, it was impossible to select an oil combination holistically for each person. The choice therefore was focused on lowering stress levels and loosening joints and muscles, with the hope also of relieving insomnia and perhaps constipation in those presenting such symptoms.

Method

All oils and/or lotions used, either for massage or self-application, were mixed at 1.5% concentration and supplied by the authors, to guarantee uniformity. Six to eight drops of the undiluted essential oil were used in the bath where possible. Out of the 52 people who volunteered for treatment (20 each in groups A and B and 12 in group C), 27 were able to complete the 9 month period. Of the rest:

- eight found the weekly recording difficult
- seven were not able to keep up the daily application (one had chosen an oil-based mix in preference to a lotion and found it difficult to remove the vegetable oil from her clothes)
- three had hospital visits, which interrupted their routine
- two changed medication, which invalidated the results
- one transferred to phase 2 after a 2 month period with no treatment
- one applied the lotion only when he remembered
- one stopped after 3 months because her speech problems showed no improvement, though she admitted to sleeping better and having less cramp during this time
- one had a mastectomy half-way through the project, but commented that her balance had improved and her GP had remarked on her increased self-confidence and positive outlook during her treatment period
- one died.

The trial was organized in the following way:

• Group A—received a weekly massage from an aromatherapist (who gave his/her time free of charge) for 12 weeks, followed by a monthly massage for 6 months, using a specific blend of essential oils. The carer applied the same essential oil blend in a lotion base daily in between treatments.

• Group B—were supplied for 9 months with pure essential oils for the bath and a lotion or oil-based mix

containing the same essential oils to be applied daily for 3 months, and every other day for a further 6 months.

• Group C—received similar treatment to group A above except that the massage was carried out with plain vegetable oil, with no essential oils added. This was difficult because, for the project to be reliable, not even the therapists were allowed to know that there were no essential oils in the mix supplied and the lack of smell could have made them suspicious. This was overcome by telling them that they were using a 0.05% concentration—even though no essential oils were present.

All participants had to obtain their doctor's permission to take part and be willing to do what was asked of them, especially with regard to home use.

Oils used

The essential oils selected were:

- *Salvia sclarea* [CLARY]—relaxant, nerve tonic; to aid general relaxation and relieve anxiety
- *Origanum majorana* [SWEET MARJORAM]—analgesic, antispasmodic, digestive tonic, hypotensor, nerve tonic, relaxant; to relieve muscle pain and insomnia and improve digestion
- *Lavandula angustifolia*—analgesic, antispasmodic, digestive stimulant, hypotensor, sedative; to relax the muscles and relieve pain, insomnia and anxiety.

Results

Ten patients in group A, nine in group B and eight in group C completed the trial. A synopsis of the results of this trial is presented here. Full details can be found in Price (1993).

The results for symptomatic relief showed very little difference between group A and group B, which points to the potential of baths and self-application for those who cannot afford weekly aromatherapy treatments. The results for group C, i.e. the patients receiving massage (and home care) with a bland vegetable oil, were as follows:

- four found the treatment relaxing and reported feeling better afterwards, although the effects did not last
- two felt brighter in themselves and in their general health

- two found the treatment itself relaxing but felt no other noticeable change.

The symptomatic improvements experienced by all three groups are shown in Table 9.1.

Conclusion

Group A: on the whole an aromatherapy treatment once a month was found to be insufficient. However:

- seven patients maintained their improvement during the last 6 months when receiving an aromatherapy treatment only once a month
- two felt able to discontinue their medication for insomnia
- two did not maintain their improvement during the last 6 months, but still felt better than before treatment commenced (beneficial effects of each treatment lasting 4–6 days).

It was felt that fortnightly (if not weekly) aromatherapy treatments would be preferable to monthly intervals.

Group B: essential oils for self-use, but without massage, appeared to be able to give relief in the same areas as in group A. Two patients felt the improvement they experienced was limited. A perceived extra benefit of group A over group B may be the complete relaxation derived from the massage, with improved circulation as a result (though this was not mentioned in the patient feedback).

Group C: massage without essential oils, although beneficial on several counts, scored the lowest in terms of lasting effects.

There follows four cases from those people who completed the above project, two from group A and two from group B; these cases have been selected at random and are not necessarily the most, or the least, successful.

Group A: aromatherapy treatment with full-body massage

- *Client W*

    Presenting symptoms:
    — tremors, weakness, stiffness, constant pain, difficulty in walking
    — (side-effects) nausea, constipation, insomnia, hypertension, weight gain, legs twitching at night

Table 9.1 Number and percentage of PD sufferers in groups A and B (combined) and group C experiencing symptomatic relief over 9 month trial period (after Price 1993). (Dashes indicate that a person was not asked by the therapist if he/she suffered from that symptom)

	Groups A and B (combined)		Group C	
	No.	%	No.	%
Anxiety	4	100	—	—
Constipation	5	83	1	33
Cramp	1	50	1	50
Depression	3	75	—	—
Energy lack	4	100	0	0
Insomnia	7	85	2	66
Memory loss	0	0	0	0
Muscular pain	8	100	3	60
Nightmares	2	100	—	—
Rigidity	2	50	—	—
Slurred speech	2	28	—	—
Stiffness	9	100	1	50
Swallowing difficulty	0	0	—	—
Tremors	4	33	1	16
Weak limbs	5	62	—	—

After 3 months (12 weekly treatments—phase 1):
— no constipation, sleeping better, fewer tremors, easier movement, dressing more easily, less stiff in the mornings

After a further 6 months (six monthly treatments—phase 2):
— improvements reversed, feeling better only for a few days after each treatment

Comments:
— 'wonderful improvement' after phase 1
— therapist felt W was missing weekly treatment in phase 2—'wish I could have treatment every week'.

- *Client X*

    Presenting symptoms:
    — tremors, joint stiffness, rigid wrists and hands (difficulty in gripping), slowness of movement
    — (side-effects) constipation, easily tired

    After 3 months (12 weekly treatments—phase 1):
    — reaction and movement better, no constipation, able to carry crockery, 'back to old self', no change in tremors

    After a further 6 months (six monthly treatments—phase 2):
    — condition more or less maintained, fewer drug side-effects

Comments:
— client very happy, goes out alone for first time in years, change more marked in phase 1.

Group B: application by carer of essential oils in lotion—no full-body massage

- *Client Y*

Presenting symptoms:
— trembling, slurred speech, poor muscle coordination, slow walking, memory loss

After 3 months (application only, once a day):
— more mobility in right shoulder, general movement improved, slight improvement in saliva control, fewer side-effects from drugs
— neurologist suggested reducing intake of Artane; he took copy of aromatherapy correspondence and at the end of 4 months took Y off this drug completely

After a further 6 months (application once every second day):
— improvements more or less maintained

Comments:
— main improvement was 'a sense of relaxation and absence of stress'.

- *Client Z*

Presenting symptoms:
— shaking in right arm (difficulty in writing), difficulty in swallowing, shuffling feet, especially at home
— (side-effects) nausea, constipation, high blood pressure

After 3 months (application only, once a day):
— constipation much better, generally better in spirits, walking a little better, no shuffling of feet—'can walk without thinking'

After a further 6 months (application once every second day):
— improvements more or less maintained, except for right hand—still shaky, constipation gone

Comments:
Delighted with general condition—'feel better most days', occasional insomnia.

The authors are pleased that some of the secondary symptoms suffered by those with PD appear to be alleviated with, or without, massage; the most effective and lasting effects seem to be due to the essential oils.

Although the study was poorly designed and therefore cannot be regarded as reliable, nevertheless the results obtained indicate that essential oils may benefit those with PD and that further work would be worth undertaking.

Summary

Essential oils can be useful in primary health care, for treating minor ailments and disorders, for prophylactic use to prevent the spread of infection, and to make the environment more pleasant.

REFERENCES

Ball J 1990 Understanding disease. Blackdown, Devon
Baly M E, Robottom B, Clark J M 1987 District nursing. Heinemann Nursing, London; p 227
Bennett G 1992 Handbook of clinical dietetics. Price, Hinckley
Bricklin M 1983 The practical encyclopaedia of natural healing. Rodale, Pennsylvania
Collin P H 1994 Dictionary of medicine. Peter Collin, Middlesex
Department of Health 1997 England: NHS: driving quality (White paper)
Donald R 1996 Multiple sclerosis; case study. Aromatherapy World Seeding (Spring): 33–35

Encyclopaedia Britannica 1996 Chronic fatigue syndrome (CD ROM)
Ersser S 1990 The use of essential oils and massage by nurses in Oxfordshire Health Authority. Essential oils in nursing project. Information pack. Institute of Nursing, Oxford
Hulmston N 1995 Case studies; multiple sclerosis. International Journal of Aromatherapy 7(2): 30/31
Livesy P 1992 Providing a source of support. Nursing Times 88(29): 26–30
Lunny V N 1997 Aromatherapy in the management of multiple sclerosis. Positive Health March/April: 40
Mutch F 1997 Case studies; multiple sclerosis. International Journal of Aromatherapy 8(2): 40/41

Parry W R 1997 Parkinson's disease. Sur in English: 11

Pénoël D 1992/3 Winter shield. Three eucalyptus essential oils which help fight winter ailments. International Journal of Aromatherapy 4(4): 10–12

Price S 1993 Parkinson's disease project: is aromatherapy an effective treatment for Parkinson's disease? The Aromatherapist 1(1): 14–21

Price S, Price-Parr P 1996 Aromatherapy for babies and children. Thorsons, London, p 66

Primary Care Nursing 1997 Nursing opportunities in primary health care. Department of Health, London

Smith I 1995 Myalgic encephalomyelitis. Aromatherapy World Harvesting (Autumn) pp 31–35

Soulisbury Report 1998

Swank R L, Dugan B B 1990 The effect of low saturated fat diet in early and late cases of multiple sclerosis. The Lancet 336(8706): 37–39

Swank R L 1991 Multiple sclerosis: fat-oil relationship. Nutrition 7(5): 368–376

Trevelyan J A 1996 A true complement? Nursing Times 92(5): 42–43

WHO 1978 Declaration of Alma Ata. World Health Organization, Geneva

Wingate P, Wingate R 1996 The Penguin encyclopaedia. Penguin, Middlesex

Pregnancy and childbirth

Introduction

A wide range of conditions occurring from the onset of puberty to beyond the menopause respond well to the use of essential oils. There is little published scientific research regarding the use of essential oils in any hormonal context apart from pregnancy, but many aromatherapists in private practice have used them to good effect with their female clients' (or their own) problems.

This chapter concentrates on aromatherapy with regard to pregnancy and childbirth. In this context essential oils can be very powerful and must be used with great care. On the one hand, gross misuse has lead to documented cases of abortion and death; on the other hand, as is shown in Reed & Norfolk's pilot study (see p. 194), correct use of oils in labour can reduce a woman's need for drugs such as pethidine. This chapter aims to identify which oils are safe to use with women in various stages of pregnancy and which should be avoided. It also explains which oils can be used safely by the lay person, and which only by qualified professionals. For ease of access, essential oils of the following types are listed: those which are emmenagogic, abortifacient, hormonal or uterotonic. Additionally, oils to be used for specific conditions arising during pregnancy are given.

Clearly the use of essential oils during pregnancy requires great expertise, and in a midwifery setting only those qualified in aromatherapy should use such oils, always in strict adherence to existing protocols and guidelines. Qualification results only from courses accredited by the aromatherapy umbrella body, the AOC (Aromatherapy Organisations Council—see Appendix C), although 'several articles in nursing journals give the impression that nurses can consider themselves competent to practise aromatherapy and use essential oils after a brief training period lasting days rather than months' (Holder 1995).

POWERFUL OILS IN PREGNANCY

There are several essential oils which may have unwanted therapeutic effects during the first trimester of pregnancy, e.g. they may be emmenagogic and are therefore best avoided at this time, especially as, once in the body fluids, they may pass through the placenta. It is known that, although the placenta acts as a barrier against both neutral and positively charged molecules, those which are negatively charged can cross it fairly easily (Maickel & Snodgrass 1973); it is also known that small molecules with a molecular weight of less than 1000 are able to pass through the placenta (Baker 1960). Therefore, as many essential oil molecules are negatively charged and all have molecular weights of less than 250, it can be assumed that essential oils do pass through the placenta. Their effects on a newly formed fetus have not yet been studied. However, essential oils may be used correctly and safely later in the pregnancy, and it is our wish to try and clarify this potentially confusing situation. 'Crossing the placenta does not necessarily mean that there is a risk of toxicity to the fetus; this will depend on the toxicity and the plasma concentration of the compound' (Tisserand & Balacs 1995).

Many books on aromatherapy are derivative and consequently few authors are able to explain their recommendations of particular oils. This lack of firm information has led many aromatherapists to avoid using any allegedly unsafe oils during the whole gestation period, even though some of the proscribed oils are not necessarily unsafe in relation to pregnancy.

For example, essential oils which appear on a general 'never to be used' list are sometimes conflated with those oils which may need to be used during pregnancy, but with care. Also, many lists of oils to be avoided during pregnancy include those containing aldehydes and phenols (such as *Cymbopogon citratus* [LEMONGRASS] and *Syzygium aromaticum* [CLOVE BUD], whose toxicity is mainly a potential irritant effect on the skin), and contraindications do not specifically relate to pregnancy (see Appendix B.6). Some oils listed contain coumarins and are therefore photosensitizers (Appendix B.7), but again this does not affect their use with particular regard to pregnancy. The essential oils listed in Appendices B.6 and B.7 should be treated with caution by *everyone*, not just those who are pregnant. Balacs (1992) began the clarification of this area by giving reasons for his list of oils to be avoided in pregnancy. His article and *The Aromatherapy Workbook* (Price 1993 p. 123) are intended to be more informative and to put back into perspective the use of powerful and extremely useful essential oils during pregnancy. Another interesting point to consider is that a woman is often unaware of being pregnant at first—sometimes for up to 4 weeks (or more, in certain cases) and could be using several essential oils regularly during that time! Where this is known to have happened, no ill effects have been reported.

To save confusion and misuse, members of the general public (and inadequately qualified aromatherapists) are best advised not to use an essential oil appearing on *any* restrictive list during pregnancy without having been given advice by a competent aromatherapist; there is a number of essential oils which can be used by them with safety during this 9 month period.

Importance of appropriate training

Restrictions directed at the general public should not be used as the blueprint for qualified aromatherapists; therapists should use their knowledge conscientiously to select essential oils at this time and, until pregnancy is well advanced, should avoid entirely the use of certain oils (see Appendices B.4 and B.5). Pharmacists and doctors are trained to prescribe powerful drugs, unlike the lay person who is simply told how much or how many to take and how often.

Likewise, it is crucial that aromatherapists learn how and when some of the powerful essential oils may be used, in specific circumstances. They should also be aware of the difference between those essential oils which are neurotoxic and abortive, those which stimulate the uterus to contract or are emmenagogic, and those which affect the hormonal balance in the body.

Proficient aromatherapists (nurses, midwives or otherwise) should know about all possible toxic effects and pertinent contraindications, so that they can select the most beneficial essential oils with discrimination and confidence. This means that if a potentially hazardous oil is required during the early gestation period for a one-off administration (e.g. a 50% dilution of *Hyssopus officinalis* on a bruise, or the inhalation of *Mentha × piperita* for nausea) it can be used without fear of adverse effects.

Effects of gross misuse of essential oils

Because of the complexity of essential oil chemistry, a number of essential oils are labelled as toxic without any evidence of their causing harm to human beings, *except by gross misuse*. Toxicity of the main component of an essential oil does not always constitute proof that the whole essential oil is toxic to humans, whatever the results of research on rats and mice (which are injected with or made to ingest essential oils—see Ch. 3). Other research has shown that the results of animal testing cannot be directly extrapolated to humans and that because of the small amounts used in aromatherapy massage the effects of the essential oils would be 100 000 times less hazardous than the amounts used in animal testing (Tisserand & Balacs 1991).

Empirical evidence accumulated over many years would seem to be a truer test than animal research. Such evidence illustrates that when used in small doses (and for a restricted length of time), even the so-called toxic oils on the lists referred to do not normally present a hazard. However, the dangers of gross misuse of essential oils—whether generally considered to be safe or toxic—are also amply documented. Take

Mentha pulegium [PENNYROYAL], which is reputed to be a strong abortifacient and a much impugned oil so far as pregnancy is concerned. The following cases of women who took large doses of pennyroyal deliberately are all recorded in medical journals.

• To induce menstruation, one woman took about 15 ml of pennyroyal and suffered acute gastritis, recovering fully (Allen 1897).
• Another made herself an infusion with about 15 ml of pennyroyal and 'threepennyworth of rum'. She felt sick after 10 minutes and later became unconscious; she vomited when roused shortly afterwards and recovered by the next day (Braithwaite 1906).
• To induce abortion, a 22-year-old American took approximately 10 ml of pennyroyal and felt dizzy within an hour, recovering the same day. Tests showed her liver and renal functions to be normal and she was discharged 2 days after admission (Sullivan & Peterson 1979).
• A 24-year-old mother of two, taking an unknown amount of pennyroyal in two separate doses (evening and the following morning) succeeded in aborting on the second day but was admitted to hospital seriously ill. Towards the end of 10 days her general condition was recorded as being satisfactory—all damaged tissues seemed to have recovered fully, except the kidneys. However, she developed pneumonia and died 3 days later (Vallance 1955).
• An 18-year-old American girl took about 30 ml of pennyroyal, thinking she was pregnant. After severe vomiting and vaginal bleeding, she suffered a cardiopulmonary arrest 4 days after ingestion. She died 2 days later following a second cardiopulmonary arrest (Sullivan & Peterson 1979).

M. pulegium can contain anything from 26.8–92.6% of the powerful ketone pulegone (see Potential toxicity below) depending on the country of origin and whether it is cultivated or wild. Lawrence (1989) quotes the pulegone content found in *M. pulegium* from the following countries:

• Uruguay (1985)   26.8%
• Angola (1976)   42%

- Greece (1972)   61.9%
- Chile (1986)   92.6%.

The average content is normally around 65%, but it is not known what percentage of pulegone was in the oils used by the women quoted above. It is difficult therefore to be certain about what dosage level is safe and when the amount begins to pose a danger. What is clear is that swallowing large quantities (15–25 ml) of any essential oil, even one considered to be safe, constitutes gross misuse, and may cause significant side-effects (see Ch. 3).

Potential toxicity

Oils that are generally regarded as neurotoxic and abortive contain a high percentage of certain ketones (e.g. (+)-pulegone), oxides (e.g. 1,8-cineole—syn. eucalyptol, also regarded as a bicyclic ether) or phenolic ethers (e.g. myristicin, found in nutmeg oil) (see Ch. 3). Whilst not all of these are emmenagogic it is nevertheless thought prudent to be cautious during the whole of pregnancy with all oils which have a high content of these powerful constituents (see Appendix B.5). They should be used only by professionals and with extreme care—possibly in emergencies only. Such professionals should become familiar with the quantity and effect of each specific component in the oils needing caution. For example, the very toxic *Artemisia absinthum* [WORMWOOD] contains only 35–45% of ketones (thujones); the less toxic *Foeniculum vulgare* var. *dulce* [SWEET FENNEL] by contrast has an approximate 65% phenolic ether content (*trans*-anethole). Another example is *Eucalyptus smithii* [GULLY GUM], one of the gentlest and safest essential oils, yet it contains 70–80% 1,8-cineole.

In order to establish definitively the toxicity of specific essential oils, reliable and repeatable research is needed. In all such research the proportions as well as the names of the ketones or phenolic ethers responsible for the neurotoxicity (and hence the abortifacient effect) should be given for each essential oil tested. For example, the ketone thujone (said to be abortive and neurotoxic) in *Salvia officinalis* [SAGE] can vary with each harvest from 15–70%. Suppliers of this oil to aromatherapy users should ask the distiller to make a test run on 1 kg of plant to check the ketone content before harvesting, as the ketone content, as well as the yield of oil, varies throughout the season, becoming higher as the season progresses. (Most farmers naturally prefer to harvest their plants when the yield is at its highest, which explains why an essential oil with a low ketone content may be more expensive.) It will be seen therefore that the properties of an essential oil depend on its total make-up, i.e. the quantities and types of ketones, oxides and phenolic ethers it contains. Even then, synergy within the plant can alter the whole oil's effects: 'Although sage has more thujone than wormwood, it seems a far safer plant' (Mabey 1988).

CAUTIONS FOR PREGNANT WOMEN
Emmenagogue or abortifacient

Before discussing which essential oils should or should not be used in pregnancy, the terms 'emmenagogue' and 'abortifacient' need to be differentiated. Valnet (1980 p. 268) defines an emmenagogue as 'a substance which induces or regularises menstruation' and an abortifacient as a substance 'capable of inducing an abortion'. It follows that an emmenagogue stimulates an occurrence which is natural in a woman but which, perhaps through emotional upset or other causes, is delayed (Wingate & Wingate 1988 p. 21), whereas an abortifacient is a toxic substance, necessarily powerful, because it has to *fight* nature, not gently help it.

This is a difficult area to clarify, but there is a definite difference between the condition of the uterus in secondary amenorrhoea and its condition during pregnancy. In the former, progesterone is produced by the ovary in order to stimulate the thickening of the uterus lining and when the supply of progesterone ceases because of non-fertilization the lining is shed. In pregnancy, the placenta, which is completely formed and functioning 10 weeks after fertilization (Myles 1993), takes over the production of progesterone and also secretes hormones into the mother's circulation to maintain the pregnancy (Wingate & Wingate 1988 p. 376). 'Even if an essential oil is proven to have an emmenagogic action, this does not necessarily mean it is a potential abortifacient' (Balacs 1992). Although there is insufficient research yet to confirm this, the experience of many aromatherapists (including the authors) would seem to indicate its truth.

Cautions

Notwithstanding the above, there are cautions which should be strictly observed with pregnant women, even when using very dilute essential oils for short periods of time. These cautions are listed below. (**NB.** Very dilute = high dilution = a low percentage of essential oils in the mix; low dilution = a higher percentage of essential oils in the mix.)

- In the case of women with poor obstetric history it is advisable to avoid using all emmenagogic or abortive oils—even if only because, should an abortion threaten, the mother (and perhaps the nurse/midwife, aromatherapist or aromatologist) may feel psychologically that an essential oil used, however sparingly or dilute (and however unlikely), may have been the cause.
- The patient's medical history should always be referred to in case of possible further contraindications, e.g. epilepsy, significant rise in blood pressure, kidney damage, etc.
- Nurses not adequately qualified in aromatherapy or aromatology (i.e. aromatic medicine) should work with essential oils only under the direction of a qualified aromatherapist or aromatologist (see Ch. 16). Midwives should follow the United Kingdom Central Council (UKCC) rules for midwives (see paras 40.2, 41.1), the Standards for the Administration of Medicines (SAM) (paras 38 and 39) and the Code of Practice (Introduction and para. 3.3.3), where they are applicable to aromatherapy and aromatology. They should also abide by any locally agreed policies, protocols or guidelines, many of which have already been drawn up by various midwifery and gynaecological services (e.g. the Ipswich Hospital).
- Essential oils should always be used on pregnant women at a maximum of 50% normal strength, both in the bath and for application or massage, e.g. eight drops in 50 ml carrier oil or lotion (this is barely one drop in 5 ml, which is about a teaspoonful), i.e. just under 1% dilution. Half strength is used for two reasons:
  - pregnant women often have a heightened sense of smell
  - normal strength could be too potent for a fetus (essential oils will pass through the placenta and their effect, especially on a newly formed fetus, is not known).
- If a breastfeeding mother uses essential oils on the breasts to stimulate lactation or clear mastitis, the oils should be used immediately after feeding; the nipples should be cleaned with a bland oil before putting baby to the breast at the next feed. (**NB.** Half normal dilution should be used also when breastfeeding.)

For a list of neurotoxic and abortive oils which should not be used during pregnancy or in general aromatherapy use, see Appendix B.4. (**NB.** Some oils listed there may be used (except during pregnancy) by aromatologists and herbalists who have received the appropriate training.)

Emmenagogic essential oils

Emmenagogic essential oils are recommended to promote menstrual flow in non-pregnant women suffering from amenorrhoea, or irregular or scanty menstruation. The oils listed below are considered by the majority of writers to be emmenagogic. Such oils should not be used in the first trimester of pregnancy, unless needed in an emergency or for a short period of time. In such instances they should be used exclusively under the direction of an aromatherapist or aromatologist. Where there is a history of miscarriage, they should not be used at all.

- *Achillea millefolium* [YARROW] contains little or no thujone as opposed to sage oil, which may contain 50% (Leung 1980), but the plant has been used as an abortive in the past (Chandler, Hooper & Harvey 1982) and so the essential oil must be regarded as emmenagogic until proven otherwise. There is also a taxonomic problem with yarrow; Lawrence (1984) speaks of yarrow being a complex of hardly separable species, which is another reason for caution.

• *Foeniculum vulgare* var. *dulce*—also hormone like, diuretic and galactogogic, facilitates delivery (average phenolic ether content 60%).

• *Myristica fragrans* [NUTMEG]—also facilitates delivery; is hallucinogenic in overdose (average phenolic ether content 6%).

• *Pimpinella anisum* [ANISEED]—also hormone like; facilitates delivery (average phenolic ether content 83%).

• *Salvia officinalis*—also hormone-like; prepares uterus for labour (average ketone content 35%).

The following essential oils are those which some books, but not all, suggest are emmenagogic and should be used with caution during pregnancy. No evidence has yet been produced to support or refute these suggestions and, under the guidance of adequately trained aromatherapists, it would appear from the facts below that their use may not be detrimental to the well-being of a pregnant woman. However, this does not necessarily mean that all of them should automatically be regarded as safe oils, because even safe oils can be used wrongly, and far from safely.

• *Chamaemelum nobile* syn. *Anthemis nobilis* [ROMAN CHAMOMILE] (contains around 13% of a ketone). The link to amenorrhoea is due to nervous problems (Valnet 1980 pp. 104–105).

• *Chamomilla recutita* syn. *Matricaria recutita* [GERMAN CHAMOMILE]—hormone-like (Franchomme & Pénoël 1990) (contains around 20–30% oxides).

These two essential oils are recommended for amenorrhoea, but their emmenagogic properties are generally considered to be very mild.

• *Commiphora myrrha*, *C. molmol* [MYRRH]. Myrrh is thought to be an emmenagogue perhaps because it is hormonal; in Grieve (1991 p. 572) it is not made clear whether the plant or the essential oil is responsible for the therapeutic action (see *Levisticum officinale* below). As a result it appears in many British aromatherapy books as a proven emmenagogue. None of the French books cites it as such and Balacs (1992) considers it to have 'doubtful toxicity'.

• *Juniperus communis* (fruct. ram. fol.) [JUNIPER BERRY, TWIG, LEAF]—diuretic. Formacek &

Kubeczka (1982) found *J. communis* to contain approximately 87% terpenes, with a small percentage of alcohols and no ketones, yet a *J. communis* cited in Franchomme & Pénoël (1990 p. 361) is given as containing two ketones (percentages not given). It is cited occasionally as an essential oil to be avoided in pregnancy, yet Franchomme cites no contraindications for this oil. Valnet (1980) gives it as an emmenagogue, though he does not cite amenorrhoea as an indication for its use—only painful menstruation, and it is not clear whether he means the essential oil or a decoction of the berries; this is crucial, as larger plant molecules can have different effects from the smaller volatile molecules. Franchomme makes no reference to the reproductive system whatsoever, nor do four other French aromatherapy books. The property of *J. communis* upon which all are agreed is its diuretic effect. This is sometimes suggested as the reason to avoid its use during early pregnancy, though it is an accepted fact that the baby draws all its needs from the mother, sometimes at her expense.

• *Levisticum officinale* [LOVAGE]—diuretic (contains around 50% phthallides, about which not much is known). The essential oil is distilled from the roots. The leaves were once used as an emmenagogue (Grieve 1991 p. 500), which may be the reason why the essential oil has been assumed to be emmenagogic also.

• *Melaleuca cajuputi* [CAJUPUT]—hormone-like (contains around 30–40% oxides). Franchomme (Franchomme & Pénoël 1990 p. 369) is the only person to advocate this essential oil needing care in use during pregnancy. He does not give it as emmenagogic.

• *Mentha × piperita* [PEPPERMINT]—hormone-like (contains 20–50% alcohols, 15–40% ketones). Like several essential oils, the main constituents in peppermint essential oil are variable, making decisions regarding its emmenagogic properties difficult. The pulegone content is usually 0.3–0.6%, though American peppermint may be just under 3% (Gilly, Garnero & Racine 1986). Peppermint is sometimes distilled after drying the plant, when the ratio of menthone (16–36.1%) to menthol (46.2–30.8%) is radically different (Fehr & Stenzhorn 1979). Valnet (1980 p. 173) and

Tisserand (1977 p. 269) list it as an emmenagogue, though Franchomme (Franchomme & Pénoël 1990 p. 374) lists it as a hormone-like oil which regulates the ovaries; he does not contraindicate it for pregnant women. Bardeau (1976 p. 216) states that it calms painful periods.

• *Ocimum basilicum* [EUROPEAN BASIL]. Because of its phenolic ether content (methyl chavicol), which varies within wide limits, depending on the species, the origin and the time of harvesting, basil is often cited as an emmenagogue. Valnet (1980) cites it as such, though Franchomme (Franchomme & Pénoël 1990) gives no mention of its use for any gynaecological condition and states that regardless of the percentage of methyl chavicol there are no known contraindications. Most of the basil oils available to aromatherapists contain a high percentage of methyl chavicol, the lowest being around 50% (and often as high as 75–80%). The plants from which the authors obtain their European basil oil have a very low methyl chavicol content, usually around 12%.

• *Origanum majorana* [SWEET MARJORAM] (contains around 40% terpenes and 50% alcohols). When this essential oil is contraindicated for pregnancy it is no doubt being confused, by the use of the common name, with *Thymus mastichina* [SPANISH MARJORAM]. The latter essential oil is a species of thyme and has totally different constituents, with an oxide content of 55–75%. There is no mention of any emmenagogic effect or of having to treat *O. majorana* with caution in any of the French aromatherapy literature (including Franchomme & Pénoël 1990, Valnet 1980) and no evidence has yet been produced to support the contraindication of *T. mastichina*, despite its high oxide content. Until there is, it may be prudent to use this latter oil with care. 'Marjoram' essential oil should not be purchased without knowing its botanical name.

• *Rosa damascena, R. centifolia* [ROSE OTTO]—hormone like (contains over 60% alcohols). Rose otto is cited several times as being antihaemorrhagic (Bardeau 1976 p. 268, Franchomme & Pénoël 1990 p. 392, Roulier 1990 p. 298), but no sources mention its having any emmenagogic properties. Wabner (1992 personal communication) states that it regulates menstruation

because of its hormonal influence, but that it is not emmenagogic.

• *Rosmarinus officinalis* [ROSEMARY]—different chemotypes (ketone content 14–35%, oxide content 18–40%). The chemotype labelled by Franchomme (Franchomme & Pénoël 1990 p. 393) as an emmenagogue is the camphoraceous rosemary. He cites the verbenone chemotype as neurotoxic and abortive (which would indicate care when used with pregnant women), but gives no contraindications regarding the reproductive system for the cineole chemotype. Roulier (1990 p. 298), on the other hand, gives no contraindications regarding the verbenone chemotype, yet warns against use of both the cineole and the camphoraceous type on pregnant women. He gives neither of them as an emmenagogue. The rosemary quoted in Valnet (1980 p. 177), which is not given as a specific chemotype and does not appear to contain verbenone, is given as an emmenagogue.

• *Salvia sclarea* [CLARY]—hormone like (contains 60–70% esters). The French authors metioned above cite clary, referring only to its hormonal properties (Roulier 1990 p. 302) specifically in regard to amenorrhoea, but with no mention of its being emmenagogic. It is considered emmenagogic by Holmes (1993), although no authority is given. According to Culpeper (1983), the juice of the herb (not the essential oil), drunk in beer, accelerates menstruation. This could be due to its hormonal properties, as sclareol (the diterpenol responsible for the hormone-like property of clary) is present in the juice in a much higher quantity than in the essential oil, due to its molecular weight (see Ch. 1).

• *Vetiveria zizanioides* [VETIVER] (average ketone content 22%). Only one source has been found to cite *V. zizanioides* as an emmenagogue, i.e. Franchomme & Pénoël (1990 p. 405).

Hormonal essential oils

A few essential oils which are hormonal but not neurotoxic or abortive are sometimes contraindicated during the first half of pregnancy, e.g. *S. sclarea, R. damascena* and *R. centifolia* (see above), but it is our belief and that of Balacs

(1992) that this is not necessary. Indeed, many of the authors' clients before 1985 used these and other now contraindicated oils such as *J. communis* in an informed manner during their pregnancies with only positive results.

This is undeniably a complex and perplexing area, and books on aromatherapy and essential oils do not always agree with each other. For example, *C. myrrha* and *C. molmol* yield hormone-like essential oil, high in terpenes—all are agreed on that. Its phenol content, when mentioned, is extremely low—some authors give ketones present and no phenols and some vice versa. In no book does it appear to contain anything untoward in the way of toxic chemicals, yet it is cited as toxic in Opdyke (1979). (Acute oral LD_{50} is equivalent to $1.65\,\text{g/kg}$ of subject's weight; in tests, no irritation or sensitization was noted.)

Hormone-regulating oils do not necessarily affect the uterus in the same way as an emmenagogue. Instead they are oils which stimulate the endocrine system, some being effective for many women's hormone-related problems such as primary or secondary amenorrhoea, irregular or scanty menstruation, PMS, pregnancy and menopausal difficulties (Price 1993 pp. 220–235). However, several of the hormonal oils contain not only emmenagogic properties but also a ketone or phenolic ether (marked with an * below). These oils should be used with prudence during pregnancy.

Essential oils with hormonal properties come into their own not only to assist uterine contractions (see Uterotonic essential oils in labour, below) but also after the birth, to support the production of prolactin. *F. vulgare*, for example, is known to promote lactation (Franchomme & Pénoël 1990 p. 354, Valnet 1980 p. 125).

The following are hormone-like, hormone-regulating essential oils (see Table 4.8):

- *Chamomilla recutita*
- *Commiphora myrrha, C. molmol*
- *Foeniculum vulgare* var. *dulce**
- *Melaleuca cajuputi*
- *Melaleuca viridiflora* [NIAOULI]
- *Mentha × piperita*
- *Pimpinella anisum**
- *Pinus sylvestris* [PINE]

- *Rosa damascena, R. centifolia*
- *Salvia officinalis**
- *Salvia sclarea.*

Uterotonic essential oils in labour

Oxytocin, the hormone which stimulates the uterus to contract, can be supported by a few essential oils which are uterotonic, even though these may be neurotoxic/abortive. By virtue of their ability to stimulate the uterus to contract, they are recommended for use in the last stages of labour to facilitate the birth. Essential oils containing ketones and phenols are also useful during this time because of their analgesic properties—the analgesic effect of the terpenes is not as strong (Price 1993 p. 53). (For oils with analgesic properties see Analgesic oils in Ch. 4 and Appendix B.9.)

Franchomme (Franchomme & Pénoël 1990 pp. 347–402) gives the essential oils listed below as being oestrogen-like or uterotonic. Their stimulating action on the uterus can facilitate the birth better than simple 'relaxing' oils such as 'lavender' (unspecified) or *S. sclarea*. That is not to say that an essential oil from one of the *Lavandula* species (or *S. sclarea*) would not be supportive: enabling the mother to relax is of prime importance, and results not only in less pain being felt during labour (Reed & Norfolk 1993—see Trial on p. 194), but also allows the mother to maintain awareness and enjoy the last unique and precious moments of birth. However, it would make sense to include a little of one of the following more strongly uterotonic oils in a mix in order to add to the benefits.

The following are essential oils which facilitate delivery (i.e. are uterotonic):

- *Cymbopogon martinii* [PALMAROSA]
- *Syzygium aromaticum* (flos) [CLOVE BUD] (difficult deliveries)
- *Foeniculum vulgare* var. *dulce* [FENNEL]
- *Mentha × piperita* [PEPPERMINT]
- *Myristica fragrans* [NUTMEG]
- *Pimenta dioica, P. racemosa* [BAY] (difficult deliveries)
- *Pimpinella anisum* [ANISEED]
- *Thymus vulgaris* ct. geraniol [SWEET THYME].

These oils should be employed during the last 2–3 weeks of pregnancy, massaged into the abdomen and the lower back twice daily. They may also be useful during labour itself.

Aromatherapists who can prescribe essential oils for internal use may recommend a weak tea made with *Salvia officinalis* two drops, one tea bag (preferably tannin-free China tea) and 0.75 litres (four cups) water. The tea bag should be removed after a short, quick stir. One cup, three times a day is recommended during the last 3 weeks, and each cup will contain less than one drop of essential oil. Bernadet (1983 p. 120) recommends a tea made with the leaves of *S. officinalis* for the same purpose, and peppermint tea may also be helpful. Other essential oils mentioned above may also be administered in this way, but always under the careful direction of an aromatologist or consultant.

Analgesic oils

It would be interesting to carry out a study similar to the one described in the trial study carried out at Ipswich Hospital (p. 194) using analgesic essential oils (high in terpenes, ketones or phenols—perhaps phenolic ethers also), to determine the pain relief and relaxation benefits for women in labour, since the relief of pain would automatically induce relaxation (Franchomme & Pénoël 1990). The following list shows the percentage of these components present in analgesic essential oils (all figures are approximate):

- *Lavandula angustifolia* [LAVENDER]—8% terpenes, 6% ketones
- *Coriandrum sativum* [CORIANDER]—25% terpenes, 12% ketones
- *Eucalyptus smithii* [GULLY GUM]—20% terpenes, 70% 1,8-cineole
- *Juniperus communis* [JUNIPER] (fruct. ram.)—60% terpenes
- *Syzygium aromaticum* [CLOVE BUD]—15% terpenes, 70% phenols
- *Melaleuca alternifolia* [TEA TREE]—55% terpenes
- *Mentha × piperita* [PEPPERMINT]—25% terpenes, 25% ketones (rectified oil can contain 60% ketones)
- *Myristica fragrans* [NUTMEG]–70% terpenes, 3% phenolic ethers

- *Origanum majorana* [SWEET MARJORAM]—40% terpenes, 0.5% phenolic ethers
- *Piper nigrum* [BLACK PEPPER]—85% terpenes
- *Zingiber officinale* [GINGER]—75% terpenes.

MIDWIFERY AND ESSENTIAL OILS

Many conditions occurring during pregnancy and childbirth, from backache and heartburn to oedema, stretch marks and uterine inertia, can be relieved or sometimes prevented by the use of various essential oils. This is being increasingly recognized by midwives. According to Sue Lundie, a midwife and aromatherapist working for Derby City General Hospital Trust, midwives working with both hospital and home deliveries are 'finding aromatherapy a useful adjunct to the range of options they are able to offer their clients to assist them in their efforts to make pregnancy, labour and the puerperium a natural and enjoyable experience' (Lundie 1993a). With this welcome entry of aromatherapy into midwifery, it is imperative that essential oils be administered by properly trained staff, working to well thought-out guidelines and protocols (see Ch. 16). This is not always the case, however. Many nurses and midwives (not qualified in aromatherapy or aromatology) are using essential oils on their own initiative, occasionally with unfavourable results.

Health Care Professionals working in areas where no policies or guidelines exist on the use of essential oils, and who are approached by women requiring advice on their use in pregnancy, should direct them to a qualified aromatherapist.

(Lundie 1993b)

This is a view shared by many aromatherapists in the nursing profession, whether or not they are practising midwives. It is reassuring to know that Community Health Sheffield (a NHS Trust), which was the first UK health authority to appoint a clinical aromatologist, does not allow any nurse unqualified in the use of essential oils to administer these except under the direction of the aromatherapist, and only she can be responsible for making up the essential oil prescriptions.

A good example of a practice guide for the use of aromatherapy in midwifery is provided by the Ipswich Hospital Practice Group in midwifery,

T is aged 39—fit and healthy, with two children aged 6 and 2. She was disappointed with her lack of control over the induced birth of the elder child. The younger one was born naturally, with the help of aromatherapy. Drugs were not used, resulting in T being fully alert and in control throughout her labour and delivery.

She came to see me 8 weeks into her third pregnancy, feeling nauseous and very tired. I gave her a full treatment, using two drops *Citrus aurantium* var. *amara* (fol.) (balances and uplifts the nervous system), one drop *Citrus paradisi* (per.) (for debility) and two drops *Citrus sinensis* (per.) (digestive stimulant, relieves nausea). I gave her the same mix of essential oils to use in the bath.

12 weeks. She had felt less fatigued after the first treatment and had slept well. As she was still experiencing some nausea, I added *Zingiber officinale* to the mix, and gave her some to use at home as an inhalation. After this, she was not so tired, slept well and her nausea was much improved.

17 weeks. She had haemorrhoids, for which I made up a lotion for daily application containing *Cupressus sempervirens* (vasoconstrictive), *Pelargonium graveolens* (decongestive, cicatrizant) and *Santalum album* (soothing). I also gave her a mixture of sweet almond and avocado, with essential oils of *Chamaemelum nobile*, *Citrus reticulata* (per.) and *Lavandula angustifolia* to apply daily to her abdomen, breasts and thighs to help avoid stretch marks. I would have liked to add *Boswellia carteri* but she did not like its aroma.

22 weeks. Feeling well, quite energetic, no sickness. Haemorrhoids were still a slight problem, but had improved. No digestive problems and her pregnancy was progressing well. Her treatment oils were two drops *C. aurantium* var. *amara* (per.) (uplifting and relaxing), one drop *P. graveolens* (hormonal balancing) and one drop *Rosmarinus officinalis* (stimulates nervous system). She responded to this treatment with increased energy and a sense of well-being.

35 weeks. Still feeling well, but rather tired and a little emotional. No evidence of oedema or heartburn, blood pressure normal. Relaxed and positive approach towards the birth. Treatment: one drop *Chamaemelum nobile*, one drop *Melissa officinalis* (relaxing), one drop *L. angustifolia* (backache), one drop *Salvia sclarea* (in preparation for the birth). Felt 'wonderful' following her treatment; was not tired, despite a restless night. I mixed a combination of cold pressed sweet almond and wheatgerm oils for her to massage her perineum daily to encourage elasticity, prevent tearing, to nourish any previously damaged tissue and to prepare this area for the impending birth.

37 weeks. Feeling rather uncomfortable: the baby's head had engaged, causing some pressure on her bladder, and there was flatulence and some lower backache. Despite this, still optimistic, no anxiety. I massaged her back and legs using one drop *C. nobile*,

one drop *L. angustifolia*, one drop *Z. officinale* (these three to soothe the digestive system, relieve flatulence and backache) and one drop *P. graveolens* (stimulates digestion and circulation). Following the massage, she felt relaxed with renewed energy—the backache eased.

During this period I massaged her back, legs and abdomen each week. The selection of oils included *S. sclarea* (imparts optimism and euphoria). The main consideration was in keeping her as relaxed and comfortable as possible, considering the increasing size and pressure of the fetus.

41 weeks. The consultant confirmed that T and baby were still well, and told her that if the baby had not arrived at 42 weeks, she would be admitted to hospital to be induced. She had been assured that this method would be used only as a last resort. As the baby was a week late, T was quite agitated and worried about the prospect of a further week's wait. To help allay her fears, I massaged her back, legs and abdomen, using two drops *Melissa officinalis* (uplifting, balancing), one drop *C. sempervirens* and one drop *P. graveolens* (circulatory system, leg cramps and haemorrhoids, which T was worried would recur, owing to pressure in the bowel area). T became noticeably calmer and more relaxed with the pressure in her back eased. The baby seemed so familiar with my hands and oils that as I worked on the abdomen, I could feel it moving and responding to the calming oils and the gentleness of the massage, reacting in the same way as T does.

42 weeks. T was admitted to hospital, where she had a Prostin pessary inserted in the vagina. Fetus heartbeat and uterine action were monitored for the first 30 minutes, registering a strong and steady heartbeat and some uterine activity. She was feeling rather anxious and a little nauseous, so I massaged her feet and back with *L. angustifolia* (nausea, relaxation). Although this maternity unit does not use aromatherapy, they were quite happy for us to proceed as we wished, using the oils. The Prostin pessary resulted in T getting irregular contractions and backache. After 6 hours she had only dilated to 2–3 cm. I again massaged her back, applying hot compresses and using a mixture of *Jasminum officinale* and *S. sclarea*.

T's progress was slow but natural. She chose not to have her membranes ruptured or to be induced intravenously. At 10 p.m., some 13 hours following admission, she was still making very slow progress. Her contractions were not very strong, but enough to prevent her from sleeping and she was beginning to feel tired and despondent. Throughout this period her blood pressure, pulse and fetal heartbeat were good. She was offered temazepam to help her sleep or pethidine to ease the pain, but she declined both. I then massaged her feet with a mixture containing three drops *S. sclarea*, paying special attention to massaging very firmly the reproductive area reflexes. The massage and oils were used to help speed up and regulate contractions.

Case 10.1   Aromatherapist: Beryl MacInnes MISPA, ITEC, SPDA, SPCD, UK (*contd*)

She began to progress more quickly and at 1 a.m. she had an extremely strong contraction: her membranes ruptured and strong and regular contractions continued. She remained totally focused and committed, breathing deeply, inhaling *L. angustifolia* on a tissue and having the same oil in cold compresses applied to her forehead and back of neck.

By 3.30 a.m. she had fully dilated, to the amazement of the nursing staff, who had predicted that she would not give birth until the following day and would almost certainly need further medical intervention. T was taken to the delivery suite, still very much in control over her own labour. She spent 2 hours in the final stages, using only gas and air and still totally focused on what she had to do. The delivery midwife gave her freedom of choice in the position she wished to deliver. T's beautiful baby boy eventually emerged at 5.45 a.m., weighing in at 8 lb 12 oz (almost 41 kg) (well over 2 lb or 1 kg heavier than her previous two children). She delivered in the squatting position, immediately cradling her baby and even cutting her own umbilical cord. She had experienced only a superficial tear, which needed a few stitches.

gynaecology and neonatal care. It begins by quoting the following from the Handbook of midwives rules (UKCC 1993 41.1):

A practising midwife shall not on her own responsibility administer any medicine, including analgesics, unless in the course of her training, whether before or after registration as a midwife, she has been thoroughly instructed in its use and is familiar with its dosage and methods of administration or application.

The Ipswich midwifery guide specifies dilutions and lists essential oils which may be used with safety and those with possible hazards. These last contain essential oils with risk of skin irritation, the restricted use of which would apply to all users of these oils and may be contraindicated for people other than pregnant women (see Appendix B.6). It then sets out the possible uses for lavender oil (type not specified) as a sedative, in labour and postnatally, in baths and by inhalation. It gives the aims of using essential oils in labour as being to:

- ease tension
- induce relaxation by relaxing the muscles
- improve the circulation
- lower the blood pressure
- provide the therapeutic benefits of touch
- strengthen the rapport between client and midwife
- give the birthing partner (if participating) a positive role to play.

There then follows a list of precautions and local contraindications plus procedures for treating four common occurrences during labour and breastfeeding (included in the lists in the next section).

GENERAL INDICATIONS FOR USE DURING PREGNANCY

The lists below show which essential oils have been used up to the present to alleviate a pregnancy-related condition. For ease of access, the conditions have been organized into four sections: antenatal, preparation for labour, labour and postnatal. The oils in each list are referred to by their common names, as they appeared in the literature from which they have been collected, viz.: Burns (1992), Cornwall & Dale (1988), Fawcett (1993), Guenier (1992), Lundie (1993a), MacInnes (1993), Norfolk & Reed (1994 personal communication), Price P (1994 personal communication).

Appendix B.1 lists further essential oils which can facilitate delivery, suggested in sources other than those included here. For methods of use of all the oils listed below, see Chapter 5.

Antenatal

Backache

- lavender, ginger, Roman chamomile—bath, massage
- Roman chamomile, lavender, rosemary— bath, application
- sweet marjoram, rosemary—bath, application in a carrier
- black pepper, sweet marjoram, Roman chamomile—bath, massage
- chamomile (type not specified), rosemary— massage, compress
- lavender, chamomile (type not specified), frankincense, eucalyptus.

Constipation

- lavender
- black pepper, sweet orange—abdomen massage, Swiss reflex
- orange (type not specified), Roman chamomile, black pepper.

Cramp

- marjoram (type not specified)
- sweet marjoram, cypress—massage, bath.

Emotional upsets

- Douglas pine, juniper, geranium, rose otto, cedarwood, clary
- clary, rosewood—inhalation from tissue.

Fatigue

- coriander, grapefruit, lavender, neroli, rosemary
- lemon, rosemary—inhalation
- grapefruit, bergamot, geranium.

Haemorrhoids

- cypress—bath, compress
- cypress, geranium—bath, compress
- cypress, geranium and sandalwood— application
- cypress, frankincense—application in a lotion
- cypress, lavender, frankincense, myrrh.

Headaches

- lavender (one drop neat)—massaged into temples or in cold compress
- basil—inhaled.

In a research study carried out at the Neurological Clinic of the Christian Albrechts University in Kiel, Germany, a significant analgesic effect with a reduction in sensitivity to headaches was produced by the combination of peppermint oil and ethanol (Göbel et al 1995). Both eucalyptus and peppermint have been used therapeutically for various pain conditions, particularly headaches (Saller, Helstein & Hellenbrecht 1988).

Heartburn and indigestion

- Roman chamomile, mandarin, orange, peppermint, petitgrain, sandalwood— application
- Roman chamomile, ginger—five drops each coriander, cardamom, dill in 50 ml carrier lotion—application
- coriander, ginger, lavender, lemongrass
- sandalwood, fennel—application in a lotion
- ginger one drop, in a teaspoonful of carrier oil
- peppermint.

Hormone balancing

- geranium (see Table 4.8 on p. 80).

Hypertension

before 36 weeks
- rosewood, sandalwood, ylang ylang.

after 36 weeks
- lavender, sweet marjoram, ylang ylang—five drops in total in bath.

pregnancy induced
- stress-relieving oils in general
- ylang ylang—bath; lemon one drop—tea (see Ch. 5)
- ylang ylang, marjoram (type not specified), lavender.

Insomnia

- lavender one to two drops— pillow/nightclothes
- Roman chamomile, lavender, sweet marjoram, mandarin, patchouli, sandalwood, ylang ylang—bath, inhalation (pillow, vaporizer)
- sandalwood, ylang ylang—on nightclothes during whole 9 months
- lavender, sandalwood, ylang ylang.

Nausea/vomiting (morning sickness)

- peppermint one to two drops—inhalation (tissue)
- petitgrain, orange, lavender, ginger, lemon—inhalation

- ginger, rosewood, petitgrain—inhalation
- lavender, ginger
- petitgrain, rosewood—inhalation; ginger—ingestion (one drop in a teaspoonful of vegetable oil). [**NB**. Unrefined hazelnut oil has a pleasant taste.]

Oedema

- lemon, orange, geranium, lavender—upward massage only
- patchouli, petitgrain—upward massage only.

Perineal tears (prevention)

- lavender, geranium—daily massage of the perineum and posterior vaginal wall with two fingers
- lavender, tea tree six to eight drops—bath or cold compress
- frankincense, German chamomile (in wheatgerm oil)—daily massage.

A study was carried out which looked at 29 first time mothers who performed 6 weeks of daily massage of the perineum against a control group of 26 women who did not. Episiotomy and second degree tear occurred in 48% of those massaging compared with 77% in the control group (van Arsdale & Avery unpublished work 1987).

Pregnancy rashes

- Roman chamomile six drops, rose otto one drop, in 50 ml carrier lotion (more quickly absorbed than oil)—application
- peppermint one drop, Roman chamomile four drops, sandalwood two drops, in 50 ml carrier oil or lotion
- chamomile (type not specified).

Stress and tension

- lavender
- ylang ylang, rose, neroli, rosewood, sandalwood, cedarwood
- bergamot, frankincense, geranium.

I have found frankincense of great use ... for anxiety and stress in women hospitalised with antepartum haemorrhage or threatened premature labour.

(Lundie 1993a)

Stretch marks

- lavender, Roman chamomile, mandarin—application
- geranium, frankincense, lavender
- rosewood, carrot seed, rose otto
- frankincense, German chamomile, neroli—massage.

Urinary tract infections

- bergamot, Roman chamomile, sandalwood—sitz baths, washes (bath)
- juniper berry, sandalwood, cedarwood—bath.

Vaginal infections

- bergamot, lavender, tea tree—sitz bath, washes
- tagetes, tea tree, rose otto one drop each—bath.

Varicose veins

- cypress, lemon—gentle massage upwards only, compress
- cypress, lavender, lemon—bath, careful massage.

Labour preparation

- clary, rose otto, sage—last 2–3 weeks
- clary—massage twice daily
- sage and fennel (to strengthen womb and Braxton Hicks contractions—bath, application, sage tea (one teaspoonful fresh, or one half teaspoonful dried, sage to one cup boiling water).

Uterine tonic

See Uterotonic essential oils in labour page 182.

Induction

- Any essential oil with relaxing properties.

Case 10.2 Aromatherapist: Kate Stockbridge, UK

Mrs E, who was at that time 36 weeks pregnant, had been admitted to hospital owing to bleeding from a low-lying placenta, a large baby and polyhydramnios (an excess of amniotic fluid surrounding the baby).

24 November. At her request, I gave her a relaxing full-body massage on the ward using jasmine, lavender and rose otto in grapeseed with calendula and wheatgerm carrier oils. She reported feelings of 'floating' for 4 hours post massage.

29 November. Due to the complications of her pregnancy she was to be induced on the following Tuesday so we arranged for a more stimulating massage. I used a blend of lavender, geranium, rose and clary.

30 November. She informed me that, although the massage was relaxing, 2 hours later she had noticed the Braxton Hicks contractions becoming more regular and more intense. This tailed off 2 hours later.

1 December. Mrs E's labour was induced for artificial rupture of the membranes. I joined her at 4.30 p.m. when she was in early labour. She was connected up to a monitor which shows a variation in the fetal heartbeat and muscular tension in the uterus (demonstrating contractions).

One indication of fetal well-being is the presence of beat-to-beat variability on the heart trace. (Beat-to-beat variability means the alteration of speed of the baby's heart rate, which should be greater than five beats per minute; a reduction is an indication of low oxygen supply.) This was the case prior to the massage and the baby's condition started to cause some concern.

Permission from the hospital was obtained and the massage was begun at 5.11 p.m. to the delight of the attending hospital staff who commented on the wonderful aroma. I gave Mrs E a full-body massage (suited to pregnancy) using jasmine, lavender and rose otto. Mrs E was turned to her right side at 5.23 p.m. The final part of the abdominal massage finished at 5.40 p.m. It was interesting to note that the beat-to-beat variability improved to a point of acceptability at 5.47 p.m., and was subsequently maintained for a further 20 minutes until 6.05 p.m. when Mrs E used a bed pan (possibly the stimulating effect of the massage caused the bladder to fill). Gravity acted on the weight of the uterus, then suppressed the blood supply to the placenta and in conjunction with the contractions led to a marked deceleration in fetal heartbeat, a result of an even lower level of oxygen getting to the placenta, a more severe indicator of fetal distress.

Mrs E also had an epidural, which was only effective on one side, despite adjustment. In advanced labour there was increased pain, which progressed round the back and into the pelvis with contractions. This area was massaged further and with increased pressure during the contractions when the pain intensified. Mrs E felt great relief from this and benefited from the physical and moral support At 10.58 p.m. a baby boy was assisted (due to fetal distress) into the world, weighing 9 lb 4 oz (4.2 kg).

Since the birth Mrs E has used an essential oil mix of cypress, jasmine and lavender in the bath to help tighten up the perineum and heal the episiotomy, which has been consistently clean and dry.

Retrospectively, Mrs E felt she had benefited enormously from my attendance and on discussion with the hospital practitioner it was felt that the blend of aromatherapy and midwifery practice was to the patient's benefit.

Case 10.3 Aromatherapist: Lynne Reed, UK

Antenatal
a. A Gravida 5 Para 3 with hyperemesis gravidarum: this lady had suffered with hyperemesis during all of her previous four pregnancies and had even undergone a termination previously because of this condition. She was admitted to hospital for intravenous therapy to correct her electrolyte balance and after several days was discharged. She was readmitted a few days later still unable to keep any food down. It was at this time that I was asked whether I thought aromatherapy could help her.

She was offered various oils to smell to ascertain how well they would be tolerated. The ones she felt most happy with were *Citrus aurantium* var. *amara* (per.), *C. paradisi* (per.), *C. sinensis* (per.) and *Mentha × piperita*. Lemon was not well tolerated as she associated it with the lemon squash that she had been drinking, which had made her sick. I gave her a drop of peppermint oil in a glass of water to sip occasionally when she felt queasy, to settle her stomach. The orange and grapefruit oils were inhaled from a tissue.

The following morning she said that she felt a bit better and that she had remembered that in the past citrus fruits were the one thing that she could eat without feeling or being sick. We decided therefore that, as soon as she felt able, these were the foods she should try to begin with.

I arranged to see her 2 days later, only to find that she had been discharged, requiring no further admissions.

Labour
b. A Primigravida: this lady made good use of *Lavandula angustifolia* baths in early labour to aid relaxation. She had one dose of pethidine 100 mg when the contractions became too much for her. She wanted a water birth (contraindicated within 3 hours

Case 10.3   Aromatherapist: Lynne Reed, UK (contd)

of having pethidine) so was anxious not to have more.

05:00   6 cm dilated and an ARM (artificial rupture of membranes) was performed. She commenced on Entonox and back massage was given. We made use of a long footstool which she could sit astride with myself behind her, her upper body being supported with a beanbag on the bed.

05:30   Fully dilated.

05:45   Entered the bath for delivery (no lavender because of the baby's eyes) and the vertex was visible.

05:55   She had a normal water birth.

Essential oils used: two drops *L. angustifolia*, two drops *Chamaemelum nobile*, one drop *Salvia sclarea*.

c.   Primigravida in early labour.

16:15   2 cm dilated.

20:05   3 cm dilated.

21:30   Coping quite well.

23:15   Persuaded to take a bath with five drops *L. angustifolia*. This was enjoyed but she could not get really comfortable in the bath.

23:45   5 cm dilated. Pethidine requested and 100 mg given.

00:45   6 cm dilated; spontaneous rupture of membranes occurred.

01:00   A back and gentle abdominal massage were given using one drop each of *C. nobile* and *Chamomilla recutita* and two drops each of *Cananga odorata* and *L. angustifolia*.

01:30   Fully dilated.

02:54   Normal delivery.

d.   Primigravida. 36 week gestation with spontaneous rupture of membranes due for induction because of prolonged rupture of membranes.

04:00   1 cm dilated, with weak to fair contractions every 5–10 minutes. She was offered a relaxing bath with essential oils of *L. angustifolia* and *S. sclarea*. She stayed in the bath for 1 hour.

06:00   Contracting fairly strongly, once every 5 minutes.

07:00   Fully dilated, with an urge to push.

07:15   Confirmation of full dilation was made and good progress was continued.

07:40   Normal delivery.

Total length of labour: 3 hours 45 minutes.

e.   Primigravida. Had made use of TENS (transcutaneous electrical nerve stimulation) machine at home. Admitted to hospital for delivery.

23:30   2 cm dilated with intact membranes.

00:30   Given bath with five drops *L. angustifolia*.

02:30   9 cm dilated; requested additional pain relief. Reluctant to leave the bath, so vaginal examination carried out in the bath. An ARM was performed and Entonox commenced.

03:30   Vertex was visible, but progress in the second stage was slow. Advised to get out of the bath.

04:30   Transferred to a delivery bed. A gentle abdominal massage was given using two drops each of *C. nobile* and *L. angustifolia* and one drop of *S. sclarea*.

05:00   Normal delivery. No other form of pain relief.

f.   Primigravida.

01:00   5 cm dilated. ARM performed.

01:45   Bath with five drops *L. angustifolia*.

02:15   Full dilation confirmed. Urge to push.

03:00   Vertex visible on the perineum.

03:10   Normal water birth.

The delivery took place in the same bath water containing lavender because it would have had time to either evaporate or blend well in the water.

Various combinations of essential oils were used for massage in labour. In 50 ml of carrier oil were blended (number of drops of each oil in brackets):

• *Chamaemelum nobile* (3), *Lavandula angustifolia* (1), *Salvia sclarea* (3) in 50 ml carrier oil
• *Cananga odorata* (3), *Lavandula angustifolia* (1), *Pelargonium graveolens* (3) in 50 ml carrier oil
• *Cananga odorata* (2), *jasminum officinale* var. *grandiflorum* (1), *Lavandula angustifolia* (2) in 25 ml carrier oil

The main aim was:

• To stimulate the pituitary and thalamus to encourage the secretion of endorphins and encephalins to reduce pain.
• To utilize the sedative properties of lavender and Roman chamomile to aid relaxation.

Labour

Contractions

• lavender
• clary, geranium
• clary—inhalation.

See also Uterotonic essential oils in labour page 182.

Discomfort, pain

• lavender five drops—bath
• bergamot, geranium, lavender, palmarosa, rose otto
• black pepper, sweet marjoram—massage.

Case 10.4 Aromatherapist: Noel Hulmston MBRCP, MGCP, UK

Diastasis symphisis pubis (DSP) is a relatively uncommon problem which can occur in pregnancy as a consequence of the ligaments in the pubic joint failing to perform as normal, probably as a result of hormonal changes, which (particularly in the case of progesterone) can have a softening effect on ligaments. The main symptom is severe pelvic pain, with possible associated symptoms such as neck pain, headaches, dizziness and a general malaise.

M had been diagnosed as having DSP 36 weeks into her pregnancy, the lower back pain having commenced at the end of her first trimester. Following a normal birth, the pain had relented for a couple of days, before returning intensely. Previous X-rays had revealed a gap in the symphysis pubis and one side of the joint lower than the other, which latter characteristic was not noticeable on examination. Physiotherapy, involving heat and mechanical traction, had resulted in her being confined to bed for a week. At the time she came to see me she had been registered as permanently disabled.

After the consultation, M's GP was approached and he approved the treatment plan I suggested, which included M's husband being shown some elementary techniques to use as 'first aid' measures if required. In addition, an hourly pain diary was maintained and some relaxation techniques were suggested.

Treatment 1: This was a back massage using a base vegetable oil, with the addition of equal quantities of *Mentha* × *piperita*, *Pelargonium graveolens* and *Lavandula angustifolia* to a 2.5% dilution. There was considerable tenderness over the left side of her lower back and, following the application of the oils, warm towels were placed over the whole of the back. A 3% blend of *M.* × *piperita*, *Cinnamomum zeylanicum* (fol.) and *Melaleuca viridiflora* in the same carrier oil base was then massaged carefully into the lower abdominal area and the upper groin on both sides. The differential in the two halves of the symphysis pubis was obvious, with the left side being noticeably raised.

For this first treatment I had decided to use hot and cold compresses directly over the pubic bone after the massage—three applications, ending with a cold pack. The essential oils used in the abdomen massage were added to the hot compress; no oils were used with the cold compress. On this occasion pain and some of the debilitating side-effects were the targets.

Amongst the latter were the depressive element, reduced muscle function and some sluggishness in the body systems. Each oil was chosen mainly for its analgesic properties; in addition, peppermint is a multifaceted oil with wide-ranging properties and geranium added diuretic, tonic and antidepressive elements. Niaouli was included to provide a benefit to the local circulation, particularly around the pubic area and for the power it has to strengthen the immune system. Cinnamon leaf was used for its warming and tonic properties.

Treatment 2: This was 2 weeks later, when identical protocols were used. M reported that she felt relaxed and appeared to be sleeping better since her first treatment.

Treatment 3: This was a further 2 weeks later. At this visit, her husband was shown how to make and apply compresses.

Treatment 4: This was 3 weeks later, when the usual pattern was followed. On this occasion there was noticeably less tenderness in the lower back and the left side of the pelvis. M reported that the intense pelvic pain, normally associated with menstruation, had gone. Always conscious of the risk of making a client 'therapist dependent', the next treatment was set for a month ahead, when the following results were reported:

- still no pain during menstruation
- the ability to stay up each evening with her husband rather than having to go to bed 3 hours before him
- reduced levels of pain (shown by the pain diary)
- reduced tenderness in lower back and rear of pelvic area.

Treatment has continued at monthly intervals with the same protocol being used. The most startling change has been in the presentation of the pubic bones, where the left side now appears to be matching the right—M also feels 'more balanced' on either side.

M continues with her regime for relaxation including having a lavender bath before retiring each night. She will remain registered disabled and possibly constantly at risk of increased pain. However, she feels that aromatherapy has helped her considerably.
[This case appeared in the International Journal of Aromatherapy: 8 (3)]

Hypertonic uterine action

- geranium, lavender.

- clary, frankincense, neroli—inhalation, massage.

Puerperal depression

- bergamot, clary, grapefruit, mandarin, neroli, rose otto, vetiver

Ruptured membranes

- lavender three drops—bath.

Stress and anxiety

- clary, lavender, rose otto, ylang ylang
- lavender
- clary, rose otto, ylang ylang—inhalation, massage
- lavender, petitgrain, ylang ylang
- benzoin, frankincense, rose
- clary, chamomile (type not specified), lavender.

Uterine inertia

- clary, lavender.

See Uterotonic essential oils in labour page 182.

Postnatal

Anxiety

- lavender—bath/tissue.

Blood loss minimization

- cypress, lavender—baths.

Breast engorgement

- geranium six drops—in bath or warm compress.

Caesarean section wounds

- lavender, tea tree—baths/compress
- frankincense, neroli, rose otto—bath.

Cracked nipples

- lavender, Roman chamomile, rose otto
- frankincense, myrrh, patchouli—lotion.

Despondency

- bergamot, clary, neroli, ylang ylang
- clary, geranium, juniper.

Emotional imbalance

- geranium, Roman chamomile, rose otto—inhalation, bath.

Fatigue

- bergamot, geranium, lavender, mandarin, petitgrain, rosemary, rose otto.

Grief following stillbirth

- frankincense, melissa, rose otto—inhalation, massage, bath.

Haemorrhage

- cypress, sweet marjoram—compress
- cypress, lavender.

Lactation

To increase:
- fennel tea—one teaspoonful crushed seeds to one cup boiling water; fennel seven drops, geranium two drops in 30 ml carrier—massage
- seven drops fennel in 50 ml carrier—massage
- aniseed and lemongrass—massage.

In the United States, the use of fennel as an oestrogenic agent persisted into the 20th century; in 1916, it was described in the National Standard Dispensatory that an infusion of fennel 'is occasionally given to increase the lacteal secretion, and to establish the menstrual flow' (Hare, Caspari & Rusby 1916). Fennel was found in subsequent studies to have oestrogenic activity (Albert-Puleo 1979).

To decrease:
- geranium—bath or compress
- peppermint—bath or compress
- geranium, lavender—compress
- geranium, lavender, peppermint—compress
- peppermint and sage—bath, compress.

In Kerala, southern India, bandaging the breasts with jasmine flowers (*Jasminum pubescens*) to suppress lactation is a common procedure, though there is very little written down to support it. Contact with jasmine flowers was found to suppress milk production in mice; exposure to the smell only of the flowers produced similar changes, though to a lesser extent (Abraham, Sarada Devi & Sheela 1979). In another part of southern India, Vallore, a study was carried out at the Christian Medical College Hospital on two groups of women who had experienced a fresh stillbirth or early neonatal death to determine whether or not jasmine (in this case *Jasminum sambac*) was as successful as bromocriptine (Group 1) in suppressing puerperal lactation; the latter was limited in its use owing to its high cost. 50 cm of stringed jasmine flowers were kept in place on the breasts (Group 2) with loosely applied adhesive tape and changed every 24 hours for 5 days (paracetamol tablets were available to both groups if needed). The results of both groups were fairly similar and it was concluded that jasmine flowers 'seem to be a clinically effective and inexpensive method of suppression of puerperal lactation with good patient acceptance' (Shrivastav et al 1988).

It may be interesting to carry out a study using a compress with jasmin absolute (*Jasminum grandiflorum* or *J. officinale*) to see whether these would have a similar effect. However, attention would have to be paid to the quality of this much adulterated oil as one containing residual solvent or any synthetics could cause irritation on the skin surface.

Mastitis

- lavender, geranium (decongestant), peppermint (cooling)—compress.

Perineum

Bruised
- cypress two drops, lavender two drops, sweet marjoram three drops, in 50 ml wheatgerm oil.

Infected
- lavender, tea tree four drops each—baths or compress
- cajuput, pine, sandalwood two drops each—bath, compress.

Painful
- lavender six to eight drops—bath
- juniper, lavender, marjoram

- neroli, tea tree four to six drops—bath
- cypress, frankincense, lavender, myrrh.

Trauma
- lavender eight drops in 50 ml cold water—compress.

Swollen ankles following delivery

- geranium—massage
- geranium, patchouli, petitgrain—massage.

Baby

Colic

- fennel—tea for mother if breastfeeding; ginger, Roman chamomile one drop each in 25 ml carrier oil—massage baby
- dill, mandarin, Roman chamomile.

Cradle cap

- cedarwood one drop in 10 ml carrier oil
- eucalyptus, geranium, lavender.

Crying unduly

- sandalwood, ylang ylang—on a tissue
- chamomile (type not specified), lavender.

PILOT STUDIES

The use of essential oils to assist labour has been well documented. In a hospital in New South Wales, Australia, for instance, clove and lavender are used to intensify contractions. 'Feedback indicates that these oils (clove oil with lavender) are particularly valuable in strengthening and enhancing contractions, whilst at the same time easing the pain and discomfort of labour' (Cutter 1992). At the onset of labour, a warm bath is taken with one or two drops of clove oil added; for massage one drop of clove oil is added, together with lavender, to make a 1% concentration and used 1 week before labour is expected.

The two pilot studies presented here were carried out in British hospitals, and their results are very encouraging.

PILOT STUDY USING ESSENTIAL OILS DURING LABOUR

Midwives in the John Radcliffe Maternity Hospital under the care of Ethel Burns (lecturer practitioner delivery suite) undertook a pilot study in 1990 to find a way of relieving pain and keeping mothers calm during labour and delivery (Burns & Blamey 1994). In this 6 month study 585 women took part (91% had full data recorded), and 10 different essential oils were used. It is important to bear in mind, when considering the data below, that this hospital is a regional referral unit, with a significant number of women with complicated pregnancies.

The oils were chosen according to the qualities attributed to each of them in aromatherapy literature, e.g. relaxing, sedating, antispasmodic, uterotonic, oestrogen-like, cooling, refreshing, antiinflammatory, antidepressant. The oils were:

- chamomile (unspecified)
- clary
- eucalyptus (unspecified)
- frankincense
- jasmine absolute (not a distilled oil)
- lavender (unspecified)
- lemon
- mandarin
- peppermint
- rose absolute.

Different oils were chosen and used for specific purposes:

- the reduction of maternal anxiety—used 321 times (predominantly lavender)
- to relieve nausea—used 130 times (predominantly peppermint)
- to increase contractions—used 111 times (predominantly clary)
- pain relief—used 88 times.

An evaluation sheet was devised to record the following data: parity, fetal distress, labour onset; analgesia before and after oils, which oils were used, how often, for what reasons and at what stage in labour, and type of delivery. Both the mother's and the midwife's evaluation of the effectiveness (and side-effects if any) were recorded.

Methods of use

The following range of methods of use was used:

- two drops essential oil in 100 ml water, sprayed on to a face flannel, pillow or bean bag
- four to six drops in a bath
- two to three drops in a foot bath
- one drop onto absorbent card for inhaling
- two drops in 50 ml almond oil for massage
- one drop peppermint directly on the forehead
- one drop frankincense directly on the palm.

All women had given their consent and were defined as being 'in labour' when contracting regularly and painfully, with a cervical dilation of at least 3 cm.

Results

Labour

80% of the women started with essential oils without any form of analgesia and of these:

- 13% used no other form of analgesia
- 67% were given essential oils first, before any other analgesia.

Delivery

The percentages of different types of deliveries were:

- 71% spontaneous vaginal delivery
- 20% instrumental delivery
- 8% Caesarean section
- 7% emergencies
- 1% elective
- 1% unrecorded.

Effectiveness

The number of essential oils employed in different combinations in this study makes it impossible to arrive at any definite conclusions about the effectiveness of any one particular essential oil. However, the overall effects of essential oils recorded by the women themselves are given below.

- 62% found them effective
- 12% did not
- 17% were unsure
- 9% did not record a decision, but 27% of these made positive comments.

Side-effects

3% (16 people) recorded transient side-effects and of these:

- eight comments were about peppermint—five said the drop placed on their forehead had had a burning effect. [authors' comment: peppermint is an essential oil best not used neat, especially near the eyes. In dilution (even 20%) this oil may retain its cooling qualities, but in concentration it often has the opposite effect to that desired. For example, it is antiirritant in low concentration (1% or less) but can be irritant if used in high concentration (above 10–20%, depending on the individual).]
- two comments were about lavender—it had exacerbated the nausea of one woman and made the husband of another feel sick.
- six comments were regarding clary: two did not like the aroma, two felt nauseated and two did not feel it worked.

Conclusions

Burns & Blamey (1994) concluded that 'The results indicate a high degree of overall satisfaction in using aromatherapy during labour/delivery, on the part of women and midwives … A relaxed woman in labour is empowered to have greater control over what happens to her'. The John Radcliffe Hospital has recently completed another pilot study, this time with 7000 women taking part. The data is currently being analysed (January 1999) and the report is expected to be published at the end of the year.

TRIAL USING LAVENDER (UNSPECIFIED) DURING LABOUR

A survey using lavender baths during labour was carried out in 1992 by Lynne Norfolk and Lynne Reed, aromatherapist/midwives at Ipswich Hospital (Reed & Norfolk 1993), with the support of their Director of Midwifery Services and using the practical procedure written by her (Fern 1992) to protect both clients and midwives from any possible misuse of oils. All midwives worked under the direction of Norfolk and Reed. The aims of the survey were:

- to determine whether there was any pain relief and relaxation to be gained from lavender baths
- to ensure there were no adverse side-effects from them.

Clients taking lavender baths (using five drops of lavender oil) and their midwives were asked to complete a questionnaire. The questionnaire covered five areas: Apgar score, type of delivery, length of labour, additional pain relief, and midwife and client perception of the effects of lavender baths. A total of 38 questionnaires were handed in (19 primigravidae and 19 multigravidae clients).

Results

Apgar scores

On this assessment of neonatal condition:

- three women scored 10
- 30 women scored 8 or 9
- two women scored 7 (one had a total of 250 mg pethidine and one had 150 mg shortly before delivery)
- one woman scored 6 (stale meconium was present)
- two women did not have the score recorded on the questionnaire.

NB. Those scoring 7 or below had other associated contributing factors.

Types of delivery

The deliveries were as follows:

- 34 normal
- two forceps
- one LSCS (failure to progress)
- one ventouse extraction (suction cup).

Length of labour

The length of labour of each of the 38 women in the trial is shown in Table 10.1. The shortest primigravidae labour was 3 h 10 min, the longest 22 h 37 min. The shortest multigravidae labour was 40 min, the longest 12 h 47 min.

Additional pain relief

Altogether, 18 out of the 19 primigravidae clients required additional pain relief during labour, contrasting with 12 of the 19 multigravidae clients. The amount and type of additional pain relief required by these clients are shown in Table 10.2.

Perceived benefits

Table 10.3 shows the benefits the midwives and their clients felt they gained from taking lavender baths.

Table 10.1   Length of labour (in hours) of 38 women taking lavender baths (after Reed & Norfolk 1993)

	Primigravidae *	Multigravidae
Up to 4 hrs	—	8
Up to 5 hrs	—	5
Up to 6 hrs	8	2
7–13 hrs	4†	4
14–22 hrs	5	—

* 2 primigravidae replies not received
† all under 10 hrs

Table 10.2   Additional pain relief required during labour by 38 women taking lavender baths (after Reed & Norfolk 1993)

	Primigravidae	Multigravidae
Entonox	3	6 (1 plus massage)
Pethidine 100 mg	5	3
Pethidine 150 mg	8 (7 one dose)	3 (1 plus massage)
Epidural	2	0
TENS	0	0
Massage only	1	0

Table 10.3   Results of questionnaires given to 38 midwives and their clients assessing effects of taking baths, with five drops unspecified lavender oil added, during labour (after Reed & Norfolk 1993)

	Midwives			Clients		
	Helped	Did not help	No reply	Helped	Did not help	No reply
Relaxation	36	0	2	31	2	5
Pain relief	30	'4	4	23	7	8
Enjoyment	34	1	3	30	1	7

Conclusions

Fetal well-being

The good Apgar scores would suggest that five drops of lavender in baths present no risks to the baby.

Type of delivery

34 of the 38 clients achieved a normal delivery.

Length of labour

It is not possible to assess whether or not labour was shortened by having lavender baths, but some appeared to progress very rapidly. However, two facts became obvious. Progress was better:

- in those who used the lavender bath when a 2+ dilation or more was established
- in those who spent more than 30 minutes in the bath (this may be due in part to the hydrotherapy effect).

Relaxation and pain relief

The majority of clients found the baths to be helpful and enjoyable. Over half felt that the baths helped with pain relief.

Perineal management

Aromatherapy can also be used to reduce any perineal trauma and discomfort which may be suffered as a result of childbirth. Perineal management is increasingly becoming part of the midwives' role as it is not uncommon for women to experience perineal trauma to some extent during the childbirth process, especially those having their first baby (Labrecque et al 1994). Many of those qualified in aromatherapy are now advising their clients to massage their perineums from 16–34 weeks onwards (the starting time varying from therapist to therapist) with a carrier oil, some using essential oils for the added benefits these can bring. Women naturally prefer an intact perineum and preventing tears and other damage saves the midwife from having to suture perineums after the birth. Apart from this saving in time, savings can also be made in cost (of suture packs); both are important considerations for the Health Service (Feasey unpublished work 1998).

Using massage 6 weeks before childbirth— with vegetable oil and with essential oils

Avery & van Arsdale are believed to be the first to carry out a study involving essential oils and the perineum. The study, which took place in 1987, involved 55 mothers-to-be: 29 who gave themselves a daily massage for 6 weeks prior to the expected date of delivery, and 26 who did not, acting as a control group. Episiotomy and second degree tears occurred in 48% of the first group, compared with 78% in the second group (Guenier 1992). Guenier herself has recommended perineal massage (using lavender and geranium) to her antenatal groups, with beneficial results.

It would be interesting to do further studies, this time with three groups: one using massage alone (known from the study above to be effective), one using massage and essential oils (to see if the effectiveness is improved by the addition of essential oils), and one control group.

Using essential oils *during* childbirth

In 1996, a small randomized pilot study was carried out by community midwife Rosemary Feasey to ascertain whether one or more pads soaked in a solution of warm water and essential oil of *Lavandula angustifolia* would help prevent injury to the perineum of labouring primigravida women when applied as active pushing commences.

Three groups of women (25 in each) took part and each group had a different perineal pad:

- group A—dry
- group B—warm and wet
- group C—warm and wet but with the addition of lavender.

Although the study was inconclusive, the majority of women found the lavender pad soothing on their perineums, and because the aroma helped them to relax, they were able to listen more carefully to the midwives' instructions (regarding when, and when not, to push) so that the perineum stretched more slowly and easily.

Feasey would like to continue with further studies, improving the protocol to take into account different factors that came to light during the trial.

Using essential oils *after* childbirth

Claims are presently made that the use of lavender in the bath after childbirth reduces perineal discomfort. Lavender was used in the bath water on a postnatal ward at Hinchingbrooke Hospital, and 85% of the mothers who used it (and answered a questionnaire) felt it had reduced perineal discomfort (Mulgrew 1989). This result was subjective and there was an absence of adequate controls; for example, there is no way of knowing whether a bath alone would give equal relief.

Subsequently Dale & Cornwall (1994) carried out a trial to assess the efficacy of lavender oil in the bath to reduce perineal discomfort after childbirth. It was a single-blind randomized clinical trial involving three groups of mothers (635 in total): one group used lavender oil (scientific name not given), one a synthetic lavender oil (for which no claims are made regarding the relief of perineal discomfort, but which has a similar chemical composition) and one an inert but aromatic substance; these additives were used in the bath for 10 days following normal childbirth. When mothers returned home, daily visits by the community midwife enabled assessment of the perineum to be continued until the 10th day.

Statistics were found to be more stable during the first 5 days when the mothers were under supervision at their daily bathing. Although women in the group using pure lavender oil showed lower mean discomfort scores during these first 5 days after childbirth, any differences failed to achieve statistical significance, therefore it cannot be concluded that using lavender in the bath eases perineal discomfort. However, there were some consistently lower mean discomfort scores in the pure lavender oil group, particularly between days three and five. This is not unexpected as perineal discomfort decreases in any case over time.

This trial raises some queries:

1. Can we be sure that an aromatic compound is inert and would not have any effect?
2. Synthetic lavender may have had some effect, as the synthetic chemicals used would be similar in structure to the compounds occurring in natural lavender.
3. The scientific name of the lavender was not given, but from the constituents quoted it appears that it was not *Lavandula angustifolia*.

The importance of accurately identifying the substance used in trials cannot be over emphasized; there is a doubt here because three of the 'main' components listed, of which camphor was one, do not exist in *L. angustifolia*. It would be worth repeating this trial with only two groups, one using *L. angustifolia* and one using water (in an essential oil bottle), though it is appreciated that the lack of aroma can present difficulties (see Parkinson's disease study in Ch. 9).

Summary

The majority of female admissions to hospital are connected with pregnancy and birth, which are not health problems unless there are complications. Pregnancy is an area of great interest to aromatherapists, nurses and midwives and consequently a great deal of experience has been accumulated in maternity wards and by visiting midwives all over the UK. Small scale trials of essential oils used in labour have given encouraging results. It is hoped that larger controlled studies will endorse these findings, and that the use of aromatherapy (including some of the more powerful oils) by qualified professionals in antenatal, maternity and postnatal settings will increase accordingly.

REFERENCES

Abraham M, Sarada Devi N, Sheela R 1979 Inhibiting effect of jasmine flowers on lactation. Indian Journal of Medical Research 69: 88–92

Albert-Puleo M 1980 Fennel and anise as estrogenic agents. Journal of Ethnopharmacology 2: 337–344

Allen W T 1897 Note on a case of supposed poisoning by pennyroyal. The Lancet i: 1022–1023

Baker J B E 1960 The effects of drugs on the fetus. Pharmacological Reviews 12: 37–90

Balacs M A 1992 Safety in pregnancy. International Journal of Aromatherapy 4(1): 12–15

Bardeau F 1976 La médecine aromatique. Laffont, Paris

Bernadet M 1983 La phyto-aromathérapie pratique. Dangles, St-Jean-de-Braye

Braithwaite P F 1906 A case of poisoning by pennyroyal: recovery. British Medical Journal 2: 865

Burns E 1992 Dedicated to better birth. International Journal of Aromatherapy 4(1): 9–11

Burns E, Blamey D 1994 Using aromatherapy in childbirth. Nursing Times 90(9): 54–60

Chandler R F, Hooper S N, Harvey M J 1982 Ethnobotany and phytochemistry of yarrow, *Achillea millefolium*, Compositae. Economic Botany 36(2): 203

Cornwell S, Dale A 1988 Aromatherapy in midwifery practice. Hinchingbrooke Hospital, Huntingdon

Culpeper N 1983 Culpeper's colour herbal. Foulsham, London, p 47

Cutter K 1992 Dedicated to better birth. International Journal of Aromatherapy 4(1): 11

Dale A, Cornwell S 1994 The role of lavender in relieving perineal discomfort following childbirth: a blind randomised clinical trial. Journal of Advanced Nursing 19: 89–96

Fawcett M 1993 Aromatherapy for pregnancy and childbirth. Element Books, Shaftesbury

Fehr D, Stenzhorn G 1979 Untersuchungen zur Lagerstabilität von Pfefferminzblättern, Rosmarinblättern und Thymian. Pharmazeutische Zeitung 124: 2342–2349

Fern E 1992 The Ipswich Hospital directorate of maternity and gynaecological practice group midwifery, gynaecology and neonatal care). Aromatherapy, Midwifery Procedures nos 23A, 23C, 23D, 23E

Formacek K, Kubeczka K H 1982 Essential oils analysis by capillary chromatography and carbon-13 NMR spectroscopy. John Wiley, New York

Franchomme P, Pénoël D 1990 L'aromathérapie exactement. Jollois, Limoges

Gilly G, Garnero J, Racine P 1986 Menthes poivrées— composition chimique analyse chromatographie. Parfumerie Cosmétiques Aromates 71: 79–86

Göbel H, Schmidt G, Dworschak M, Stolze H, Heuss D 1995 Essential plant oils and headache mechanisms. Phytomedicine 2(2): 93–102

Grieve M 1991 A modern herbal. Penguin, London

Guenier J 1992 Essential obstetrics. International Journal of Aromatherapy 4(1): 6–8

Hare H A, Caspari C, Rusby H H 1916 The national standard dispensatory. Lea & Febiger, Philadelphia, p. 63

Holder R 1995 Aromatherapy in hospitals—a study in acceptance. The Aromatherapist 2(2): 11–19

Holmes P 1993 Clary sage. International Journal of Aromatherapy 5(1): 15–17

Labrecque M, Marcaux S, Pinarlt J J, Laroche C, Martin S 1994 Prevention of perineal trauma by perineal massage during pregnancy. A pilot study. Birth 21(1): 20–25

Lawrence B M 1984 Progress in essential oils: yarrow oil. Perfumer & Flavorist 9(4): 37

Lawrence B M 1989 Progress in essential oils: pennyroyal. Perfumer & Flavorist 14(3): 71

Leung A Y 1980 Encyclopedia of common natural ingredients used in food, drugs and cosmetics. John Wiley, New York, p 409

Lundie S 1993a Aromatherapy in maternity care. Unpublished paper

Lundie S 1993b Introducing and applying aromatherapy within the NHS. The Aromatherapist 1(2): 30–35; 1(3): 32–37; 2(1): 34–38

Mabey R 1988 The complete new herbal. Elm Tree Books, London, p 72

MacInnes B 1993 The use of aromatherapy in pregnancy and childbirth. Unpublished dissertation, Shirley Price International College of Aromatherapy, Hinckley

Maickel R P, Snodgrass W R 1973 Physiochemical factors in maternal-fetal distribution of drugs. Toxicology and Applied Pharmacology 26: 218–230

Mulgrew M 1989 Mothers' experience of post natal care. Internal report, Hinchingbrooke Midwifery Service, Huntingdon, Cambridgeshire

Myles M 1993 Textbook for midwives, 12th edn. Churchill Livingstone, New York, p 43

Opdyke D L J (ed) 1979 Monographs on fragrance raw materials. In: Food and Cosmetics Toxicology. Research Institute for Fragrance Materials, Pergamon Press, New York, p 581

Price S 1993 The aromatherapy workbook. Thorsons, London

Reed L, Norfolk L 1993 Aromatherapy in midwifery. Aromatherapy World (nurturing issue, Summer): 12–15

Roulier G 1990 Les huiles essentielles pour votre santé. Dangles, St-Jean-de-Braye

Saller R, Helstein A, Hellenbrecht D 1988 Klinische Pharmacologie und therapeutische Anwendung von Cineol (Eukalyptus) und Menthol als bestandteil ätherischer Öle. Internistische Praxis 28(2): 355–364

Shrivastav P, George K, Balasubramaniam N, Jasper P, Thomas M, Kanagasabhapathy A S 1988 Suppression of puerperal lactation using jasmine flowers (*Jasminum sambac*). Australian and New Zealand Journal of Obstetrics and Gynaecology 28: 68–71

Sullivan J B, Peterson R G 1979 Pennyroyal poisoning and hepatoxicity. Journal of the American Medical Association 242(26): 2873–2874

Tisserand R 1977 The art of aromatherapy. Daniel, Saffron Walden

Tisserand R, Balacs M A 1991 Research reports. International Journal of Aromatherapy 3(1): 6

Tisserand R, Balacs M A 1995 Essential oil safety. Churchill Livingstone, New York, p 105

UKCC (United Kingdom Central Council) 1993 Handbook of midwives' rules. UKCC, 23 Portland Place, London

Vallance W B 1955 Pennyroyal poisoning: a fatal case. The Lancet ii: 850–851

Valnet J 1980 The practice of aromatherapy. Daniel, Saffron Walden

Wingate P, Wingate R 1988 The Penguin medical encyclopaedia. Penguin, London

People with learning difficulties

Introduction

Therapy using essential oils with massage has had considerable success in one of the least responsive therapeutic areas—the treatment of people with learning difficulties; touch and essential oils have been shown to help develop trust as well as to ease tension, reduce aggression and improve general health (Alexander 1993). Several case histories will be presented, along with advice about the need for particular caution in the selection and presentation of oils in this context.

Special needs

Since the 1970s there has been a markedly positive change in understanding and attitudes towards adults and children whose mental or physical attributes are retarded in some way. Treated as outcasts from society before then, there was little regard for their needs as individuals, nor much attempt to improve their happiness and well-being. They were rarely touched, except possibly to receive rough treatment, and it is believed that the lack of positive tactile stimulation could lead to the rocking, hand wringing and head banging that play such a large part in the behaviour pattern of many people with learning difficulties.

Touch is a basic behavioural need in much the same way as breathing is a basic physical need. When the need for touch remains unsatisfied, abnormal behaviour will result.

(Montagu 1986)

Fortunately, such people are now being recognized in their own right:

Mentally disordered people should be treated with the same respect for their dignity, personal needs, religious and philosophical beliefs, and accorded the same choices, as other people. Special consideration should be given to those with particular cultural and communication needs.

(Mental Health Act 1983)

People with learning difficulties require the same (and probably more) care, love, touch and attention as a person whose illness or disability takes a different form. Terms like 'challenging behaviour' and 'learning difficulties' have replaced words like 'mentally deficient' and 'backward' and, instead of keeping patients away from contact with the outside world, every effort is made to help them to achieve as normal an everyday life as possible. This is brought about primarily by using and developing the sense of touch (and also, in many instances, the sense of smell):

Touch is central to our work with people who have severe learning difficulties ... addressed by considering the quality of touch which people receive

---

Case 11.1   Aromatherapist: Mary Anna Hanse SPDipA, UK

I was asked if I would visit a busy ward of a hospital for mentally handicapped people in the Midlands, to see if my work had any relevance to the severely disturbed, deaf and blind residents there with severe mental handicaps, and with whom nurses wanted to improve communication. The visit was a most rewarding experience, because it really did show the value of touch. I spent about 4 hours in a ward and worked with three patients.

The first person is a man called M, who goes around on all fours and likes to bash his head on the tiled floor. The staff said that when they intervened and tried to stop the bashing it made matters worse: M accelerated the behaviour and they had to leave him to work through the self-mutilation. When I saw him rhythmically hitting his forehead on the floor until the sores he had accumulated on his forehead bled onto the tiles, I suggested that I try to massage his back to see what would happen. I used a carrier oil with relaxing essential oils and started first to introduce the aroma near his face for him to inhale. I talked to him as I worked, in case some vibration could be picked up, or something communicated. I worked in large circles on his back, first very gently, and as his response was immediate and positive, I used a firmer stroke. The instant I started, M straightened up and stopped the head banging. He sat on his knees, fully absorbed and not moving an eyelash, for the 10 minutes or so that I worked on his back. M remained peaceful for the rest of the afternoon.

The second person I worked with was a young man, G, with severe nasal congestion who refuses to be touched by anyone apart from two or three staff he knows well. Staff had been using the usual drugs, which did not seem to clear the congestion, and G was keeping others as well as himself awake at night. Recently he had been taken to see a specialist in another hospital because the congestion was so troublesome, but G would not let the consultant near him and they had to bring him back unhelped. I put some essential oils for sinusitis and catarrh on a tissue and, while a nurse held them near his face, I worked

on his feet, using a Swiss reflex cream containing the same essential oils. Before starting on his feet I chatted to him and very gently first touched and stroked his hands and face. On his feet I worked on the sinus reflex points. After a while his sinuses started running and he was needing to spit, etc. The staff were surprised not only at the blockage moving, but at G allowing touch from a stranger.

Finally, the most moving and surprising, was the response of a 19-year-old girl called F. This young woman is very disturbed. When I saw her, the word that came to my mind was torment. She was continually thrashing backwards and forwards, punching her head with her fists, slapping her head and face, sticking her fingers into her eyes, pushing away hands that tried to touch her. She ceaselessly thrashed around. I was told that she refused to let people touch her. Her carers and parents, who show so much concern for her, never have the satisfaction of knowing whether she appreciates it. She does not communicate this.

I stayed with her for about 2 hours. At first with total rejection, and then ever so slowly, there was a gradual acceptance of my presence and then of my touch. The last half hour or so, F was relaxed and lying back on the bean bag, sometimes with her arms behind her back with a little smile and sometimes giving a gurgling laugh of pleasure. I held her on the solar plexus area between ribcage and stomach, with the other hand on the adrenals at the back. It seemed that there was a healing calm produced by hands placed on the body, combined with the effect of the relaxing essential oils and the total effect was dramatic. The nurses were wishing that it could have been photographed or better still, videoed, as they had never seen F like that. There was a concentration on what was going on in the ward; a focus and a quiet calmness—the nurses said that all the residents seemed more calm than usual.

I believe that there is much useful work that could be done in the area of profound handicaps, using essential oils and having the confidence to use hands for communication and healing.

in everyday interactions. … Gently holding a hand, a kind touch on the arm, a pat on the back or holding someone who is crying can often convey silently but more clearly and easily than words how people really feel.

(Sanderson, Harrison & Price 1991 p. 11)

Both children and adults need to feel loved and to be completely accepted, including the acceptance of any particular physical impairment or negative emotional behaviour. Aromatherapy offers the rare opportunity to develop a professional empathetic rapport with patients, hopefully with the culmination of trust building, sharing and gently guiding the patient towards wellness again (Garnett-Ore 1996). A feeling of being loved will help to increase a person's feeling of self-worth, as will praise when something positive is achieved or the person's hair or other grooming features are pleasing to the eye. Also, 'it is important that tasks which are given should be attainable with short term goals, so that there is early reward, for nothing breeds success more than success itself' (Bischoff 1992) and success will boost a person's self-belief.

TREATMENT

Massage, as discussed in Chapter 7, is merely an extension of touch, which relaxes the muscles and 'encourages the mind to take a break from its usual frenetic activity' (Bischoff 1992). The addition of essential oils to a bland massage oil broadens massage into a therapy which can have profound effects on the mind, thus beneficially affecting the emotional and physical behaviour of the person with learning difficulties.

The fact that aromas can trigger the memory (Van Toller & Dodd 1988 p. 153) suggests that, on the second and subsequent occasions when the same oil is used, memories of the first occasion are aroused. If these memories are happy ones, treatment will be enhanced each time, building on any therapeutic benefit generated by the first treatment and this has, indeed, been found to be the case (Price 1987).

It is believed that, as with most health problems for which essential oils are used, stimulation and/or relaxation are prime factors in the initiation of the healing process—whatever the health problem. This is remarkably evident in the case of those with learning difficulties: their power of communication is considerably increased, and challenging behaviour is decreased. The use of essential oils accelerates any progress being made—and a positive constructive circle is begun, resulting in the person becoming independent in small personal tasks previously attended to by a carer (Sanderson, Harrison & Price 1991 pp. 80–81).

The cost of essential oils compares favourably with the cost of orthodox drugs; however, staff time devoted to aromatherapy can be identified as the most costly part of the treatment (Hydes 1997)

Essential oil range and selection

The range of oils from which selection is made is very important in the case of people with learning difficulties and should not include those containing aldehydes, ketones, oxides, phenols or phenolic ethers as principal constituents. The oils to avoid are listed in Appendices B.4–8 and it is recommended that these are not even kept on the premises.

The selection of the two or three oils to be presented to each person or child should not be undertaken at random. The medical details of each case should first be studied, and then oils pre-selected which will influence the symptoms presented. From these, two to three oils are chosen for their relaxing or uplifting properties (whichever is felt to be the effect required). This means that, although the selection has been made primarily to affect the mental and emotional side of the client, it will also alleviate any symptoms being suffered, such as constipation, insomnia, rheumatic pain, poor circulation, respiratory disorders, etc.

For example, someone who cannot sleep well and who suffers from rheumatism could be offered *Citrus limon*, *Origanum majorana* and *Chamaemelum nobile* as the selection of oils from which to choose. (For a full list of oils to help insomnia see the comprehensive list on page 213.)

Case 11.2 Aromatherapist: Lucile Bischoff SPDipA, South Africa

R is 21 years old, with mild to borderline mental retardation and suspected temporal lobe epilepsy, for which he is prescribed Tegretol 200–300 mg. His mother disappeared soon after his birth, and his father is an alcoholic who was battered himself as a child and physically and sexually abused R and his 3 brothers. The children were removed and placed in a home. R can look after himself and works in sheltered employment at the home.

Aromatherapy was introduced to try and help with his erratic mood swings, which fluctuate from sulking, or very aggressive behaviour with self-abuse. It is not known to what extent his retardation is related to the emotional factors. He does have a 'girlfriend' at the home but there are frequent arguments, some of them quite physical.

Treatment 1. On my first visit to the home I brought some plants to show the children where the oils came from. R recognized the lavender and said that you could make tea from it, much to the surprise of Mrs S (the helper assigned to help me). I think this boosted R's ego quite a bit as he stated that he was very clever. He showed considerable interest in the oils and enjoyed smelling them. I decided to let him dictate the course of treatment, allowing him to choose his own oils. Any communication was directed at Mrs S and not to me. He was very curious but also nervous about the massage so I first worked on the other children so that he could see exactly what it involved. By the time it was his turn he was very eager and stated that if I did the same on him he might just fall asleep. I gave him a back massage and a gentle foot massage, which he enjoyed. Deciding to let him

choose his own oils and length of treatment broke the ice and helped to build his confidence and trust. He enjoyed the treatment and said he felt quite sleepy afterwards.

Treatment 2. I was greeted with a smile; he was in a good mood as he had helped on the switchboard that morning, which I think made him feel important. The results from the previous treatment were favourable. He had slept in the afternoon and also been in a good mood with no fighting. This time, our conversation was a bit better and we chattered about a geranium plant I had given him on the previous visit, as I felt that something of his own to look after might help with his moods. Although there was an improvement in our conversation, I felt that most of the time he was being polite. He enjoyed his back massage the most.

Treatment 3. R was waiting for me to arrive this time. He seems to be a happier person, smiling more and seeming to be content. He brought his own music for the session, which we played while I was working on him, but he soon realized that it was too fast and asked me to change it as it was making a noise. He is relaxing far more during treatments. I noticed that he was closing his eyes and dozing on and off during the treatment.

Matron and the staff are extremely pleased at the change in his behaviour; he was easier to control and not losing his temper as often. I made up an oil for him to use in his bath or to rub on to his hands and arms if he was feeling cross. I also showed him a few breathing exercises. The essential oils used were *Boswellia carteri*, *Cedrus atlantica* and *Citrus aurantium* var. *amara* (flos).

Having selected the essential oils which would be most helpful to the person concerned, the way in which these are presented is of great importance. The aim is to select an aroma which is acceptable to and appreciated by the person for whom it is intended, so time should be taken when introducing the essential oils. Never offer more than three and offer them one at a time, noting the reactions carefully: Did the hand push it away? Was the head averted? Did the person come closer? Did he or she reach out for the hand holding the aroma? The end result will be enhanced when an oil favoured by the person is used and the preferred one, on its own, should be used first in whatever method of treatment is adopted.

In visualization therapy, if a colour is introduced by the therapist while the subject has already begun to visualize one of his or her own

choice, confusion disrupts the relaxation (Van Toller & Dodd 1988 p. 152). The same potential for confusion (and reduced benefit) applies to the choice of essential oils for those with learning difficulties: if the therapist decides to mix together two that the person favoured, this is not the same thing as using one which the client has actually smelt, unless the mix has also been presented.

Presentation of aromas

The essential oils can be presented in two ways:

- one drop on a spill or tissue—neat for smelling
- ready mixed in a carrier oil on the back of the therapist's hand. Using the hand sometimes enables the therapist to make physical contact with a client who previously has not been enthusiastic about being touched.

Case 11.3   Clinical aromatologist: Barbara Payne SPDipA, SPCD Aromatology, UK

During a visit to one of the Mencap homes in Bridlington I was asked if there was anything I could do to help J, a 30-year-old resident of the home, with learning and physical disabilities, and very bad bouts of depression. She had always found communication to be problematic, particularly with visitors. She had hardly ever slept right through the night, which sometimes made her tired and irritable the next day.

J looked continually at the floor. I offered her a choice of three oils to smell and she looked intently at the bottle containing sandalwood essential oil. This was taken to be an indication that she liked the smell. I mixed the oil into a balm base and asked her if she would like me to massage her feet. Again, although interest was shown in the massage offered, she looked intently at the jar and reached out to touch it. I gently started to massage her foot and she was clearly delighted. Her gaze at the jar slowly rose until she was looking straight into my eyes while at the same time stretching out her toes for more. The staff were amazed at the eye contact as they had never seen her do that before. I spoke gently to her and let her hold the sealed jar, whilst massaging the other foot (which she had eagerly pushed into my hands). I demonstrated to staff how to massage the foot slowly and gently and suggested they might use the cream at J's bedtime. The next day I received a phone call from J's carer to say that J had slept well the whole night and was in a very happy frame of mind. Treatments with the foot balm have continued and so has the improvement in J. She now sleeps through every night and consequently life has improved both for her and everyone around her.

If the diluted method is preferred, small bottles of each essential oil diluted in jojoba oil can be kept for this purpose alone. (Jojoba keeps well because it is a liquid wax resistant to oxidation.)

Should the person appear to like more than one (or all) of the offered oils equally, this is not necessarily a sign to blend these together (see above): a different aroma will be produced. Simply select one of the favoured single oils for the first few treatments, or offer a mix or blend of two or three of the oils on the first list as one more possible aroma to be offered to the client.

Should none of the aromas offered gain a positive reaction, rather than change to yet another oil, a drop of *Lavendula angustifolia* can be added to each spill or tissue, and one of these offered again. The blend offered is still a single aroma, but may be more acceptable. Where there is a large number of clients or patients, and time permits, it is useful to keep second sets of neat (and diluted) trial bottles which contain *L. angustifolia* together with an equal amount of a single essential oil. A third set using *Santalum album*, *Pelargonium graveolens* or another popular oil, such as *Citrus reticulata*, in place of *L. angustifolia* is another possibility.

Norfolk Park School, Sheffield, uses essential oils together with massage throughout their school on children with severe learning difficulties, and have produced a video and small book designed to assist anyone working with handicapped adults on a one-to-one basis. Also available is Aromatherapy for people with learning difficulties (Sanderson, Harrison & Price 1991), which is helpful for those working in this field.

LEARNING DIFFICULTIES TRIAL

Lucile Bischoff, principal of an aromatherapy school in South Africa, carried out a trial study on three children with learning difficulties at the San Michelle Home for the mentally and physically handicapped. Because different essential oils were used for each child and there was no placebo, the study does not show any particular essential oils effecting an improvement. Nevertheless, it is of value in showing that essential oils, together with massage, did have a positive effect on the children concerned. Even though the trial was terminated two treatments short of the set number, the six treatments carried out are still useful, as they show definite improvements in the behaviour of the children. It would be worth doing further controlled studies in this area, this time with named botanical species.

The aims of the study were to see how aromatherapy and massage could benefit people with learning difficulties by:

- promoting self-awareness and trust
- increasing communication
- providing tactile and sensory stimulation.

Lucile encountered a few obstacles and limitations. Space was a problem at the home and cooperation and feedback from the staff were not very forthcoming. An epidemic of hepatitis unfortunately broke out before the end of the scheduled number of treatments, prematurely ending the study.

Evelyn

Evelyn was 7 years old, blind and mildly mentally retarded, a suspected syphilis baby. She was incontinent, unable to speak, wash, dress or feed herself. The oils selected (no botanical specification given) were: one drop each lavender and geranium essential oil in 10 ml grapeseed carrier oil.

Treatment 1. Evelyn's behaviour was very erratic, changing from extreme excitability to crying and refusal to have a massage. She eventually tolerated a back massage for a full minute while sitting on Lucile's lap.

Treatment 2. Her behaviour was far better, although still resisting and frequently asking to be taken to the bathroom. A short foot, hand and back massage was managed.

Treatment 3. Evelyn recognized Lucile's voice and was happy to 'see' her. Although she resisted lying down, a breakthrough was felt regarding communication and acceptance.

Treatment 4. Evelyn allowed the massage of her feet, legs, arms and hands for a short while, plus a 2 minute back massage lying down.

Treatment 5. She was still resisting a little, but the length of each massage session increased and Evelyn lay down again for her back to be massaged.

Treatment 6. Evelyn was beginning to relax more; lavender and geranium have been placed in her room and on her clothes for identification.

Walter

Walter was 7 years old at the time of the study, hyperactive and on medication for severe mental retardation. His IQ is under 40 and he was considered untrainable. His brother (with whom he has a good relationship) is in the same home and his mother is institutionalized. His medication was Catapres and Melleril.

The oils selected were: one drop each of chamomile and lavender essential oil in 10 ml grapeseed carrier oil.

Treatment 1. A short foot massage was managed without resistance (except for asking the helper to hit Lucile if it hurt him). When asked if he would like a back massage he jumped onto the bed face down and thoroughly enjoyed one. He asked for oils to be put on his face and stomach.

Treatment 2. He was very eager and lay still for a 15 minute massage of his feet, legs, stomach and back. At the end of the treatment Lucile asked for a hug, which he allowed, but with no response on his part. There was no eye contact or communication.

Treatment 3. The helper said that Walter had been talking much more, and after treatment 2 had sat down with crayons and scribbled for the first time. While being massaged, Walter smiled often and was quite chatty, but before and after his treatment, he refused to communicate or respond to a hug.

Treatment 4. Walter was very quiet and refused to communicate, though apparently still enjoying the massage.

Rachael

Rachael was 8 years old, with quadriplegia (which presented the biggest problem), cerebral palsy due to birth trauma, profound mental retardation and epilepsy. Rachael comes from a very loving family. Her medication was Epilim, Tegretol and Valium.

The oils selected were: one drop each of chamomile and lavender essential oil in 10 ml grapeseed carrier oil.

Treatment 1. Difficulty was experienced with handling, but Rachael's legs and feet (perhaps sensitive as she kept pulling them away) were massaged; she enjoyed the head massage.

Treatment 2. Handling was easier this time—and there was much smiling and laughing.

Treatment 3. Rachael was much more relaxed. There was no feedback from her mother, which was disappointing.

Treatment 4. She still enjoyed the head massage the most. She enjoyed watching Lucile's shadow on the wall.

Treatment 5. Rachael showed a definite response to the music being played, trying to find it with her eyes when it was switched off. Still no feedback from her mother.

Results

Unfortunately, the hepatitis outbreak prevented further treatments for all three children.

Evelyn

- Massage tolerance increased from 1 minute to 15.
- There was an improvement in relaxation.
- There was ready acceptance of sensory stimulation through touch.
- There was improvement in communication.

Walter

- There was a definite improvement in behaviour patterns.
- There was more cooperation with tasks performed at home.
- There was an improvement in communication, especially speech.
- He showed an interest in objects around him (this was previously non-existent).

Rachael

It was difficult to assess any improvement as there was no feedback from her mother and no cooperation from the staff. However, she was progressively easier to handle and Lucile felt it was worth it for the enjoyment Rachael derived from the treatments. Her circulation must have benefited also.

Even though, so far as the authors are aware, there have been no trials or studies carried out on people with learning difficulties in Britain, a tremendous number of individual cases have been recorded. Peg Holden-Peters, who gives aromatherapy treatments (and uses vaporized essential oils) at Grove Park, a school for children with special needs, as well as at a special unit in Wadhurst Primary School (both in East Sussex) says that:

Out of the 26 children that I have massaged regularly, 20 have been able to relax thoroughly (9 of these quite deeply) and the other 6 have achieved relaxation for short spells of from 2–5 minutes. ... Children who spend most of their days in a wheelchair benefit from having their limbs loosened up by gentle aromatherapy massage. The leg and arm muscles of one child were fiercely resistant, but since aromatherapy began, her hands are no longer tightly clenched and she opens them easily.

(Holden-Peters 1993a)

Other benefits noticed include sleeping more soundly on nights after treatment. Within 2 weeks a 12-year-old child who used to whimper when touched was tapping his teacher on the shoulder to request a cuddle and his challenging behaviour was considerably reduced. Other reports from teachers and conversations with parents have shown the benefits possible by using essential oils with massage on children with special needs.

Severely physically disabled children have been loosened up by aromatherapy sessions. Since receiving aromatherapy, two girls with cerebral palsy, who always had their fists tightly clenched, now open them and keep them loose most of the time.

(Holden-Peters 1993b)

Summary

In spite of the anecdotal nature of aromatherapy's reported successes with people with severe mental and physical handicaps, it is clear from these few studies and case histories that it would be worth holding properly conducted trials. Not only could more be discovered about the benefits of aromatherapy, but much could be learned about the nature of learning difficulties themselves.

REFERENCES

Alexander B 1993 The place of complementary therapies in mental health. A user's experience and views. Nottingham Advocacy Group, pp. 3–4

Bischoff L 1992 How aromatherapy can help people with learning difficulties. Treatise, Clinical Practitioner's Diploma, Shirley Price International College of Aromatherapy, Leics.

Garnett-Ore X 1996 Aromatherapy within mental health services. The Aromatherapist 3(1): 17–29

Holden-Peters P 1993a Aromatherapy and special needs children. Treatise, Clinical Practitioner's Diploma, Shirley Price International College of Aromatherapy, Leics

Holden-Peters P 1993b Grove Park. The Aromatherapist 1(1): 22–24

Hydes S 1997 Establishing aromatherapy as a complement to traditional treatment in the mental health services. Treatise, Clinical Practitioner's Diploma, Shirley Price International College of Aromatherapy, Leics

Mental Health Act 1983 Draft code of practice. General principles of care and treatment: 1

Montagu A 1986 Touching: the human significance of the skin. Harper and Row, New York

Price S 1987 The effect of essential oils on the memory. Aromanews 6: 6–7

Price S 1993 The aromatherapy workbook. Thorsons, London

Sanderson H, Harrison J, Price S 1991 Aromatherapy for people with learning difficulties. Hands On, Birmingham

Van Toller S, Dodd G 1988 Perfumery: the psychology and biology of fragrance. Chapman & Hall, London

12

Stress

Introduction

This chapter examines the phenomenon of stress in modern life. It looks at natural therapies used to combat stress in the hospital environment, and explores in depth the role of essential oils. A trial study is cited which demonstrates that massage with essential oils can significantly reduce stress levels in the patients of GPs. This is followed by a guide to the selection and combination of essential oils for the relief of stress, which is accompanied by illustrative examples.

THE EFFECTS OF STRESS

Stress is an important concept in nursing for two reasons: first, because it has been shown to be an important causative factor in illness and, secondly, because illness itself is a stress-producing event. At a commonsense level most people would define stress as a 'feeling' which is provoked by any situation which is too much for the person to cope with (Baly, Robottom & Clark 1987 p. 41)

In the last few years the word stress has almost become synonymous with substandard health, assuming such significance that it has now been adopted as a medical term. A current definition of stress is given by Wingate & Wingate (1988) as: 'Any influence which disturbs the natural balance of a person's body or mind', including 'physical injury, disease, deprivation and emotional disturbance'. There is no doubt that much stress today is due to the modern society in which we live—city and motorway driving, environmental pollution, divorce (which completely changes the traditional form of family life), unemployment, the threat of being mugged or burgled, flying, hospitalization—the list is endless. For many, the last is the most stressful thing which could happen to them (Jamison, Parris & Maxon 1987). In hospital, patients lose their identity and become a number, exchanging their daily attire for nightwear—and taking on a new role as a 'condition' in a bed (Buckle 1997 p. 165). Stress connected with hospitals is not confined to those who enter as patients—they are tended by nurses and doctors who themselves are under stress. Aromatherapists working in hospitals often have to treat the staff to help relieve the pressures they are under. Doctors in particular are often unduly stressed, by the very nature and responsibility of the work they do; GPs are no exception. However, some do not give themselves the treatment they prescribe for their patients, often turning to alcoholism and drug abuse, which are both on the increase in the medical profession (Bennett 1987).

The emotions associated with stress can include deep anxiety, depression, desolation, grief, heartache, pain and mental torment. There are various forms and degrees of stress, defined only by each individual's ability to cope with a specific situation. These are normally categorized as belonging to one of two groups—positive and negative stress. Both of these involve a response by the body to internal or external demands made upon it (see Ch. 8).

The right amount

Stress is like a violin string: too much tension and the string will snap, too little and it will not produce any music. However, just the right amount of tension produces vibrant energy. Without a certain amount of stress none of us could function positively. The stress before a race or a job interview is a kind of challenge—to win, or be successful—just as the stress of cooking daily for the family can be a challenge to satisfy the family appetite at specific times and to meet their nutritional needs. These are positive stressors without which we cannot function to our best ability. However, stress, which is not merely nervous tension (Selye 1956), can build up to an excess level—one of negative stress or distress—through physical injury, illness, work overload, emotional disturbance and even lack of a challenge.

According to Selye (1956) there are three stages in the development of the body's response to stress:

1. The initial direct effect of the body exposed to a stressor, bringing about the alarm stage, where:

   a. a temporary cessation of digestive juices occurs
   b. the respiratory and heart rates increase
   c. extra oxygen is transported to the brain and the muscles (in preparation for strenuous action or emotional strength)
   d. energy is released quickly from stored fats and sugars
   e. extra adrenalin is produced
   f. the immune system shuts down.

2. The resistant stage, where the extra oxygen, energy and adrenalin are brought into action to enable the body to cope with this unacceptable situation (expected to be temporary). With isolated occurrences the body is able to rid itself of the stress and the body functions return to normal. However, in the absence of help in or release from the situation, the responses in stage 1 above are continuous and the body tries to adapt itself to the stressor in an effort to reach a balanced state. If the level of stress is prolonged or becomes chronic and is allowed to continue without help, the body reaches the third stage (below).

3. Exhaustion, with reversion to the alarm stage, resulting inevitably in eventual health problems. These may manifest as headaches, inability to sleep, digestive problems, skin disorders, susceptibility to infections, etc. owing to the closing down of the immune responses.

Breakdown

Early on in stage 3, people may become irritable, even aggressive, critical, restless, inefficient, withdrawn, moody and with an uncontrollable urge to cry at the least setback. They may find that coffee, cigarettes or alcohol give temporary

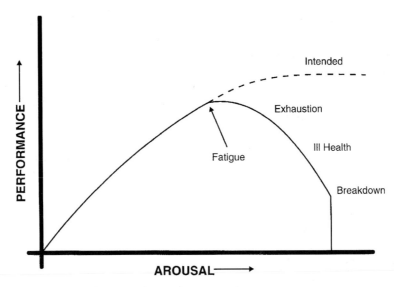

Figure 12.1   The effect of stress on performance (Dr Peter G F Nixon).

relief to their mental stress, or they may take tranquillizing medication, any of which may eventually add to their discomfort.

The combination of several ongoing stressors can result in a nervous breakdown, or what is sometimes termed 'burnout'. The nervous system, influenced so strongly by the mind (see Ch. 8), is unable to cope, and lethargy, inactivity, apathy and indifference set in. In this state, almost a 'waking coma', nothing seems possible to the sufferer, i.e. there is a breakdown in nervous energy. As the English philosopher John Locke put it (at the end of the 17th century): 'Though the faculties of the mind are improved by exercise, yet they must not be put to a stress beyond their strength'.

It is important to be able to recognize the danger signals and find a natural method of combating them, so that severe consequences can be avoided. Figure 12.1 illustrates the relationship of stress to performance: when stress goes beyond a certain level, fatigue sets in and the performance level drops.

Natural methods of stress relief

Of the numerous ways of reducing stress, the following are the most frequently practised in hospitals in the UK and USA:

- *Relaxation.* For instance, the Northern View Day Hospital in Bradford successfully uses muscle relaxation techniques combined with a self-hypnosis tape and relaxing music to reduce levels of stress in the elderly (Harrison & Skinner 1992).
- *Counselling.*
- *Reflexology and/or Swiss reflex massage.*
- *Massage (without oils).*
- *Therapeutic touch, or the laying on of hands.* This is used by nurses belonging to the American Holistic Nurses Association as well as by many nurses in England (Krieger 1979).
- *Hydrotherapy* (often followed by massage).

Case 12.1   Aromatherapist: Lynne Reed SPDipA, UK

This was an antenatal case, a primigravida lady resting in hospital with pregnancy-induced hypertension. The evening that I saw her, her diastolic blood pressure was in the region of 110 mmHg. This was being recorded at 15 minute intervals using a Dynamap. She was obviously anxious and during the course of our chat, I asked her if she would like me to massage her feet for a little while. This I did, using Swiss reflex cream with three drops each of *Cananga odorata* and *Lavandula angustifolia*. We continued this for a little over half an hour, during which time her diastolic blood pressure dropped gradually by 10 mmHg. The last recording before she settled down to sleep was 95 mmHg.

- *Laughter.* Worwood (1990) advises patients to laugh as much as possible since it boosts the endorphin level and makes them feel good. She goes on to say that several hospitals in the United States take the physiological effects of laughter so seriously they have designated 'laughter rooms' where patients can have their prescribed fun. Michigan psychologist Zajonc maintains that even fake smiling triggers a reaction in the brain, making a patient feel better (cited in Price 1993).
- *Essential oils.* A large number of essential oils are stress reducing and to this end can be used independently on a paper tissue, in the bath and in a vaporizer. Also, the effects of massage are enhanced when essential oils are added to the basic massage oil, as discovered by Passant (1990).

ESSENTIAL OILS IN THE RELIEF OF STRESS

The main function of aromatherapy as introduced in the 1960s, i.e. with obligatory massage, was to relieve stress. The first aromatherapists were taught to concentrate only on relieving the stress, so that the body's own healing mechanism would be brought into play to alleviate symptoms brought on by the stress, such as migraines, problems related to menstruation, eczema, etc. Aromatherapy as practised today combines several aspects of healing which enhance each other's effects. Time is spent observing and listening to the patients, who often unburden themselves of their problems when encouraged by a skilful listener. Simple dietary advice is offered, such as cutting out coffee, tea and caffeinated soft drinks, and relaxing tapes have been introduced by some into their treatments.

A community psychiatric nurse in Leeds remarked to the authors in 1993 that 'therapies such as massage and aromatherapy are being seen more and more in the treatment of depression and anxiety, often being seen as an alternative rather than a complementary therapy'. While many of the drugs used can have a therapeutic part to play, they can also have

unpleasant side-effects. Indeed, the anxiolytic group of drugs such as Valium, Librium, etc. have such addictive qualities that they are seldom prescribed today except in extreme cases of sudden trauma, and then only with caution and for short periods (Kirk unpublished work 1993).

Essential oils have not been clinically tested in the same way as drugs but they are potentially less dangerous and far less damaging to the body (see Ch. 3). Their benefits have led to their increasing use by health professionals who have recognized the major role they can play in the reduction of stress.

STRESS PROJECT ON GP REFERRALS

In 1991 a project was carried out by Jean Gonella (unpublished work 1993) over a period of 6 months, on 16 women suffering from severe stress. The aim was to try and reduce the need for medication such as tranquillizers, antidepressants and hypnotics. Each woman was referred by her GP and fulfilled the following criteria;

- stress level above that acceptable to client/family
- disruption/dysfunction to client/family.

Clients were accepted on the project with:

- physical symptoms such as backache, headaches, etc.
- experience of panic attacks
- unresolved or prolonged bereavement
- hormone-related problems.

The treatment given was full-body massage with the essential oils *Lavandula angustifolia* [LAVENDER], *Pelargonium graveolens* [GERANIUM] and *Santalum album* [SANDALWOOD]. *Salvia sclarea* [CLARY] was added where there were hormonal problems.

Results

The clients had to rate the severity of their problem on a scale of severe, medium, negligible or non-existent. The results collated from individual questionnaires show the average percentage of problem severity before treatment, with the level after treatment shown in brackets (see Table 12.1).

Although the results are impressive, Gonella would like to see 100 clients given treatment together with an equivalent control group in order to prove that aromatherapy could reduce drug therapy (Gonella unpublished work 1993).

Selection of essential oils

The essential oils in this section are those recommended by Franchomme & Pénoël (1990), Roulier (1990) and Price (1993). Up to four different essential oils may be needed to treat stress holistically. Together they will enhance each other's effects, i.e. a synergy will be created. Oils are chosen according to the particular stress symptoms presented by the patient. The symptom lists below can be used in the following way to make the appropriate choices. First, decide which if any of the circumstances and symptoms heading the numbered lists 1–13 below apply to the patient. Secondly, decide whether the patient's symptoms are due to deep anxiety or to depression. Then select from the anxiety or depression lists oils also appearing in the more specific lists 1–13 below. It is important to note that only a selection of the possible essential oils will be given here in order to illustrate the method of selection; for complete lists see Appendix B.9.

Anxiety

- *Cananga odorata* [YLANG YLANG]
- *Chamaemelum nobile* [ROMAN CHAMOMILE]
- *Citrus aurantium* var. *amara* (flos) [NEROLI BIGARADE]
- *Citrus aurantium* var. *amara* (fol.) [PETITGRAIN BIGARADE]

- *Citrus aurantium* var. *amara* (per.) [ORANGE BIGARADE]
- *Citrus bergamia* (per.) [BERGAMOT]
- *Citrus limon* (per.) [LEMON]
- *Citrus reticulata* (per.) [MANDARIN]
- *Coriandrum sativum* [CORIANDER]
- *Cupressus sempervirens* [CYPRESS]
- *Lavandula angustifolia* [LAVENDER]
- *Lavandula × intermedia* 'Super' [LAVANDIN]
- *Melissa officinalis* [LEMON BALM]
- *Ocimum basilicum* var. *album* [BASIL]
- *Origanum majorana* [SWEET MARJORAM]
- *Pelargonium graveolens* [GERANIUM].

Depression

- *Boswellia carteri* [FRANKINCENSE]
- *Chamaemelum nobile*
- *Citrus aurantium* var. *amara* (flos)
- *Citrus bergamia* (per.)
- *Juniperus communis* (fruct.)
- *Lavandula angustifolia*
- *Lavandula × intermedia* 'Super'
- *Melaleuca viridiflora*
- *Ocimum basilicum* var. *album*
- *Origanum majorana*
- *Pelargonium graveolens*
- *Thymus vulgaris* ct. geraniol, ct. linalool, ct. thujanol-4 [SWEET THYME]
- *Thymus vulgaris* ct. thymol, ct. carvacrol [THYME].

1. Agitation
   - *Citrus aurantium* var. *amara* (flos)
   - *Citrus aurantium* var. *amara* (per.)
   - *Citrus bergamia*
   - *Cupressus sempervirens*
   - *Lavandula angustifolia*

Table 12.1 Problem severity before and after aromatherapy treatment. Average percentages are given, with the post-treatment level in brackets

| | Severe | | Medium | | Negligible | | |
	before	after	before	after	before	after	Non-existent
Anxiety	63%	(0%)	25%	(50%)	12%	(50%)	(0%)
Depression	43%	(5%)	30%	(18%)	10%	(52%)	(25%)
Insomnia	43%	(5%)	26%	(18%)	5%	(55%)	(25%)
Pain	55%	(20%)	38%	(25%)	2%	(50%)	(5%)
Tiredness	25%	(10%)	65%	(30%)	5%	(55%)	(5%)
Confidence	55%	(12%)	20%	(13%)	25%	(75%)	(0%)
Coping skill	50%	(8%)	25%	(22%)	25%	(70%)	(0%)

Case 12.2 Clinical aromatologist: Nicola Darrell (BSc Hons, MIAT, MISPA, MIFA, MIIAA), Eire

K, a 42-year-old woman working in a family business, was referred for treatment by her GP, with severe anxiety and stress. The root of her trouble stemmed from problems with the family business and the GP had felt that relaxation techniques would help. Used to taking an active part in the business—and socializing—she had, over the past 3 weeks, become increasingly withdrawn and anxious. As well as experiencing panic attacks (which left her clammy and freezing) in crowded places, she was also experiencing these at night. This was disturbing her sleep pattern and she found it hard to wake up in the morning. The stress was causing extreme tension in her neck and shoulders and she was suffering headaches as a consequence. Her breathing tended to be shallow and rapid and she had lost more than a stone (6.4 kg) in weight over the 3 weeks, partly resulting from lack of appetite.

At her first visit K was extremely negative. Due to the amount of anxiety she was experiencing I took her through some breathing exercises before attempting to massage her. I then carried out a full-body massage using *Chamaemelum nobile* (Roman chamomile) (this is high in esters, which have an immediate effect on the nervous system), *Rosa damascena* (rose otto) and *Origanum majorana* (sweet marjoram); the last two are both neurotonic, the latter also benefiting lack of sleep and headaches.

Initially, K opted to attend for treatment twice a week. After the first treatment K said that she felt much calmer and more relaxed. She actually looked taller, as she was standing upright rather than being

bent over with the tension in her shoulders, and she said that her head felt much clearer. I gave her a blend of essential oils to use at home in the bath and as an inhalant if required. The blend included *Valeriana officinalis* (valerian), *C. nobile*, *Lavandula angustifolia*, *O. majorana* and *Cananga odorata* (ylang ylang).

On her next visit she reported that she found inhaling the oils when particularly anxious had relieved the hyperventilation and she had started to incorporate regular relaxation and breathing exercises into her routine.

After 3 weeks (six treatments) she felt sufficiently confident to go shopping without experiencing any anxiety. She was also able to sort out some of the problems at work over this period. For the following 3 weeks, K attended for treatment once a week; she was beginning to put weight back on and her appetite had returned to normal.

After these 3 weeks, K felt able to resume some of her work duties. She continued attending for aromatherapy, coming now once every 3–5 weeks. She had not ceased taking her medication during her aromatherapy treatment time, but 6 months after her aromatherapy treatments had begun her doctor felt it was possible for her to reduce her medication, which she did over the next 3 months. At this stage, although her confidence was not completely restored, she found she was able to carry out a heavy work schedule and once again enjoy social activities.

She continues to attend for aromatherapy when she feels the need.

- *Lavandula × intermedia* 'Super'
- *Melissa officinalis*
- *Origanum majorana*
- *Pelargonium graveolens*
- *Thymus vulgaris* ct. geraniol, ct. linalool, ct. thujanol-4.

2. Emotional instability
   - *Citrus aurantium* var. *amara* (flos)
   - *Citrus aurantium* var. *amara* (fol.)
   - *Melissa officinalis*
   - *Origanum majorana*
   - *Pelargonium graveolens*.

3. Fatigue
   - *Coriandrum sativum*
   - *Cupressus sempervirens*
   - *Ocimum basilicum* var. *album*.

4. Headaches and migraines
   - *Chamaemelum nobile*
   - *Citrus limon* (per.)

- *Lavandula angustifolia*
- *Lavandula × intermedia* 'Super'
- *Melissa officinalis*
- *Mentha × piperita*—digestive
- *Ocimum basilicum* var. *album*—nervous
- *Origanum majorana*—congestive and menstrual
- *Pelargonium graveolens*—congestive.

5. Hypertension
   - *Cananga odorata*
   - *Citrus limon* (per.)
   - *Lavandula angustifolia*
   - *Lavandula × intermedia* 'Super'
   - *Ocimum basilicum* var. *album*
   - *Origanum majorana*
   - *Melaleuca viridiflora*.

6. Inability to concentrate, loss of energy (mental and physical)
   - *Citrus limon* (per.)
   - *Coriandrum sativum*.

7. Indigestion
- *Citrus aurantium* var. *amara* (per.)
- *Citrus reticulata* (per.)
- *Melaleuca viridiflora*
- *Melissa officinalis*.

8. Insomnia
- *Cananga odorata*
- *Chamaemelum nobile*
- *Citrus aurantium* var. *amara* (flos, fol., per.)
- *Citrus bergamia* (per.)
- *Citrus limon* (per.)
- *Citrus reticulata* (per.)
- *Coriandrum sativum*
- *Cupressus sempervirens*
- *Juniperus communis*
- *Lavandula angustifolia*
- *Lavandula* × *intermedia* 'Super'
- *Melissa officinalis*
- *Ocimum basilicum* var. *album*
- *Origanum majorana*.

9. Irritability
- *Boswellia carteri*
- *Chamaemelum nobile*
- *Citrus aurantium* var. *amara* (fol.)
- *Citrus aurantium* var. *amara* (per.)
- *Citrus bergamia* (per.)
- *Citrus reticulata* (per.)
- *Cupressus sempervirens*
- *Juniperus communis* (fruct.)
- *Lavandula angustifolia*
- *Origanum majorana*
- *Pelargonium graveolens*.

10. Low immunity
- *Boswellia carteri*
- *Melaleuca viridiflora*
- *Origanum majorana*.

11. Muscle tension (mainly neck and shoulders)
- *Chamaemelum nobile*
- *Juniperus communis*
- *Lavandula angustifolia*

Case 12.3 Aromatherapist: Kate Stockbridge, UK

Client background and presenting problems
A is a gentleman in his mid-sixties, referred to me by a community psychiatric nurse as he had developed panic attacks and vertigo. She felt that aromatherapy would help in relieving his stress and therefore aid relaxation. His problems had arisen as a result of the long term stress of caring, full time, for a relative with Parkinson's disease.

A was physically and mentally tired and was not sleeping well. He described himself as having a 'thickness of the head' and 'solid headaches'. Emotionally he was low—and tearful as he expressed his frustration at this situation. His arms and legs had large areas of 'shark's skin'—psoriasis and warts. He also complained of coldness in his knees, which ached.

Treatment plan
To ease anxiety and depression, promote sleep, relieve his headaches and at the same time provide warmth and acceptable physical contact. Treatments were fortnightly for six sessions.

Carrier and essential oils chosen
10 ml almond oil
5 ml evening primrose oil (for skin problems)
one drop each of:

Citrus aurantium var. *sinensis* (sweet orange)—antidepressant, sedative
Jasminium officinale (jasmine)—antidepressant, warming, euphoric, relaxant
Origanum majorana (sweet marjoram)—analgesic, warming.

Remedial massage techniques were used around the patella where there were granular deposits, also around the scapula where there was tension.

For use in between treatments, A was given 50 ml lotion containing:

20 drops *Citrus limon* (lemon)—warts, anxiety, depression, immunostimulant
five drops *Juniperus communis* (juniper)—anxiety, skin problems, detoxifying
five drops *Chamaemelum nobile* (Roman chamomile)—skin problems, headaches, insomnia, anxiety.

This was applied twice daily to the affected areas.

Results
After the first session A was more relaxed, although he still had some tension in the shoulder region. He appreciated the treatments, which relaxed and rejuvenated him. By the third treatment the discomfort in his head had cleared; he began to feel brighter and more able to cope. After his sixth and final session he said he no longer experienced vertigo, the headaches had gone, his skin was much improved and he felt less tense in his shoulders. Emotionally, he was better able to relax at home and felt more positive about the future.

- *Lavandula × intermedia* 'Super'
- *Origanum majorana*
- *Eucalyptus smithii* [GULLY GUM] can be added to increase the synergy of any mix (Pénoël 1992, 1994).

12. Nightmares
   - *Boswellia carteri*
   - *Citrus limon*
   - *Melissa officinalis*.

13. Sadness
   - *Boswellia carteri*
   - *Citrus aurantium* var. *amara* (fol.)
   - *Citrus reticulata* (per.)
   - *Melaleuca viridiflora*.

Combination of essential oils

Although more than four essential oils may be found which are common to, or suitable for, the symptoms suffered, the choice is best restricted to three or four. Once chosen, it is advisable and time saving to make up a dropper bottle of the selected essential oils, which should be labelled and used in whichever method is thought most appropriate (see Ch. 5). The relative proportions of each essential oil should be influenced by the aroma preferences of the patient concerned.

Practical examples

The method of selecting and combining essential oils described above is illustrated by the following examples.

Depression due to grief, with nightmares. *Boswellia carteri* is the only common denominator, therefore half the number of drops used should be of this oil. *Melissa officinalis* would be a good second oil, to relieve both the nightmares and the depression.

Depression, with headaches and insomnia. Use *Chamaemelum nobile, Lavandula angustifolia* and *Origanum majorana*. If the immune system is felt to be low, *O. majorana* should be present in the highest proportion in the mix. Should the aroma need adjusting, select any other essential oil from the antidepressive range.

Case 12.4 Aromatherapist: Sandra Agnew, Australia

A 58-year-old male was admitted to hospital on 25 November 1993 in a semicomatose state after a drinking session, diagnosed as alcoholic cirrhosis of the liver. Clinical signs were disorientation, extreme jaundice, indicated by his eyes (which were bright yellow), distorted and puffy facial features, bloated abdomen and uncontrollable tremors. Biochemical and haematological pathology tests showed grossly impaired liver function, e.g. enzyme 60 times greater than normal values. The family was informed by the medical officer that due to the severity of his conditions he was unlikely to survive.

Two days after admittance he was lucid, uncomfortable, apathetic and immobile. His skin was flaky and extremely itchy, especially on his arms and legs. He was given Valium and diuretics to sedate and get rid of excess fluid, and consequently he was drowsy, but aware of his surroundings and recognized his family. The tremors had diminished considerably and he was agitated and worried about his condition.

His daughter, a regular client of mine, approached me to see if aromatherapy was a possibility. I contacted the medical officer who confirmed the prognosis and willingly gave permission for an aromatherapy massage, implying that any treatment would be beneficial.

His daughter was shown some basic massage techniques and began massaging daily, starting on 28 November. After 2 days he commented that he was sleeping soundly because the itchiness was relieved—previously the itch had been waking him. On 10 December the pathology tests were repeated: the liver enzymes, although still elevated, were decreasing and coagulation studies were normal. His mental attitude was greatly improved and he was enthusiastic about the daily massage to the extent that visitors were asked to massage his hands, legs and feet. Mobility and appetite were improving and he wanted to go home.

The following oil blend was used in an almond and avocado oil as a carrier base (for quick penetration and skin-healing properties): Roman chamomile (calming to the central nervous system, a liver stimulant, relieves pruritus), frankincense (uplifts, soothes, aids digestion), lavender (relieves anxiety, stimulates cell renewal), rosemary (a liver decongestant, activates metabolism, stimulates the nervous system), clary (calms the central nervous system, and panic state, helps withdrawal symptoms of alcohol, strengthens the immune system).

He was discharged from hospital on 20 December into the care of his family who continued the daily massage with essential oils. A biochemical test on 5 January 1994 showed liver function to be almost normal. The patient looks and feels well, is in great spirits, eating well and generally enjoying life.

Anxiety, with emotional instability and insomnia. Use *Citrus aurantium* var. *amara* (flos), *C. aurantium* var. *amara* (fol.), *M. officinalis* and *O. majorana*.

Anxiety with agitation, and high blood pressure. Use *Cananga odorata, L. angustifolia, L. × intermedia* 'Super' and *O. majorana*.

Anxiety with agitation and indigestion. Use *C. aurantium* var. *amara* (per.) and *M. officinalis*. Should a third oil be desired, one may be selected for whichever symptom is strongest.

Low immunity, with sadness, high blood pressure and indigestion. The only common denominator here is *Melaleuca viridiflora*, which should be present in the mix in the highest proportion. *O. majorana* can help to control the hypertension and stimulate the immune system. *B. carteri*

uplifts, easing sadness and stimulating the immune system.

Summary

This chapter has examined the phenomenon of stress in modern life, and the role essential oils can play in reducing its effects. Gonella's 1991 trial project (Gonella 1993) clearly demonstrates that massage with essential oils can significantly reduce stress levels in the patients of GPs. The guide presented here to the selection and combination of stress-reducing oils is intended to enable readers to choose and administer appropriate oils for their patients, with a view to achieving similarly beneficial results.

REFERENCES

Baly M E, Robottom B, Clark J M 1987 District nursing. Heinemann, London
Bennett G 1987 The wound and the doctor. Secker & Warburg, London
Buckle J 1997 Clinical aromatherapy in nursing. Arnold, London
Franchomme P, Pénoël D 1990 L'aromathérapie exactement. Jollois, Limoges
Harrison L, Skinner R 1992 Relax for health. Nursing Times 88(49): 46–47
Jamison R N, Parris W C V, Maxon W S 1987 Psychological factors influencing recovery from outpatient surgery. Behaviour Research Therapy 25: 31–37
Krieger D 1979 The therapeutic touch. Simon & Schuster, New York
Passant H 1990 A holistic approach in the ward. Nursing Times 86(4): 26–28
Pénoël D 1992 Winter shield. International Journal of Aromatherapy 4(4): 11
Pénoël D 1994 Eucalyptus smithii. The Aromatherapist 1(2): addendun
Price S 1993 The aromatherapy workbook. Thorsons, London
Roulier G 1990 Les huiles essentielles pour votre santé. Dangles, St-Jean-de-Braye
Selye H 1956 The stress of life. McGraw Hill, New York
Wingate P, Wingate R 1988 Medical encyclopedia. Penguin, London
Worwood V 1990 Fragrant pharmacy. Macmillan, London, p 109

Intensive and coronary care

Introduction

This chapter presents the results of several clinical trials which show the value of essential oils in significantly reducing patient stress levels in coronary and intensive care contexts. The treatment of severe burns with essential oils is briefly discussed, and illustrated by anecdotal evidence. It is suggested that further studies to corroborate this evidence should be undertaken.

LIFE-THREATENING SITUATIONS

It is difficult to talk generally about the use of aromatherapy in intensive care, because the reasons for needing it are many and often sudden— breathing difficulties, lung viruses (see Case 13.1), strokes, heart attacks, heart surgery, road accidents, etc.

It was suggested almost 40 years ago (Meyer, Blacher & Brown 1961) that being in an intensive care unit (ICU) could be a depersonalizing experience, leading to demotivation, apathy and withdrawal. This is not necessarily true today and the level of attention and expertise given nowadays in most hospital ICUs makes this less than likely. Nevertheless, the acute emotional and psychological trauma patients still endure in what is to them a strange and unfamiliar place (often without their loved ones beside them) can leave them with an intense feeling of loneliness and isolation. It has been found that a nurse who is able to take the time to touch patients who are critically ill—holding their hand, even without talking—could establish, in a relatively short time, an empathetic relationship with them (McCorkle 1974).

Many factors need to be addressed when looking after the intensive care patient. These include the possibility of further invasive infections, and the severe stress experienced by patients and relatives. Factors such as these respond to aromatherapy, which is used now in many intensive and coronary care wards throughout the UK.

The overriding concern of the aromatherapist in these environments is patient stress, because 'anxiety can precipitate life threatening arrhythmia and extend infarction areas, if not allayed quickly enough' (Harris 1993). Patients' anxieties have been found to be centred on their personal illness rather than on the hospital surroundings (Rowe 1989), and even though frequent nursing reassurances may prevent intimidation by the high-tech environment, their state of mind can be calmed further by the use of essential oils. However, the ICU can still be 'a hostile environment to patients, who are surrounded by a bewildering array of monitoring and support equipment and who are subjected to a variety of invasive therapeutic techniques' (Waldman et al 1993).

The clinical trials which follow show the effectiveness of aromatherapy in coronary and intensive care contexts. However, the authors are concerned that only common names are given for the oils used in most studies and trials, especially when there are so many varieties of 'chamomile', 'eucalyptus' and 'lavender', for instance. Full botanical and analytical identification is essential if such trials are to be taken seriously.

Trial studies

BATTLE HOSPITAL, READING

Christine Dunn, a senior nurse at Battle Hospital, Reading, began to explore massage as a means 'to help patients immobilised by drugs and equipment to relax' (Wilkinson 1991). Being interested also in essential oils, Dunn, Sleep & Collett (1995) set up a randomized, controlled trial to attempt to evaluate the effectiveness of aromatherapy and massage in the nursing care of patients in an ICU. Prior to the trial, six

---

Case 13.1 Aromatherapist: Elizabeth Sonn, UK

Suddenly, my father, normally fit and healthy, was taken seriously ill overnight with an unknown lung virus. He was rushed to hospital, put on a life support machine and the family was told it was only a matter of time!

After 3 days I suddenly awoke to the fact that, if the hospital would allow it, I might be able to help. I approached the consultant, who was amazed that I had not spoken up before, and he agreed that I could do whatever was needed.

For the first 2 days I used two drops each of eucalyptus and benzoin (in about a teaspoonful of grapeseed oil) for his lung congestion, rubbing it on to his chest wherever the life support equipment would allow! The reflex points on his feet were massaged, using the Swiss reflex method and concentrating mainly on the lung and lymph areas. This was accompanied by gentle music to help relax the mind and balance the emotions. Peace and a wonderful aroma emanated from the room.

Mother did not go unprotected either. She received a massage of lavender and marjoram for her aching legs, emotional exhaustion and stress, and jasmine to give her the courage needed. A mix of Bach flower remedies were taken also.

I continued to massage my father in the intensive therapy unit at every available time. After 3 days, tea tree was added to assist with the viral infection. X-rays taken on the 4th day showed a slight improvement. The doctors and nursing staff were impressed, and such was their interest, that their support increased—along with their curiosity regarding aromatherapy.

Two days later, following a couple of nasty scares, hyssop was added to father's treatment to help normalize the fluctuating blood pressure. Improvement continued.

One week later the consultant thought that my father would survive, but that the oxygen level had to be down to 35% before they would remove him from the life support machine, and this would be a critical phase of his recovery. It could take up to a couple of weeks and at this stage there was a possibility that he would react with panic, fear and irritability. I changed the oils at this point in his recovery to jasmine (confidence booster), rosemary (for clear thinking) and clary (calming). Bach flower 'Rescue Remedy' was used between his lips.

Within 2 hours of removal from the machine, father was sitting up. The medical staff remarked with amazement at his speedy recovery. He was removed from the intensive therapy unit within 24 hours and was home within a fortnight, although the prediction had been 8–10 weeks. Once home the massage with essential oils, Swiss reflex treatment and music were gradually stopped. Within 3 months father was once more to be seen playing golf and swimming a couple of times a week, none the worse for his traumatic experience.

members of the nursing team undertook training in massage and aromatherapy techniques with an aromatherapist staff nurse at the same hospital. The aspects of the proposed study were fully explained to patients and their relatives and their formal consent to taking part obtained. The study protocol was approved by the Research and Ethics committee for the West Berkshire Health District.

In the study, each patient selected was to receive one of the three treatment schedules:

• massage, on areas of the body available to the therapist (e.g. back, outside of limbs, scalp), using a standardized technique of light effleurage strokes with grapeseed oil only. The period of massage was between 15 and 30 minutes and three treatments were given within the 5 day period that the patients were there. Conversation was limited to responding rather than initiating contact.

• aromatherapy: as above, but using essential oil of *Lavandula vera* (a synonym for *L. angustifolia*) in a 1% dilution. Although the same supply of oil was used throughout the trial, it does not appear to have been analysed before the test commenced, which is imperative in a research study because essential oils vary with season, place and possible adulteration.

• undisturbed rest, for 30 minutes. Each patient was informed before the rest period that, although they would be undisturbed, they would continue to be observed by the allocated nurse. Areas to be assessed:

• behavioural: on non-verbal patients, this was scored using a modified assessment tool developed specifically for patients unable to respond verbally (O'Brien & Alexander 1985). The range of behaviours was categorized into a four-point scale, which was used on conscious patients.

• physiological: the variables measured were systolic and diastolic blood pressure, heart rate and rhythm, and respiratory rates

• psychological: four-point scales were used here also for patients to self-assess their level of anxiety, mood and ability to cope with the present situation.

Results

• Behavioural analysis: the majority of patients remained in the same behavioural category as before treatment.

• Physiological analysis: in session one aromatherapy appeared to reduce both systolic blood pressure and heart rate, although it was not so clear for patients receiving rest alone. The effectiveness of the treatments was less marked in sessions two and three.

• Psychological analysis: 76% of patients were able to complete this assessment. From the data the proportion of patients who showed an improvement in each of the three treatment groups and sessions was able to be calculated. The resulting percentages are given in Table 13.1.

Aromatherapy proved more effective than both massage and rest in reducing reported anxiety. It was also rated higher at improving mood and coping ability, with the exception of results from session two, when rest was marginally better at helping to cope.

Conclusion

The evidence suggests that massage can offer a useful therapy from a psychological point of view in an ICU setting and this was found to be enhanced by the addition of true lavender essential oil, which may also have contributed to the patients' emotional well-being.

Table 13.1	Percentage of patients whose psychological assessment improved as a result of treatment				
Session	Treatment	No. of patients	Anxiety	Mood	Coping
1	Aromatherapy	36	72	56	50
1	Massage	39	59	49	46
1	Rest	36	44	42	42
2	Aromatherapy	29	76	69	55
2	Massage	32	69	56	41
2	Rest	30	67	60	57
3	Aromatherapy	21	70	55	45
3	Massage	23	65	43	39
3	Rest	22	50	45	36

ROYAL SUSSEX COUNTY HOSPITAL

Trials were carried out at the Royal Sussex County Hospital early in 1992 (Woolfson & Hewitt 1992) showing that foot massage with essential oil of lavender (botanical name not given) could lower the blood pressure, heart and respiratory rates of people in intensive care. Two treatments a week were given for 5 weeks to patients in both intensive and coronary care units. All treatments were given at the same time of day and observations recorded at the beginning, end and 30 minutes after each session.

The trial, carried out by Woolfson & Hewitt, consisted of three groups, each of 12 people, receiving treatment as follows:

- group 1: 20 minute massage using lavender in a vegetable oil
- group 2: 20 minute massage using only vegetable oil
- group 3: 20 minute undisturbed rest period only.

The results showed a consistent decrease in blood pressure, heart rate, pain, respiratory rate and wakefulness in all three groups, with the greatest benefits experienced by patients in group 1 (see Table 13.2).

Averaging the totals in Table 13.2, the overall benefits to each group were as follows:

- group 1: 63.32%
- group 2: 43.28%
- group 3: 22.85%.

Conclusion

This trial bears out the theory that although massage alone is beneficial, the greatest benefits in all areas tested here are experienced when essential oils are used as well.

Table 13.2 Number and percentage of patients experiencing reductions in physiological stress indicators after: massage with lavender (Group 1); massage alone (Group 2); undisturbed rest (Group 3)

Reduction in:	Group 1 % (No.)	Group 2 % (No.)	Group 3 % (No.)
Heart rate	91.6 (11)	58.3 (7)	41.6 (5)
Pain	50.0 (6)	41.6 (5)	16.6 (2)
Blood pressure	50.0 (6)	41.6 (5)	16.6 (2)
Respiratory rate	75.0 (9)	41.6 (5)	16.6 (2)
Wakefulness	50.0 (6)	33.3 (4)	25.0 (3)

MIDDLESEX HOSPITAL, LONDON

A similar trial to the one carried out at the Royal Sussex County Hospital (see above) was undertaken in 1992 (Stevensen 1994) at the Middlesex Hospital, London. Intensive care patients were given foot massage using *Citrus aurantium* var. *aurantium* (flos) [NEROLI BIGARADE]. Neroli was chosen for its calming, antispasmodic, antidepressant and gentle sedative actions. It also has antiseptic qualities and there are no known contraindications to its use in physiological doses.

The trial consisted of four groups of 25 cardiac patients in intensive care. They all fulfilled the following criteria:

- only requiring oxygen through a mask
- no mechanical blood pressure support
- not receiving cardiac pacing during time of procedure
- be English speaking (for speedy communication)

and with regard to the feet:

- no pedal arterial line for blood pressure monitoring
- no suppurating or infected skin conditions.

Each patient was given an information sheet and a consent form to sign. The treatment received by each group was as follows:

- group 1: 20 minute standardized foot massage with 2.5% neroli in apricot kernel vegetable oil
- group 2: 20 minute standardized foot massage using only the apricot kernel oil
- group 3: 20 minute conversation with a nurse, without tactile input or formal counselling
- group 4: 20 minute period with routine care, but without intervention of any kind.

Each group was assessed physiologically and psychologically five times the day after cardiac surgery (referred to as day 1) and again 4 days later (referred to as day 5). The physiological measurements were heart rate, respiratory rate and blood pressure. To assess both positive and negative aspects of the patients' psychological state, a modified Spielberger questionnaire was given, verbally on day 1, with a written one on day 5. The negative aspects were pain, anxiety, tension; the positive ones, calm, rest, relaxation. The four options for patients' replies were: not at all, slightly, moderately, very.

Additional questions asked the subjects to relate:

- their perception of the massage
- its benefits to date (if any)
- the length of time they perceived the duration of the effects to have lasted, over the 4 day period
- comments on the frequency and timing of the massage
- suggestions regarding future or added treatments
- other comments.

Five assessments took place on day 1 at the following times:

- 1 hour before the intervention period
- immediately before the 20 minute intervention period
- immediately after the intervention period
- 1 hour after the intervention period
- 2 hours after the intervention period.

Results

The physiological results showed statistically significant differences between groups 1 and 2 and the two control groups 3 and 4 in the respiratory rates immediately after the intervention.

No difference was seen at the next measurement period.

The psychological results were as follows:

- On day 1, groups 1 and 2 had statistically significantly better psychological results than the control groups, 3 and 4.
- On day 5, there was a significant difference in psychological benefits between groups 1 and 2; 82% of groups 1 and 2 remembered having the massage and all of these had found it beneficial. Group 1 had a marked reduction in anxiety compared with group 2, but the perceived difference in pain reduction between the two groups was minimal. Group 1 found the effects more relaxing, restful and calming than did group 2 and, generally, found the effects to be longer lasting.

This trial shows that touch and massage give positive psychological results to patients in intensive care. It also confirms the findings of the Royal Sussex County Hospital's trials that, while massage alone is beneficial, massage with essential oils gives enhanced and longer-lasting effects.

ROYAL SHREWSBURY HOSPITAL

Most of the recorded uses of aromatherapy in intensive care are concerned with heart surgery, and another such study was carried out in 1992 at the Royal Shrewsbury Hospital on the effectiveness of essential oils in reducing the anxiety level of patients admitted to the coronary care unit, and afterwards in the post-coronary care ward (Harris 1993). In this study, the method used was inhalation of plant oils from an electric vaporizer. Patients were monitored on admission, 12 hours later, and then prior to discharge to the post-coronary care ward. There were four groups of five people, three groups each being given a single essential oil chosen from lavender, ylang ylang and the absolute of jasmine respectively, the fourth being a control group, inhaling water vapour only. The trial took place over a 4 week period and results were obtained by questionnaire. One person in each of groups 2 and 4 did not return the questionnaire.

The reduction in anxiety experienced by patients was as follows (number of patients shown in brackets):

- group 1: 60% (three out of five)
- group 2: 75% (three out of four)
- group 3: 80% (four out of five)
- group 4: 25% (one out of four).

Of the 14 people receiving essential oils who returned the questionnaire, 10 (71.4%) experienced a reduction in anxiety. All patients showed a lowering of blood pressure from their initial admission levels and within 12 hours of the study.

Harris contends that: 'though a significant drop in blood pressure was noted on the majority of patients, this cannot be wholly attributed to the inhalation of essential oils'. However, even with such small groups, the results appear to show that some benefit was gained.

The Royal Shrewsbury Hospital trial described above shows that positive results can be obtained by inhalation of essential oils without massage. A further trial would determine whether neroli, administered by massage in the London Middlesex Hospital trial, can give 100% reduction in stress levels by inhalation only. Our expectation is that it would. Such a trial would prove interesting, more so if it were to use the three oils employed in the Shrewsbury Hospital and with 20–25 people in each group, as in the Middlesex Hospital trial. A trial of this type would give a fuller picture of the efficacy of essential oils in the reduction of anxiety in an intensive care situation.

Severe burns

Essential oils can also be used to treat emotional shock and to minimize the risk of infection. This is especially so in the case of severe burns. Damaged tissue is a good incubator for bacteria, and essential oils can play a potentially life-saving role in such cases by sanitizing the microenvironment.

In 1988 essential oils were used in intensive care for a woman with extensive severe burns at the University College Hospital, London (Price 1989). The authors' blended oils were to be vaporized in her room, to keep the air aseptic. The oils selected were *Pinus sylvestris* [SCOTS PINE], *Citrus limon* [LEMON] and *Eucalyptus globulus* [BLUE GUM]. *Lavandula angustifolia* [LAVENDER] and *Boswellia carteri* [FRANKINCENSE] were supplied in a base oil for areas of the body which could be touched. Essential oils that were regenerating to skin tissue were put into a cream base (containing plant extracts) for use on the patient's face and neck burns. These, although not as seriously affected as other parts of her body, were of great concern for the once attractive female patient. She not only survived, but the skin on her chest (the worst-affected area) became more elastic and supple than the consultant had thought possible (Parkhouse 1988 personal communication). The facial and neck skin improved dramatically.

Case 13.2   Aromatherapist: Anna Hanson, Sweden

H, a 36-year-old male, had been checking the gas stove, which kept leaking gas in the air space around it. When H lit a ring the whole space exploded into flames, burning his face and neck. Although he had managed to put some cold water on his face, he had to put out the fire and comfort four children, so some time had passed before I was called, arriving half an hour after the burning occurred. H was in great pain, but refused to go to the hospital, which was in any case over 25 kilometres away, and without immediate treatment the burn would have worsened.

H's face and neck were burned, and burned hair was sticking to the whole area. He was in shock. I filled two basins with ice-cold water and ice cubes into which I poured pure lavender. I dipped wash cloths in the water and applied them to H's face. They were constantly changed since they immediately turned warm on his burn. The oldest child helped me to change the iced water every now and then. This went on for 2 hours, and I used 10 ml of *Lavandula officinalis* during this time.

Treatment
I gave him a strong painkiller and mixed a gel for his face of fresh aloe vera—25 ml (direct from the plant), 10 drops *L. officinalis* and 20 drops *Melaleuca alternifolia*. H felt immediate relief and after 5–10 minutes the pain lessened. After 1 hour the gel had formed a strong film (stronger than that on healthy skin) and the pain was gone.

H's eyes and lips were very swollen, his face a little red and on his upper lip blisters were forming where he had licked off the gel. I took a photograph of H after which he went to bed and slept soundly.

Day 2—morning: the whole face was sore. The nose had an open wound where the skin was burned off. It was not bleeding though it was very weepy and swollen. Under the eyes were brown dry patches which would probably break to form wounds. His eyelids were swollen and red, his lips swollen and cracked and his cheeks streaked in red and white. I washed the area with a hydrosol of rose (I had no lavender hydrosol), putting it also on compresses to try and remove the burned hair—still stuck on the skin. When the skin was dry I applied the gel blend again.

I applied the second gel blend to nose and upper lip.
Day 2—evening: during the day the brown patches had paled somewhat. His chin and neck were still painful. The nose had dried up and a scab was forming around the edges of the wound. H had slept during the day.

The washing and compress treatments were repeated, using the hydrosol, and more of the burned hair was removed. I made a weaker gel blend, since the emergency was over, using fresh aloe vera gel (25 ml) with only five drops of *L. officinalis*.
Day 3—morning: I cleansed the skin with hydrolat to remove the last of the burned hair. Although the wounds looked as though they may become infected, the nose and lip had started to dry up, the area was less swollen and the patches under the eyes were almost gone. The whole area was still sensitive.
Day 3—evening: the whole area was incredibly sensitive, so the hydrosol was sprayed on. At this point everything stung, everything seemed too strong. Even the cooling and soothing gel stung. The nose and lip started bleeding slightly and the risk of infection was still overhanging. Although the area

was still sensitive to the touch, the face and neck showed only a faint redness now. The gel blend was applied to the nose and lip and jojoba oil to the rest of the area.

Day 4—morning: turning point! No pain, only itching. Nose and lip had little scabs and looked clean, without any suggestion of impending infection. A doctor representing the insurance people arrived. He said the nose and lip had second-degree burns; the face and neck were first degree. He did not believe the burn had been as bad as I reported, but he changed his mind when I showed him the photographs.

H took a lukewarm shower and the gel dissolved in the water. I applied the jojoba oil to the whole area except nose and lip, which was given the gel blend.

In the evening the procedure was repeated.

Day 5—morning: this was the same procedure as yesterday evening. Some areas in the face were a bit red and tender, though the rest of the face was fine. The nose had a strong scab, which was already beginning to come off. The lip was healing well, with the wound diminishing. It was all very itchy. The procedure was repeated in the evening.

Day 6—morning: H went to work after the procedure from yesterday was repeated. During the day half of the nose scab came off, showing healthy new pink skin underneath; there was no bleeding. Although the skin looked a bit powdery, it was not peeling and appeared to be almost back to normal—no itchiness, tenderness or redness.

The procedure was repeated in the evening, using carrot oil instead of jojoba. More of the nose scab had come off, and the powdery look had gone.

Conclusion

On the 8th day the last of the nose scab came off, showing new skin. There was no peeling, and no scars. H looked well and strong, with no indication that he had been badly burned only a week previously. He used the carrot oil blend for some weeks and took care to avoid heat and the sun.

Had H gone to the hospital, some 20–25 kilometres away, the timespan alone would have made the burn much more serious; a bigger part of the face and neck could have turned into second-degree burns. We were able to cool the wound faster since we stayed at home.

Summary

The research studies presented in this chapter clearly demonstrate the efficacy of essential oils in significantly reducing patient stress levels in coronary and intensive care contexts. It is interesting to note that both the inhalation of oils and different forms of massage with them produce beneficial results. Further studies that directly compared the efficacy of different methods of administration would be welcomed. The evidence regarding the efficacy of essential oils in the treatment of severe burns, though powerful, is still largely anecdotal. Proper clinical studies in this field are needed to corroborate the existing evidence.

REFERENCES

Dunn C, Sleep J, Collett D 1995 Sensing an improvement: an experimental study to evaluate the use of aromatherapy, massage and periods of rest in an intensive care unit. Journal of Advanced Nursing 21: 34–40

Harris C M 1993 Is there a benefit to patients in using aromatherapy oils in a coronary care unit? Pilot study results (Copies available from The Royal Shrewsbury Hospital)

McCorkle R 1974 Effects of touch on seriously ill people. Nursing Research 23(2): 125

Meyer B C, Blacher R S, Brown F 1961 A clinical study of psychiatric and psychological aspects of mitral surgery. Psychosomatic Medicine 23(3): 194–218

O'Brien D, Alexander S 1985 High dependency nursing care. Churchill Livingstone, New York

Price S 1989 Essential oils in a burns unit. Aromanews 16: 4

Rowe L 1989 Anxiety in a coronary care unit. Nursing Times 85(45): 61

Stevensen C J 1994 The psychophysical effects of aromatherapy massage following cardiac surgery. Complementary Therapies in Medicine 2: 27–35

Waldman C S, Tseng P, Meulman P, Whitter H B 1993 Aromatherapy in the intensive care unit. Care of the Critically Ill 9(4): 170–174

Wilkinson M 1991 The healing touch in an age of technology. The Independent. October 15: 17

Woolfson A, Hewitt D 1992 Intensive aromacare. International Journal of Aromatherapy 4(2): 12–13

14 Care of the elderly

Introduction

Some of the greatest benefits to both patient and carers come from the use of essential oils with the elderly, since quality of life is improved for all concerned. Studies are presented which show definite reductions in the need for medication for sleep disturbances in settings where aromatherapy has been tried. Treatments for a variety of conditions often associated with old age are given, with particular reference to rheumatology.

THE EVE OF LIFE

Care of the elderly has always been regarded as one of the least glamorous sides of nursing. It is also one of the richest areas of care, and can make the difference between a winter of discontent and an Indian summer.

Aromatherapy enhances the holistic framework in caring for elderly persons: I find a number of cases where they are not at peace with themselves, the reason being a lot of unfinished business within themselves and their family. The psychological pain this generates, at times causes these physical symptoms to be uncontrolled, despite the use of orthodox medicine. Combine the two, orthodox and complementary, and the outcome is what is termed ideal for patient and carer. Families who sit with loved ones, or not so loved ones, are at a loss what to say and what to do. The three simple words 'I love you' or 'I am sorry' are at times difficult for them to say. At this juncture touch is encouraged as a form of communication and with this communication, essential oils are used.

(Tattam 1992)

The nursing home houses 21 residents with various degrees of senile dementia, as well as the degenerative physical conditions and limited or no mobility apparent with many elderly persons. The staff at the home are relaxed in their approach and aim to create an atmosphere of a home environment for all the patients. Medication is kept to a minimum and an activities coordinator is involved with the patients every weekday for group and one-to-one sessions. Family and friends are welcome to participate in the care-giving at any time and as often as possible.

The director of nursing selected eight patients who would benefit from the type of care Incare offers, and access was given to all relevant medical files and nursing and consultants' notes. A period of 10–15 minutes was to be spent with each individual during a 2 hour weekly visit. I decided to use only one essential oil to start with—to prevent confusion, to gather detailed results and acquaint the staff and residents with the benefits of each oil as it was introduced. The blend used was 2.5% dilution of *Lavandula angustifolia* in sweet almond oil.

The areas to be worked upon were mutually agreed: hands, feet, shoulders, face, etc. Those who were bedridden generally received foot massage as a means of stimulating circulation there.

The observations after 10 weeks were positive. Lavender was vaporized in a ceramic vaporizer all day and into the evening. The staff enjoyed the pleasant fragrance and the oil masked the constant odour of urine. The staff reported back on the pleasant environment the vaporized essential oil created—for themselves, for the visitors and mainly for the residents.

Of the patients receiving weekly treatment, all have responded to greater or lesser degrees to the aroma, the contact and the one-to-one communication. A reduction in emotional outbursts has been noted for those that are disturbed or disruptive, both during the day and during the night. Recognition of both the oil and the treatment is acknowledged by the majority of the patients. All responded positively to the contact, finding an increase in mobility and decrease in pain. Some individual reactions are reported below.

a   TM: severe Alzheimer's with emotional disturbances
Had required an increase in night medication owing to nocturnal disturbance. TM's partner spends 4 hours per day in physical exercise and social contact, and when the partner was not there TM exhibited aggressive verbal abuse of other residents. TM showed decreased ability to remember short term events and seemed to have difficulty recognizing people. After 10 weeks of aromatherapy, the emotional disturbances had decreased dramatically and nocturnal disruption ceased after using lavender on TM's pillow. I was greeted recently by TM using my first name and giving me compliments.

b   JR: alcohol-induced dementia, blind, reduced mobility
With no family, friends or relatives interested in visiting, JR had regressed to internalization, with little communication or interest in others around. Within two to three sessions his severe depression seemed to disappear, with an increase in conversation, attention to surroundings and interaction with other residents.

c   OC: senile dementia, lives in the past, very confused
Initially OC was reluctant to allow contact or even to converse with a stranger. OC now looks forward to the weekly sessions and jokes about family and events of the past. Conversation is more coherent and recently, through the massage session, OC will massage my hands.

Helen Passant, now retired, was one of the first nurses to introduce massage into a hospital, shortly after she became sister of what was then called the geriatric ward at the Churchill Hospital, Oxford in the 1980s. It soon became apparent to her that with massage the patients' skin became stronger and more resistant to bruising and tissue damage.

Later, essential oils were introduced into the vegetable oil the nurses were using, and it was found that the added benefits of these enabled the levels of conventional sedative drugs administered to be reduced. Other effects were soon noticed and, through the support of the consultant and the professor of geriatric medicine, herbal and essential oil remedies were included on the drug charts.

When all the above is taken into account, massage has been shown to bring great comfort to the elderly. It was found that therapeutic touch and essential oils can benefit and uplift both patients and nurses, giving the latter a more satisfying role. It can open the doors to a closer relationship, 'allowing patients to speak of their dreams and hopes, of their fears and pleasures. To relieve stress and pain on all levels was something I had not thought possible—but it is' (Passant 1990).

Not all elderly people in care want to be touched (McCann & McKenna 1993) and there are nurses who find physical contact with their patients in this way difficult. An excellent way to establish a touch relationship is to reach for the patient's hand as though about to give a simple handshake, placing the other hand on top (to form a 'sandwich') (Price 1993 pp. 211–212) (see also Ch. 7). When touch itself has been established, progress could be made to a simple massage, otherwise a patient unfamiliar with massage could become agitated or further confused (Horrigan 1995).

Mark Hardy, working with the elderly mentally ill at The Old Manor Hospital, Salisbury, expressed his concern regarding the 'almost habitual way in which night medication is prescribed' (Hardy 1991). Although not every patient experiences side-effects (notably ataxia, confusion and constipation plus other unwanted effects such as dry mouth and incontinence due to abnormally deep sleep), the use of certain essential oils can induce sleep easily. In many cases there is no need for hypnotics, or a reduced dose only. Many of the other side-effects can be alleviated with essential oils. However, when using vaporized oils for this purpose, all people in the room will be affected, with perhaps an occasional, but rare, adverse reaction. Fowler & Wall (1997) emphasize that this is an important point when treating people with cognitive impairment and advise that regard for personal choice should be exercised when treating patients with aromatherapy in nursing homes.

Dr Park, director of the ITU at Addenbrooke Hospital, states that aromatherapy has helped to reduce the need for expensive sedation and painkilling drugs on account of the relief obtained from constipation and general aches and pains by the application of this therapy (Macdonald 1993).

Dosage for the elderly

When determining the dosage of essential oils to be used, the weight, age and health (both mental and physical) of the person should always be taken into account (Price 1993 p. 154). With children, and older people whose bodily systems have begun to slow down, only half the normal concentration of essential oils is needed, i.e.

12–15 drops per 100 ml of carrier oil or lotion. The exact number of drops is rarely crucial (except where internal use is concerned) and is usually given as a range. For patients who need to use the oils over a long period of time, it is best to keep to the lower end of the range. *Eucalyptus smithii* [GULLY GUM] is one of the exceptions to this rule as it is extremely gentle in action and should always be used in preference to *E. globulus* [TASMANIAN BLUE GUM] on elderly and children alike (see Respiratory problems p. 234).

As in all use of essential oils, synergy within and between essential oils is an important consideration (see Ch. 3). Two oils are always more effective than one, and up to four oils, when selected with knowledge, can be even more so. Each person is an individual, and one essential oil may not have the required effect on everyone—as with drugs, where one brand is not necessarily appropriate for each person.

TREATMENT OF SPECIFIC CONDITIONS
Circulation

Case 14.2 Aromatherapists: Eleni Hajisava and Mary Ann Gardner, Australia

Hajisava and Gardner visit Lara Lodge in Oakleigh, which provides special accommodation for men. The residents are elderly, and a number of them are former alcoholics. They concentrate on foot treatments, using foot baths and massage.

a A man with a past history of a stroke had poor circulation to his feet and tended to develop gangrenous spots on his toes. These spots had to be surgically removed when they appeared. He was given foot baths using essential oil of pine, and his feet were massaged with a blend of niaouli for its antiseptic effect. Since starting weekly treatments no further spots have occurred.

b This man was very immobile and as a result had such poor circulation to his lower extremities that his legs were blue. He was given foot baths using lavender (occasionally with small amounts of rosemary) and mandarin for its antispasmodic effect. As a result the circulation to his legs and feet has been very much improved.

Another benefit to these elderly men, who otherwise tend to be isolated, is that Incare visits give them an opportunity to get together as a group. When Hajisava and Gardner arrive, the residents gravitate to the day room, evidently looking forward to their treatments.

Digestive disorders

Currently, the aromatherapy organizations do not allow their members to give essential oils internally and their insurance does not therefore cover this activity. This can be frustrating to many aromatherapists, because complaints involving the digestive system often respond more rapidly to ingestion. Studies in aromatology (in addition to an accredited aromatherapy course—the two together give a qualification in aromatic medicine) can be undertaken in order to qualify for this insurance and in the UK the Institute of Aromatic Medicine (IAM) gives cover for internal use to aromatologists who have qualified on an accredited course (for information, contact the IAM — see Useful addresses, p. 376).

When adequately qualified and suitably insured to prescribe and administer essential oils internally in accordance with the protocol, eight drops in total of the selected essential oils should be well mixed into 50 ml of vegetable oil (as suggested by Sassard 1932) or liquid honey, and one teaspoonful of this mixture administered three times a day, or morning and night depending on the needs of the patient. Suppositories for the elderly should contain no more than two drops of essential oils.

The essential oils suggested for each digestive condition below may be:

- administered internally, per os diluted as above, or per rectum in a suppository
- applied to the abdomen in a carrier lotion or oil
- massaged in a clockwise direction into the abdomen.

Should a consultant or doctor disapprove or be wary of using essential oils to treat anything but stress and anxiety, select those essential oils from the suggestions which are recommended also for stress relief (see Ch. 12 in conjunction with the different digestive oils mentioned in this section).

Constipation

Many elderly people suffer from constipation, often as a result of medication taken or a poor or overrefined diet. Despite the best efforts of the nutritionists even younger people in hospital can become constipated owing to a change in environment. As with everything, constipation should be treated in a holistic fashion, endeavouring to discover the cause, and treatment should include regulating the diet.

Essential oils can be effective for constipated patients when used with massage of the abdomen and/or the feet. With the feet, the area to concentrate on is the soft tissue just below the level of the sesamoid bones and above the calcaneus, on the plantar surface of the foot. If not trained in Swiss reflex treatment (see Ch. 7) or reflexology, start with the right foot and massage in large firm circles in the direction from the lateral to the medial side; the left foot should then be massaged in firm circles from the medial to the lateral side. This directional massage of the colon reflexes, with pressure, helps peristalsis, as does movement 3 of the abdomen massage, carried out firmly and slowly with the heel of the hand, shown in Chapter 7, page 142.

The most effective oils for constipation are: *Citrus aurantium* var. *amara* (per.) [ORANGE BIGARADE], *Rosmarinus officinalis* [ROSEMARY] (camphor and cineole chemotypes), *Ocimum basilicum* var. *album* [EUROPEAN BASIL], *Piper nigrum* [BLACK PEPPER] and *Zingiber officinale* [GINGER].

The last is cited for constipation by Franchomme & Pénoël (1990 p. 406) and for diarrhoea by Valnet (1980 p. 135). Like *Foeniculum vulgare* var. *dulce* [FENNEL], it may be a balancing oil in this direction.

Diarrhoea

This condition can sometimes be just as upsetting to a patient as constipation, and in this case, and where the diarrhoea is of nervous origin, the tranquillizing effects of *Origanum majorana* [SWEET MARJORAM] and *Citrus limon* [LEMON] are effective, together with antiinflammatory oils such as *Melaleuca viridiflora* [NIAOULI], *Mentha* × *piperita* [PEPPERMINT] (which in addition, will help against nausea) and *Pelargonium graveolens* [GERANIUM]—this last oil is also tranquillizing. These antiinflammatory oils are also useful for colitis and gastroenteritis, whilst *Syzygium aromaticum*

This case history took place at a private nursing home in Hull as part of a project to see the difference aromatherapy could make to some of the clients there. It was conducted with the consent and backing of the client's family and the doctor in charge.

K suffers from Alzheimer's disease, which started 3 years ago, and she has been blind for 6 years. She also suffered a stroke 5 years ago, which left her with a right-sided weakness. Although K has periods of aggression, followed by times of normality, she is a delight to care for and has a lot to contribute towards society. She loves music and can recall the words of songs long forgotten by most people. However, she has many problems for, as well as the Alzheimer's disease, she suffers from insomnia, chronic constipation and loss of appetite, among other discomforts.

On my first visit we spent the time in the home's garden as I wanted to give K the opportunity to smell some flowers. Afterwards, over a cup of tea, I introduced her to the essential oils and we had a 'sniffing session'. She instantly recognized the fragrance of rose so we decided, whatever else we would use, rose would be one of the oils in the blend for the massage.

Armed with her favourite music hall tape I gave K her first massage. She loved every minute of the experience and sang all the words to the songs during her massage! I asked for K to be given a nightly bath containing five drops of lavender, plus one or two drops of the same oil to be sprinkled on her pillow before going to bed. She enjoyed a tot of whisky, so I suggested that this, together with the bath and pillow use of lavender, be given eventually, instead of her temazepam medication, which was reduced gradually. She was eager to receive this more acceptable nightcap.

I mixed some base cream with a few drops of *Lavandula angustifolia* to be applied to her forehead when she became aggressive; the nursing staff observed and documented the reactions. The baths and lavender on the pillow were daily treatments, the massage treatments being conducted on a weekly basis. After 8 weeks she was almost off temazepam; after 12 weeks it was completely stopped with no adverse reactions.

K's life is now much improved and happier. Her right side is stronger now, with more mobility, the constipation problem is under control owing to the abdominal massages, the insomnia has been almost eradicated and she responds well to the lavender cream on her forehead. Each time K heard my voice, she started to get ready for her massage and, although blind, she very much enjoyed the oils through her sense of smell, which in turn provoked happy memories from the past. K, her family and all the nursing staff, including the doctor, all feel this has become a worthwhile project.

(flos) [CLOVE BUD], *Pimpinella anisum* [ANISEED], *Melaleuca cajuputi* [CAJUPUT] and *Myristica fragrans* [NUTMEG] relieve the spasms (Valnet 1980 pp. 95, 101, 114, 161).

Diverticulitis (diverticulosis)

Diverticulosis, the harmless presence of small bulges in weak points in the large intestine, exists in most elderly people (Wingate & Wingate 1988 p. 147). It is only when one or more of these diverticula becomes inflamed that chronic diverticulitis can set in and constipation, slight abdominal pain and bleeding may manifest. The diet should be changed to one rich in fibre, and massage with the antiinflammatory essential oils (under Diarrhoea above) would be beneficial, with those effective for constipation incorporated where necessary, such as *C. aurantium* var. *amara* (per.), which is also antiinflammatory.

Other antiinflammatory oils which act on the digestive system are *Commiphora myrrha* [MYRRH] (distilled only), *Chamomilla recutita* [GERMAN CHAMOMILE], *Juniperus communis* (fruct.) [JUNIPER] and *Melissa officinalis* [MELISSA].

An elderly woman at the Queen Elizabeth Centre, Ballarat, was unable to open her bowels owing to atrophy of the large intestine (colon), and required admission to hospital every 3 weeks for a colonic washout. Doctors were planning to perform a total colectomy (surgical removal of the large intestine), which would have left the woman with a colostomy.

I made a blend of fennel, patchouli, sandalwood and black pepper in vegetable oil, and this blend was massaged gently into the woman's abdomen several times that evening. Next morning she had a normal bowel action. Ongoing care consists of daily abdominal massages and an oral aperient nightly. Other staff members have been taught how to do this massage so that it can be performed daily and not just when I am on duty. Best of all, the woman's bowels are opened regularly, and surgery has been avoided.

Indigestion (dyspepsia)

Chronic indigestion can be due to many causes. Common physical reasons, if there is no gastritis or ulcer present, may be eating too quickly, too much or swallowing air with the food. Medication or heavy smoking may also be responsible (Wingate & Wingate 1988 p. 256). In many cases stress can be implicated and this should be treated as well by abdominal and/or foot massage with relaxing essential oils 30 minutes before a meal.

As a preventive measure and to help those who are eating incorrectly (e.g. too fast, poor diet), a teaspoonful from a mix of digestive oils in a vegetable oil (see above for quantities) taken 15 minutes before a meal would be an effective measure. If this is not possible, then the abdomen should be massaged with the same mix 30 minutes before the meal. *Carum carvi* [CARAWAY], *C. aurantium* var. *amara* (per.), *F. vulgare* var. *dulce* and *P. anisum* are the most effective oils. *O. basilicum* var. *album* can be added if the indigestion is of nervous origin and *O. majorana* if gastritis or an ulcer are present.

To ease indigestion once present, the same oils can be used. Also effective at this stage are *Citrus reticulata* [MANDARIN], *C. limon* (per.) [LEMON] (analgesic and antacid), *M. officinalis*, *M. × piperita* and *R. officinalis* (camphor and cineole chemotypes).

Headaches and migraines

These can occur for a number of reasons, which are not always apparent, especially in the elderly. Because of this, it is important to make use of the synergy between essential oils and mix two or more together.

The oil most often used to combat headaches and migraine is *Lavandula angustifolia*. Equally effective are *Chamaemelum nobile*, *M. × piperita*, *O. basilicum*, *O. majorana* and *R. officinalis*. The choice of oil may depend on the cause, for example *M. × piperita* works well on a headache caused by digestive disorders. Inhalation from a tissue (or by other means—see Ch. 5) gives the speediest reaction, though massage of the neck and face, particularly the forehead (using two or three of the above oils in a carrier oil), gives the patient the additional relaxing and soothing benefits of massage. Anyone not fully qualified in massage should limit this to gentle strokes with the whole hand, as described in Chapter 7.

Pressure sores

This is an area where traditional medicine has limited success, and nurses using aromatherapy have been rewarded by the healing which has occurred with the use of essential oils. Cicatrizant oils together with those which are strongly antiseptic can be used in a spray with water when the sores are suppurating—10 drops in 100 ml water, shaking well each time before spraying the area. If it can be touched, gently apply a little from a mix made from five to six drops in 50 ml oil of *Calendula officinalis* (macerated carrier oil), which itself has cicatrizant effects on wounds and persistent ulcers (Price 1993 p. 172). Calendula oil will also help to strengthen the skin if the mixture is massaged in gently twice a day. Compresses may be useful (see Ch. 5), but check that the dressing used is non-stick. Passant (1990) frequently used a combination of rose, geranium, lavender and marjoram (all unspecified) in inhalations to calm and comfort her patients before changing dressings (Wise 1989).

Recommended essential oils include *Boswellia carteri* [FRANKINCENSE], *Chamomilla matricaria* [GERMAN CHAMOMILE], *L. angustifolia* [LAVENDER], *Lavandula × intermedia* 'Super' [LAVANDIN] and *P. graveolens* [GERANIUM]. The cicatrizant qualities of the resinoid *Styrax tonkinensis* [SIAM BENZOIN] could also play a part in healing.

Insomnia

The problem of helping an elderly patient achieve a good quality, refreshing night's sleep is a bigger problem in hospitals than when the patient is at home.

Hospital admission can disrupt sleep patterns to such a degree that a useful night's sleep can become impossible. This is especially true in the elderly, whose normal sleep pattern may already be erratic. Factors such as anxiety, lack of privacy, noise and ward activity are all contributory factors, not all of which can be totally eliminated. Often the usual nursing practices are still not sufficient to correct the problem, even when noise levels and lack of privacy are reduced to a minimum. As a result, we often find that the use of drugs is resorted to.

(Cannard 1994)

Lavender (expected to be *L. angustifolia*), is the usual essential oil used to induce sleep, although Macdonald's (1995) finding, that 'a few drops of the appropriate oils on the pillow helped to induce a peaceful sleep in many patients', implies the use of more than one, which is always an effective measure. Without accurately specifying lavender the type used is unknown and separate varieties of both lavenders and lavandins can give very different results. Hospital pharmacists often supply the more camphoraceous *L. latifolia* [SPIKE LAVENDER] rather than the French *L. angustifolia* (Buckle 1992).

Since the reduction in production of French lavender (see Ch. 1), much of the essential oil sold by that name is in fact lavandin. The variety of lavandin closest to true lavender is *L. × intermedia* 'Super', though it has fewer constituents. True lavender contains more terpenes, alcohols and esters and *L. × intermedia* 'Super' contains more camphor (around 5%). See Chapter 1 for details of the differences in properties and effects of these two plants.

Franchomme & Pénoël (1990 p. 364) indicates *L. × intermedia* 'Super', *M. officinalis* [MELISSA], *Citrus bergamia* [BERGAMOT] and *O. majoran* [MARJORAM] for insomnia. Other effective oils are *C. nobile* [ROMAN CHAMOMILE], *C. aurantium* var. *amara* (flos) [NEROLI BIGARADE] and *C. reticulata* (per.) [MANDARIN], plus *O. basilicum* var. *album* [EUROPEAN BASIL] for nervous insomnia (Valnet 1980 p. 97). Some sedative and calming essential oils seem to possess sleep-inducing properties, e.g. *Santalum album* [SANDALWOOD] and *Valeriana officinalis* [COMMON VALERIAN], as do some hypotensors, such as *Cananga odorata* [YLANG YLANG] and *C. limon* [LEMON]. The essential oils can be vaporized, used on a tissue, put in the bath or applied in massage.

PROJECT USING LAVENDER TO PROMOTE SLEEP

A 6 week project using vaporized essential oils to relieve insomnia was carried out at the Old Manor Hospital in Salisbury (Hardy 1991). The aim of this project was to find a natural replacement for night medication, and after consulting relatives and ward staff the project was begun. Lavender (unspecified) was used in a vortex unit, which was activated during the last 2 weeks of the project for three periods a day: 9 p.m.–10.30 p.m., 2 a.m.–3 a.m. and 5.30 a.m.–6.30 a.m.

Four male residents (referred to in this text as A, B, C and D) took part, their ages ranging from 67 to 88. Their normal medication (length of time on named medication in brackets) was as follows:

- A—promazine 25 mg (3 years)
- B—Heminevrin (chlormethiazole) 1 cap (7 months)
- C—temazepam 10 mg (1 year)
- D—no medication (nor previously).

The four men's sleep patterns were assessed over a 6 week period:

- weeks 1 and 2—normal medication given
- weeks 3 and 4—no medication was given
- weeks 5 and 6—no medication given, but lavender oil was used.

Results

The results were split up into day and night periods, each giving the average number of hours sleep (see Table 14.1).

The total number of hours slept by the four men over the 6 week period is shown in Table 14.2. From Tables 14.1 and 14.2 it can be seen that:

- All four men slept approximately the same number of hours with lavender oil as with medication.
- B slept longer with lavender and was originally the worst sleeper, with noisy, aggressive periods during the day. These moods improved considerably towards the end of the project.
- C and D no longer felt the need to sleep so much during the day, perhaps indicating that their quality of sleep during the night was improved with lavender; 4 days after the lavender was administered C reported

Table 14.1 Average number of hours slept during night and day by four subjects (A, B, C and D) with medication (weeks 1 and 2), without medication (weeks 3 and 4), and without medication but with vaporized lavender oil (weeks 5 and 6)

	With medication (weeks 1 and 2)	Without medication (weeks 3 and 4)	With vaporized lavender (no medication) (weeks 5 and 6)
Night			
A	8.9	7.1	8.8
B	6.6	5.2	7.4
C	9.3	7.8	9.3
D	8.5	8.0	8.3
Day			
A	1.5	1.0	1.6
B	0.5	0.5	0.5
C	2.8	2.0	1.9
D	1.1	0.4	0.2

Table 14.2 Total number of hours slept by four subjects (A, B, C and D) over the 6 week period of the project

	With medication (weeks 1 and 2)	Without medication (weeks 3 and 4)	With vaporized lavender (no medication) (weeks 5 and 6)
A	125	100	123
B	94	78	103
C	132	110	130
D	117	108	116

that he had not had such a good night's sleep for years.

• The cost of essential oils was found to be 60% less than the cost of conventional drugs.

Conclusion

Lavender oil used in this manner can successfully replace medication to relieve insomnia.

Oldham Cottage Hospital conducted a similar small scale study on the possible use of lavender to encourage rest and relaxation in elderly patients, thus stimulating the healing process (Hudson 1996). The study took place over 14 days and the sleep patterns, the amount of dozing and the daytime alertness of the patients taking part were monitored and recorded.

• On days 1–7 the only difference in the patients' normal daily routine was the monitoring—no lavender was used.

• On days 8–14 one drop of lavender was put on each patient's pillow at night—no other changes were made.

At the end of the 14 days the records were analysed and it was found that all patients had reacted favourably to the treatment. There was increased alertness during the day and improved sleep patterns; in those patients who had previously been confused there was an almost 50% decrease in their symptoms. These are probably not the only studies to have been carried out on small numbers of people and this illustrates the importance of small scale trials, which can then stimulate controlled research in this sphere.

ESSENTIAL OILS AS AN ALTERNATIVE TO TEMAZEPAM

The Tullamore Nursing Development Unit (NDU), the General Hospital, Tullamore, Southern Ireland has also looked at the use of aromatherapy in sleep disturbance in the elderly. In this unit, drugs are used as a last resort but, where necessary, the drug of choice for a patient with sleep disturbance is temazepam (an intermediate-acting benzodiazepine). This drug certainly has its place in the treatment of short term sleep disturbances. However, if drugs can be avoided, especially in the elderly, then any adverse reactions, interactions and dependency can also be avoided (Reynolds 1993 p. 590, Storrs 1980 p. 17). Graham Cannard, coordinator in this NDU, together with his team of nurses, decided to look for an alternative to conventional medication and selected aromatherapy to augment the nursing practices already employed in an attempt to reduce the use of night sedation.

Methods

The first step was to assess the amount of night sedation being prescribed. Of the 10 patients in the NDU at that time, eight were prescribed sedation each night. These eight patients were a combination of respite and acute medical patients over the age of 70. One was a long stay patient. Christine Dalton, a nurse and qualified aromatherapist, was enlisted to help implement the programme. Dalton undertook the training of the NDU nurses in the correct use of one blend of essential oils to reduce levels of insomnia. Shirley Price's 'Care for Sleep' oil was used, a pre-mixed blend of oils containing European basil (low in methyl chavicol), lavender and sweet marjoram.

The other three nurses on the team (Clarke, Caffrey and Tracey) were taught the various methods of administration and the team decided that the two methods upon which they could concentrate were vaporization into the atmosphere and a 5 minute hand massage using the oils for those patients for whom the vaporization alone was not successful. Under the guidance of Dalton, guidelines for the use of aromatherapy were drawn up.

The team explained their aims and proposed methods to the consultant physician and received his full support. As they were concerned that the patients might be adversely affected if aromatherapy did not work for them, and the night sedation had been deleted from their prescription chart, the consultant agreed that the prescription for night sedation would be rewritten as an 'as required' medication so that if the patient were distressed by still being awake at midnight, then the medication could be administered. Because of the potential for withdrawal symptoms, the team was advised by Dalton that for the first two nights the patients would be given their usual sedation (as prescribed) together with aromatherapy, in order to

establish a response to the oils before withdrawing the medication. The nursing team began by surveying the medication charts of all the patients in the NDU prior to the introduction of aromatherapy (some were on regular night sedation—usually temazepam). The sleep patterns of those patients were charted and 94 patient nights were recorded over 2 weeks without aromatherapy.

Following the introduction of aromatherapy, sleep patterns were again recorded over 94 patient nights. Sedation was administered only when requested by the patient but treatment with essential oils was ongoing. A record was maintained for each patient, showing the name of the oil used, the amount, the method of administration and the night sedation given (if any). An evaluation of the sleep pattern was carried out and charted the following morning. The sleep pattern was assessed by the nurse, asking the patient how he/she slept and if he/she felt refreshed. The nurse's observations of the sleep patterns were also charted. These records were filled in each night for each patient and were used to obtain the data.

Results

Prior to the introduction of aromatherapy the situation was as follows:

- patients reported a good night's sleep for 69 of the 94 patient nights (73%)
- night sedation was given on 85 of the 94 patient nights (80%) to help achieve this quality of sleep.

After the introduction of aromatherapy the situation changed as described below:

- during the two nights where night sedation and aromatherapy were given simultaneously, all patients slept well (100%)
- following this, night sedation was given only when requested by the patients and was necessary on 34 patient nights (41%)
- the number of patients reporting a good night's sleep improved to 91 out of the 94 patient nights (97%)
- a reduction in night sedation of 49% was achieved
- some patients needed no sedation at all whilst using aromatherapy, whilst some required it periodically
- only one patient requested sedation on a regular basis.

Table 14.3 Percentage of patients sleeping well and needing medication before and with introduction of *Care for Sleep* essential oil mix

	Before essential oils	With essential oils
Slept well (%)	73	97
Needed medication (%)	80	31

This information is summarized in Table 14.3. The figures in this table show an overall 24% improvement in sleeping and a 49% reduction in medication as a result of the use of essential oils.

Conclusion

Apart from the obvious effect on the sleep patterns of the patients, other benefits of using aromatherapy were noted. These were:

• The homely and fresh smell of the ward was very comforting; the usual 'hospital smell' that is often present had been disguised.

• Patients received more physical contact with the nurse owing to receiving hand massage with the diluted essential oils. The importance of touch is recognized as being therapeutic in itself (Byass 1988, Price 1993 p. 196) This is especially true for the elderly hospitalized patient who may receive very little physical contact that is not associated with a nursing procedure.

• It was noted that the use of the 'Care for Sleep' essential oil mix was much less expensive than the use of temazepam.

This small scale study has certain limitations. It did not show how much the psychological effect had on improving sleep patterns in the patients, nor did it show whether massage or vaporization was the more effective method of administration. There was also some difficulty in assessing sleep patterns: occasionally the patients and the nurses' comments were at variance.

However, the study did show that the use of this blend of oils for sleep disturbance in the elderly is of definite benefit. It is a useful adjunct to the usual nursing care given to the patient and is free of side-effects. The team are hoping to expand their knowledge of aromatherapy so that they can offer essential oils to patients with other problems, in the hope that the use of drugs may be reduced and the quality of care improved.

Respiratory problems

A subgroup of the volatile oils listed in textbooks of materia medica, pharmacology and therapeutics as having expectorant properties includes a number of oils obtained chiefly from members of the conifer family (Boyd & Pearson 1946). Oils from other families are reputed (from anecdotal evidence) to have expectorant properties also.

Elderly people suffering from catarrhal problems, such as chronic bronchitis or asthma, can benefit from a daily application of essential oils in a carrier lotion on to their chest and neck. The thin skin behind the ears also facilitates penetration by essential oils. Suitable anticatarrhal, expectorant and mucolytic oils include:

• *Boswellia carteri* [FRANKINCENSE]—also antitussive
• *Cedrus atlantica* [CEDARWOOD]
• *Eucalyptus smithii* [GULLY GUM]—also antiviral (common cold and influenza)
• *Hyssopus officinalis* [HYSSOP]—also antiinflammatory and antitussive (but suitable only for non-epileptic patients)
• *Melaleuca viridiflora* [NIAOULI]—especially in chronic cases
• *Mentha × piperita* [PEPPERMINT]—also antiinflammatory
• *Origanum majorana* [SWEET MARJORAM]—also antispasmodic
• *Pimpinella anisum* [ANISEED]—also antispasmodic
• *Pinus sylvestris* [SCOTS PINE]
• *Salvia officinalis* [SAGE]
• *Styrax tonkinensis* [STYRAX BENZOIN] (a resinoid, so quality is of paramount importance).

If any respiratory infection is present *Thymus mastichina* [SPANISH MARJORAM] and/or *T. vulgaris* ct. geraniol or ct. linalool [SWEET THYME] (the latter is both antiinflammatory and antispasmodic) should be added to the mix, unless *E. smithii*, which has powerful disinfectant properties (Pénoël personal communication 1993), is one of the oils used. Eight drops of essential oils in total should be added to 50 ml carrier lotion.

E. smithii is an excellent preventive measure for winter coughs and colds because it increases the resistance of the respiratory system to infection. It has a pleasant aroma, is inexpensive and can be vaporized daily in the lounge area of the ward, and/or in the ward (or bedrooms, as many of the newer hospitals name the rooms of the elderly or patients with learning difficulties).

Rheumatism and arthritis

Rheumatism is a vague term which covers various types of conditions involving pain in the muscles. The two main types are rheumatoid arthritis, which involves inflammation of the joints, and osteoarthritis. Rheumatoid arthritis is more common in women and involves chronic inflammation of the connective tissue around the joints (normally attacking them in symmetrical pairs), which causes pain, swelling and stiffness, frequently accompanied by weight loss and fatigue. In osteoarthritis there is a progressive wearing away of the cartilage, the connective tissue thickens and any fluid which may fill the joint causes swelling, resulting in severe pain and reduced movement. Wingate & Wingate (1988 p. 349) suggest that, because there is no inflammation, the term 'osteoarthrosis' is preferred.

A change in diet has been known to bring about a noticeable improvement in people with rheumatoid arthritis and essential oils have been used successfully for many years to reduce inflammation and pain in the fibrous tissues around the joints (Price 1992), giving increased mobility. There are many different varieties of arthritis and there is no specific evidence as yet that the bone pain in osteoarthrosis can be alleviated.

Choice of oils

Although there are many essential oils indicated for muscular pain and arthritis, if it is not possible to discover the cause and deal with that first, the individual needs to be examined in terms of the symptoms displayed in order to make full use of the properties of the essential oils.

Pain is perhaps the most important symptom to consider and 'while conventional analgesics give some relief, they seldom give complete or sustained relief. Furthermore, where there is

chronic pain, the stress associated with the anticipation of pain can increase the sensation of pain' (Macdonald 1995). It follows that stress-relieving essential oils which are also analgesic may have the strongest effect, because they deal with mind-initiated pain as well as the physical pain from the joints themselves. *Origanum majorana*, *Pelargonium graveolens* and essential oil from the branches of *Juniperus communis* [JUNIPER] have both analgesic and stress-relieving properties; juniper is also antiinflammatory (Roulier 1990 p. 268) as is geranium. Many of the antiinflammatory essential oils seem to be mainly indicated for inflammation of the digestive tract, e.g. *Coriandrum sativum* [CORIANDER]. For arthritis, essential oils are required which primarily affect inflammation of the connective tissue. However, *C. sativum*, like *Melaleuca cajuputi* [CAJUPUT] does possess antiinflammatory properties that are effective on connective tissue, thus indirectly dulling arthritic pain (Franchomme & Pénoël 1990 p. 343).

Essential oils which are both stress relieving and antiinflammatory include *Chamaemelum nobile* [ROMAN CHAMOMILE], *Cymbopogen citratus* and *C. flexuosus* [LEMONGRASS], *Lavandula angustifolia*, *Lavandula × intermedia* 'Super' and *Aloysia triphylla* [LEMON VERBENA]. *Pinus sylvestris* [SCOTS PINE] and *Cymbopogon nardus* [CITRONELLA] (Franchomme & Pénoël 1990 p. 348) are antiinflammatory. *Melaleuca viridiflora* [NIAOULI] is both antiinflammatory and analgesic; where the patient is also depressed, this is a valuable oil to use.

Other essential oils with analgesic properties are *Piper nigrum* (Roulier 1990 p. 295) and *Zingiber officinalis*. *Rosmarinus officinalis* [ROSEMARY] is an effective muscle relaxant in stronger doses (Franchomme & Pénoël 1990 p. 393), and for temporary relief (but not as a regular measure) can be applied undiluted on a small area. For severe pain, *Syzygium aromaticum* (flos) [CLOVE BUD], *M. cajuputi* and *Myristica fragrans* [NUTMEG] may have a stronger effect.

J. communis and *R. officinalis* also help to reduce any fluid around the joints.

The most effective method of using the essential oils (diluted for regular use) is applying them directly to the affected area or with a compress. They can be applied with or without massage, although massage can help to relax the muscles. A warm bath containing essential oils also relaxes the muscles and reduces the pain.

STUDY USING AROMATHERAPY IN RHEUMATOLOGY

A hospital study carried out in 1990/91 at the Devonshire Royal Hospital in Buxton, Derbyshire, included only patients at a non-inflammatory stage of their arthritis, owing to the understandable scepticism of the doctors, who were unsure of the effects of aromatherapy (Cawthorne 1991). Although it was difficult to draw conclusions from this small study, because so many different essential oils were used, it resulted in recommendations for a follow-up study to be undertaken, with patients selected at random. In the original study, out of the 10 patients who returned the questionnaires:

- 10 enjoyed using the oils
- seven experienced pain relief (two were able to reduce their analgesics)
- six were sleeping better (one decreasing his night sedation)
- nine felt more relaxed.

It was interesting to note that the nurses had used all the oils in combinations of two or three oils. They were chosen in partnership with the patients. The aim was to match the patient's problem with a smell they liked. For example, if a patient was tense and depressed then both relaxing and uplifting oils were used.

(Cawthorne 1991)

Although the specific oils used on each patient were not given, the results appear to demonstrate the multi-therapeutic action of essential oils and their effectiveness when selected for the individual.

SINGLE-CASE SUBJECT PROJECT ON RELIEF OF ARTHRITIC PAIN

Macdonald (1995) carried out a single-case subject project at Duncuan (Care of the Elderly Unit), Lochgilphead, Argyll, not only as a pilot study for future work but in order to see how aromatherapy could be incorporated into her working day. She states that: 'large numbers of subjects are not required for single case research, where generalisability (sic) is achieved through replication studies … Le Roux & Lyne (1989) have argued that single-case research designs provide firm foundation for developing sound nursing practices … It was decided that three patients would be a manageable number in the first instance'.

Project aim

The aim of Macdonald's project was to discover whether the use of aromatherapy enhanced conventional methods of pain relief. Informed consent was sought from the patients (three females aged between 60 and 90 selected at random), who were given written details of the intervention in addition to a verbal account. The UKCC Code of Conduct was adhered to at all times.

Method

A simple two-phase design was used alternately. Phase A lasted 3 weeks and conventional analgesics only were given. Phase B lasted 2 weeks, and as well as conventional analgesics incorporated the topical application (without massage) twice daily of 5–10 ml of essential oils in a carrier lotion. The oils selected were eucalyptus, juniper, marjoram and rosemary (botanical names unspecified) in a 1.5% dilution. Phase A and phase B were then repeated. The extra week in phase A was to allow for any carry-over effect of the treatment. The Scott & Huskisson (1976) pain scale was used to measure change in the condition of the patients. Lack of time and resources prevented the measurement of pain experienced in walking, dressing or sleeping. The pain scale, which ranged from 0 (no pain) to 10 (worst possible pain) was used at each drug administration.

Results

Barthel index scores for self-care (maximum possible score 53) and mobility (maximum possible score 52) were taken on admission for assessment and again after the 10 week period (mobility score shown in brackets). The results of these are shown in Table 14.4.

For simplicity's sake, the pain scale figures are shown as an average (PSA) for each week. Table 14.5 also shows the number of times medication was administered, week by week.

Conclusions

Some interesting conclusions can be drawn from this project, and some of them are presented below.

Patient A. In week 6, as expected, there may have been some effects of the essential oils remaining, shown by the average reduced pain scale figures compared with weeks 1–3 and 7 and 8. Less medication was needed during weeks 4, 5, 9 and 10, when essential oils were applied daily. Strangely, medication in week 3 was lower than when essential oils were introduced in week 4. Could it be psychological, in that she was anticipating being helped by the essential oils? Immediately the treatment stopped, the patient was in need of medication (week 6).

Weeks 9 and 10 show an accelerating reduction in both medication and pain scale readings, and it is interesting to speculate what the results would have shown had the project been extended for a further 5 weeks.

Patient B. During the whole of weeks 6, 7 and 8 without essential oils, B's medication and pain scale readings were lower than during the first 3 weeks, reducing to 0 on both counts after the second intervention with essential oils. It could be that B's faith in aromatherapy after the first application period was a contributory factor (see Ch. 7).

Patient C. C's medication did not alter, although the pain scale readings were considerably reduced at each aromatherapy intervention. The reduction to 0 on the pain scale during the second intervention may suggest that C's medication could be reduced if the topical application of essential oils were to be continued permanently.

Many further interesting observations were included in this project, full details of which can be found in Macdonald (1995).

Dementia

Some elderly people suffer from organic deterioration of their mental faculties. They are unable to think clearly or to concentrate for any length of time, their memories may be confused and unreliable, some may hallucinate sights and sounds and others may have difficulty with their speech. The commonest type of physical change is seen in Alzheimer's disease, where nerve tissue throughout the brain withers and dies. Alzheimer (1864 to 1915) described characteristic changes in the brains of patients who had died with "presenile" dementia, that is, people in their

Table 14.4 Barthel index scores for self-care and mobility for three patients (A, B and C), assessed on admission and after 10 week project

	Self-care		Mobility	
	Week 0	Week 10	Week 0	Week 10
A	24	27	10	10
B	4	7	3	10
C	53	53	28	42

Table 14.5 Weekly pain scale averages (PSA, where 10 = worst possible pain) and number of weekly medications (Meds) administered to patients A, B and C over course of 10 week project, without and with essential oil use

Week	A		B		C	
	Meds	PSA	Meds	PSA	Meds	PSA
1 } Medication only	14	5.28	10	5.85	21	2.14
2	12	5.71	10	5.85	21	3.71
3	8	4.71	8	5.28	21	3.71
4 } Medication plus	9	4.71	4	2.28	21	0.28
5 } essential oils	6	2.57	1	0.28	21	0.00
6 } Medication only	11	3.71	5	2.71	21	1.85
7	11	5.71	5	3.00	21	1.00
8	12	5.42	7	3.57	21	2.85
9 } Medication plus	7	3.00	1	0.57	21	0.00
10 } essential oils	1	1.57	0	0.00	21	0.00

50s and 60s, but similar changes in older people are common and account for many if not most cases of "senile" dementia' (Wingate & Wingate 1988).

Demanding illness is common in 20% of over 80 year olds; two-thirds of the 20% of elderly people over 80 who have an illness requiring care may suffer from Alzheimer's disease and it has been suggested that in the 40- to 60-year-old age group there may be 15 000 cases.

For patients with Alzheimer's, who are robbed of not only their memory but also their awareness, scented oils may have the ability to act as a trigger and help them recapture some of their past experiences (Brett 1997). Essential oils best known for stimulating the mind and improving the memory are *Rosmarinus officinalis* [ROSEMARY] and *Mentha × piperita* [PEPPERMINT] (Van Toller & Dodd 1991). Passant (1990) used cardamom, geranium and lavender (unspecified) and Franchomme recommends *Syzygium aromaticum* (flos) [CLOVE BUD]. For those who are depressed, essential oils which are a tonic to the nervous system may be used, such as *Boswellia carteri* [FRANKINCENSE], *Citrus aurantium* var. *amara* (flos) [NEROLI BIGARADE], *Ocimum basilicum* var. *album* [BASIL] (with a low phenolic ether content—see Ch. 8), *Origanum majorana* [MARJORAM], *Rosa damascena* [ROSE OTTO] and *Salvia sclarea* [CLARY SAGE]. All the oils in this section can be given by inhalation, in the bath or by scalp, hand or foot massage.

Although Horrigan (1995) stressed that massage could be startling, or even cause further confusion in demanding patients, Miller (1995) felt that it could provide a meaningful communication tool.

Summary

Essential oils have wide application in the treatment of the elderly (and other) hospitalized patient, and nowhere more so than for sleep disturbance. Small scale studies have shown the effectiveness of aromatherapy in this situation, and it is to be hoped that their conclusions (and the less unequivocal results of rheumatology trials) will be corroborated by further controlled studies.

Case 14.5   Aromatherapist: Marlene Cadwallader (BAppSciNursing), Australia

I provide care in Heyfield Bush Nursing Hospital, which is a 13 bed rural hospital providing care for the elderly, acute medical paediatric casualty, outpatients clinic, and day surgery neonatal and palliative care. The hospital manageress, staff and doctors accept and support the provision of care using essential oils and massage and Reiki channelling, appreciating the benefits of tactile therapies. Although there is no written policy for the use of essential oils within the hospital, there is often the aroma of lavender, geranium or rosemary wafting from a vaporizer in the secretary/manager's office.

a   One elderly resident always appears sleepy and lethargic. A combination of orange, lemon and lavender in a base oil has helped her immensely and other nursing staff have commented on her increased alertness and sense of humour, showing the effects of the uplifting properties.

b   An elderly male patient aged about 85 years, who had experienced several strokes, was self-caring, possessed a tremendous sense of humour and always had a smile on his face. He loved chatting, but always forgot what he was saying in the middle of a sentence, much to his annoyance. An oil blend of lemon (to uplift his spirits as he tended to fall asleep frequently), lavender and rosemary (to assist his memory) was made up in a carrier of grapeseed oil and calendula oil (to nourish his dry skin). Foot, hand and back massages were given when time permitted—mostly foot massages, which he looked forward to with a cherubic grin. As time progressed, he developed more movement in his legs and feet, permitting increased mobility. His family were amazed at the improvement in his general health.

c   A middle-aged gentleman was admitted with an allergic reaction. Welts and rashes appeared over his body, as well as recurring swelling of his throat and lips. He was most unwell and intramuscular medication was administered on a regular basis to reduce the swelling, with cold packs, showers and calamine being applied externally to relieve the itch. I happened to be working on a night shift when we met, and he said 'this itch is driving me mad'—he was speaking literally. I made up a solution of three drops of lavender, two drops of tea tree and one drop of peppermint, putting one drop into a small bowl of water for sponging off his body. He claimed the solution soothed his body and he certainly appeared more relaxed.

Case 14.6   Aromatherapist: Brenda Weston SPDipA, MISPA, SRN, SCM, UK

Mrs P had suffered a severe stroke the previous September, leaving her left arm completely paralysed and with only partial recovery in her left leg. She had always been a very independent and strong-willed lady, lived alone, and at the age of 89 still ruled her children with a rod of iron. During her hospitalization, Mrs P had taken her disability very badly, resenting the loss of her independence. She became so depressed, almost suicidal, that she required the assistance of a psychiatrist.

On admission to my nursing home, she initially settled very well, enjoying the home's Christmas festivities, outings at the local church and day centres, and days out with her family. Then, during January, she became very unsettled and unhappy, realizing she was never going to go back to her own flat. She became very angry with her family for forcing her into this decision, and for selling her flat and belongings. She became determined to leave us, and actually wandered off, twice falling badly. This resulted in two periods of hospitalization for a fractured pelvis and femur.

The psychiatrist periodically reviewed Mrs P's case and changed the medication to sedate her and to relieve her depression. Mrs P became very apathetic,

and due to the effects of the medication slept 20 hours out of 24, resulting in dehydration, loss of weight, anorexia and incontinence. I could not bear to watch Mrs P's condition deteriorate and decided to 'interfere'. My care plan involved daily massage of hands, legs and face with melissa (an antidepressant), lavender and geranium. These were blended in a base of grapeseed oil with 25% hypericum (a restorative to the nervous system). The same mixture of essential oils was used in Mrs P's bath, and periodically placed on her bed linen prior to her returning from the bath.

Prior to starting this treatment, Mrs P's mood and behaviour was monitored for 7 days, using the Beck inventory for measuring depression, to see whether there was any pattern to her distress and mood. It was noted that she appeared worse in the late mornings and in the evenings before bed. Treatments were therefore given mid-morning and at bedtime.

After 4 weeks Mrs P was more content and alert, her medication had been reduced, and she was eating and drinking well, gaining weight in the process. She has even begun to take outings with her family again and is more positive about the future, planning to enjoy life as best she can.

REFERENCES

Boyd E M, Pearson G L 1946 The expectorant action of volatile oils. American Journal of Medical Science 211: 602–610

Brett H 1997 Alzheimer's disease. Aromatherapy World Winter: 31–33

Buckle J 1992 Which lavender oil? Nursing Times 88(22) (August 5): 54–55

Byass R 1988 Soothing body and soul. Nursing Times 84(24): 39–41

Cannard G 1994 On the scent of a good night's sleep. Trial project. Midland Health Board News January: 3

Cawthorne A 1991 Aromatherapy on trial. Aromanews 30: 7–8

Fowler P, Wall M 1997 COSHH and CHIPS: ensuring the safety of aromatherapy. Complementary Therapies in Medicine 5: 112–115

Franchomme P, Pénoël D 1990 L'aromathérapie exactement. Jollois, Limoges

Hardy M 1991 Sweet scented dreams. International Journal of Aromatherapy 3(2): 12–13

Horrigan C 1995 In: Rankin-Box D (ed) The nurse's handbook. Churchill Livingstone, Edinburgh

Hudson R 1996 The value of lavender for rest and activity in the elderly patient. Complementary Therapies in Medicine 4: 52–57

Le Roux A A, Lyne P A 1989 Firm foundations: applying the results of research based on the clinical trial design to nursing practice. RCN Research Society Conference, Cardiff. RCN, London

McCann K, McKenna H 1993 An examination of touch between nurses and elderly patients in a continuing care setting in Northern Ireland. Journal of Advanced Nursing 18: 838–846

Macdonald E M L 1995 Aromatherapy for the enhancement of the nursing care of elderly people suffering from arthritic pain. The Aromatherapist 2(1): 26–31

Macdonald K 1993 Orange blossom cure for heart patients. Daily Mail March 16

Passant H 1990 A holistic approach in the ward. Nursing Times 86(4) (January 24): 26–28

Price S 1992 Arthritis and rheumatism. Yoga and Health, February: 37–38

Price S 1993 The aromatherapy workbook. Thorsons, London

Reynolds J E F 1993 Martindale: the extra pharmacopoeia. Pharmaceutical Press, London

Roulier G 1990 Les huiles essentielles pour votre santé. Dangles, St-Jean-de-Braye

Sassard P 1932 Essai de synthèse sur les propriétés et applications thérapeutiques du Sapolinol. Bulletin Medical. Février: 32

Scott J, Huskisson E C 1976 Graphic representation of pain. Pain 2: 175–184

Storrs A M F 1980 Geriatric nursing. Baillière Tindall, London

Tattam A 1992 The gentle touch. Nursing Times 88(32): 16–17

Valnet J 1980 The practice of aromatherapy. Daniel, Saffron Walden

Van Toller and Dodd 1991 Perfumery. Chapman & Hall, London

Wingate P, Wingate R 1988 Penguin medical encyclopedia. Penguin, London

Wise R 1989 Flower power. Nursing Times 85(22) (May 31): 45–47

15 Palliative and terminal care

Introduction

Complementary therapies have become increasingly popular since the mid 1980s, with a growing number of the general public and the nursing profession becoming aware of alternative and complementary methods which can be beneficial to the patient in palliative or terminal care. With the help of aromatherapy, hundreds of people faced with possible terminal illness have enjoyed a quality of life better than they might otherwise have experienced.

INTRODUCTION OF AROMATHERAPY INTO TRADITIONAL SETTINGS

Although palliative care may involve care of the terminally ill, it is not quite the same as terminal care. 'Palliative means caring for someone who may not get better, but who is nevertheless not at death's door, and may live for many years.' (Buckle 1997 p. 227). It is that which alleviates pain and gives temporary relief, and is often needed for people with chronic though not necessarily life-threatening problems.

Many people needing palliative or terminal care are looked after in their homes through the informal carer network, and a great number are cared for in hospices. Hospices were the first health care establishments in Britain to welcome aromatherapy as a possible mode of relief to their patients. When the therapy was relatively unknown, aromatherapists found hospices to be the easiest point of entry for the introduction of the use of essential oils into an NHS situation.

This may have been because hospices often have good resources of time and money (many being funded by charities), although most of the therapists offered their services voluntarily. It may also have been because those in charge (who had no first hand knowledge of the efficacy of massage or the use of essential oils) felt that at least it could do no harm!

The help aromatherapy can offer in this field has been warmly received and much appreciated by both patients and staff. It has helped staff on oncology units and in hospices to provide the enhanced quality of care they seek to give their patients. In many ways it has also been the way of entry into wider acceptance in the Health Service as a whole.

(Lundie 1994)

With both palliative and terminal care, one of the primary aims is to bring about an improvement in the quality of life of the patient, and essential oils have been found to be capable of this, by relieving stress, raising the spirits, strengthening and revitalizing the mind and providing comfort to the body by easing some of the distressing effects of the illness. In fact, the Director of Nursing Services at Compton Hospice stated that 'we often wonder how we coped without the aid of aromatherapy' (Kensey personal communication 1986).

In achieving this aim there is no doubt that the relief of stress is beneficial, not only for the patients themselves, but also for the relatives and loved ones who can only watch and support. The use of essential oils by an aromatologist or aromatherapist can improve the outlook and mood of patient and relatives alike. Moreover, the nurses and carers can also benefit, for they too are under a certain amount of stress owing to working continually among those who may not have long to live, and having to cope with the inevitable fears, anxieties and questions of both patients and visitors.

Selecting the most effective essential oils

An important consideration when selecting essential oils holistically is that the patient should like the aroma. Always let him or her smell a mix before using it, adjusting the aroma if

necessary with an extra drop of one of the prescribed (or other) essential oils. The psychological effect of a welcomed aroma can do much to begin the healing process.

Stress

Many essential oils have the ability to relieve stress (see Ch. 12). The most popular one used by nurses in the last few years has been lavender, almost to the exclusion of others. No doubt this is on account of its pleasant aroma, long list of therapeutic effects, known low toxicity (except *Lavandula stoechas*, which is high in ketones) and reasonable cost. There have been a few studies carried out on the stress-relieving effects of lavender, but the specific variety of lavender used is not usually given—it may not even have been known (see Ch. 1 under Clones of lavender and lavandin). Other essential oils with a wide range of therapeutic effects are being introduced more and more, sometimes in synergy with lavender, and include oils such as:

- *Chamaemelum nobile* [ROMAN CHAMOMILE]
- *Citrus limon* (per.) [LEMON]
- *Origanum majorana* [SWEET MARJORAM]
- *Pelargonium graveolens* [GERANIUM].

Stress may have different consequences for different people and when determining which essential oil(s) to use for stress the consequential symptoms presented (e.g. insomnia, constipation) must also be borne in mind (see Ch. 12).

Stress and insomnia

- *C. nobile* (also helpful in cases of nervous shock)
- *Cananga odorata* [YLANG YLANG]
- *Citrus reticulata* (per.) [MANDARIN]
- *Lavandula angustifolia*, syn. *L. officinalis*, *L. vera* [LAVENDER]
- *O. majorana*.

The use of more than one of these essential oils will increase the synergy. Experience shows that the effect of two (or three) oils blended together is usually greater than that of one used alone (see Ch. 3).

Depression

The depressed state of mind, particularly that of a terminally ill person, may have a more detrimental effect on the body than stress, and more appropriate oils to use under these circumstances would be:

- *Ocimum basilicum* var. *album* [EUROPEAN BASIL].
- *Thymus vulgaris* [THYME], preferably one of the sweet (alcohol) chemotypes. The geraniol chemotype has a particularly gentle aroma, which may be more acceptable to the patient than the harsher phenolic chemotypes. A sweet thyme would blend well with *Citrus bergamia* [BERGAMOT], which is also an uplifting essential oil.
- *Citrus aurantium* var. *amara* (flos) [NEROLI BIGARADE], a nerve tonic and antidepressant (Franchomme & Pénoël 1990 p. 338) is a useful essential oil to include in the mix and significantly improves the aroma, especially if one of the phenolic thymes is being used.

Depression and the immune system

It is believed that the use of certain oils may strengthen the body's resistance to secondary infection. This is an important consideration for those living with HIV-related immunodeficiency, and something for which allopathic medicine has no answer as yet (see immune system list on p. 356 in Appendix B.9). Essential oils which may be effective for both depression and lowered immunity are:

- *Boswellia carteri* [FRANKINCENSE], an uplifting essential oil which helps to strengthen the immune system. It also relieves arthritic pain and inflammation.
- *C. bergamia* [BERGAMOT], which will recharge the central nervous system with energy (Roulier 1990 p. 243), therefore indirectly helping to strengthen the immune system. It is also a good digestive oil.
- *Melaleuca viridiflora* [NIAOULI], which is uplifting and an immunostimulant as well as being radioprotective (Roulier 1990 p. 288).

Chapter 5 gives methods of use and percentages of essential oils to be used, though these are best used at half the normal strength on very sick people.

The few examples above should give some indication of how to select essential oils. Always make the first selection according to the emotional state of the patient concerned. From this, two or three oils may then be selected for the more specific symptoms portrayed. This synergistic selection will then have positive effects on the whole person—i.e. the choice is holistic.

Imagery and positivity

Some patients who already know a little about complementary therapies and who have not reached the final stages of their illness (and those who can take on—with help—some responsibility for their own health) may be able to apply some of the principles of visualization and the ability of the body to heal itself through positive thoughts, helped by determination, a caring therapist and supportive relatives.

The success of a positive attitude and visualization has been observed by many nurses and aromatherapists working with different complementary therapies on patients living with cancer and HIV-related immunodeficiency. A change of attitude is naturally easier for someone in the earlier stages of a disease to accomplish, when they can learn about improved diet, positivity, reflex therapy, massage and aromatherapy before the disease has got too firm a hold (Machin 1989). Laughter therapy is also an excellent aid to health recovery, as Norman Cousins found when he was unable to find pain relief through drugs (Cousins 1979).

The use of touch and massage

Aromatherapy with massage is particularly suited to those in palliative care and the terminally ill, who have a profound need for the caring and loving touch of gentle hands. Massage conveys warmth, comfort, pleasure and safety (McNamara 1993 p. 13). For these people, the use of essential oils to enhance the massage can relieve some of the anxiety in a caring way and perhaps bring about deeper, more relaxed sleep. Such treatment inspires patients (when asked to describe their reactions to their aromatherapy treatment) to utter words such as 'remarkable', 'marvellous', 'cheering', 'soothing', 'reassuring', 'comforting', etc. (Phillips 1989). As a general rule, these reactions are heard after the use of essential oils together with massage—but comfort, touch and massage *without* essential oils would also result in the expression of similar comments.

A trial carried out to assess the value of massage for patients with breast cancer showed an improvement in concentration and lessening of fatigue and stress, as well as generally feeling better, compared with a control group (Sims 1986). The most recent study into the benefits of aromatherapy massage in palliative and terminal care was undertaken by the Centre for the Study of Complementary Medicine at Countess Mountbatten House (Evans 1995). The study ran for a period of 6 months, 1 day a week, 4 hours per session. The oils chosen depended on the presenting symptoms and were diluted to half the strength normally used. The oils most frequently used had balancing, soothing and calming properties (see Table 15.1). Sixty-nine patients received massage and completed a questionnaire. Although there was a difficulty in providing substantial data from this study, it achieved an 80% success rate in that almost all the patients treated derived benefit in some way. Of those, all

were specific about the areas in which they gained the benefit or relief. It could be debated, however, whether the benefit was derived from:

1. the patient being given individual attention for a period of time
2. someone talking to the person
3. use of touch and massage
4. use of essential oils.

A more fully controlled study would need to be carried out to distinguish between these possibilities.

Although massage is much used in aromatherapy treatments, the use of essential oils in appropriate healthcare situations can (and should) be extended wherever possible to include other equally beneficial methods such as inhalation and compresses (see Ch. 5).

With bedridden patients a full massage is not always possible or necessary to bring about the desired improvement. The outcome of a specific-area massage (e.g. the feet) *with* essential oils may almost be compared to that of a full-body massage *without* them, and takes much less time out of a busy nursing schedule. Any massage done should be modified to suit the needs of each individual patient, taking into account the stage of development of their illness and, in the case of people with cancer, whether or not they are receiving radiation treatment.

Table 15.1 Oils commonly used in palliative care				
Diagnosis	Age Male (M) Female (F)	Reason for referral	Site of massage	Oils used
Ca breast	F-69	Bereavement, low mood	Face, hands/arms	Marjoram/lavender/rose
Ca lung	F-52	Relaxation	Hands/arms, legs	Eucalyptus/lavender
Oesophagus	M-55	Back pain	Back/hips	Lavender/marjoram
Ca ovary	F-50	Anxiety	Hands/arms/feet	Geranium
Ca stomach	M-57	Relaxation	Face/hands/arms, legs/feet	Camomile/lavender
Ca breast	F-37	Relaxation	Face/hands/arms, back/buttocks	Camomile/lavender/neroli

From Evans 1995.

The essential oils and/or the massage may bring hidden emotions to the surface, even tears. Carers should be aware of and prepared for this possibility and be confident that they can handle it successfully, using any counselling skills they may have or referring the patient on if they feel they cannot deal with the situation themselves.

Terminally ill patients need strong support to be able to cope with the reality (and sometimes the apparent injustice) of their illness. When it comes to understanding and soothing their fears and alleviating their mental suffering, essential oils too can play an important part. Examples of oils said to relieve fear and despair are as follows:

- *Boswellia carteri* [FRANKINCENSE]
- *Citrus reticulata* (per.) [MANDARIN]
- *Citrus aurantium* var. *amara* (fol.) [NEROLI]
- *Cananga odorata* [YLANG YLANG].

Nurses who can carry out only a simple treatment with essential oils still have an effective tool at their disposal, which has already achieved a measure of success. Cadwallader (1993 personal communication) finds working with selected essential oils in appropriate ways to be very valuable with terminally ill patients and their families; it especially assists with coping abilities and allaying the distress and anxiety associated with dying.

CANCER

Cancer has been recorded since Egyptian times, and treatment for cancer using aromatic plants was mentioned 2000 years ago by Dioscorides in his Materia medica (Elliott 1991). Cancer is widespread today, and although more than 200 different types have been diagnosed the reasons for its development and spread are unknown (McNamara 1993). This is in spite of great advances in the treatment of many types of cancer, and extensive research worldwide.

Fear of being diagnosed as having cancer is one of the great stresses in the lives of those who have already lost one of their family through this disease, and those with no family history of cancer can suffer shock, confusion and fear after diagnosis. Statistics show that one in four people will develop cancer at some stage, which unfortunately increases any anxiety already experienced regarding the disease.

A change in health status will result in emotional conflict which may be expressed as psychosomatic-related symptoms which may increase distress. A person's loss of control over his or her emotions may worsen feelings of hopelessness and helplessness and inhibit normal coping strategies which motivate moves towards recovery.

(Crowther 1991)

Suggestions for treatment

There are no precise guidelines on the employment of aromatherapy for cancer, and normally no specific oils are used by therapists, because they are generally selected by taking a holistic view of each patient. Dr Valnet, considered to be an authority on the subject of aromatherapy, gives a selection of essential oils for the prevention and treatment of cancer. The oils he cites are as follows (Valnet 1980):

- *Syzygium aromaticum* (flos) [CLOVE BUD]
- *Cupressus sempervirens* [CYPRESS]
- *Pelargonium graveolens* [GERANIUM]
- *Hyssopus officinalis* [HYSSOP]
- *Salvia officinalis* [SAGE]
- *Artemisia dracunculus* [TARRAGON].

He also cites the essential oils of garlic and onion, but these are not generally used in aromatherapy because of the impossibly strong odour. Aromatherapists today may be wary of using the essential oils of *H. officinalis*, *S. officinalis* and *A. dracunculus*. The first two contain neurotoxic constituents and are contraindicated in pregnancy; the third has a high content of methyl chavicol, although one source states that no contraindications to the essential oil are known (Franchomme & Pénoël 1990 p. 326). In the appropriately controlled dosage (usually very low in aromatherapy—especially on the extremely ill) these oils may in future come to be accepted as useful in the treatment of cancer, when our knowledge is more advanced than it is at the moment. Certainly, the fears (after tests on animals) that tarragon and basil might be carcinogenic (because of the similarity of the safrole molecule to that of methyl chavicol) have proved unfounded (Caldwell 1991). Well-trained aromatherapists and aromatologists need have no fears about the safe use of these oils (i.e. in low concentration), with due respect to any contraindications.

As well as Valnet, other writers mention essential oils they believe are effective against cancer:

• Bernadet (1983) recommends the internal use of *C. sempervirens*, *S. aromaticum* and *P. graveolens* for the prevention of cancer. He also states that people with cancer can use plants to act on their general state.
• Gattefossé (1993 pp. 72, 84) cites Professor Cabassè as suggesting that *Boswellia carteri* may be used for the prevention of smoker's cancer, and Sassard as recommending *H. officinalis* (five drops in olive oil) three times daily for cancer of the liver.
• Bardeau (1976) mentions *Citrus limon*, *Commiphora myrrha* [MYRRH], *Lavandula officinalis* and *L. latifolia*, *Melaleuca viridiflora*, *Rosa damascena* and *R. centifolia* [ROSE OTTO] and *Styrax benzoin* [BENZOIN].
• Roulier (1990 p. 230) suggests that certain essential oils can help to improve the immune system and eliminate abnormal cells. He states that they should be determined and used by the aromatherapy practitioner following laboratory tests, and includes *S. aromaticum*, *Lippia citriodora* [TRUE VERBENA], *M. viridiflora* and *Pogostemon patchouli* [PATCHOULI].

Osato (1965) carried out research on people with cancer using the isolates of citral (by injection) and citronellal (by mouth). The results were not conclusive and the percentage of people in remission after 15 years was 5%. It may be that the whole essential oils rich in citrals (neral and geranial), such as *Cymbopogon flexuosus* [LEMONGRASS], *Aloysia triphylla* [LEMON VERBENA] and *Melissa officinalis* [TRUE MELISSA], could be added to the list of possible oils to try.

Some patients with cancer can acquire a deficiency in the immune system, especially those on chemotherapy or undergoing radiation. For these people, essential oils which are believed to strengthen the immune system, such as *B. carteri* cited previously (Franchomme and Pénoël 1990

p. 328), *M. viridiflora* and *S. aromaticum* (flos) (Roulier 1990 p. 230), may be useful. (See also p. 242 and Appendix B.9.)

Regarding the use of essential oils, Franchomme & Pénoël (1990 p. 88) say that it is not a question of aiming at using them to break down a malignant tumour. Nevertheless, the antitumoral properties of certain sesquiterpenic lactones, sesquiterpenic ketones and benzaldehyde (as well as the antiviral properties of certain ketones) can be useful, in expert hands, to assist the prevention of certain degenerative states.

Benefits

Patients vary in their aromatherapy needs and each of the following must be considered for each person requiring treatment:

• amount of pain suffered
• site and extent of any tumours
• tenderness of specific areas
• frequency of radiotherapy, if being treated
• rate of the circulation
• ability to sleep
• condition of the skin
• medication taken
• whether or not the person is on chemotherapy
• state of the person's morale, etc.

Those who elect to receive aromatherapy treatment may benefit in one or more of the following ways:

• a reduction in anxiety, stress and tension (which in turn helps to reduce high blood pressure), fear (which keeps the body in a permanently tense condition) or shock
• a feeling of well-being, which counteracts an inability to cope, strengthening self-belief
• relief of constipation, headaches, muscular pain and insomnia, resulting in an improvement in the quality of life, often followed by a reduction in medication for these secondary problems
• elevation of the pain threshold level (Barker 1993), sometimes enabling a reduction in analgesics
• improvement in the circulation of both blood and lymph, helping to eliminate unwanted toxins more efficiently

- stimulation of the immune system. 'There is ample evidence of the overall increase in immune functioning when relaxation is achieved by soft tissue massage' (Chaitow 1987), which is believed to be enhanced by the appropriate essential oils.

Safety

There are differences in opinion over whether or not full-body massage in the early and middle stages of cancer should be carried out. However, in all cases where full-body massage has been used during these stages, with or without essential oils, only beneficial results have been obtained. There is abundant empirical evidence from the many aromatherapists presently working with patients living with cancer, and there is certainly no evidence after many years of aromatherapy use to substantiate the theories of opponents. Most doctors agree that, although massage with essential oils cannot cure cancer, its advantages outweigh any risks (see also p. 125).

The aromatherapist's first concern is to treat the *person*, not the disease, and a person receiving radiation treatment or chemotherapy certainly needs help to cope during this stressful time.

Case 15.1   Aromatherapist: Jeannie Maher, Australia

a   This lady in her 50s had had a brain tumour removed—she still had a malignant tumour level 4 which was growing deep into the middle of the brain. She had received 6 weeks of radium treatment and was on a lot of medication. On first seeing her, she was partly paralyzed down the left side and was using a walking frame. Circulation and lymph were poor, broken sleep pattern due to arm and leg twitches, general health not good, having seizures at least once a week increasing as time went on. She became dehydrated easily and had a very itchy scalp where her hair was growing back and the skin was very dry.

She was having physiotherapy treatments up to 3 times a week, which she found made her very tired, so they cut them back to once or twice a week. These were concentrated on exercising the partly paralyzed limbs. She was a healthy hard-working lady. The first symptoms of her disorder were loss of balance and migraines which she did not normally suffer. On visiting the doctor, he immediately did tests and referred her to a neurosurgeon. They operated—this was not only a shock to herself but also to her family. Her daughter contacted me a few months after her mother's operation, having heard of aromatherapy in England.

Treatments were given weekly, then twice-weekly, using a base which included 5% avocado and 5% calendula to help her dry skin, with lavender essential oil (central nervous system, sedative, antiseptic, bactericidal and balancing). She was more relaxed afterwards and it helped to give her a better quality of sleep as the treatments stopped the nervous twitching of her arm and leg. On different occasions I would alternate essential oils, sometimes using mandarin for its balancing and uplifting effects, and sedative effect on the nervous system.

Her general condition was becoming worse and it was decided that aromatherapy and physiotherapy treatments should cease for a period of 1 month. At this time they also found the tumour had spread and seizures were becoming more frequent. The doctors suggested she recommence aromatherapy treatments because she had commented that they assisted in her feeling of well-being. Also, it had been found that during the course of my treatments the seizures had been of shorter duration and less violent; the treatments had also relieved some of the pain.

b   This elderly lady had lost her first husband and her son became a paraplegic at the age of 17 after being in an accident. She had remarried a few years ago. In 1977 she was diagnosed with diabetes and in December 1992 was discovered to have cancer. The scan showed a large mass in the head of the pancreas obstructing the common bile duct.

I was asked to do a treatment just before Christmas when the cancer was in the final stages. She had been given only a few weeks to live. Circulation was poor, skin dry and she was having trouble swallowing. The nail of her big toe had infection around it. For this treatment I mixed one drop each of frankincense and lavender in a base of almond oil and applied tea tree to the infected toe. I massaged mainly her feet, lower legs and hands, and the neck and shoulders to help with the swallowing. It was around lunchtime when I was there during the treatment—her husband and son were having a prawn sandwich. One of her greatest desires was to be able to eat a prawn sandwich—she had been eating mainly liquid foods.

Her desire was fulfilled as she got to eat and swallow her prawn sandwich following the treatment, as it relaxed the muscles with the massage. She found this very special as she had thought that would never be possible. She passed away several days later.

One of the problems we have had in offering aromatherapy here at the Neil Cliffe Cancer Care Centre is that of demand from the clients compared with the time therapists have available, so we devised a way of offering aromatherapy to many clients within these time constraints, while maintaining high standards.

Our aims for using aromatherapy are to enhance the relaxation process and promote a sense of well-being. We offer hand or foot massage, and feel that the one-to-one contact of patient and therapist is intrinsic to the therapeutic process. Relaxation is taught in a group room, with up to eight clients, and takes about 30 minutes. Aromatherapy massage is then offered on an individual basis, which takes about 15 minutes each person. There are usually three aromatherapists and an appointment system is organized so that everyone has a treatment.

Essential oils are selected and blended with a carrier oil by a qualified member of staff—a nurse or occupational therapist with qualifications in aromatherapy and/or massage. Lavender is used the most because of its safe reputation, its relaxing qualities and its appeal to clients, who actually ask for it. Peppermint is used occasionally because of its antispasmodic action on the digestive system, easing nausea and vomiting. Bergamot and geranium are occasionally used for their uplifting qualities.

a A gentleman with cancer of the colon, with recurrent disease and also a colostomy. In an attempt to control symptoms of nausea, antiemetic drugs were given via syringe driver. However, the problem persisted. He agreed to attend the centre for relaxation and aromatherapy. We decided to use

Mentha × *piperita* to settle his stomach and apply this by a hand massage. The next week he reported that the feelings of nausea were eased on the evening of the treatment, and requested it again.

He attended on a weekly basis and always requested peppermint as he felt he was benefiting from it. The one-to-one attention gave him the opportunity to discuss his frustrations in no longer being able to follow his interests, and the opportunity to replace these by joining in other activities at the centre—which he did!

b An elderly lady with a diagnosis of head and neck tumour. Unfortunately, side-effects of the treatment caused a degree of deafness and she was also partially sighted. She chose to have a hand massage with oil of *Lavandula angustifolia*. The aim of this treatment was to stimulate her sense of smell as her other senses were depleted. The one-to-one contact allowed her to discuss her own agenda; she used the time well knowing she had the therapist's individual attention. She said she felt more relaxed and comforted at the end of the massage. She looked happy and cheerful, as if she had had a special treatment.

Evaluation
The way in which we offer aromatherapy massage could be classed as therapeutic massage with essential oils, rather than aromatherapy. This description better reflects the fact that presently we cannot undertake pre-treatment individual assessment or use specific oils to treat specific symptoms. However, the current system enables us to ensure that many people benefit from a therapeutic massage with essential oils.

Chemotherapy

The use of essential oils with massage alongside chemotherapy treatment is an area of uncertainty. As massage helps to release and eliminate toxic waste, it could be assumed that, provided the massage given is of the right type, pressure and location, it would be beneficial. For people undergoing chemotherapy, it may be preferable to administer only specific-area massage. This releases fewer toxins into the bloodstream at a time and at a slower rate—an important factor, as even people without cancer and on high medication may feel unwell for up to 48 hours after a full aromatherapy massage. A full-body massage is therefore recommended for people on chemotherapy only if it is extremely gentle and brief.

According to a study carried out on people with Parkinson's disease (Price 1993), patients receiving specific-area application of essential oils (without massage) derived more benefit than did those receiving full-body massage without essential oils.

To the patient receiving chemotherapy, therefore, the benefits of specific-area massage with essential oils should also be no less than those gained by full-body massage, and nothing extra would be achieved by the latter (apart from the patient experiencing a caring touch for a longer period of time). When the toxic residues begin to clear after the course of chemotherapy, the area of the body massaged can be increased, slowly building up to a full-body massage (with the consent of the patient).

When using essential oils with chemotherapy, a low concentration of essential oils in a blend is recommended: about four drops of essential oils in 50 ml carrier oil (or lotion) is enough. Only distilled oils should be used during this time, as solvent-extracted oils (absolutes) with their impurities could produce an adverse reaction, especially on the skin. In all cases it is advisable to carry out a patch test on the client before any massage, because of possible sensitivity of the skin (Horrigan 1991). There seems to be no substantiation for the view that essential oils should not be used at all during chemotherapy treatment, nor in fact before all the residues are cleared from the body, although erring on the side of caution is commendable (McNamara 1993 pp. 46/47).

Radiotherapy

Radiotherapy is another area where people are hesitant to use essential oils. For some years now essential oils have reportedly been used in France for the purpose of mitigating the side-effects of this treatment; the essential oils are used on the area to be irradiated to reduce deep burning and scarring. Pénoël suggests *Melaleuca viridiflora* (Franchomme & Pénoël 1990 p. 282) and Franchomme ascribes this property to most of the *Melaleuca* oils, i.e. *M. alternifolia* [TEA TREE], *M. cajuputi* [CAJUPUT] and *M. viridiflora* ct. cineole (Franchomme & Pénoël 1990 pp. 368–371). This is also mentioned elsewhere.

In cases where radiotherapy is necessary, the skin can be protected by the use of niaouli on the treated areas. This essential oil minimises the severity of burning in the skin. The oil is applied neat, undiluted before the irradiation sessions, and after the session a mixture is applied. This mixture may be either a) *Melaleuca viridiflora* 50% in *Hypericum perforatum* (St John's wort) 50% or b) *Melaleuca viridiflora* 50% in *Rosa rubiginosa* (rosehip) 50%.

(Roulier 1990 p. 230)

It may take some time before this can be accepted in Britain, but many aromatherapists (including ourselves) recommend the application (not massage) of essential oils to people undergoing radiotherapy. The oils can be applied routinely on a daily basis in between radiation treatments (excluding the day of the treatment), with no adverse results. The authors doubt that French doctors would recommend neat or 50% dilution of essential oil if it were to be harmful, and as aromatherapists use only 2–5% any worry of risk is considerably reduced. Massage of any kind, however, is contraindicated.

One of the side effects of radiotherapy is that the skin may become very tender and fragile and massage could cause the skin to break. This is where the application of oils rather than massage is very useful, and is used in France. The diluted essential oils (niaouli and/or tea tree) can also be sprayed onto the irradiated area. Other areas of the body may receive massage (with oil if desired).

(McNamara 1993 p. 48)

One of the authors' clients with breast cancer used a mix of *Lavandula angustifolia*, *Rosa damascena* (distilled) and *Boswellia carteri* (distilled), which was blended for her using the dilution mentioned above in calendula carrier oil. This was not to help prevent scarring (I had no knowledge then of what was happening in France), but to lift the client out of her depression after being told she would need radiation therapy, and to help recover the positive attitude she had had towards her cancer previously. The oil mix was used on her breasts at her own request (and with the permission of her doctor) twice a day in between her radiotherapy sessions, with what she felt were positive results regarding her depression.There were no adverse effects after radiation, and although one case does not constitute conclusive evidence there appears to be no evidence that the use of essential oils on someone receiving radiation treatment may be harmful, especially on parts of the body not being irradiated.

As with most other essential oil treatment, there is only empirical knowledge in this area to date, and very little even of that. In low concentrations, most essential oils can be used beneficially on a person receiving radiation treatment, provided that any contraindications are observed.

Cautious conclusions regarding use of essential oils on cancer patients can therefore be formulated:

• In the case of weak general health, the elderly or advanced cancer, half the normal strength of oil blends should be used (i.e. 30 drops in 100 ml).

• Massage with normal pressure (never heavy) may be used on specific restricted areas—shoulders (except on patients with breast cancer), feet, hands, scalp, face, depending on the individual case.

• Only very gentle massage should be used for a full-body treatment.

• Permission must be sought from the doctor in charge to use essential oils on a person with cancer.

• Massage should not be given on an area receiving radiotherapy.

• For a person receiving chemotherapy, specific-area or full-body massage may be given, bearing in mind the precautions indicated by the type and site of the cancer; the massage blend should be at quarter normal strength.

• Any suspected cancerous site should be avoided; Swiss reflex therapy (see Ch. 7) should be used instead.

Complementary approaches

One organization dedicated to helping people with cancer is Wirral Holistic Care Services, which carried out a study on cancer and complementary therapies between 1984 and 1987. The aim was to identify the specific needs of people with cancer and to emphasize the need for patients to take control of their treatment back into their own hands. The study used a basic question-and-answer format with time evaluation tools and self-selected participants came via local cancer self-help groups or direct contact with the researchers (Crowther 1991). The average time spent in questioning was 1 hour, depending on the identified needs of each person, which included the following, in order of importance:

• emotional support
• counselling
• education on self-care
• dietary advice
• education on the disease

Case 15.3 Therapist: Lai Fong Cox, Hong Kong

A patient who had been admitted with a suspected bowel obstruction was vomiting heavily, producing nearly 3 litres a day. He had had a laparotomy and was found to have bowel cancer, which necessitated a further operation. The operation itself had no complications and the patient recovered.

By the 3rd or 4th day postoperation, the patient started having diarrhoea, producing 3 litres a day. To begin with, the doctors thought that this was due to the patient fasting for some time and having intravenous fluid. The patient was therefore started on a liquid diet, gradually progressing to a soft diet. The patient tolerated the diet plan very well for 4 days, with no complaints of nausea or vomiting, but the diarrhoea did not subside, and he continued passing 3 litres of faecal fluid every day. Following this, the doctors changed the diet back to intravenous infusion and the patient was given total parenteral nutrition (TPN) in order to give his bowels a rest and cease the diarrhoea. The TPN feed was carried out for another 3 days with no improvement in the patient's frequent diarrhoea and he was put back on a normal diet. By then it was more than 10 days since his operation.

I asked the primary nurse to let me try aromatherapy with him. The request was granted and I also received permission from the patient and his wife. Due to the surgical operation, I could not perform any type of body massage so I carried out Swiss reflex therapy. I prepared the reflex massage cream, adding eucalyptus, lavender and chamomile. These three essential oils are able to ease diarrhoea and relax the nerves. After the first session the patient said that he had a good sleep and after six daily sessions said that he had not felt so well for a long time.

The amount of faecal fluid gradually reduced from day to day until the 6th day, when it was down to 900 ml. The primary nurse, patient and I were very pleased with the result.

I then had a change of duty rota and a week later, when I went back to work, I was disappointed that the patient's diarrhoea had returned to 3 litres a day. I started the therapy again and managed to do three daily sessions, during which time some improvement was evident to the primary nurse. Unfortunately, she could not convince the doctors of this and the patient was discharged. I could not help him further owing to the distance, though I was told the he was looking for further complementary therapy to help with his cancer. About 9 months later, he was readmitted and died soon after.

Case 15.4   Aromatherapist: Marlene Cadwallader (BAppSciNursing), Australia

a   A 60-year-old male had a pancreatic cancer. His pain was managed with analgesia and nausea treated by Maxolon; 9 litres of fluid had been withdrawn from his abdomen (paracentesis).

I used a blend of chamomile (which is calming and antinausea), lavender (also with a calming, all-round effect) and geranium (which is balancing, correction of fluid retention).

I noted that the next paracentesis produced a much smaller volume of fluid—2 litres or less. He looked forward to his massages over a period of a couple of months. In that time he was able to eat a light diet, relax to music and come to terms with his coming death.

Lavender was altered to neroli when signs of distress were showing. This provided a calming and peaceful effect, which was useful for the family when provided with a drop on a tissue. A tissue with neroli was also placed on to shelves and drawers and one was placed inside the sphygmomanometer situated at the head of the bed. The family were at ease, feeling that the oils, massage and Reiki made the transition easier.

It was also noticed that the nursing staff were much happier and cheerier amongst themselves. Was it the neroli?

b   Patient B, a 61-year-old male who was battling severe pain from cancer of the lung, was slowly coming to terms with the fact that his life would not be prolonged. I worked closely with him and his family in the hospital setting. His feeling of relaxation and peace was evident as he would say 'I feel really good', and he claimed he also slept well for a couple of nights after a treatment.

The essential oils I used to assist comfort were frankincense, chamomile and rose as a pure oil blend for placing on the soles of his feet and to inhale. The same mix was used in a reflex base cream mix for hand, foot and back massages.

The monoterpenes and esters in rose oil are balancing and calming, the sesquiterpenes and aldehydes in the chamomile easing anxiety, tension, anger and fear, calming the mind and providing peace. The sesquiterpenes, terpenes and alcohol in frankincense would be sedative and analgesic, creating a balance by soothing the mind, providing a feeling of calm, allaying fear and anxiety. It is possible that frankincense may have been helpful in easing his shortness of breath (Sellar 1992).

His wife carried a tissue on which was a drop of rose—she claimed it helped her accept the inevitable. To help with the bereavement I provided a mix of one drop melissa, three drops marjoram and one drop rose blended in 8 ml of carrier oil, which was used by the family as a self-massage around the neck and shoulders

Marjoram was chosen as it contains terpenes, alcohols, ketones and sesquiterpenes, providing an analgesic and calming effect, relieving anxiety, strengthening the mind to confront situations. It seemed to be very helpful in providing a comfort in grief.

Melissa, with its alcohols, esters, aldehydes and a high percentage of monoterpenes, has a calming and 'pick-me-up' effect on the emotions. It is good for shock, panic and hysteria, helping the bereaved to face situations of loss and promoting positivity. Rose oil was chosen for the reason stated above; it was generally felt that the oils were effective in providing peace and acceptance.

- education on the treatment modalities and complications and/or side-effects
- information on complementary therapy (seen as non-invasive)
- information on alternative therapy (may be invasive).

The Bristol Cancer Help Centre, set up in 1980, also gives help and encouragement to many sufferers of the disease. Despite criticism from time to time, a tremendous amount of comfort, hope and relief from pain has been given by the centre over the years. There have been positive improvements in health in a number of patients, including some unusual remissions. As Burke & Sikora (1992) point out, 'If complementary and orthodox cancer care can be provided together, it is possible that the consequent benefits would be greater than the sum of the two'. The vast majority of patients in hospices suffer from cancer, though there is a steady increase in the number of patients with HIV-related illness being admitted. Jill Baxter was possibly the first person to work with essential oils on the terminally ill, offering her services voluntarily. R. Kensey, Director of Nursing Services at the Compton Hospice in Wolverhampton, wrote to the authors' college (where Baxter trained) about the benefits her patients received from aromatherapy:

The fact that someone cares helps patients and relatives alike to learn to accept their illness. Feelings of isolation, loneliness, depression and fear are reduced through the relaxation afforded by the gentle massage with essential oils. Pain in the bone and muscles is also relieved and we have found that movement of the limbs is easier after a treatment. Jill has certainly made a difference to our hospice.

(Kensey 1986 personal communication)

HIV/AIDS

Since its appearance in the 1980s the human immunodeficiency virus (HIV), which causes a defect in the human immune system, has spread at an alarming rate, ruthlessly attacking even infants and the unborn (who may contract the disease in the womb or from breastfeeding). At the 9th International Conference on AIDS in Berlin in June 1993 it was revealed that one million babies had been infected by then. Two real needs were identified:

- to develop a vaccine that is effective and available to all
- to develop effective barrier methods under the control of women, for example a vaginal viricide (International Conference on AIDS 1993).

Conventional drugs have so far been generally unsatisfactory against viruses and, although several essential oils are effective on some of them, no research has yet been carried out regarding their effect on HIV in particular (see Ch. 4). None are claimed by aromatherapists to treat the infection itself; nevertheless, aromatherapy can do much to improve the quality of life, as it can for people living with cancer, and several essential oils have been found to boost the immune system (see below).

Maintaining the immune system must be of paramount importance, and therapies aimed at re-establishing the unique functional integrity of the total human being should be used. Certain essential oils … are powerful in supporting the immune system, … particularly so if used early in the treatment. This in itself could turn the tide and tip the balance between maintaining well-being or developing the opportunist infections that lead to full blown AIDS.

(Burnett 1992)

A study of the chemistry of individual essential oils is a great help in making the choice of what to use on people with HIV, because the effects of certain chemical constituents have been researched. As with cancer patients, a holistic choice of essential oils should be made, starting in this case with those which may stimulate the immune system into action, then selecting from these the essential oils which could have a beneficial effect on other prevailing symptoms.

Immunostimulants

Essential oils which may benefit the immune system include:

- *Boswellia carteri* (Franchomme & Pénoël 1990 p. 328)
- *Syzygium aromaticum* (flos) (Roulier 1990 p. 230)
- *Inula graveolens* [INULA] (Roulier 1990 p. 230)
- *Melaleuca alternifolia* (Franchomme & Pénoël 1990 p. 369)
- *Melaleuca viridiflora* (Roulier 1990 p. 230)
- *Pogostemon patchouli* (Roulier 1990 p. 230)
- *Thymus vulgaris* (thymol, linalool and geraniol

Case 15.5 Aromatologist: Alan Barker, UK

This is a difficult case to relate but the basic problem is that A is in the last stages of full-blown AIDS. He cannot cope with baths or massage owing to the onset of Kaposi's sarcoma. Added to this there is evidence of infiltration of the nervous system, due to the virus, which has at this point become phagocytosed by the macrophages allowing these cells to cross the normally impervious blood–brain barrier.

The options open to the team are very limited, but not beyond helping. There needed to be a way to get the oils into the lymphatic system in order to stimulate the growth of T-helper cells and white blood cells. We devised an effective way of applying the oils by introducing them in a lotion carrier and applying this to the main lymph nodes, i.e. the armpits, thorax and groin area. The method in which the essential oils are applied may seem unorthodox, but it was necessary to adapt to the needs of the client. It is only by taking these unprecedented steps that we may be able to connect with this new challenge in healthcare and aromatherapy. The oils we are using are 10 drops each of *Citrus limon* (per.), *Thymus vulgaris* ct. alcohol and *Melaleuca alternifolia* in 30 ml carrier lotion. The lotion, applied in a thick smear, is easily absorbed into the skin and lymph node area without too much effort on the part of the client or therapist.

At the time of writing, A is stable and very well able to cope with the applications, and his T-helper cell count is rising.

chemotypes). Franchomme & Pénoël (1990) give the thujanol chemotype, but this is very difficult to cultivate from cuttings (Lamy 1989).

Should any oil not on this list be thought to be holistically helpful for the patient, it should be added, to increase the synergistic effects.

Psychological factors

The factors of stress and depression need also to be considered in oil selection and *Thymus vulgaris* (particularly the geraniol and linalool chemotypes) is known to stimulate the immune system as well as uplift the nervous system (Franchomme & Pénoël 1990). In spite of the lack of research studies on essential oil activity against the HIV virus, there is empirical evidence from many aromatherapists and aromatologists who have had encouraging results using widely differing oils—due to the nature of holistic selection for each individual.

The psychological state of the client's carers is important too. Alan Barker (1994 personal communication) has this to say:

It is vital that we care for the carers—their 'burn out' can break a vital link in the chain of care, and to show the partners and the carers how to administer a simple massage or application of an essential oil prescription is a wonderful way of creating a bond or link with care. All too often the partners of patients feel left out and this is a great opportunity for them to be again a part of this person's life/death.

ARC symptoms

Symptoms which present themselves as a result of the progression of the virus (known as the AIDS-related complex or ARC) are such things as infected and swollen glands, recurrent fevers, sore throat (caused by the presence of an additional virus, herpes or candida), coughing (sometimes with sputum) and severe shortness of breath (Barker 1993).

An area not often considered in connection with the HIV virus is the skin, which is very often badly affected by seborrhoeic dermatitis, atopic dermatitis, psoriasis, Kaposi's sarcoma and drug-induced eruptions (Burnett 1992). Carrier oils such as calendula, rosehip and hypericum have a beneficial effect on the skin, and should be used in conjunction with essential oils known for their

---

Case 15.6   Aromatologist: Alan Barker, UK

Mr A was diagnosed with the HIV virus (body positive) in 1988, and has for the most part been cared for in the community by a designated community-based nurse. On the occasion of any opportunistic infection that could not be dealt with within the confines of the community (through the genitourinary outpatient department), admission to the hospital was needed.

A wide range of drug therapy has been employed, depending upon the needs of Mr A, and opportunistic infections have for the most part been kept under control. This, as in many other cases, often requires long spells in hospital and, depending upon the infection or problem, may require compound drug therapy, e.g. chemotherapy or radiation therapy. Mr A had had the offer of complementary therapy in various forms (one being aromatherapy) both in the community and in a hospital situation. The aromatherapy in the home setting has been of great value, not only to Mr A but also to partners and carers.

With the amount of chemotherapy being used, Mr A was suffering from an itching dermal reaction and insomnia. Conventional options were having very little effect, apart from putting more chemicals into his body. After being asked by the consultant if I could do anything, we tried a bath oil containing five drops

each of *Pelargonium graveolens* and *Chamomilla recutita* in 100 ml vegetable oil (90% grapeseed, 10% unrefined macerated oil of calendula—i.e. low concentration). As well as this, a cream was made up (15 drops of *C. recutita* in 30 g base cream), to apply as needed to any itching part of the body.

Because of respiratory problems Mr A (together with conventional antibiotic therapy) had a diffuser in his own room (both at home and in hospital) using *Boswellia carteri*, *Cinnamomum camphora*, *Eucalyptus smithii* and *Satureia montana*. These were varied according to his needs. Essential oils were given in a shampoo base to help his itching scalp: *Chamaemelum nobile*, *Melaleuca alternifolia*, *Rosmarins officinalis* and *Thymus vulgaris* ct. alcohol. Generalized relaxing baths and massage (clinical areas only, i.e. foot, legs, neck and shoulder) were given, using numerous relaxing, calming and soothing essential oils.

Mr A died of *Pneumocystis carinii* infections and progressive multifocal leukoencephalopathy, amongst other complications, but his quality of life in the final stages was of the very highest, owing in part to dedicated staff administering aromatherapy prescriptions and to a positive attitude by health care professionals to the use of this complementary medicine.

Case 15.7   Aromatherapist: Joy Burnett Borneo, UK

S is 37 years old and was diagnosed HIV positive in 1986. He developed *Pneumocystis carinii* infection, pneumonia and various other infections early in 1991. I was contacted by the Cleveland Aids Support who had been asked by the patient's consultant if any help was available.

6.11.91   S was very depressed, angry and unable to handle his own sense of helplessness. His whole body was covered with atopic dermatitis. He was unable to walk because of pain in his legs and ankles—he scratched constantly and legs, ankles and bottom are scratched raw. The essential oils used for his back massage were bergamot (to uplift, and to help his depression, emotional and mental weariness), German chamomile (for impatience and irritability) and sandalwood (for repressed anger, emotions and fear). I mixed an oil for him to apply to himself daily (to relieve the itching and help combat the dermatitis) containing lavender, German chamomile and patchouli.

13.11.91   The skin on his legs was much improved (S applying the oil up to six times a day). I massaged his back, arms and hands with the same mixture as last week as he reported feeling so good after the first aromatherapy treatment. I gave him a blend of lavender, geranium and sandalwood for his bath.

27.11.91   His temperament seemed to have improved (his mother's comment). His skin was much better but the pain and swelling in his feet were considerable so I concentrated on these. I used juniper (for the oedema), chamomile (an antiinflammatory) and geranium (for the circulation). This was gently applied to his legs and a mixture was left for him to apply himself.

12.12.91   The massage was as before, concentrating on his legs and feet. He stated he generally felt much better and had managed to walk a bit this week. His skin had continued to improve and he was applying his original mix regularly.

27.12.91   His skin was much better; his ankles were still red and itchy but he was no longer scratching. He was feeling generally a lot better and had been away for Christmas. His legs were less painful and he was managing to walk a little. Massage this week included frankincense to help with the scarring.

Treatment continued successfully through the early months of 1992 and the skin problem erupted again only when he was taken into hospital in May, just before he died.

---

affinity with the particular skin symptoms as well as stress and depression.

Once the considerations above have been noted, the treatment by aromatherapy of a patient with HIV-related symptoms can follow the normal pattern. The treatment's effectiveness lies in the fact that the essential oils trigger natural homoeostatic principles in the body to create a healing process (see Ch. 8).

One of my HIV positive patients cried for quarter of an hour after his second aromatherapy massage and reported feeling 'as if he had let out a can of worms'. He slept better than he had since before he was first diagnosed.

(Burnett 1992)

Summary

Complementary medicine has been able to offer much in the way of support to those living with diseases such as cancer and HIV-related illness. This is increasingly backed by the medical profession despite the fact that there is little in the way of published research results on the use of aromatherapy in this field. However, a few studies have been carried out which show positive results with regard to the improvement of life quality and a greater acceptance of death.

REFERENCES

Bardeau P 1976 La médecine aromatique. Robert Lafont, Paris, p 313

Barker A 1993 The clinical use of aromatherapy and the AIDS virus. Unpublished dissertation, Shirley Price International College of Aromatherapy, Hinckley, Leics

Bernadet M 1983 La phyto-aromathérapie pratique. Dangles, St-Jean-de-Braye, p 158

Buckle J 1997 Clinical aromatherapy in nursing. Arnold, London

Burke C, Sikora K 1992 Cancer—the dual approach. Nursing Times 88(38): 62–66

Burnett J 1992 Using aromatherapy to enhance the immune system and alleviate symptoms for those affected by HIV and AIDS. Unpublished dissertation, Shirley Price International College of Aromatherapy, Hinckley, Leics

Caldwell 1991 Research reports. International Journal of Aromatherapy 3(1): 6

Chaitow L 1987 Soft-tissue manipulation. Thorsons, Wellingborough

Cousins N 1979 Anatomy of an illness as perceived by a patient. Norton, New York

Crowther D 1991 Complementary therapy in practice. Nursing Standard 5(23): 25–27

Elliott C 1991 Cancer was a killer in the dark ages. Sunday Telegraph, December 29: 9

Evans B 1995 An audit into the effects of aromatherapy massage and the cancer patient in palliative and terminal care. Complementary Therapies in Medicine 3: 239–241

Franchomme P, Pénoël D 1990 L'aromathérapie exactement. Jollois, Limoges

Gattefossé R-M 1993 Aromatherapy. Daniel, Saffron Walden

Horrigan C 1991 Complementing cancer care. International Journal of Aromatherapy 3(4): 15–17

International Conference on AIDS 1993 The HIV/AIDS pandemic: global spread and global response. Berlin

Lamy R 1989 The cultivation of chemotypes of thyme and rosemary. Riverhead Publishing, Hinckley

Lundie S 1994 Introducing and applying aromatherapy within the NHS. The Aromatherapist 1(1): 283

Machin M 1989 Advanced cancer. International Journal of Aromatherapy 2(1): 19

McNamara P 1993 Massage for people with cancer: a working paper. Wandsworth Cancer Support Centre, London

Osato S 1965 Chemotherapy of human carcinoma with citronellal and citral and their action on carcinoma tissue in its histological aspects up to healing. Tohoku Journal of Experimental Medicine 96: 102–123

Phillips A 1989 Advanced cancer. International Journal of Aromatherapy 2(1): 18

Price S 1993 Parkinson's disease project: is aromatherapy an effective treatment for Parkinson's disease? The Aromatherapist 1(1): 14–21

Roulier G 1990 Les huiles essentielles pour votre santé. Dangles, St-Jean-de-Braye

Sellar W 1992 The directory of essential oils. Daniel, Saffron Walden

Sims S 1986 Slow stroke back massage for cancer patients. Nursing Times 82(13): 47–50

Valnet J 1980 The practice of aromatherapy. Daniel, Saffron Walden

Policy and practice

Aromatherapy in the UK

Introduction

Complementary therapies have grown in importance within the National Health Service (NHS) during the 1980s and 1990s. There have been increasing demands that they should become regulated and observe similar ethical and practical constraints to those of orthodox medicine. This chapter reports recent developments within the field of complementary medicine and aromatherapy in particular; it also proposes a model set of policies and protocols for the professional practice of aromatherapy in UK healthcare settings.

THE GROWTH OF COMPLEMENTARY THERAPIES IN THE NHS

The ever-increasing interest by the nursing profession in complementary therapies, especially aromatherapy, has raised several issues of importance to the nursing profession. As a result, a forum within the Royal College of Nursing (RCN) introduces nurses to the various complementary therapies available, with a steering committee set up to compare results of their use by nurses in hospital situations. Where the benefits to patients can be quantified, it is hoped to use this evidence to persuade more hospital managers to fund natural therapies—including aromatherapy. The RCN has also compiled a Statement of Beliefs (see p. 265), which reflects the principles which should be observed by nurses practising complementary therapies.

At the same time a directive entitled the Liability of Suppliers of Service makes it clear that 'individuals should be able to justify their actions should any malpractice claim be made against them by clients' (Rankin-Box 1992). Clearly, aromatherapy as it has been implemented to date—by any nurse in any circumstance thought to be valid—cannot continue, and a number of hospital authorities have already set up criteria for the practice of complementary therapies (or are in the process of doing so).

Complementary medicine is being used increasingly within the National Health Service; almost 40% of GP partnerships in the UK will refer their NHS patients to complementary therapists where they feel it would be of benefit (Thomas et al 1995) and about 75% of the public presently use complementary therapies through the NHS (RCCM 1997).

New developments

In 1997, a discussion document was published by the Foundation for Integrated Medicine. This document summarizes the conclusions of four working groups, under the guidance of a steering committee set up at the suggestion of HRH the Prince of Wales, to consider the current position of orthodox, complementary and alternative medicine in the United Kingdom (Integrated Healthcare 1997).

The aim of the discussion document was to investigate the possibility of the public having access to a wider range of effective and safe forms of treatment. Suggestions reflecting the views of practitioners of differing disciplines (and the possibility of their working effectively together) are made within it for potential further action in the fields of research, regulation, education and training and the delivery of integrated care in all forms of proven complementary and alternative medicine. At the launch of the report, it was mentioned within the regulation section that aromatherapy is one of the therapies where impressive developments have been made in terms of self-regulatory structures, improved standards of training and greater public recognition (Baker 1997). Also in this category are acupuncture, healing, herbal medicine and homoeopathy; in all cases progress was due to

intraprofessional cooperation. Of special note were the osteopathic and chiropractic professions, which have now attained statutory self-regulation (Integrated Healthcare 1997 p. 29).

Although professional bodies are introducing more efficient systems of regulation, there is unfortunately an overabundance of different representative bodies in most complementary therapies. This can be confusing to the public, who have no way of knowing which therapies are safe and appropriate in the circumstances of their particular condition or what qualifications and level of skills an individual therapist in any one discipline possesses (Integrated Healthcare 1997 p. 5).

The discussion document identifies the call for 'a common body of knowledge and skills which all health-care practitioners need'. This echoes the view the authors have had for 3 years or more that there should be a basic curriculum which all would-be complementary practitioners should complete before studying the discipline or disciplines of their choice. This would ensure uniformity in the basic skills required by all complementary practitioners in order to practise their therapy or therapies efficiently and knowledgeably. It would also simplify the study of further therapies, not only saving repetition of certain modules in each discipline studied, but enabling the extra time thus gained to be spent on more in-depth knowledge of the therapy in question. At the moment, non-medically qualified practitioners of complementary and alternative therapies are free to practice under common law, irrespective of their levels of training or clinical competence. The elements common to all therapies proposed by the discussion document and hoped to be covered in the curriculum are:

- basic anatomy, physiology and pathology
- fundamentals of orthodox medical diagnosis and guidelines for patient referral
- complementary and alternative medicine (CAM) therapies and their potential uses, including the principles of diagnosis and practice
- holistic models of healthcare
- professional ethics
- the therapeutic relationship

- impact of social, cultural, economic, employment and environmental factors on health
- counselling skills
- principles of quality management and audit
- organizational skills, including record keeping
- technical skills ranging from prevention of cross-infection to information management.

The discussion document also proposes that a single, leading, voluntary, self-regulatory body should be established for each of the CAM professions and therapies and, although this may be seen to be an ideal situation, the proliferation of complementary and alternative medicine associations makes it a potentially awesome task. Aromatherapy is one of the few therapies to have an umbrella body (see AOC in Appendix C), despite its many associations.

Art or science?

Aromatherapy is the most widely used complementary therapy in the NHS (Lundie 1994), and many nurses are now taking up training in the subject. Cawthorne (1991) states that: 'aromatherapy allows nurses to practise the *art* of nursing, which over recent years, due to the increase in medical technology, has taken a secondary role to the *science* of nursing. The relaxing nature of the massage also has a calming effect on the nurse who gives it. In addition, it allows them to give true holistic care'.

In the UK aromatherapy is becoming increasingly regarded as a balance of both art and science. The French origin, from which the UK version was born, was mainly scientific, as can be seen from both Gattefossé's book *Gattefossé's Aromatherapy* (1993) and Valnet's book *The Practice of Aromatherapy* (1980), where the emphasis is on internal and external use (without massage) of essential oils, the choice being based mainly on the chemical components of the oils and their effects on human systems of the body. The British origin was mainly non-scientific, the use of essential oils with massage being regarded as more art than science. The effect of essential oils on the nervous system and individual prescription was the emphasis in Madame Maury's

book, published first in English under the title *The Secret of Life and Youth* in 1964 (republished in 1989 as Marguerite Maury's *Guide to Aromatherapy*) and all subsequent books published in the UK. The first book to be published in English was entitled *The Art of Aromatherapy* (Tisserand 1977).

Massage at that time became the most important feature of the teaching in the early aromatherapy schools, with essential oil chemistry hardly mentioned. However, a balance of science and art is as essential in aromatherapy (see Ch. 17—France) as in any subject; in the case of aromatherapy, without a good scientific knowledge, treatments cannot be of the most effective calibre and in recent years chemistry has become a prominent feature in aromatherapy courses, the length of training having been increased and standards put in place by the professional associations. As more research is done it is imperative that aromatherapists (and particularly aromatologists) understand the chemistry behind the oils and the relationship (if any) between these and the effects of the oils on the body. However, holism, the theory that a complex entity, system, etc. is more than merely the sum of its parts, has still to play a major part in aromatherapy treatments for the scientific application to be truly successful.

Human beings have an interdependent relationship with plants, depending on them for oxygen, food and energy: the human and plant ecosystems rely intimately on each other, and are part of the whole which is life itself ... As we know, essential oils have been proving their ability to influence human health on physical, emotional and mental levels ... It is this emotional dimension that confirms aromatherapy as an art, and lifts it up from a mere interaction of plants and human chemicals.

(Eccles 1997)

Growth in acceptance

Several hospitals, including the Ardenlea Marie Curie Centre and Help the Hospices, are funding nurses on aromatherapy courses, many of these being run specifically for the nursing profession. In 1994 the RCN, in conjunction with the Shirley Price International College of Aromatherapy, produced a video which emphasized the need for adequate training for nurses and knowledge-able use of essential oils.

Consultants and GPs today certainly have a more sympathetic and cooperative attitude towards aromatherapy than when the authors came into the profession in the 1970s; only since the late 1980s and early 1990s has there been a growth in the willingness of the medical profession to listen seriously to claims of the positive and sometimes dramatic effects that essential oils can have on people's overall health (see Ch. 4). One of the reasons for the previous reluctance was the understandable reaction to the short length of training formerly required—only 5 or 6 days, compared with the same number of years for medical training! It was never put across clearly or knowledgeably enough in those days by enthusiastic aromatherapists that aromatherapy was not intended to supplant allopathic medicine, but to supplement it and enhance the caring work carried out by nurses—to reintroduce natural healing agents into hospitals perhaps suffering from an overdose of synthetic drugs. Another off-putting factor could have been the aromas—how could pleasant smells affect the health in a positive way? Finally, the word 'massage' with its then sleazy connotation did not help, particularly at a time when touch was being ousted from nursing care and machines were largely replacing the healing hands of the physiotherapist. Now, however, clinical successes in hospitals where essential oils have been used and the results of projects and trials (albeit not of rigorous research standard, which is very difficult in the case of essential oils) have led to a greater willingness to listen and to utilize aromatherapy in hospitals and community care. The change in status of NHS hospitals in 1990 is thought to have been a contributory factor to the increase of complementary therapies being practised in healthcare:

Self-governing status for NHS hospitals—NHS Trusts—was created in the 1990 NHS and Community Care Act. These were set up to manage hospitals and other NHS services. Since 1990 all providers in the NHS have opted for NHS Trust status and there are no longer any hospitals which are directly managed by Health Authorities.

(Farrer 1997 personal communication).

At first, therapists found it easier to obtain permission to work in hospices with the terminally ill, usually on a voluntary basis (it was often the opinion that at least no harm could be done!), but now aromatherapy is welcomed in general hospitals, and a number of therapists also work in conjunction with their local GP on minor health problems which can be helped by essential oils. A major breakthrough occurred in 1993, when GPs were empowered to refer patients to complementary therapists for treatment on the NHS, provided that the GP concerned remained clinically accountable for the patient.

An understanding of the attitudes of the medical and nursing profession, and of the legal and professional issues which govern their practice, is important as they all play a part in the acceptance and use of complementary therapies generally, and aromatherapy specifically. This even before consideration is given as to whether the necessary pennies are available to spend on what at first may appear to be an aromatic luxury.

(Lundie 1994)

The University of Exeter survey (1997) revealed that, although the number of members from complementary therapy associations working in the NHS was very low in most disciplines, aromatherapy, healing and reflexology associations indicated the highest numbers—with 'up to half'. 'Aromatherapy and reflexology are popular with nurses and this is likely to account for much of their involvement.' (University of Exeter 1997 p. 60).

The professionalization of aromatherapy in the UK

Aromatherapy was introduced originally through the beauty therapy world in the 1960s. Massage therapists became aware of it in the first half of the 1980s, by which time only four aromatherapy books had appeared—*The Art of Aromatherapy* 1977 (Robert Tisserand); *Aromatherapy: The Use of Plant Essences in Healing* 1979 (Raymond Lautié & André Passebecq); *The Practice of Aromatherapy* 1980 (Jean Valnet) and *Practical Aromatherapy* 1983 (Shirley Price).

In the late 1980s and early 1990s many books on the subject appeared, and nurses from all backgrounds—including those working in primary healthcare, community and mental healthcare, private healthcare and Social Services day and residential care—became conscious of the immense possibilities of this gentle therapy. Aromatherapy began creeping into the health professional's practice without due attention to the training of those using the essential oils—and without Health Authority policies or hospital protocols from which to work (as is the case at present in many other countries—see Ch. 17). This was perhaps due in part to the great number of aromatherapy books written for the general public, which emphasize the ease of use and the successful effects of essential oils. However, it was also due to the strong desire of nurses to give their patients help in an area which had begun to be neglected by 20th century medicine. Many of the original nurses who trained in aromatherapy were leaving, or were about to leave, the nursing profession because they felt their caring skills were being pushed into the background. Less and less time was available in hospital settings for the personal contact which used to be a key element of their chosen profession. There was also the hope (which has since been proved, albeit only by anecdotal evidence) that the use of essential oils could perhaps help to reduce the need for secondary medication given to cope with the side-effects of primary treatment.

Professional aromatherapy associations

In response to these trends, in 1985 10 aromatherapists, including the authors, met to discuss the inauguration of the first worldwide aromatherapy organization—the International Federation of Aromatherapists (IFA)—which created the first set of standards for aromatherapy in this country. In 1988 a special group within the IFA was established in what must be regarded as a unique endeavour by a non-medical profession to introduce aromatherapy into medical establishments. Aromatherapy-in-Care (AIC) therapists introduced themselves first into hospices, as did a number of independent aromatherapists, where they all used their skills initially on patients with cancer. Their voluntary services were much appreciated and soon extended into NHS hospitals, self-governing cancer care organizations, centres for people with learning difficulties and other support groups.

A second major aromatherapy association (of which again the authors were founder members), the International Society of Professional Aromatherapists (ISPA), was launched in 1990 to give qualifying aromatherapists a choice of membership and insurance benefits as well as a choice of venues for meetings. Also launched in 1990 was the Register of Qualified Aromatherapists (RQA). These associations offer legal support and insurance, providing cover for malpractice, public and product liability. Their aims are to develop and maintain high standards of qualification and to provide a forum for the development and exchange of knowledge and skill. Annual general meetings (in ISPA's case a weekend seminar) are held with speakers appropriate to the requirements of professional aromatherapists. There is also a number of smaller associations; one of these, the Institute of Aromatic Medicine (IAM) (formerly the Institute of Aromatic Therapists), is unique in that it can give insurance cover for the intensive topical application and the internal use of essential oils to those accredited aromatherapists who have studied the properties and effects of essential oils for a further 2 years and attained the required standard by examination.

There are a few associations which accept therapists of various disciplines, e.g. the Guild of Complementary Practitioners, formed in 1995.

Members of all aromatherapy associations have together been instrumental in arousing the interest and acceptance of the British medical profession, who can see for themselves the advantages of touch and essential oils. This has been supported by aromatherapists who, like the authors, have lectured in hospitals, presented papers at nursing conferences to create an awareness in this field and encouraged trials and research studies within healthcare settings, always emphasizing the necessity of informed consent. Although referring to research in allopathic medicine, the extract below could apply to treatments, trials and research studies in aromatherapy too (perhaps without the word 'discomfort'!).

The Declaration of Geneva of the World Medical Association binds the physician with the words 'The health of my patient will be my first consideration'. … In any research on human beings, each potential subject must be adequately informed of the aims, methods, anticipated benefits and potential hazards of the study and the discomforts it may entail. He or she should be informed that he or she is at liberty to abstain from participation in the study and that he or she is free to withdraw his or her consent at any time. The physician should then obtain the subject's freely given informed consent in writing.

(Declaration of Helsinki 1996)

Training

Lannoye Report. In April 1994, a Belgian MEP, Paul Lannoye, put forward a report in which he reminded the Committee of the immense and growing interest in complementary therapies throughout the EU. The report called for the adoption of a number of aims, including:

- the recognition of complementary medicine and harmonization of teaching
- the encouragement of research programmes, taking into account the holistic nature of complementary medicine
- the establishment of a European committee of experts to rule on clinical effectiveness of treatment
- the establishment of a European committee to consider the training and experience of complementary practitioners (Baker 1995)

He called for freedom of choice in healthcare for EU members, saying that safety in these disciplines could be provided by improved standards of training, as it was illegal practice and lack of proper training which was putting patients at risk. At the first presentation it was bitterly opposed; however, Lannoye revised it substantially and it was re-presented (Griggs 1997 p. 307). The report eventually went through the European Parliament but with so many amendments that Lannoye removed his name from it and it is now called the Collins report, after the present chairman of the Environment, Health and Public Safety Committee (Miller 1998 personal communication). If the report achieved nothing else, it certainly highlighted the urgency of appropriate training for future practitioners of complementary medicine.

Short courses, workshops and seminars. Health professionals without recognized training in aromatherapy or aromatology (complete aromatic medicine) should use essential oils only under the direction of, or after consultation with, a qualified aromatherapist or aromatologist; 1 and 2 day seminars in aromatherapy may be adequate for such health professionals but it should be made clear that more rigorous training is required in order to practise independently and prescribe essential oils for individual patients.

Accredited training. Aromatherapy training establishments approved or accredited by an aromatherapy association to the minimum standards of the Aromatherapy Organisations Council (AOC—see Appendix C) teach detailed chemistry and properties of a minimum of 30 essential oils, their actions on the body and mind and how to use them accurately. When a knowledgeable aromatherapist dispenses appropriate essential oils there should be little likelihood of any adverse effects. It is a question of being aware, as with any medicine, of what and how much should be administered and for how long.

National Occupational Standards. National Occupational Standards (NOS) are agreed basic specifications of performance, describing current and desired levels of competence in the workplace. They are different from a job description, as competence in the workplace demands more than just the necessary technical skills. Other requirements include 'people skills', the ability to communicate effectively, assessment and evaluating skills, etc., all of which are incorporated into a set of occupational standards. The government aims to introduce these for the majority of occupations by the year 2000.

The purpose of having national occupational standards is that they can be used to develop education and training standards to promote therapists who are able to offer high quality services. The units selected and the level of learning required will clearly depend upon the nature of the qualification, i.e. a degree will demand much greater depth of study than a course in basic practical skills.

There are moves to establish a nationally recognized award based on NOS, and the most likely form is as a National Vocational Qualification (NVQ), known as the Scottish Vocational Qualification (SVQ) in Scotland. The development of NVQs and SVQs would be the responsibility of an appropriate National Training Organization (NTO) which would take on the responsibilities of the Occupational Standards Council from the OSCHSC (see Appendix C).

Designing and preparing the necessary assessment systems would be the responsibility of awarding bodies. These awarding bodies would then have to submit their qualifications to the Qualifications and Curriculum Authority in order to gain accreditation. It is likely to be well into 1999 before aromatherapy NVQs/SVQs are in place.

Not all aromatherapy associations are in favour of aromatherapy going down the NVQ route, many preferring self-regulation through application for a Charter, as achieved by the physiotherapists some years ago. It is important also to recognize that the current NVQ level 3 Beauty Therapy Aromatherapy Massage, which is offered by many colleges of further/higher education is for *aroma massage* and it is not a qualification in aromatherapy as a form of complementary medicine. Higher level NVQs are expected to be put in place for the complementary therapy of aromatherapy.

There is a growing interest in university-validated courses, though these are not yet to degree standard. Undoubtedy an undergraduate award will be available in the very near future, but at the moment university courses are at diploma standard and do not include the facets of knowledge included in aromatology training, despite one giving the name 'Aromatic medicine' to its course.

RCN Complementary Therapy Forum

In 1991, a Special Interest Group was set up by the RCN to look into complementary therapies. The group developed a Statement of Beliefs, together with guidelines for nurses looking for a complementary therapy course or practitioner. The group has now been renamed the RCN Complementary Therapy Forum (CTF) and it focuses on how to introduce complementary therapies into the workplace and on the standardization of nurse education in this field.

One of its objectives is to make nurses aware of the need to check the credentials of any course in which they are interested, including the tutor: student ratio and the qualifications of the tutors. It suggests asking whether or not there is supervised practice, an anatomy and physiology examination and a practical examination in the therapy. Counselling, communication and self-development skills should be included along with support for the trainee therapist.

RCN Statement of Beliefs

The RCN Statement of Beliefs for the practice of complementary therapies (to be revised as necessary and on the advice and suggestion of members and other interested parties following discussion by the steering committee) reads as follows:

1. We believe that nurses using complementary therapies as part of their care should know and understand their responsibilities to the patient/client and the United Kingdom Central Council for Nursing, Midwifery and Health Visiting. Further we believe that the UKCC code sets the professional requirements to be met by all registered nurses using complementary therapies.

2. We believe that all patients and clients have the right to be offered and to receive complementary therapies either exclusively or as a part of orthodox nursing practice.

3. We believe that all patients have the right to expect that their religious, cultural and spiritual beliefs will be observed by nurses practising complementary therapies.

4. We believe that all complementary therapies available to patients must have the support of the collaborative care team.

5. We believe that a registered nurse who is appropriately qualified to carry out a complementary therapy must agree and work to locally agreed protocols for practice and standards of care.

6. We believe that the patient/clients, in partnership with the nurse complementary therapist, should determine the suitability of any proposed complementary therapy. Informed, documented consent should be obtained and detailed records kept with the patient/client's care record.

7. We believe that, where possible, research-based complementary therapy practices should be used. Where this is not possible then nurse complementary therapists, as accountable professionals, must be able to justify their actions.

8. We believe that nurse complementary therapists should, when appropriate, be prepared to instruct significant individuals in the patient/client's life (including the patient/client) so that they can learn basic complementary therapy skills for self-care.

9. We believe that nurse complementary therapists should seek to develop their self-awareness and interpersonal skills and so enhance their role as reflective practitioners.

10. We believe that nurse complementary therapists have a responsibility to collect detailed information on all therapy sessions and to evaluate the outcomes of therapy on the patient/client.

11. We believe that the practice of complementary therapies by nurses should be the subject of at least an annual review by an appropriately constituted multidisciplinary committee. The review should take into account patient measures of satisfaction and benefit.

It is not easy to quantify complementary therapies working exclusively with energies, e.g. acupuncture or spiritual healing. Aromatherapy, however, is a multiple therapy embracing energies, therapeutic touch, massage and the administration of remedies—not to mention the pleasing aroma, which could be partly responsible for aromatherapy possibly being the most popular complementary therapy which nurses wish to study.

The United Kingdom Central Council for nursing, midwifery and health visiting

It is advisable that nurses, as professional and accountable practitioners, should take into account the UKCC Code of Professional Conduct (CPC) (1992a), Scope of Professional Practice (SPP) (1992b) and Standards for the Administration of Medicines (SAM) (1992c), since these documents govern all nursing activities. A booklet entitled 'Guidelines for professional practice' (GPP) was produced by the UKCC in 1996 to provide a guide for consideration of the statements within the CPC and to provide information on the specific circumstances, safeguards, policies and procedures needed to provided treatment or care relevant to each area of practice.

The guidelines contain several pages on the importance of obtaining consent before giving any treatment or care. This consent must be based on adequate information being given on exactly what is involved and should be 'shared freely with the patient or client, in an accessible way and in appropriate circumstances' (GPP pp. 17–20). This consent may be given verbally, in writing or by implication and may be withdrawn or refused in the same way at any time. Confidentiality is important and any information which has been given in confidence should be used only for the purposes of the treatment.

The UKCC documents, together with appropriate and well-thought-out policies and local protocols for the use of aromatherapy (see below), are designed to lead to informed professional functioning by nurses who choose to include aromatherapy in their work. Many issues covered in these UKCC documents are directly applicable to nurses working with essential oils, and the relevant points will be brought into focus for the purposes of this chapter. For ease of reference each document quoted will be referenced by its initials in brackets.

'The range of responsibilities which fall to individual nurses, midwives and health visitors should be related to their personal experience, education and skill' (SPP Introduction p. 2). Experience and skill should be built upon education—a comprehensive and detailed learning base is essential.

'Just as practice must remain dynamic, sensitive, relevant and responsive to the changing needs of individual patients and clients, so too must education for practice' (SPP 3).

Many practitioners of different disciplines do not regularly update their knowledge. This is unwise since updating is of paramount importance, especially in a world where ideas and accepted behavioural patterns are changing fast. 'The practice of nursing takes place in a context of continuing change and development' (SPP Int. 1).

The CPC states that:

'As a registered nurse, midwife or health visitor you are personally accountable for your practice and, in the exercise of your professional accountability, must:

- promote and safeguard the interest and well-being of patients and clients;
- ensure that no action or omission on your part, or within your sphere of responsibility, is detrimental to the interests, condition or safety of patients and clients;
- maintain and improve your professional knowledge and competence;
- acknowledge any limitations in your knowledge and competence and decline any duties or responsibilities unless able to perform them in a safe and skilled manner.'

The registered nurse, midwife or health visitor must:

- 'take steps to remedy any relevant deficits in order effectively and appropriately to meet the needs of patients and clients' (SPP 9.3)
- 'recognise and honour the direct or indirect personal accountability borne for all aspects of professional practice' (SPP 9.5)
- 'avoid any inappropriate delegation to others which compromises those interests' (SPP 9.6).

The last two points, when applied to aromatherapy, emphasize the need for suitable insurance cover specific to the use of essential oils. RCN members are covered exclusively when on duty; if cover is required out of official working hours it can be obtained from one of the professional aromatherapy or aromatology (i.e. aromatic medicine) associations on becoming a full member. ISPA and the Institute of Aromatic Medicine (IAM) also insure student aromatherapists during their time of study.

The UKCC acknowledges that nurses require support staff in their work and, although it does not have a direct role in the training of healthcare assistants, it states its position in relation to support roles:

- 'patients and clients require skilled care from registered practitioners—and support staff require direction and supervision from these same practitioners' (SPP 11)
- 'healthcare assistants to registered nurses, midwives and health visitors must work under the direction and supervision of those registered practitioners' (SPP 23.1)
- 'healthcare assistants must not be allowed to work beyond their level of competence' (SPP 23.3).

In conclusion, the UKCC declares that the framework and principles of SPP reflect the personal responsibility and accountability of individual practitioners, entrusted by the Council to protect and improve standards of care.

With this amount of responsibility and accountability applying to the practice of aromatherapy and aromatology in hospitals, it is time for nurses suitably qualified in these professions to have the courage to say, with the following writer, 'I am an aromatherapist' first and foremost.

All too often I hear the same cry—'I am a qualified nurse using aromatherapy' ... A nursing qualification does not make you a better aromatherapist—indeed, to some, it can be a disadvantage. We should be proud of our profession in the use of essential oils and not need to use another profession as a crutch. Many people may say 'But a nurse will have a greater understanding of clinical matters'—this is not true at all! ... If we feel inadequate with the essential oil training we have had—if it has not covered the areas needed in a clinical field—then find a course which does.

If we are insecure with our training and wish to hide behind the apron strings of another profession, this is not acceptable to either discipline; in fact, the one will strangle the other.

(Barker 1994)

Barker goes on to say that we are competent and appropriately trained professionals in our own right, and do aromatology/aromatherapy a great disservice by tagging it on to another discipline to give it credibility when it is already a valid system of medicine.

AROMATHERAPY, AROMATOLOGY AND AROMATIC MEDICINE

Aromatherapy is 'the *controlled* use of essential oils to promote the health and vitality of the body, mind and spirit by inhalation, baths, compresses, topical application and full-body massage'—not merely 'a massage using essential oils' (see Ch. 5) (Price 1985).

The definition of aromatology (i.e. complete aromatic medicine) is 'the *controlled* use of essential oils to promote the health and vitality of the body, mind and spirit by inhalation, baths, compresses, topical application (as above) and selected area massage, plus external intensive use of undiluted oils and internal use via rectum, os and vagina'. The difference in massage and additions to aromatherapy which require more in-depth training, are as follows:

- massage of different parts of the body as applicable in healthcare situations (full-body massage is not taught as an integral part of the training)
- the external intensive use of essential oils for a strong healing action (i.e. infections, acute conditions)
- internal use:
  - suppositories and pessaries using suitably diluted essential oils
  - ingestion, using suitably diluted essential oils (mainly for digestive conditions).

In France, essential oils are administered internally (pessaries, suppositories and injections as well as by mouth) by medical doctors and phytotherapists, since oral ingestion is an extremely effective method for disorders of the digestive tract, reaching the site of the problem by a direct route. Topical applications (without massage), usually using undiluted oils, inhalation and compresses, are the other methods generally used by French medical aromatologists.

The first British aromatherapists to write books on aromatherapy were Tisserand (1977) and Price (1983). Apart from Lautié & Passebecq (1979) and Valnet (1980) (both translated from French) no other books were published for a further 5 years. Tisserand was not in the beauty business and although Price was originally a beauty therapist, she found her vocation in the kind of aromatherapy advocated by Lautié & Passebecq and Valnet, and later Gattefossé, accepting ingestion, as did Tisserand, as an appropriate method of use.

The first aromatherapy organization comprised mainly beauty therapists, and the beauty therapy code of practice was therefore taken into consideration. Since this disallows oral administration of anything, even vitamin tablets, it was written into the association's code of practice (and therefore that of every subsequent aromatherapy association) that internal use was not allowed. In one way this was providential, because there soon appeared on the market a plethora of both partly 'trained' people and commercial 'essential oils', most of the latter being of a standardized perfume quality (many still are), and therefore not ideal for therapeutic use (see Ch. 2) and definitely not suitable for internal use. For this, only essential oils which are known not to be adulterated, standardized or 'ennobled' in any way, from plants grown organically or naturally (i.e. free from harmful herbicides and pesticides) may be ingested. Wild, naturally and organically farmed plants are the only suitable sources—and oils from these should be used for all methods of therapeutic use.

Volatile (essential) oils appear in the British Pharmacopoeia and have traditionally been used orally in medical practice for many years as expectorants (Boyd & Pearson 1946), carminatives and for digestive disorders generally (May et al 1996). In this respect they are used as medicines, conform to certain standards and can be found in formulations within a recommended dose range (Farrell 1994 personal communication)—but they are not administered by the British medical profession as medicines in their own right. However, at the time of writing there are a few hospitals in the UK which do administer essential oils orally (diluted in a suitable medium), with the consent of the consultants concerned. Some of these hospitals come under the Community Health Sheffield (NHS Trust), which employs a clinical aromatologist.

Aromatherapists give essential oils mainly by massage and inhalation; nevertheless the oils access all parts of the body:

- in inhalation, essential oils have direct access to the lungs
- in massage, essential oils pass the skin into the bloodstream and the surrounding tissues
- in gargles, pessaries and suppositories. Suppositories act directly on the rectum as a treatment for anal fissures and haemorrhoids or by absorption via the blood supply to the colon for systemic use. This route, giving direct access to the blood supply, avoids 'first pass' metabolism in the liver and is rapid in effect (Buckle 1997 p. 42).

Oral ingestion should not be dismissed—or feared—but to use this method (or indeed any internal method) the specialized training given on an aromatology (complete aromatic medicine) course is essential. The very mention of the ingestion of essential oils has most English speaking aromatherapists throwing up their hands in horror and a resounding 'no' fills the air. ... It may well be that our lack of knowledge is leading to a closed mind attitude on the legitimate therapeutic use of essential oils as ingested agents. Aromatherapists trained to current standards may not have the necessary knowledge to use essential oils in this manner, but it may not be quite the minefield that is envisaged.

Let's not ignore the interest in oral ingestion simply because we fear the unknown. There are many issues within the world of aromatherapy today. Ingestion of essential oils is just one. ... The road to understanding is through education. If you take that road and come to a decision regarding the ingestion of essential oils, the real outcome is not whether you agree or disagree, it is the fact that you have made an informed decision.

(Byrne 1997)

Standards for the administration of medicines

With respect to the above, nurse or midwife aromatherapists using essential oils, whether for baths, inhalations, topical application (including compresses), suppositories, pessaries and/or massage, should accept that they are administering medicines. Therefore, some of the SAM, written by the UKCC for its members, indirectly apply to them, emphasizing yet again the need for professional training or supervision: 'The administration of medicines is an important aspect of the professional practice of persons whose names are on the UKCC register. It requires thought and the exercise of professional judgement' (SAM Introduction p. 2). 'The Council expects that, in this area of practice as in all others, all practitioners will have taken steps to develop their knowledge and competence' (SAM Introduction p. 4). The document goes on to reiterate that all registered nurses, midwives and health visitors must recognize the personal professional accountability which they bear for their actions.

Medicinal preparations are prescribed by a physician, checked and dispensed by a pharmacist and administered by a nurse. An essential oil prescription is prescribed by a competent aromatherapist or aromatologist and administered by that practitioner, or by a nurse suitably trained in the method of administration, and in ideal circumstances the prescriber should not be the dispenser and the dispenser should not administer (Farrell 1994 personal communication). The prescription of essential oil massage mixes should nevertheless satisfy the following criteria:

- 'that it is based, whenever possible, on the patient's awareness of the purpose of the treatment and consent' (SAM 6.1)
- 'that the prescription is either clearly written or typed, and that the entry is indelible and dated' (SAM 6.2)
- 'that the prescription provides clear and unequivocal identification of the patient for whom [it] is intended' (SAM 6.5).

The UKCC SAM states that the nurse, midwife or health visitor must apply knowledge and skill to the situation at hand, whether administering, assisting with administration or overseeing self-administration of medicines (in this instance, essential oils). The practitioner must be confident that she or he:

- 'has an understanding of substances used for therapeutic purposes' (SAM 9.1)
- 'is able to justify any actions taken' (SAM 9.2)
- 'is prepared to be accountable for the action taken' (SAM 9.3).

All of the above is, strictly speaking, applicable to orthodox medicinal products. However, it is the present authors' belief that it should also apply to the administration of essential oils, by whatever method.

The section in SAM dealing specifically with complementary and alternative therapies summarizes very well our selection from the documents above:

Some nurses, midwives and health visitors having first undertaken successfully a training in complementary or alternative therapy which involves the use of substances such as essential oils, apply their specialist knowledge and skill in their practice. It is essential that practice in these respects, as in all others, is based upon sound principles, available knowledge and skill. The importance of consent to the use of such treatment must be recognized. So, too, must the practitioner's personal accountability for her or his professional practice.

(SAM 39)

The hazards of unqualified practice

Many aromatherapy books give the impression that the reader can fully understand the subject after reading only one book, and the fact that local colleges offer 24 hour courses (over 12 weeks) seems to support this theory. Accredited aromatherapy schools and some NHS units using aromatherapy offer 1 or 2 day seminars for healthcare professionals. This is acceptable, provided that adequate emphasis is placed on the necessity for such healthcare professionals to work under the supervision of a professional aromatherapist or aromatologist.

Regrettably, there are many health professionals not qualified in aromatherapy or aromatology who, because the therapy appears to be uncomplicated, have been (and in some hospitals still are) using essential oils without adequate training, insurance or supervision by an aromatherapist or aromatologist. Lundie, a midwife and aromatherapist, states (1993 personal communication) that this state of affairs:

has resulted in some rather worrying situations and incidents arising. This has caused concern among those members of the nursing, medical, pharmaceutical and aromatherapy professions, who are well aware that essential oils are highly concentrated and potent herbal preparations which should be used with the same caution as any other medicinal or pharmaceutical product.

Professionals from all areas now feel that aromatherapy (without being medicalized—which would be undesirable and regrettable) must be placed within a well-structured framework.

Some instances which have arisen owing to lack of qualification have led some hospitals to forbid the use of aromatherapy totally. One example occurred in a hospital before the appointment of a clinical aromatologist. A nursing assistant considered two to three drops of essential oil of *Mentha × piperita* [PEPPERMINT] to be inadequate in a bath of water, so (without consulting anyone) put in more than 20, resulting in unpleasant tingling sensations in the patient's legs and burning in the genital area (Barker 1992 personal communication). The patient could not be persuaded to try essential oils again, even after explanations from the qualified aromatologist. Similar stories are common, but the authors are unaware of any lasting harm from such incidents.

It is not unreasonable to ask health professionals wishing to use essential oils on their own initiative (particularly in healthcare settings where the condition of patients may be very poor), to receive the necessary training to the standard required by a professional association.

AREA HEALTH AUTHORITY POLICIES

In order to obtain permission from the hospital management board for the practice of aromatherapy or aromatology on the wards, a nurse should be well prepared—if necessary with research references—to demonstrate the efficacy of essential oils and a draft protocol to prove that the nurse concerned is responsible, knowledgeable and keen to proceed in a correct and competent manner. She should be able to answer confidently any questions on why the therapy is viable and how the essential oils will affect the patient, e.g. what effects the constituents have on the body and what, if any, are the contraindications. A stress-relieving treatment (not necessarily full-body massage) could be offered to a surgeon or senior consultant so that first hand experience is available to them. A policy document can then be prepared to serve as a basis for the individual hospital protocol.

The Bath District Health Authority is believed to have been the first to produce a policy statement and it has been used by many health authorities as a basis for their own, adding to it or enlarging it as they saw fit. The authors have combined all points from the Bath District Health Authority Policy, Dewsbury Health Authority (DHA) Policy (based on the Bath District Policy) and the Community Health Sheffield (NHS Trust) Policy 1993 and 1994 (based exclusively on aromatherapy). Each reference to the UKCC principles will be given in full, to give as complete a picture as possible to those wishing to introduce aromatherapy into their hospitals. Where a single authority expresses a statement, the initials of the authority concerned appear in brackets.

Policy statement

Complementary therapies

These are natural and holistic therapies which may be used exclusively or in harmony with recognized nursing practice.

It is recognized that complementary therapies may enhance patient care (DHA), but only those approved after agreement with the Complementary Therapies Steering Committee may be used on a register held by the Steering Committee (DHA).

Some registered nurses, midwives and health visitors, having first undertaken successfully a training in complementary or alternative therapy which involved the use of substances such as essential oils, apply their specialist knowledge and skill in their practice. It is essential that practice in these respects, as in all others, is based upon sound principles, available knowledge and skill. The importance of consent to the use of such treatments must be recognized. So, too, must the practitioner's personal accountability for her or his professional practice (UKCC SAM 39).

Recognized practitioners

Those who may practise are as follows:

• Accountable practitioner: a registered health-care professional holding a recognized qualification, such as a

— medical practitioner (DHA)
— first level nurse—RGN, RMN, RSCN, RNMH, RM
— second level nurse—EN(G) or EN(MH)
— occupational therapist (DHA)
— physiotherapist (DHA)

who has undertaken a recognized training course leading to competence in a specific complementary therapy.

• Assistant (if appropriate): a healthcare worker who has attended an introductory programme in a specific therapy by a qualified practitioner employed by the health authority concerned. All participants who have completed the basic programme will be obliged to undertake training at yearly intervals to keep them up to date with developments and research in complementary medicine. The assistant will work only under the guidance of an accountable practitioner.

Criteria for practice

The criteria for the practice of complementary therapies are listed below.

Authorization. The accountable practitioner must have been given authorization to practise by his or her service manager (see Nurse management responsibility below).

Permission needs to be sought from the relevant medical practitioner before establishing a specific complementary therapy in a particular area. Should any medical practitioner refuse permission, his or her patients will be excluded.

Consultation. The accountable practitioner must practise the specific complementary therapy in consultation with relevant medical practitioners of the multidisciplinary team. The practitioner should have full knowledge of the patient/client's past and present medical history.

Consent. The patient/client/relative/carer must give informed consent for the accountable practitioner to practise the specific complementary therapy in accordance with the UKCC booklet Exercising accountability (United Kingdom Central Council 1989).

Documentation.
• The accountable practitioner must demonstrate and document within the patient/client care plan or notes the relevance of the complementary therapy being used.
• The accountable practitioner should keep a record of patients/clients and the treatments given according to the training given in each specific complementary therapy (British Complementary Medicine Association (BCMA) Code of Conduct).

Evaluation.
• The accountable practitioner must evaluate and document the effectiveness of the specific complementary therapy being used.
• The final decision on a treatment plan when approved by all parties will be officially documented in the nursing care plan of the named patient/client.

Competence

The attention of accountable practitioners will be drawn to specific UKCC Professional Codes of Conduct, as well as those of the Chartered Society of Physiotherapists (DHA) and British Association of Occupational Therapists (Professional Standard 16) (DHA) where applicable:

• 'Ensure that no action or omission on your part, or within your sphere of responsibility, is detrimental to the interests, condition or safety of patients and clients' (SPP 6.2).
• 'Acknowledge any limitations in your knowledge and competence and decline any duties or responsibilities unless able to perform them in a safe and skilled manner' (SPP 6.4).

Accountability

The UKCC Exercising accountability principles (1989) can be summarized as follows:

• The interests of the patient are paramount.
• Professional accountability must be exercised in such a manner as to ensure that the primacy of the interests of patients or clients is respected and must not be overridden by those of the professions or their practitioners.
• The exercise of accountability requires the practitioner to seek to achieve and maintain high standards.
• Advocacy on behalf of patients or clients is an essential feature of the exercise of accountability by a professional practitioner.
• The role of other persons in the delivery of healthcare to patients or clients must be recognized and respected, provided that the first principle above is honoured.
• Public trust and confidence in the profession is dependent on its practitioners being seen to exercise their accountability responsibly.
• Each registered nurse, midwife or health visitor must be able to justify any action or decision taken in the course of her or his professional practice (UKCC 1989).
• The practitioner must accept accountability for improving and maintaining an appropriate level of knowledge and skill for the specific complementary skill practised:
— Patients and clients require skilled care from registered practitioners, and support staff require direction and supervision from these same practitioners (SPP 11).
— Healthcare assistants to registered nurses, midwives and health visitors must work under the direction of these registered practitioners (SPP 23.1).

— Healthcare assistants must not be allowed to work beyond their level of competence (SPP 23.3).

• A practitioner, in the exercise of professional accountability, must act always in such a manner as to promote and safeguard the interests and well-being of patients and clients (SPP 6.1).

• The interests of the patient or client must be paramount.

Nurse management responsibility

The manager for the clinical area will be accountable for ensuring that:

• Authorization has been obtained for the use of specific complementary therapies by staff.

• Any complementary therapy used is one approved by the health authority concerned.

• The accountable practitioner has undertaken a recognized training course at an accredited training institution, to a standard entitling that practitioner to full membership of the relevant professional association.

• The manager and accountable nurse make an agreement with regard to the level at which that nurse practises the specific complementary therapy (and this to form part of the individual hospital's protocol).

• Permission has been sought from appropriate medical practitioners before establishing a specific complementary therapy in a particular area.

• Assistant practitioners have received an approved level of training by an accountable practitioner before assisting with a specific complementary therapy.

• A list of assistant practitioners is maintained for reference (DHA).

• The manager and accountable practitioner review the practice of the specific complementary therapy on an annual basis (or more frequently if appropriate) to ensure: (a) a quality service and (b) that administration of prescription treatments is carried out in a professional manner and to the benefit of the client.

Service provision

Arrangements for the involvement of accountable practitioners in complementary therapies is subject to the needs of the service and availability of resources. Responsibility for resourcing therapies lies with individual managers (DHA).

Research

It is anticipated that clinical areas in which complementary therapies are practised will encourage a research-based approach to practice.

COST B4. European Cooperation in the field of Science and Technology (COST) aims to coordinate national research projects at a European level.

The European Research Action COST B4 was launched in 1993, in order to harmonize the research into the therapeutic significance of unconventional medicine and the associated cultural, psychological, legislative and economic aspects; this to be used as a basis for evaluating its possible usefulness or risks in public health. By 1995 14 countries had signed the Memorandum of Understanding, in which the signatory countries agree to cooperate in research into the above aspects.

Following its first meeting in October 1993, the Management Committee of the Action prepared a brochure of their current research projects including details of those involved. This was circulated in summer 1994 and has been updated annually during the 5 year programme, with the final report being due in July 1999. Several studies involving the use of aromatherapy appear in the COST B4 responses to the questionnaire; these included projects on dementia, Parkinson's disease (see Ch. 9), learning disabilities and cancer.

COST B4 includes projects from the USA and Israel, but is not linked to the listed research centres in these two countries, but 'any of their institutes interested in this cooperation can apply to participate' (Riek 1994). The advantage of this approach lies in a quick and easy information exchange between the scientists involved, and in the distribution of tasks for the research work involved in the Action.

The first COST B4 workshop took place in 1994, with delegates from 19 countries. The presentations included an overview of research currently taking place in the COST countries, which was followed by others covering several different modes of research. The second day covered conditions such as pain, therapies such as homoeopathy, practical considerations such as the interface between orthodox and complementary medicine and research issues such as methodology. 'Delegates reported that the structure of the workshop and of the seminars in particular, was useful for information exchange and for networking. It is hoped that more specialised working groups will tackle specific research issues in considerably greater depth.' (Vickers 1995). A future aim is to make a bridge between conventional and unconventional medicines, creating an open forum for official medicine of the various unconventional approaches to disease, illness and care. (See also Research Council for Complementary Medicine in Appendix C.)

Prescription of oils

The Medicines Act 1968 does not allow natural therapists to prescribe or supply substances freely simply because they occur naturally. In the main it is herbalists who are affected but aromatherapists and aromatologists come under the same heading, since they too prescribe herbal substances (Sheffield Health Authority, SHA). The Act defines a herbal substance or herbal remedy (section 132.1) as 'a medicinal product consisting of a substance produced by subjecting a plant or plants to drying, crushing, or any other process, or of a mixture whose sole ingredients are one or more substances so produced, and water or some other inert substance'. This of course includes plant oils.

Conditions

The conditions of prescribing are:

- the remedy must be a herbal remedy as defined above
- the herbal remedy may be sold, supplied, manufactured or assembled without a licence in a shop or a consulting room provided that the occupier supplies to a particular person in that person's presence after being requested to use his/her own judgement as to the treatment required.

This means that a practitioner cannot supply a person, even without charge, an oil or mixture of oils without a licence—unless that person has consulted that practitioner and he or she has actually seen the person (SHA).

Labelling regulations

Since July 1977, regulations control the dispensing of products for medicinal use. The mandatory requirements for every container of medicine, lotion, ointment, tablet, etc. are as follows:

- It must have a label.
- The label must contain:
  - the name of the patient for whom the medicament has been prescribed
  - the name and address of the practitioner who has supplied the product
  - directions for use and dosage, which may be omitted if the use has been explained to the patient and substituted by: 'to be used as directed'. (However, the authors feel that directions for use should always be written down.)
  - 'for external use only' if it is a liquid preparation for topical use.
- Bottles must be fluted (ribbed) when dispensing remedies prescribed for external use only.

Summary

- A licence is necessary to supply a medicinal product unless:

  - the remedy is a herbal remedy and
  - the remedy is prepared for administration to a particular person who has consulted the practitioner and been personally seen by them, or
  - the product is supplied in the original wrappings of the manufacturer without any claims being made by the supplier, e.g. as in a shop.
- All products supplied by the practitioner should be labelled. Labels should be typed or indelible ink used. The label must contain the following information:
  - name of the patient

— name and address of the practitioner

— directions for use

— 'for external use only' if it is a liquid preparation for topical use.

• Liquid preparations for topical use must be dispensed in a fluted (ribbed) bottle.

HOSPITAL PROTOCOLS AND GUIDELINES

A protocol, directorate or set of guidelines for the practice of aromatherapy and the specific use of essential oils within that practice is a key document required by each hospital. This document should set out which essential oils are to be used, how they are to be used, by whom and for how long.

The following, adapted from the Community Health Sheffield (NHS Trust) protocol will give the nurse aromatherapist or aromatologist wishing to prepare such a document the general guidelines to be observed. For the purposes of this document, 'accountable practitioner' refers to the professional aromatherapist or aromatologist and 'healthcare assistant' refers to the person working under the supervision of the said professional aromatherapist or aromatologist.

Local protocol

1. Permission to use essential oils on a patient or client must be requested from that patient or client's GP or consultant before commencement of the treatment and may be requested by the on-site nursing staff.

Other members of the multidisciplinary team will be made aware that aromatherapy is being used as part of a treatment plan agreed with the patient/client and carer.

2. All patients or clients must be referred to the accountable practitioner. After receipt of the referral a letter of confirmation will be sent to the patient or client giving details of the consultation date.

3. It is essential that accountable practitioners and healthcare assistants are aware of and have studied their Health Authority policy document.

4. Persons using aromatherapy or aromatology must be one of the following:

a. an accountable practitioner, i.e. a healthcare professional who is a full member of an aromatherapy or aromatic medicine association, or

b. a healthcare assistant, i.e.:

— a healthcare professional who has attended an introductory programme on aromatherapy of at least 2 days if external to the hospital plus extra tuition by the accountable practitioner, or

— a healthcare professional who has attended an introductory programme on aromatherapy of at least 2 days run by an accountable practitioner.

A healthcare assistant may give massage to the parts of the body listed in 7d below, except for the back, face and full-body massage, which may be given only if the said assistant already holds a qualification in full-body massage.

5. The patient/client approach must satisfy or include all of the following points:

a. Aromatherapy treatments will be offered only after full consultation with and acceptance by the patient/client; together with the healthcare assistant if required.

b. An assessment, including the plan of treatment, will be offered and fully explained to the patient/client; this may include any one or more of the methods of approach mentioned in 8 below. The final decision on a treatment plan, when approved by all parties, will be officially documented in the nursing care plan of the named patient/client.

c. Before using any essential oils on a client or patient, they should be tested on that patient/client in the dilution—and carrier—which will be used for the treatment. To do this, place a small amount of the mix on one of the following places: inner elbow, inside wrist, in the groin, behind the knee or just behind the ear. It should be left for 12–24 hours, covered with a light porous dressing if necessary. If there is no irritation or reddening of the skin, treatment may proceed.

d. At all times the dignity of the patient or client shall be respected. When giving massage, any part of the body not being massaged shall be covered in accordance with the ethics and code of professional conduct set out in the professional practice document of the ISPA, IAM and BCMA Codes of Practice.

e. The location of treatment will vary according to each patient/client's needs. If a full-body massage is entailed this should normally be given in the patient/client's private room (using curtains in a ward situation). The possible exception to this may be a hand massage, but the wishes of the patient/client should be respected with regard to privacy if required.

6. The treatment should be allocated for each named client for a period of no more than 3 weeks, when the prescription/treatment should be reassessed.

7. Types of treatments will be selected from the following list according to the individual patient or client's needs, using essential oils appropriate to that patient/client:

a. inhalation (dry or with steam), with or without an electric room diffuser. Electric diffusers must meet the requirements of the Health and Safety at Work Act. No night-light vaporizers or ceramic rings are to be used because of fire risk.

b. baths—foot, hand, sitz or full-body. Oil prescriptions should be added after the bath has been run.

c. topical application, without massage.

d. massage—full-body, arm, hand, leg, foot, back, face, neck, shoulders, scalp. Relevant contraindications to full-body massage will be taken into account.

e. compresses.

f. ingestion.
   — anal suppositories
   — vaginal pessaries
   — orally for digestive disorders: only with the consultant's permission and only if insured for the internal use of essential oils with the IAM or the RCN.

8. Essential oil prescriptions must satisfy the following requirements:

a. Only genuine therapeutic quality essential oils are to be used, i.e. not essential oils of perfume quality, but only those which can be traced to source and which originated from plants grown by natural farming methods or from biologically grown or wild plants—this is the responsibility of the accountable practitioner.

b. Only unrefined or cold-pressed and unrefined carrier oils are to be used, from plants grown using natural farming methods.

c. The accountable practitioner will use the number of drops and amount of carrier oil laid down by the accredited aromatherapy or aromatology course followed.

d. The prescription bottle must be made up only by the accountable practitioner for a named patient/client's use only—it is not to be used on any other patient or client.

e. A prescription card must be allocated to each patient or client, recording the following:
   — name of patient or client
   — address or ward number/name
   — date of birth
   — name of GP/consultant
   — details of prescription, including carriers where used
   — details of administration of prescription
   — frequency of administration of prescription.

The prescription/administration card must be signed on application of the prescription, by the authorized accountable practitioner or healthcare assistant.

f. The bottle label must contain:
   — the name of the patient or client
   — the date of expiry (i.e. 3 weeks)
   — the directions for administration.

The prescription will not be added to, substituted nor changed in any way without consultation with the accountable practitioner.

g. Any change of prescription must be noted on the prescription card by the accountable practitioner; and the old treatment bottle is to be returned to the accountable practitioner.

h. Reassessment of all aromatherapy prescriptions must take place within the 3 week period of the prescription date on the label.

i. All treatment bottles are to be returned to the accountable practitioner (regardless of a review) after the expiry date.

9. Recording of clinical data.

Patient or client response (positive and/or negative) to the prescription is to be clearly and informatively recorded on the named patient or client's nursing care plan.

10. The safety aspects of using essential oils must be observed (see also COSHH regulations, Ch. 3):

a. Storage of all essential oil prescriptions must take place in
   — the locked external medicine/dangerous drug cupboard, or
   — the locked external preparations cupboard, or
   — a locked cupboard in the occupational therapy department.

All essential oil prescriptions must be treated with the same respect as any other prescribed medicine.

b. The toxicity of, and reactions to, essential oils must be borne in mind at all times by accountable practitioners and healthcare assistants who must be aware of the following possible hazards and the consequences of their abuse:
   — neurotoxicity
   — dermal toxicity
   — dermal sensitivity
   — possible respiratory sensitivity
   — phototoxicity.

[Author's note: see Ch. 3 and Appendix B.]

c. In incidents with essential oils requiring first aid, the following points must be observed:
   — should a patient or client accidentally swallow any pure essential oil, contact the emergency services (999) then contact the accountable practitioner at once
   — should a patient or client get any pure essential oil into the eye, wash the eye immediately with vegetable oil only—not saline solution—then contact the accountable practitioner at once

   — should any adverse reaction be presented, stop using the prescription and contact the accountable aromatherapist or aromatologist.

d. Prohibited or restricted essential oils. It is important that accountable practitioners and healthcare assistants are aware of essential oils which:
   — must not be used at all
   — must be used with caution. If it is found possible to purchase these over the counter, this should be reported to one of the aromatherapy trade associations.

[Authors' note: see Appendices B.4 and B.5.]

11. General points to bear in mind include the following:

a. Essential oils must not be used undiluted over a large area of skin.

b. Essential oils must never be used undiluted on or near the eyes.

c. It must be understood that excess use, i.e. too high a concentration, may lead to headaches or nausea, or can lead to the opposite effect to that intended (e.g. a high concentration of *Lavandula angustifolia* can produce insomnia instead of sleep).

d. It is suggested that a limited range of essential oils be selected carefully and specifically to cover the requirements of the health conditions and side-effects from orthodox drugs found in a healthcare situation. Further essential oils can always be added if or when found to be necessary.

The following have proved to be the most useful and cover all health topics mentioned in this book:

- *Boswellia carteri* [FRANKINCENSE]
- *Cananga odorata* [YLANG YLANG]
- *Chamaemelum nobile* (formerly *Anthemis nobilis*) [ROMAN CHAMOMILE]
- *Chamomilla recutita* (= *Matricaria chamomilla)* [GERMAN CHAMOMILE]
- *Citrus bergamia* [BERGAMOT]
- *Citrus limon* [LEMON]
- *Citrus reticulata* [MANDARIN, TANGERINE]
- *Citrus aurantium* var. *amara* (flos, fol. and per.) [NEROLI BIGARADE, PETITGRAIN BIGARADE, ORANGE BIGARADE]

- *Cupressus sempervirens* [CYPRESS]
- *Eucalyptus smithii* [GULLY GUM]
- *Foeniculum vulgare* [FENNEL]
- *Hyssopus officinalis* [HYSSOP]
- *Juniperus communis* (fruct. and ram.) [JUNIPER BERRY AND TWIG]
- *Lavandula angustifolia* [LAVENDER]
- *Lavandula × intermedia* 'Super' [LAVANDIN]
- *Melaleuca alternifolia* [TEA TREE]
- *Melaleuca viridiflora* [NIAOULI] (if genuine)
- *Mentha × piperita* [PEPPERMINT]
- *Ocimum basilicum* var. *album* [EUROPEAN BASIL]
- *Origanum majorana* [SWEET MARJORAM]
- *Pelargonium graveolens* [GERANIUM]
- *Piper nigrum* [BLACK PEPPER]
- *Rosmarinus officinalis* ct. cineole, ct. camphor [ROSEMARY]
- *Salvia sclarea* [CLARY]
- *Santalum album* [SANDALWOOD]
- *Syzygium aromaticum* (flos) (formerly *Eugenia caryophyllata*) [CLOVE BUD]
- *Thymus vulgaris* ct. alcohol [SWEET THYME]
- *Zingiber officinale* [GINGER].

Guidelines

Together with a protocol, each hospital usually has guidelines on the specific uses of essential oils within their field of care. Typical inclusions in a general set of guidelines would be:

- local contraindications
- conditions which can be treated
- essential oils which can be used for these conditions, including sample prescriptions
- methods by which, in that particular hospital, the selected essential oils can be administered for the specified conditions
- method of recording treatments and prescriptions of essential oils.

Summary

This chapter has shown the great steps that have already been taken towards self-regulation of aromatherapy in the UK, alongside the practice guidelines created by several health authorities. It is to be hoped that more health provision agencies will welcome these positive moves, and that the suggested policies and protocols will be adapted and applied where appropriate.

REFERENCES

Baker S 1995 AOC update. The Aromatherapist 2(2): 8–9 (see also pp 4–5)

Baker S 1997 AOC update November 1997. Aromatherapy World, Distillation, Winter 1997: 12

Barker A 1994 Aromatherapy in a hospital setting. Aromatherapy World, Spring: 6–7

Boyd E M, Pearson G L 1946 On the expectorant action of essential oils. American Journal of Medical Science, 211: 602–610

Buckle J 1997 Clinical aromatherapy in nursing. Arnold, London

Byrne K 1997 Ingestion of essential oils—food for thought. Simply Essential 26: 34–36

Cawthorne A 1991 Aromatherapy on trial. Aromanews 30: 7–8

Declaration of Helsinki, adopted by the 18th World Medical. Assembly, Helsinki, Finland, June 1994, as last amended at the 48th General Assembly, Somerset West, Republic of South Africa, October 1996

Eccles S 1997 [Editorial]. Aromatherapy Quarterly 55: 5

Gattefossé R-M 1993 Gattefossé's aromatherapy. Daniel, Saffron Walden

Griggs B 1997 New green pharmacy. Vermilion, London

Integrated Healthcare 1997 A way forward for the next five years? The Foundation for Integrated Medicine, London

Lautié R, Passebecq A 1979 Aromatherapy: the use of plant essences in healing. Thorsons, Wellingborough

Lundie S 1994 Introducing and applying aromatherapy within the NHS. The Aromatherapist 1(2): 30–35

Maury M 1989 Marguerite Maury's guide to aromatherapy. The secret of life and youth. Daniel, Saffron Walden

May B, Kuntz H, Keiser N M, Köhler S 1996 Efficacy of a fixed peppermint oil/caraway oil combination in non-ulcer dyspepsia. Arzneimittel-Forschung/Drug Research 46(II) 12: 1149–1153

Price S 1983 Practical aromatherapy. Thorsons, Wellingborough

Price S 1985 Aromatherapy training notes. Shirley Price International College of Aromatherapy, Hinckley

Rankin-Box D 1992 Appropriate therapies for nurses to practise. Nursing Standard 6(50) (Complementary therapies special supplement): 51–52

RCCM 1997 Public usage of complementary medicine: an overview. Research Council for Complementary Medicine Information Service, London

Riek 1994 COST B4 Unconventional medicine in Europe. Responses to the COST B4 questionnaire. European Commission, Luxembourg

Thomas K, Fall M, Parry G, Nicholl J 1995 National survey of access to complementary health care via general practice. University of Sheffield

Tisserand R 1977 The art of aromatherapy. Daniel, Saffron Walden

United Kingdom Central Council 1989 Exercising accountability. UKCC, 23 Portland Place, London

United Kingdom Central Council 1992a Code of professional conduct. June. UKCC, 23 Portland Place, London

United Kingdom Central Council 1992b The scope of professional practice. June. UKCC, 23 Portland Place, London

United Kingdom Central Council 1992c Standards for the administration of medicines. October. UKCC, 23 Portland Place, London

United Kingdom Central Council 1996 Guidelines for professional practice. UKCC, 23 Portland Place, London

University of Exeter 1997 Professional organisation of complementary medicine in the United Kingdom. Centre for Complementary Health Studies, University of Exeter

Valnet J 1980 The practice of aromatherapy. Daniel, Saffron Walden

Vickers 1995 COST Action B4 Unconventional medicine. First annual report 1993–94. European Commission, Luxembourg

Aromatherapy worldwide

CHAPTER CONTENTS

Introduction

The practice of aromatherapy varies widely across the globe. In some countries, such as France, phytotherapy (which includes aromatology—the study of essential oils) is an established branch of medicine for which essential oils may be prescribed by the doctors concerned, usually for use by application to various parts of the body (not massage), per os, rectum and vagina, compresses, gargles or in a diffuser. In other countries, such as South Africa, aromatherapy is in its infancy, and is practised in hospitals using mainly massage, and on a voluntary basis, by aromatherapists and interested nurses.

This chapter examines aromatherapy use within the healthcare systems of 16 countries, representing a range of different stages of development, implementation and styles of practice.

EUROPE

BELGIUM
Present position

In Belgium no standards or certification in aromatherapy exist at present. Although the laws are quite severe concerning the exercise of medical activities, many so-called 'therapeutes' are working illegally with different methods (homoeopathy, acupuncture, the use of more spiritual disciplines, etc.).

Recently, however, a move has been instigated by the government to legalize four former 'alternative' therapies: acupuncture, chiropractic, homoeopathy and osteopathy. It will then be more difficult for people without a medical background and the relative standard of study to exercise these four therapies.

Those more inclined to use aromatherapy are the paramedical practitioners (osteopathy, etc.) and healthcare workers (care of the elderly, etc.). However, there is a great lack of information, especially about quality and safety issues. Essential oils are now subject to the new herb regulations and need to be noted for oral use in preparations; some are not allowed for this use any more. Non-oral use is regulated by the new European Cosmetics law.

Training

The only courses that have been given during the past few years were for herbalists—mainly directed to professionals and shop owners. Recently, however, health shop organizations and suppliers of health products have managed to revive the 'herbalist' certification, which is now officially accepted.

Courses are given in official professional continuous education centres (Vlaams Institute voor het Zelfstandig Ondernemen—VISO), sponsored by the government to update the knowledge of small companies, although there is only very limited education on essential oils during this 2 year course; aromatherapy is given as an additional course for those interested in this therapy. This is also the case for other schools of naturopathy throughout Belgium, all from different organizations and backgrounds.

Many elderly care centres and beauty care institutions are starting to use essential oils intensively.

According to Michel Vanhove, who teaches aromatherapy for the VISO, the picture is similar in the French-speaking part of Belgium, although aromatherapy there is more inclined to the medical aspect, with more doctors being involved.

FRANCE

In France aromatherapy is a branch of medicine generally included with medical herbalism (phytotherapy) and used by medical doctors already involved in alternative or complementary medicine. Thousands of doctors, hundreds of pharmacies and some analytical and bacteriological laboratories are involved in aromatology and phytotherapy. The profession of aromatherapist does not really exist in France and the use of essential oils in body massage, as it is practised in the UK, has only recently started to become known.

The development of natural therapies

In order to understand its medical development, it is necessary to view the position of aromatherapy in the larger context of the range of the different natural therapies in France.

The first form of natural therapy to be practised in France was homoeopathy, and all French homoeopaths are medical doctors. Natural therapies are taught as a medical specialty, over 3 years, at Bobigny Medical University near Paris. Doctors who follow this teaching are called naturothérapeutes, in order to distinguish them from naturopaths, i.e. naturopaths who are not medical doctors. Such naturopaths, like osteopaths, are not legally allowed to practise—though many do. Several other university medical departments organize postgraduate teaching in different alternative fields, including phyto-aromatherapy.

The Institut Méditerranéen de Documentation, d'Enseignement et de Recherche sur les Plantes Médicinales (IMDERPLAM) runs regular study courses on the medicinal properties of plants, including the medicinal properties of essential oils; one of the courses covers this theory together with massage and holistic oil selection (taught by the authors). The publication in 1993 and 1994 of two of Shirley Price's books in French has aroused great interest in the UK style of aromatherapy in France. This, together with the aromatherapy taught at IMDERPLAM, the courses currently taught (in French) by the authors in the Drôme valley and the fact that many kinesothérapeutes (massage therapists) use essential oils in their treatments, suggests that aromatherapy as practised in the UK will begin to develop in France. Already the general public can buy essential oils in health food stores and from many markets in the south of France. It is mostly doctors already practising a form of natural therapy who use essential oils and, in most cases, they use them along with phytotherapy. This means that the final prescription will generally include different plant extracts (e.g. tinctures or a concentrated form in gelules) and essential oils to be taken internally (orally and/or as pessaries and suppositories) or, less often, to be applied externally. The external application usually involves much higher concentrations than are used in the UK, ranging from the neat essential oils to a 5–10% dilution for good penetration of the skin, for example on the thoracic area (see Dr Pénoël's case study in Ch. 4 p. 64).

Patients take their prescription to the local pharmacist, and phytoaromatic preparations are made up either there or by one of the larger pharmacies which supply the smaller ones. There are several hundred pharmacies which stock a range of essential oils of therapeutic quality. Homoeopathy is still largely refunded by the national health system and, although phytoaromatic preparations also used to be refunded, the law was altered in January 1991 to change this situation. The price paid by patients to the pharmacist for phytoaromatic preparations could then no longer be claimed back from the insurance system, thus the individual had to bear the total cost.

The 1991 decision was a shock not only to the patients, but also to the laboratories. However, the French pharmacists' union decided to take legal action and, after 4 years of struggle, the case was brought in front of the Supreme Court, where the government lost and the union won. The law was rescinded and the cost of phyto-aromatherapeutic preparations, when prescribed by medical doctors, could once again be claimed on the insurance system.

Interestingly, insurance companies are forced to admit that, for instance in the case of influenza epidemics, the aromatherapeutic management costs less and, where applicable, is more effective than allopathic methods.

The reinstatement of the original situation plays a significant role in presenting to the rest of the world a picture of a system that has proved its usefulness and its efficacy for more than 40 years.

Main medical applications of essential oils

Should anyone enquire about the main purpose of aromatherapy in the UK, the answer would probably be 'relief of stress and nervous tension', whereas in France that same question would elicit the answer 'infectious conditions, mainly of the respiratory system'. Other infections often treated with essential oil prescriptions in France are those of the skin, digestive system, urinary tract and genital area, and common viral diseases.

A significant step in the fine tuning of the struggle against infection was the introduction of the aromatogram. This involves the testing of individual essential oils or blends against specific strains of bacteria or fungi taken from the patient (see Ch. 4). Several bacteriological laboratories perform aromatograms and prescriptions are made in accordance with the results of the tests, ensuring that the oils used by the pharmacist are the same as those tested by the laboratory. The amount of data accumulated from aromatograms over the years sheds new light on the way microbes are considered and individual susceptibility, not only in infectious disease but also in a subtle manner in different pathologies, such as inflammatory and even autoimmune diseases, as well as psychological problems.

Another interesting approach in France involves the analysis of different blood proteins and the comparison of two tests, one taken before and the other after a period of treatment with essential oils (in this instance it is better to use one essential oil rather than a blend). Here again, a wealth of biochemical data has been accumulated by different laboratories, which confirm the powerful action of essential oils. By treating the underlying chronic and hidden infection, where present, results can be obtained in many different pathological areas.

Aromatherapy is implemented in all medical fields, including allergies, inflammatory and immune dysfunctions, rheumatology, dermatology, gynaecology and hormonal imbalances, cardiovascular disease, digestive system problems, and nervous, psychological and sexual dysfunctions. In each case, the level of action of essential oils will vary according both to the specific diagnosis and to the way the patient is prepared to become involved in the healing process itself.

Another important use of aromatherapy in France, and one where no placebo or psychological effect can be said to intervene, is in emergency situations involving burns, wounds, external trauma, etc. The successful use of essential oils in such acute cases provides strong confirmation of their efficacy.

The doctor's frame of reference

In daily medical aromatherapy practice, it is important to distinguish between the different ways of prescribing essential oils that vary according to the frame of reference chosen by the practitioner—allopathic, naturopathic, etc. Essential oils can be considered as blends of natural molecules and prescribed by a doctor in the same way as any other pharmaceutical drug. In a very first approach, any allopathic physician can be taught to use a specific essential oil for a specific condition. An acute disease, tonsillitis for example, can be successfully treated by an essential oil, e.g. *Melaleuca alternifolia* [TEA TREE]. But when dealing with chronic cases or repetitive acute ones keeping to this allopathic frame of reference, even though using essential oils, will soon reach a limit of effectiveness.

Long experience by Pénoël and Verdet, both doctors and phytotherapists, shows clearly that essential oils give the best therapeutic results when used in the frame of reference of natural medicine (see Ch. 4). Pénoël has always taught that aromatherapy is the spearhead of natural medicine, and that refusing to take a holistic approach eventually leads to disappointment. For instance, seeking to improve an allergic condition without paying attention to nutrition represents a loss of time for the therapist and a waste of money for the patient. Similarly, endeavouring to help scar tissue formation on a leg ulcer oozing pus, without understanding that this ulcer might represent an effort by the organism to expel toxins, would be tantamount to 'setting the fox to mind the geese'.

In France doctors trained as naturothérapeutes take the time to analyse all the elements of the lifestyle of their patients so that they can give advice on how to correct those that seem to play a role in the occurrence or the continuation of the disease. Their use of essential oils is part of this overall holistic approach, with great attention paid to the patient's state of mind.

The way ahead

To establish in France the profession of aromatherapist as it exists in the UK is at least as large and important a task as that of opening the British medical profession to clinical aromatherapy and aromatology. In France, however, there are certain obstacles to be overcome. For instance, the word 'massage' is reserved for those who have a diploma of physiotherapy (called masseurs/kinésithérapeutes). Graduates of IMDERPLAM and Shirley Price International College of Aromatherapy (SPICA) who already hold this qualification may practise aromatherapy legally but those without it cannot advertise their skills and may not lawfully practise.

What is needed is a change in the educational and legal systems to enable people who are neither medical personnel nor beauty therapists to receive full training in aromatherapy and to practise professionally. The successful UK model could serve as a prototype for creating aromatherapy training schools and establishing this valuable profession in France. It is to be hoped that, as a result, aromatherapy will become available in French hospitals in the same way as it is in the UK.

A close collaboration between UK and French aromatherapy professionals will be of benefit not only to those two countries, but to other countries also wishing to establish aromatherapy as part of their healthcare system.

GERMANY

The word 'aromatherapy' became known in Germany in the mid 1980s, but therapy with essential oils is still very young. Essential oils can be bought in all pharmacies and in many health shops, tea shops and markets. Many of these are of very poor quality and are used only in aroma lamps, although one or two firms do go out of their way to procure genuine essential oils. As in the UK, no medicinal claims can be made on the labels of bottles containing essential oils.

Aromatherapy association

An association, Forum Essenzia, has been set up for aromatherapists and gives therapeutic workshops on aromatherapy in which the necessity of using quality essential oils for therapeutic purposes is emphasized. Many of these workshops are directed at nurses, heilpraktikers (those qualified in natural medicine), physiotherapists, doctors and pharmacists, as aromatherapy can be practised legally only by doctors and heilpraktikers. Other health professionals, such as nurses and occupational therapists, working in hospitals are allowed to use essential oils to alleviate minor conditions, e.g. dry skin or headache, but must have permission from the doctor in charge of the patient if they wish to use essential oils for more serious medical conditions. Doctors tend to leave the choice of oils to the nurse concerned, as they themselves are unlikely to know very much about them— although there are a few doctors who use essential oils in their own practices. The nurse must keep an updated written progress report of which essential oil is used, how often and how many drops. Any changes in treatment must also be recorded and all improvements shown.

Essential oil use

Conditions treated in hospitals include anxiety, difficult breathing, pneumonia, scars and wounds, digestive problems, sleeping problems, varicose ulcers, terminal illness and birth. Nurses also work in the fields of endocrinology and psychocancer therapy and with patients in psychosomatic wards. The essential oils most often used are:

- *Aniba rosaeodora* (ROSEWOOD) for depressive sleeplessness and grief
- *Cedrus atlantica* (CEDARWOOD) for difficulty in breathing and anxiety
- *Citrus limon* (expressed) [LEMON] for fever, influenza, bronchitis and sleepiness
- *Foeniculum vulgare* [FENNEL] for flatulence
- *Lavandula angustifolia* [LAVENDER] for sleeplessness, headache, pain and shock and Dupruytren's contracture
- *Melaleuca alternifolia* [TEA TREE] for *ulcera cruris* (leg ulcers), decubitus ulcers (bedsores) and candida

- *Melaleuca leucadendron* [NIAOULI] for neuralgia, respiratory tract diseases and skin troubles
- *Mentha × piperita* (PEPPERMINT) for headaches
- *Pelargonium graveolens* [GERANIUM] for depression, pregnancy and childbirth
- *Rosa damascena* (distilled) [ROSE OTTO] for women's complaints and skin diseases
- *Rosmarinus officinalis* ct. cineole/camphor [ROSEMARY] for headaches, poor concentration, poor tone and low blood pressure
- *Thymus vulgaris* ct. linalool [SWEET THYME] for laryngitis, coughs and respiratory conditions.

Methods used

Massage is only one of the methods used in aromatherapy nursing care, and the technique is not that of classical massage but gentle stroking or embrocation. This means that nurses trained in aromacare can apply the essential oils to the body without having a recognized qualification in massage.

Other methods include inhalation, sponge baths (in cases of fever), compresses and foot massage—and foot baths for pain control.

Training and standards

By using complementary medicine in conjunction with conventional medicine, nurses hope to provide their patients with additional optimum care. Although there is no set training or general policy for nurses using essential oils and most nurses acquire their knowledge from weekend workshops and by reading aromatherapy books, a few schools for midwives and nurses now include some instruction on aromatherapy in their curriculi.

Some nurses in Munich meet regularly to work out a Code of Practice for the use of essential oils, combined with the ADL (Activities of Daily Living) code. Nursing care plans help nurses to see the patient as a holistic being and the ADL code is the basis for everyday living.

There are three levels of training in the use of essential oils:

- aromatherapy—for doctors and state approved naturopaths; this study includes the internal use of essential oils

- aromacare—for all other health professionals (such as nurses)
- aroma counselling—for students in all other professions.

Anatomy, physiology and pathology are taught only in schools for naturopaths, physiotherapists and others already having a profession in healthcare. Courses in aromatherapy independent of those within the medical profession are held in Germany, but the resultant qualification gives the status of aroma counsellor, not aromatherapist.

The way ahead

Although a new German law appears to have given the same scientific status to alternative medicinal treatments as to orthodox treatments (a fact which has angered some in the medical profession), the International Fragrance Association (IFRA) is strongly against essential oils being registered as healing agents. In the near future a meeting is to be held of national cosmetic producers, essential oil companies and lawyers to discuss the problems involved. However, so far as the therapy itself is concerned, it is generally accepted that, as alternative therapies are popular with the German public, it would be difficult for any government to remove them from the list of approved treatments.

NORWAY

Eighty per cent of the Norwegian population have tried complementary therapies over the 2 to 3 years that the government have agreed to allow complementary therapies in hospitals, should patients wish to receive it. These include aromatherapy, acupuncture, reflexology, homoeopathy, kinesiology, chiropractic and phytotherapy, among others, the first therapies to be tried being reflexology, healing and acupuncture. As in the UK, aromatherapy was introduced through the beauty therapy profession; Shirley Price, Eve Taylor and Arnould Taylor were the first to teach there in the early 1980s. After some years nurses became conscious of the immense possibilities of this gentle but effective therapy and aromatherapy began creeping into the practice of health professionals, both inside and outside hospitals, together with other complementary therapies.

Introduction into healthcare

Astrid Torgauten (a children's nurse) and Margareth Thomte (an aromatherapy teacher)—both SPICA trained—gave lectures to midwives and children's nurses in Oslo and Akershus respectively. Midwives then started to make special blends of essential oils in a carrier for pregnant women to ease back pain and neck and shoulder tension. Foot massage for swollen feet and legs, and hand massage, also became popular. Nurses are now finding that the staff are positive, and curious enough to come to the nurse aromatherapists for treatment. Many doctors are still sceptical but, of these, most allow the use of *Lavandula angustifolia* for its sedative effect in the bath, for inhalation and for short massage sequences.

Outside hospital settings, aromatherapy is beginning to make an impact in health care. Some doctors send their patients to aromatherapists for problems such as fibromyalgia, rheumatism, muscular pain and stiffness (with physical and psychological background), and headaches.

Several companies in Norway, including Microsoft Norway SA, have discovered that those of their staff who receive aromatherapy massage work more efficiently, use less medication and are off sick less frequently.

Homoeopathy has been used with aromatherapy with very good results; aromatherapy and ear acupuncture have also been found to work very well together for sinus problems and chest infections.

Aromatherapy associations

Norske Aromaterapeuters Forening (NATF)—the Norwegian Aromatherapists Association—was formed in 1990. Although this began as an association for aromatherapists trained in different schools, it gradually became an organization for aromatherapists trained in one school only. In 1994 a new NATF leader formed the Norske Aromaterapeuters Hoved Forening (NAHF).

There is an umbrella association, Norske Naturterapeuters Hovedorganisasjon (NNH), which caters for therapies such as reflexology, aromatherapy and kinesiology, and in 1997 a Norwegian association for herbal therapy, phytotherapy, aromatherapy and aromatology was formed. This is an association for aromatherapists, phytotherapists, Norwegian distillers of essential oils and doctors with an interest in complementary therapies. It is hopefully meant to be an umbrella association for everyone working with essential oils and other plant extracts.

Complementary therapy in the public health service

In 1997, the Social and Health Department officially appointed the Aarbaake committee to review questions about complementary medicine and therapy. The aims of this committee are to obtain and systemize the knowledge in the different disciplines of alternative medicine—in other words, to discover the extent to which documented effects are proven from the different forms of alternative medicine.

After viewing all documentation, the committee will evaluate what kind of role the different forms of alternative medicine may have within the public health service. The committee will also draw up a proposition as to how alternative medicine and its practitioners may eventually be regulated.

The committee is divided into three groups:

1. to view the value of alternative and complementary medicine
2. to view different documentation
3. to view the legal points.

The Aarbakke committee's report came up for consideration on 15 December 1998 and is now under discussion.

Training

Therapists within aromatherapy and other natural therapies vary in their educational training—from a workshop of 2 to 3 days up to training taking several years. Because of these large variations, an educational council of tutors in natural therapies was formed in 1993; Skolerädet i Naturterapeutisk Utdannelse (SNU), the School Council for Education in Natural Therapies. This soon split into two factions: those who believed a minimum standard of in-house training should be 200 hours over a minimum of 1 year (plus qualifications in anatomy, physiology and pathology, if not already held), and those who believed in less.

Norske Høgskoleräd for Naturmedisin (NHRN), the Norwegian College Council in Natural Medicine, an education council for complementary therapies, was formed in 1994 by those going for standards above the minimum, or more. This council has doctors on the board who are interested in complementary therapies; these doctors are also advisors for setting a qualification standard which would be acceptable to the Social and Health Department.

Research

At HIO (Høgskolen in Oslo) four medical technician students became interested in essential oils. In 1996 they researched the scientific documentation regarding the antibacterial effects of essential oils. They found several reports which concluded that essential oils have an antibacterial effect, but every one of the experiments was an in vitro study. If essential oils showed an antibacterial effect in studies in vivo, then essential oils could be an alternative to antibiotics. In the spring of 1997 these four students did some pre-experiments and discovered that none of the methods used in studies in vitro were sensitive enough to be used in studies in vivo. They therefore had to do a study of methodology. Table 17.1 shows the preliminary results which they believe can be further improved.

The way ahead

Essential oils are used in moderation but Norway still has a long way to go before aromatherapy can (if it ever will) enter the Norwegian hospitals as practised in the UK. Time alone will tell; the Aabaake committee report is awaited.

Research on attitude is already done, and within those responsible for healthcare there are different attitudes towards alternative and complementary therapies. However, more information about essential oil chemistry and the effects of these on the body must be given to professionals and others interested in using the oils.

The goal must be that orthodox medicine and complementary therapies work together in the future for the best quality of life in public health services and for the people generally.

Table 17.1 *Thymus vulgaris* ct. thymol diluted in different fluids sereus ATCC 11778				
	Diluent			
Dilution ratio	Almond oil	Absolute alcohol	0.2% Teepol	Absolute alcohol Agar with 0.2% TP
	mm	mm	mm	mm
1:1	25	27	30	40
1:2	14	24	11	32
1:4	6	41	7	27
1:8	0	14	6	22
1:16	0	8	8	17
1:32	0	6	6	11
1:64	0	0	0	7
1:128	0	0	0	5
1:256	0	0	0	0
Control	0	0	0	0

REPUBLIC OF IRELAND

Use of aromatherapy

Complementary therapies are used in Irish hospices, AIDS clinics and some hospitals. However, healthcare is to a large extent paid for by private insurance in the Republic of Ireland and as complementary therapies are not available on public healthcare their use in primary care is limited. Nevertheless, a tremendous amount of interest is shown by nurses, as in the UK, and it is appreciated that teaching/learning guidelines and a Code of Practice are needed, with direction from the Irish Nursing Board.

Regarding aromatherapy, the situation is comparable to the UK in that each hospital needs to discuss the introduction of aromatherapy with its Board of Management and Department of Nursing. Some will actively encourage patients with conditions such as stress-related complaints, back pain and oedema to attend for aromatherapy treatment. It is easier for them to see the benefits of massage, and this points to the fact that much education, with back-up from research, is called for in the field of essential oils.

As in the UK, the main areas where interest is shown in applying aromatherapy are maternity care, terminal care and care for the elderly. Public health nurses (the equivalent of health visitors) and nurses in various areas of specialty are showing a great interest in training but the majority of aromatherapy is carried out in private practice at present. There also exists the problem of inadequate, or lack of, training among nurses and therefore the attitude of doctors and consultants is very variable, many being sceptical. Some will actively encourage patients with conditions such as stress-related complaints, back pain and oedema to attend aromatherapy, whilst others can be openly cynical, especially of those practitioners whose training is short or non-existent.

Aromatherapy is used in a limited way in palliative care in both vaporizers and hand massage. A trial study was carried out by Tullamore General Hospital in 1994 regarding the use of essential oils in assisting sleep for the elderly (see Ch. 14). Another study is being carried out at O'Connell Court in Cork (a residential unit for sufferers of Alzheimer's disease); however, at the time of writing, the results are not yet published.

Many hospices have aromatherapists giving part-body treatments to the patients and using essential oils on a regular basis. There is a very positive feedback coming from the patients themselves and their families of the tremendous benefits these treatments have for the well-being of the patients.

Aromatherapy is being practised in several hospices and hospitals, among them St Patrick's Hospice in Cork and the Bons Secours hospital, where aromatherapy is mainly available in the maternity unit. Establishments in Dublin, Limerick, Tipperary and Galway, providing psychiatric services for people with learning difficulties, are all using aromatherapy, with great benefit to patients and clients.

The Roman Catholic Church

The Irish Province of the Hospitaller Order of St John of God (a worldwide religious organization within the Roman Catholic Church dedicated to service in the community) is an Order which recognizes the value of complementary medicine. The Order provides psychiatric health services, services for the elderly and those with learning difficulties and it supports, as far as is practicable, staff who wish to train in aromatherapy, massage and reflexology. These therapies are used in the Order's work and they are recognized as bringing positive benefits to patients and clients.

Training

Mary Cavanagh of Wicklow, apart from teaching in aromatherapy schools, has also been teaching, for the past 10 years, nurses, occupational therapists and care workers in hospitals and special needs residential centres throughout the Republic of Ireland. Much teaching has also been carried out throughout the country within the North Eastern Health Board by Monica Mackin, with particular emphasis on the Disability and

Psychiatric Services. The calming effects of essential oils have been particularly noticed here on clients with aggressive behaviour and tea tree oil has been used to good effect to irrigate wounds which were MRSA (methicillin resistant *Staphylococcus aureus*) positive, all swabs being negative to MRSA after treatment.

The inauguration of the Irish branch of the International Society of Professional Aromatherapists (ISPA) in 1996 was a major step forward for the therapy, which is growing rapidly in Ireland and will no doubt soon reach the same level as in the UK.

SWEDEN

Despite being introduced in the early 1980s, aromatherapy is still not very widespread in Sweden, where not many complementary therapies are practised.

The healthcare system does not yet accept nor apply complementary therapies, perhaps because there is no tradition of natural or complementary medicine. Despite this, many healthcare employees, such as nurses and people working with the elderly, children or handicapped individuals, are beginning to show a great interest in aromatherapy though they cannot use it in their work. Aromatherapists are not yet allowed in the hospitals to work, not even on their own clients who may be in there.

Complementary therapy law

Aromatherapists outside the hospital work with classical aromatherapy, mostly massage and skincare. They are subject, along with other complementary practitioners, to a law called 'the quack's law'. This law states (together with other items) that:

1. it is forbidden to treat patients within the state healthcare system unless permission has been sought and obtained
2. children under 8 years of age may not be treated, although discussions are now taking place with a view to raising this age limit
3. venereal diseases and illnesses which may occur during pregnancy may not be treated, neither may diseases such as cancer, diabetes and epilepsy
4. all treatments must be on a face-to-face basis with the client.

If any of these laws are broken, a fine or a term in prison will be enforced. Not being knowledgeable about the laws is not acceptable as an excuse. The laws surrounding complementary therapies are tightening up every year and therapists are finding it hard to work within the very limited space left to them. It appears to be a question of politics and the feeling is that the government wishes to see complementary therapies and products banned completely from the market.

One reason for this may be that there was no great demand for other therapies (there being no tradition of complementary medicine in Sweden, and the healthcare system functions exceptionally well). This is changing slowly, albeit with difficulty, mainly because of state healthcare becoming so expensive and not always bringing the desired health benefits. The population is now demanding the right to choose its own form of medicine, though at the moment the issue is something of a 'political war'.

Aromatherapy association

There is an aromatherapy association in Sweden, the Swedish Aromatherapy Association, which was founded in 1992. It is the only one in Sweden and monitors the schools and their educational levels; it also has a close relationship with companies selling essential oils. It is hoped that this kind of cooperation will advance the use and knowledge of aromatherapy in Sweden.

SWITZERLAND

Except in certain cantons (e.g. Appenzell) the term 'therapist' is reserved in Switzerland for those in a profession approved by the federal government, such as doctors and certified naturopaths (e.g. physiotherapists and psychotherapists). The term 'aromatherapist' can therefore be used only by a therapist with medical qualifications. People trained in essential oil use who have no medical qualifications are therefore called 'aromatologists' (practising aromatherapy). In 1993 an association called VEROMA was set up to provide support for both aromatherapists and aromatologists, to regulate and promote standards for these professions across Switzerland, Germany and Austria.

The general interest and acceptability of the use of essential oils is growing, with some patients now requesting treatment with essential oils. However, it is not easy to introduce aromatherapy into hospitals—which are very conservative institutions. Not even traditional therapies such as homoeopathy are available to patients in general hospitals, though some doctors practise it privately.

Hospice use

The following is an account of Ueli Morgenthaler's work as a nurse and aromatologist at a hospice for AIDS patients in Zurich where, at the time of writing (December 1997), although the SBK's (see p. 293) module of aromatherapy training is known, their official guidelines regarding complementary therapies are not in place. When starting the job in 1992, Morgenthaler put a small selection of useful oils in the physiotherapy room next to the massage table. He mentioned his wish to start some aromatherapeutic activities in the hospice, and the doctor in charge was very encouraging. Sometimes, when there was a problem that ordinary medication could not solve satisfactorily, he or other nurses would ask Morgenthaler to suggest a choice of essential oils, the methods of use and either to carry out the massage treatments or to supervise the correct administration of the mix as inhalations, compresses or skin care and aromalamps (candles are not prohibited in this hospice). Permission was given to use the oils in any external form but there was no specific policy and no written guidelines.

Problems tackled in this way included: itching and very dry skin, coughs and shortness of breath, muscular pain, fever, eczema, rampant thrush, mood changes, depression, debility, fatigue and anxiety, and diarrhoea and vomiting.

As the nurses in the hospice became more interested in the essential oils (paid for by a special donation fund), they began to use them in aromalamps for their fragrancing action and for the effect they have on the mind.

At the beginning of 1994 the doctor in charge at the hospice mentioned the need to channel the healing arts knowledge of some individuals working at the hospice, so that it could be more professionally available to the patients. As a result, a number of these individuals founded an alternative therapies project group, aimed at selecting what could be passed on to other nurses in the form of continuing education. The continuing education package formulated consists of the following: each specialist (in aromatherapy, herb teas, compresses, homoeopathy, massage and touch, and reflexology) prepares a tutorial session presenting his particular field in a simplified manner, giving examples of procedures that other nurses can implement independently with patients in their everyday work. Each field aims to create a nursing standard with guidelines to which the nurses can refer.

At first, as far as aromatherapy was concerned, 12 single essential oils were introduced and the nurses were shown how to blend them. However, working with a selection of single oils was not totally satisfactory for two reasons: the aroma of a single oil is often not as acceptable as a carefully chosen blend; the nurses were not trained in aromatherapy, and to meet this difficulty blends of essential oils were formulated for each of the most frequent problems and the most popular aroma from these was selected by the patients and nurses. The conditions chosen were: pain, skin problems including skin infections, digestive problems, fatigue, insomnia, depression, fever, respiratory disorders and anxiety. A blend was also made for freshening the air in the wards.

The following guidelines are now officially accepted for use with the above blends:

• descriptions of the blends of essential oils, including the necessary precautions, especially in potentially skin-irritating oils, as well as the normal precautions of aromatherapy

- instructions for adding the essential oil blends to a bath correctly and administering a compress and an inhalation
- a list of the most common problems and symptoms together with the suggested essential oil blend and method of use
- a special section dedicated to the mind and mental problems, using aromalamps
- descriptions of how to store essential oils correctly, and where they can be ordered.

Hospital use

Essential oils are used in some hospitals where there is no clear framework. In such instances it is most commonly nurses who introduce them, after reading about aromatherapy and using it at home. As therapeutic massage may not legally be practised by nurses, the method of use they generally choose is airborne inhalation. Most hospitals forbid the burning of candles, so aromalamps cannot be used. Instead absorbent stones saturated with essential oils are put on patients' night tables to help with conditions such as tension, anxiety, sleeplessness, fear, stress, apathy and depression.

The use of aromatherapy varies between institutions, depending to a large extent on the level of acceptance of the medical staff. Described here is one instance of its use in a hospital.

Hospitals in the Canton of Bern have introduced 'fever washing' for general well-being, reduction of fever and healthy sweating in adult patients—it is not used on children. This use of essential oils has had a very positive reaction. The essential oil mix used is one drop each of bergamot, eucalyptus, lavender and mint (Latin names were not given). The oils are emulsified (with a dispersant) in lukewarm water. For genital and thrush-like ailments, depending on the situation, a further one to two drops each of lavender and tea tree are added.

Local massage or compresses with essential oils are also offered or applied to ease insomnia, fear, stress and general pain. In the interests of general safety, the teachers instruct that the essential oils must be emulsified and that the mixes cannot be administered orally.

National procedural principles

The SBK (See Training for nurses on p. 293) has established principles of procedure and basic rules for the handling of essential oils for institutions in which aromatology—sanctioned by doctors—is allowed. A number of the areas covered by these rules are outlined here, beginning with the principles for procedure, which are as follows:

- Nurses must possess minimal technical knowledge (e.g. HöFa 1) and be able to justify nursing procedures using essential oils. Their knowledge must include the risks and limitations as well as the potential.
- There must be clarification with the nursing directors or matron and doctors. It must be clear in which areas of this special field of medicine essential oils are used in nursing.
- The patient or relatives are to decide whether or not therapy with essential oils is tried (the nurses will provide them with the relevant information).

Essential oils and methods of use

The principal essential oils to be used are (no botanical names given): bergamont, cedarwood, eucalyptus, lavender, lemon, melissa 30% [authors' note: 30% dilution], orange, peppermint, rosemary and tea tree.

Additional oils the association suggests considering are: clary, frankincense, immortelle, petitgrain, rose and sandalwood.

Nursing is to be carried out using the following methods: inhalation (oil vaporizer, handkerchief, steam), lavage/douches, baths, compresses, dressings, application, massage and swabs.

The fields of application in nursing are: disinfection of rooms; personal hygiene and hair care; fever; colds; disturbed sleep and relaxation; pain (headache, backache and stomachache); mycosis; insect bites; healing of wounds, care of scars, burns and sunburn; fear, anxiety and confusion; and comfort for the dying.

Important base rules include the following:

- No synthetic oils are to be used. Simulated oils may smell similar, but never have the same effect as pure oils and may cause side-effects such as headaches and nausea.

• An oil rejected by the patient but still used by the nurse may have no therapeutic effect; the mental processes are involved in the mode of action to a greater extent than with traditional medicine.

• Essential oils are concentrates and, although they are natural substances, they are by no means innocuous. Risks include sensitivity, irritation and possible toxic effects.

• Essential oils should never be brought into contact with the eyes.

• No oral application is permitted since this form of administration is in the exclusive domain of medically trained aromatologists.

• Essential oils should always be diluted before use—less is more. Exceptions are swabs in mycosis.

Recommended doses are:

• vaporizer: 1–5 drops in water
• massage/application: 1–3 drops emulsified [quantity of carrier not specified]
• dressing/compresses: 1–3 drops in water or oil [quantity of carrier not specified]
• inhalation: 1–2 drops in water
• full bath/douches: maximum 10 drops (adults) or 5 drops (children), always emulsified [the authors feel both these doses are too high, especially for hospital patients].

The emulsifiers to be used are: neutral liquid soap, honey, vinegar, neutral body milk, almond oil, jojoba oil or almond oil cream.

Other important base rules are listed below.

• A sensitivity test should be carried out before each application of a new oil, a small amount being applied direct to the skin inside the elbow. If the area turns red or itches after 24 hours then care should be taken.

• An essential oil should not be used continuously for more than 3 weeks, since the effect diminishes. An equivalent oil with the same effect can always be used after this time. [The authors have never found this to be the case. However, an essential oil should be ingested for no longer than 3 weeks, not

because the effect may diminish, but because of possible toxic build-up in the liver.]

• Care should be taken if the patient is taking a homoeopathic remedy, because of possible interferential action.

Training for nurses

There is an increasing interest, in particular amongst nurses, in the possible benefits of complementary forms of therapy. Those interested in essential oil use would like to see a nationally recognized training in aromatology and more research to provide a sound basis for discussion with classical medicine. The Nursing Research Institute established in Switzerland in 1992 researches exclusively areas of orthodox medicine.

The new Swiss Red Cross syllabus for nursing has now increased the choice for students and many nursing schools have therefore included aromatherapy training.

Some basic nursing courses include a general overview of complementary therapies (including aromatherapy) and some postgraduate training, such as that given in HöFa 1 schools, includes essential oil use. Where this is the case, the following points are covered:

• history of essential oils and aromatherapy— limits and potential
• properties and action of essential oils
• production and quality of essential oils
• mode of action, effects and dangers of essential oils
• nursing competency and cooperation with the doctor
• basic rules for essential oil use
• application potential in nursing practice.

The SBK (Schweizerischer Berufsuerband der Krankenschwestern and Krankenpfleger), the Swiss association of nurses, also organizes training in the use of essential oils, both at home and in hospitals (see National procedural principles above). The introduction of essential oils into nursing as promoted by the SBK has two main objectives:

1. that essential oils be used in a caring manner to support and promote the well-being of the patient
2. that the use of essential oils by nurses be understood to be complementary to orthodox medicine.

These objectives provide a clear framework within which some hospitals do allow nurses to use essential oils, though most still do not, as the SBK has not issued any official guidelines regarding nurses using complementary therapies in a hospital setting.

Training outside the nursing profession

Training in aromatherapy is available mostly through German schools, although SPICA courses are taught in Zurich (see Useful addresses p. 375). Aromatherapy bodywork forms only a part of the complete training available. The strict legal restrictions on the practice of natural therapies in Switzerland are similar to those in Germany and it is expected to be a long fight before state approval of aromatherapy is granted.

The way ahead

Essential oils are used in some hospitals and hospices, but aromatherapy as it is practised in the UK will probably not be able to enter the Swiss healthcare system before more established and widespread therapies like homoeopathy and acupuncture. Those therapies in turn can only fully enter the hospital setting when those responsible for healthcare change their attitude towards alternative and complementary therapies and show an active interest in them.

REST OF THE WORLD

AUSTRALIA

Aromatherapy has been progressing very quickly in Australia over the last 2 years. With the improvement in training standards more people are aware of the importance of high professional standards and qualifications, which has stimulated nurses, psychiatrists and doctors to show more interest in professional aromatherapy. Many nurses and doctors are seeking training themselves and both private practices and hospitals are looking to employ professional aromatherapists. For example, at the Austin and Repatriation Medical Centre in Melbourne complementary therapies have been used 'to soften the very mechanistic and stressful critical care unit and so aid patient relaxation and healing' (George 1996).

Present position

The position of complementary medicine in Australia is comparable with that in the UK: 81% of nurses interviewed in a survey by the Australian Nursing Federation said they were interested in complementary therapies, 34% of these favouring aromatherapy.

The RCN of Australia has put out a Position Statement for the whole country regarding complementary therapies, 'which are widely used in Australian society and are acknowledged as making a significant contribution to the health-care of Australians'. In this Statement, complementary therapies are understood as therapies used in holistic practice and derived from:

1. traditions of healing (e.g. aromatherapy, acupuncture, reflexology)
2. therapeutic use of self (e.g. humour, therapeutic touch, validation therapy)
3. physical therapies (e.g. massage, hydrotherapy)
4. energy therapies (e.g. meditation, guided imagery, music therapy).

The use of complementary therapies in nursing practice by registered nurses, either as private practitioners or as employees, is appropriate where the nurse:

• has a qualification appropriate to nursing practice and is competent to practice accordingly

- practices within the scope and context of a legal framework as set down in Nurses Acts, professional standards, guidelines of regulatory bodies and the policies and protocols in place in work settings
- practices within the limits of the person's knowledge and skill.

The RCN also recommends that policies are developed by employers in consultation with nurse practitioners, to provide guidelines for the use of complementary therapies in their facilities. These guidelines should include reference to client consent, documentation processes and procedures, qualifications and competency of practitioners, parameters of accountability of practitioners and employers. Nurses practising complementary therapies should obtain personal professional indemnity insurance. The nursing profession should increase its research of activity in the theoretical aspects of complementarity to increase knowledge and enhance understanding of the efficacy of complementary therapies.

A number of conferences on complementary health have been held since 1994; at the RCN conference 'Pathways to healing' several papers were presented on aromatherapy and at one of the Ausmed conferences aromatherapy was the most mentioned therapy. The first Australasian Aromatherapy Conference was held in 1996, since when this purely aromatherapy conference has become a yearly, and very popular, event. The sheer size of Australia makes it difficult to estimate the prevalence of aromatherapy and it is hoped that readers will be able to form a general picture from the states from which the authors have received a response to their requests for information.

Aromatherapy associations

Much work has been started—and is on the increase—by the Australian branches of the two international professional associations, the IFA and ISPA. The IFA formed an Aromatherapy Incare group on the lines of its mother association in the UK, and the ISPA has formed its own group, Aroma-Care, just ahead of its mother association in the UK.

Use of aromatherapy

During 1997, many hospitals in Gippsland, Victoria, introduced policies on aromatherapy use in healthcare and many workshops have been organized at the Toongabbie Wellbeing Centre for health agencies, Heyfield hospitals, the Gippsland Women's Health Service and many others. In South Australia, funding has been awarded to one hospice to do a study on the use of aromatherapy and massage on its patients. Some sections of the healthcare system, providers and consumers are looking at the therapeutic use of essential oils and their effectiveness in conditions such as skin infections, stress-related problems and pain management.

A large part of the growth in the Victoria area has been attributed as being due to the intensive lecture tour of Len and Shirley Price in Victoria, for both health professionals and the interested public (Cadwallader 1997).

Aromatherapists providing treatments for the Newry Football Club (for pre- and post-training) and the Country Fire Authority (for tension and fatigue and also for the treatment of smoke-irritated eyes with Chamomile Eye Care, a specialized aromatherapy product) have been welcomed in the rural areas.

Because hospital budgets have been cut drastically in recent times, essential oils are mostly provided by the nurse aromatherapist giving the treatment, although some nursing homes have now begun to purchase essential oils as recommended by the aromatherapist; in one, the essential oil blends are made up by the pharmacist.

In March 1998, Sale Nursing Home has provided aromatherapy funding, and the Buckland Nursing Home at Springwood, New South Wales, has introduced complementary therapies, including aromatherapy, to its daily practice. Aromatherapy has been found to be 'extremely beneficial to older patients with sleep disturbances and significantly improves mood and anxiety levels' (Roberts 1996). At this nursing home, the essential oils are used in conjunction with hydrotherapy to good effect; one resident who had severe dementia with behavioural problems greatly reduced his anxiety levels and episodes of agitation by having daily 20–30 minute sessions in the bath with essential oils (Roberts 1996). Several hospitals in Newcastle (NSW) use essential oils: Christo Road Private Hospital has a freelance aromatherapist who is paid by the patients; the John Hunter Hospital granted funds to a midwife to undertake an aromatherapy course and the Hunter Area Health Service has enrolled 12 of its nurses on to an aromatherapy course.

Aromatherapy has been enthusiastically received in nursing homes for the elderly and numerous maternity units throughout the country; many through Aromatherapy Incare and Aroma-Care programmes. Vaporization is particularly popular, for antiseptic purposes and to help insomnia. Massage of the hands, feet, shoulders and face is more customary than full-body massage, with abdominal massage being used successfully to relieve constipation. Baths, sponge bowls and compresses (e.g. for relieving headaches) are also used.

Aromatherapy Incare

The Incarers give their time voluntarily, spending whatever number of hours they can spare each week giving treatments to patients.

There is an Incare package, which gives therapists wishing to take part guidelines on what to do, a letter of introduction and copies of various articles to show how Incare is effectively used in hospitals and nursing homes.

When the programme first began, stress was the prime feature of treatments given; no doubt the aromatherapists selected oils for the physical effects each patient suffered as result of stress, but no claims were made in this respect. 'In very few cases would it be appropriate to give full-body massage—hand and arm treatments, a foot massage or scalp and neck would be the wisest way to begin. Remember, we must be seen as Carers, who are treating stress and promoting emotional well-being' (Barrett 1993).

The acceptance of aromatherapy has come a long way since then, the remedial properties of the oils being promoted and recommended in all areas where aromatherapists work. For instance, midwives at Queanbeyan District Hospital, NSW use essential oils for perineal trauma, head colds, mastitis, headaches, induction of labour, pain, etc., which are not necessarily stress related (see also below). In Sydney, the Prince of Wales orthopaedic unit vaporizes oils to minimize staff stress and the plastic surgery outpatients clinic vaporizes oils to minimize the anxiety of patients having painful dressings removed. At the Mater Private Hospital, also in Sydney, essential oils are used in various ways in the renal unit, oncology, intensive care unit and the delivery suite (anonymous 1997).

Aromatherapy has been installed into the cardiac unit of a hospital in Queensland; there is also a Health Department-funded trial using several natural therapies in a detoxifying programme for heroin addicts.

In the Australian Capital Territory, Canberra, an aromatherapy clinic has been established in the Queen Elizabeth II family centre, which caters for women and children (up to the age of 3) with problems such as: stress, postnatal depression, maternal exhaustion, breast- or bottle-feeding difficulties, babies with sleep disorders, babies with reflux, and toddler training.

Aroma-Care

Aroma-Care began its work in March 1994, mainly as a result of the invaluable help given by Marlene Cadwallader (B App Sci. Nursing, trained in aromatherapy at the Australian School of Awareness—ASA), who approached the Directors of Nursing in many hospitals. Gail Graham, the Director of Nursing at the Knox Private Hospital, Victoria, met with the Director of Studies of the ASA, together with interested therapists from this School. These therapists were asked to enter the hospital system as voluntary workers in the psychiatric ward and also in the Knox Private Hospital's 11 affiliated establishments. As well as aromatherapy support being given to intensive care units within several hospitals, work is also carried out at the Dandenong drug and alcohol abuse centres and the multiple sclerosis centre at Wahonia, where students are also invited to work under supervised guidance to relieve stress overload and fluid retention.

Cadwallader herself uses essential oils and massage in Heyfield Bush Nursing Hospital and also in Hostel Care (documented and approved by the Hostel Board) for immobility, oedema, stiffness and pain. The hostel is presently looking into funding.

Margaret Tozer, aromatherapist and teacher of aromatherapy, has worked for the last 6 years mainly with people with cancer. Her work includes many aromatherapy applications to alleviate symptoms resulting from chemotherapy treatments and emotional traumas. Some of her therapists have gained part-time paying positions through doing community work in drug rehabilitation and multiple sclerosis and in hospices and private hospitals.

Some aromatherapists are now paid for their work: in Victoria—with the mentally handicapped at the Melba Centre, Mount Evelyn and with the elderly at the Pakenham Hospital; in Tasmania—at the Launceston General Hospital, in the birthing centre.

In Queensland, Nurses-in-charge have been given permission to use essential oils on their wards at the Southport Hospital, while Monash Peninsular has an undergraduate programme for nursing students, which follows a similar pattern to the workshops held at the School of Health Sciences at Monash University, Gippsland. The Gippsland workshops aim to:

- introduce and increase the carers' understanding of complementary therapies and their uses when caring for the elderly at home, in special accommodation hostels and nursing homes
- discuss how aromatherapy, massage, reflexology, Reiki and visualization can assist the person who is confused, anxious, restless, low in spirits, constipated or nauseous
- discuss appropriate courses that carers may undertake, to develop further skills and

knowledge in aromatherapy and related complementary therapies.

Policies, protocols and guidelines

Policies and protocols have begun to be written, appearing to follow the same lines as those in the UK, not only to safeguard the interests of the patients, but also to ensure professionalism and confirm high standards by aromatherapists in their approach to aromatherapy in hospitals, hostels and nursing homes.

Each state in Australia has its own Nurses' Board and its own Act and these Acts vary in every state; e.g. nurses in Victoria must practise in accordance with the Victoria Nurses' Act 1993, while those in the Australian Capital Territory must practise in accordance with their state's Nurses' Act (1988), which is very different from that of Victoria.

The picture of complementary health practice and training is different in each; however, guidelines for complementary therapy, where they exist, are fairly comparable. The Nurses' Board of Victoria developed and endorsed Guidelines for use of complementary therapies in nursing practice in 1995; no changes have been made since that time, though they were up for review in 1998 (Anderson personal communication 1998). The guidelines so far include many points contained in UK policy documents, such as professional standards of practice, informed consent, the necessity for adequate professional indemnity cover, accountability and competency (see Ch. 16).

Northern Territory

There is no specific legislation that refers to the use of complementary therapies; nurses wishing to practise in that area would be guided by the Code of Professional Conduct and the Code of Ethics for all nurses in Australia.

New South Wales

The NSW College of Nursing has produced a general position statement for the profession on complementary therapies. The forms of therapy used by nurses in their practice is a matter for clarification between the nurse, the client and the nurse's employer; this would apply whether a proposed therapy was alternative or orthodox.

Australian Capital Territory

To date the Board has not been approached on issues relating to complementary therapies nor has it been approached to examine any curriculum on the subject. As a consequence it has not as yet developed a position in relation to the matter.

South Australia

The Nurses' Board does not give credentials to nurses using complementary therapies. However, it does recognize those who are working in non-traditional roles of nursing; such nurses are expected to complete a self-assessment package based on the Australian Nursing Council Competencies for registered and enrolled nurses.

Queensland

The Queensland Nursing Council uses a set of guiding principles for all enhancements for the role of a registered nurse. Two essential ones are:

* adoption of new, enhanced role responsibilities is based on appropriate consultation, education and assessed competence
* the Registered Nurse is jointly responsible with the employer for ensuring that continuing education and assessment of competence are undertaken for the new role responsibility.

The guiding principles, which are currently being revised, will be used until appropriate policies and procedures have been approved by the Queensland Nursing Council.

Victoria

In 1995 the Nursing Board of Victoria put forward some proposed guidelines for the practice of complementary or alternative therapies, in recognition of the increasing interest shown both by the general community and by a significant number of nurses. The Board defined these complementary therapies or interventions as 'treatments that are aimed at a more holistic approach to healing'.

The brief summary of the proposals set out below is taken directly from the Nurses' Board of Victoria Guidelines for complementary therapies in nursing practice (the Nurses' Act 1993 referred to applies only to the Nursing Board of Victoria).

1. Professional standards
   a. In using complementary therapies, a registered nurse must practise in accordance with the Nurses' Act (1993) and the Board's 'General statement to nurses undertaking clinical practice procedures'.
   b. The nurse must also take into account the profession's Code of Ethics, Code of Conduct, Professional Standards for Practice and the ANCI Competencies.
   c. This applies to all currently registered nurses whether they are working principally as nurses or as complementary therapists.
2. Responsibilities of a nurse using complementary therapies
   a. Informed consent
      (i) The informed consent of patients or clients must be sought.
      (ii) Where a therapy lies outside usual nursing practices, the nurse must ensure that the patient is able to make an informed decision to accept or refuse the therapy and such consent should be documented.
   b. Employment
      (i) Nurses working in hospitals or agencies must be cognizant of the policies of these bodies in relation to the use of complementary therapies.
      (ii) Nurses must be aware that acting within the guidelines of an employer does not absolve them of responsibility or individual immunity in cases of negligence.

c. Professional indemnity cover

Every nurse should have professional indemnity insurance and it is recommended that a nurse who practises complementary therapies regularly confirms the extent and nature of such cover as it relates to complementary therapies.

d. Accountability

In view of the wide range of complementary therapies available, nurses are advised to select and practise with care. They should take into account factors such as: evidence of the safety and efficacy of the therapy, the suitability of the therapy for combination with practice, legal and ethical implications and the availability of initial and ongoing education in these therapies.

e. Competency

(i) Nurses are responsible for ensuring that their knowledge of the therapies is at a level which ensures safe application in practice.

(ii) Courses should be carefully selected, bearing in mind the following factors:
— that the course is accredited or approved by the professional organization
— the level of practice for which the course is recognized
— the transferability of qualifications
— the recognition of prior learning
— the quality of the education, e.g. course duration and teacher qualifications.

(iii) Nurses are responsible for maintaining or updating their nursing knowledge and skills and they must be aware of the limitations of their knowledge and skills in relation to the complementary therapies.

(iv) They should function within the limits of their skills and consult or refer where necessary.

f. Collaboration

Nurses as part of a healthcare team should discuss the use of complementary therapies with the medical practitioner or any other member of the team caring for an individual patient/client.

Western Australia

The Guidelines of Western Australia (1996) are similar to those of Victoria given above.

In 1996, guideline statements were developed for nurses registered in Divisions 1 or 2 of the Register who have undertaken a recognized course in complementary therapy post-registration and who wish to incorporate complementary therapies in their practice. Within these, it is suggested that policies and guidelines (for which the employers are responsible) should include the following:

- who can practise complementary therapies; qualifications, experience, competencies, training and credentialling necessary
- type of clients, condition, assessment and referral
- type of therapies that may be practised and any limitations on the practise of those therapies
- where the therapies can be performed
- documentary, reporting requirements
- type of client consent
- information and education of clients re use of therapies—Consumer guidelines.

Consumer guidelines for the client are important for complementary therapy within nursing practice. Clients must recognize their own responsibilities and acknowledge the duty of the nurse, based on a nursing assessment to discontinue therapy and/or refer client to others. Also within the guideline statements are:

- nurses are encouraged to engage in and contribute to well-designed research studies
- nurses practising complementary therapies must maintain professional standards set by the relevant professional or regulating body for the practice of the specific complementary therapy
- in practice nurses should use therapies only where there is evidence (scientific basis) to indicate care or therapy is beneficial.

The guidelines for Western Australia also include ingestion.

Tasmania

Guidelines are in place to assist individual professional judgement and the development of local policies. They are not intended to be all inclusive and should be treated as a guide only. The guidelines cover consent and most of the other issues in the guidelines for Victoria above.

Essential oil legislation

The Australian Federal Government have created the Therapeutic Goods Act (TGA) to promote both the safe use of essential oils and truth in advertising. Despite this, companies are unfortunately (as in the UK) selling perfume quality oils (i.e. standardized or adulterated) or adding isolates to their products simply to make use of the term 'aromatherapy'. Certain oils, mainly the *Melaleuca* genus, are labelled as poisonous and cannot be sold without a licence. Essential oil companies and herb farms in Australia and Tasmania are successfully growing herbs, distilling essential oils and making carrier oils. The climate and mountainous areas in Tasmania are comparable (in beauty also) to southern France, lavender being grown from cloned *Lavandula angustifolia* originally obtained from that country.

Research

Scientists in universities continue researching the chemistry of essential oils, analysing their antimicrobial properties, searching for answers to a superbug prevalent and resistant to antibiotics.

One or two research projects in hospitals and universities are either under way or in the pipeline: these include funded research in South Australia to evaluate the use of aromatherapy and massage in improving the quality of life of clients with advanced cancer; research on the effects of aromatherapy in relation to midwifery practice in Victoria and a current trial at a nursing home in New South Wales to promote sleep in the elderly with a view to reducing sedation.

In 1997, a new alternative therapies research centre opened at the Royal Women's Hospital (NSW), which may undertake aromatherapy trials in the future.

The way ahead

Australia has a two-tiered health system, which means that privately insured patients can access therapies more readily than public patients; GPs receive Medicare rebates from the government, using provider numbers for billing the care they deliver to patients. There is an increase in GPs studying alternative therapies because they feel threatened by them; their training costs are reimbursed by the government because they are in the medical profession. Professional aromatherapists, with no provider number from the government, can administer care, either in or out of mainstream healthcare settings, for which the client or private insurance has to pay. The federal government has issued a policy statement stating that they support the right of Australians to have free choice in using nontraditional, natural or alternative medicine—it has yet to be seen how strongly they support that right. A long struggle is anticipated to convince the government to fund aromatherapy, the present funding for essential oils in public hospitals coming in most cases from the practitioner's pocket, raffles, donations and petty cash.

CANADA

Early beginnings

Aromatherapy in Canada appeared in the late 1980s as Californian (USA) products became increasingly available through mail order. The use of essential oils continues to grow at what most experts agree is between 25 to 30%. In the mid 1990s, the East Coast pioneered corporate aromatherapy with several companies vying for the inclusion of essential oils in the workplace. The West Coast continues to be developed as a result of a company which began in the early 1990s and developed a chain of retail stores dedicated entirely to aromatherapy.

Aromatherapy associations

Several associations have appeared, with the Canadian Federation of Aromatherapists (CFA) and the Canadian branch of the National Association of Holistic Aromatherapy (NAHA—America) leading the way.

Hospitals and hospices

Studies are sprouting in various healthcare facilities, particularly old folks' hospitals and hospices. A double-blind study is being set up at the time of printing with the aim of proving the essential oils to be capable of outperforming certain over-the-counter drugs.

Insurance

Government insurance companies have now accepted certain patients' requests for essential oils and essential oil natural remedies as medical support in the recovery from motor vehicle accidents. The state-run operation will reimburse customers' aromatherapy products bills. Certain private insurance companies are providing aromatherapy coverage in their plan as well as agreeing to provide liability coverage for certificated aromatherapists.

ISRAEL

Present position of complementary therapies

There are several complementary medicine units in hospitals throughout the country, including Hadassah University Hospital in Jerusalem, and Sheba Hospital in Tel Hashomer, although aromatherapy on the whole remains in a more embryonic stage within the medical system. Alternative medicine practised in hospitals does not officially include aromatherapy, although some practise it under the heading of massage. Nurses, 'birthing coaches' and midwives and physical therapists are studying aromatherapy courses on their own initiative, then introducing it individually into their professional settings. Many of these courses are taught by alternative

medicine institutes and there are also private courses. The most knowledgeable aromatherapists are those who obtained certification abroad (mostly in the UK).

Some of the alternative therapies, such as reflexology, have their own association; one has not yet been formed for aromatherapy and, because of this, aromatherapy does not have the same standing as it has in the UK. Many of the more specialist aromatherapists therefore become members of a British association.

Essential oils have been used with great success by Dr Shamai Giler to enhance the healing process following CO_2 laser surgery procedures; Dr Giler is a leader in laser surgery at the Plastic Surgery Institute, Rothschild Medical Centre. At the Natural Oils Research Association conference in the spring of 1997 in Tel Aviv he reported that, where essential oils were used, patients tended to have less scarring after operations and there was an enhancement of wound healing.

At the Herzeliah medical centre (a private hospital), the alternative medicine clinic, headed by Dr J G Zilkha, is believed to be the only clinic in Israel using aromatherapy; treatments usually include herbal medicine also. Scientific studies are presently being conducted on essential oils and aromatic plants at the Nevch Ya'ar Research Centre.

Complementary therapists are allowed to advertise, except for those working within conventional medicine. Because it is expensive to advertise, only those with money can do so; unfortunately, many of these are not adequately qualified.

Regulation of essential oils and aromatherapy

The sale of essential oils is not regulated by the Health Ministry, as they are seen as products which are used externally. It is forbidden under Health Ministry regulations to administer essential oils for internal use, as this would put them into the category of a medicine. There are many brands of oils on the market sold in body shops and perfumeries; on most products, neither the origin nor the producer are mentioned.

At the moment there are no laws regulating any complementary therapy. However, in 1988, as interest in complementary therapy began to increase, the Health Ministry established a public commission. After 3 years of investigations, it issued extensive recommendations (which were met with criticism by many in the medical field) including liberalizing the existing laws and eliminating the legal monopoly of conventional medical practitioners on medical care. A majority of the commission members said that unconventional medical techniques, including aromatherapy, shiatsu, reflexology, acupuncture, naturopathy, homoeopathy and iridology, should not be outlawed if they did not harm patients. They noted, however, that should a patient be harmed by a non-physician the practitioner would be subject to severe sanctions and malpractice suits. To date, none of its recommendations has been made law.

JAPAN

Essential oil use

The field of aromatherapy has been extended from the retail market into the market of aesthetics and cosmetics. Regarding distribution, not only specialty stores but also drugstores, supermarkets and department stores have started to deal in essential oils and mail order has also become popular. New suppliers and new brands are increasing more and more in the world and have become known rapidly in Japan; this is considered to be due to the worldwide extension of the Internet.

There is no clear regulation by the government, but recently the Health Ministry started to make a survey of suppliers who dealt in essential oils.

Aromatherapy associations

Several aromatherapy associations have been set up since 1995: the Japanese Federation of Aromatherapists (JFA), the International Federation of Aromatherapists (Japan) and the Japanese Aromatherapy Association (JAA),

followed by the Federation of Japanese Aromatherapists (FJA). The German aromatherapy association, Forum Essenzia, also has a branch in Japan. Many schools teaching aromatherapy have been opened in quick succession, and one or two organizations have been established by some of them specifically for their own therapists, e.g. the Japanese Aroma-Artist Association, the Japanese Aromacoordinator Association and others.

During 1997 the interest in essential oil use increased within the medical profession, and in order to contribute to the advancement of aromatherapy in this field, the Japanese Society of Aromatherapy (JSA) was founded at the beginning of 1998. This society was set up by doctors, nurses, midwives, dentists, pharmacists, acupuncturists, dieticians, etc.

KOREA

Complementary therapies already established in Korea are oriental systems of herbalism, acupuncture, and related techniques. The first form of Western natural therapy to be practised was aromatherapy, having been introduced by Dr David Oh (MD, ND, PhD) who was trained in Canada. The Korean Association of Naturopathic Medicine was established by him in January 1997 and over 100 medical doctors are now members. Apart from monthly academic meetings, the association runs various seminars and workshops where naturopathic modalities like aromatherapy, homoeopathy, hydrotherapy, chiropractic and qi (chi) energy medicine are introduced. As a result, Dr Oh then founded the Korean Aromatherapy Association in April the same year, its members (who are not allowed to prescribe essential oils internally) being mainly medical doctors and beauty therapists. There is no licensing system established yet for professional aromatherapists, but the use of essential oils in the aesthetical field, including skin care shops, has recently started to become popular and aromatherapy is expected before long to be one of the most popular natural therapies in Korea.

Essential oil use

The general public can already buy essential oils in herb shops and department stores and use them to reduce stress, nervous tension and other small daily problems. Aromatherapy treatments they have experienced were considered to be positively beneficial to various conditions. The main medical applications of essential oils are neuropsychiatric disorders including: depression, anxiety, headaches and migraines, insomnia and general stress, together with respiratory infections, skin problems and cardiovascular disorders. The clinical methods used are inhalation and massage (particularly combined with meridian acupoint massage). Clinical data and results from experimental studies have been accumulated from a few hospitals, including some using EEG, EAV, Doppler and thermographic devices.

Training

Although several medical doctors are responsive to aromatherapy, most are still slightly sceptical. Nevertheless, despite the fact that it is not widely used in Korean hospitals, there are a few doctors who are interested enough to attend workshops and seminars. Most of these are organized by the Institute of Naturopathic Medicine in conjunction with the Korean Aromatherapy Association.

NEW ZEALAND

The undeniable increase in popularity of, and interest in, aromatherapy in New Zealand during the last 5 years has, as yet, not been accompanied by general acceptance in hospitals. However, there is evidence that rest homes, hospices and centres for people with disabilities enthusiastically offer aromatherapy as a complementary therapy, supported by medical staff. From a survey done of all the institutions in the New Zealand Hospice Directory, 34 out of 35 centres replied, all of whom stated they use or are interested in using complementary therapies; 19 said they offer aromatherapy through volunteer and visiting practitioners.

For those keen to see an expansion of the use of aromatherapy as an adjunct to traditional methods of care and treatment there are signs of progress and, in a few institutions, programmes have been established; these should provide models which can be used to encourage further expansion and acceptance.

Aromatherapy programmes

Scattered mainly through the North Island, there are relatively new programmes in operation in at least four hospices and a number of nursing homes, and students attending an aromatherapy training course at one polytechnic are accepted for periods of clinical placement in a local healthcare institution.

Programmes vary in intensity and scope according to the qualification of the aromatherapist involved. In two cases the work is dependent upon volunteers, while in four others trained aromatherapists are either employed on contract or retained as consultants. There is considerable interest among nurses to practise aromatherapy as part of their work, but nurse aromatherapists have little or no time to practise aromatherapy after their nursing duties are done. As in other countries, expenditure on healthcare in New Zealand has been reduced, so a further problem arises of finding funds to pay for aromatherapy supplies. In some cases the authorities have approved payment for oils from general funds. In other cases oils are chosen and donated by the aromatherapist. Sometimes donations are made towards purchase of essential oils either by patients or by their relatives.

Protocols and the NZROHA

Protocols are in place in two instances and are being formalized in others, where currently the programmes follow established formal guidelines and those of the New Zealand Register of Holistic Aromatherapists (NZROHA), the professional body of aromatherapists in New Zealand. A discussion paper on protocols in healthcare institutions is about to be published. The Register was formed in 1993 originally as a support group for aromatherapists and to inform the public of the benefits of consulting an aromatherapist. Professional membership of the Register requires an applicant to satisfy his professional standards of training. The level of current professional membership stands at 83. There is also a student category of membership. A quarterly magazine 'Sharing aromatherapy' is produced, which contains a list of trained aromatherapists throughout the country. The Register has set professional standards for its practising members including the requirement that they abide by its Code of Ethics and Code of Practice.

The NZROHA was a founding member of the NZ Charter of Health Practitioners Inc. and has developed a syllabus and examination structure which is currently awaiting approval by the NZ Qualifications Authority, a government body, before it becomes operative nationally.

Treatments and essential oils

Use of diffusers in rooms and of lavender to enhance sleep is common among the institutions. Where a professional aromatherapist with several years' experience is in charge, the range of treatments includes baths, foot baths, massage of hands and feet, backs, necks and shoulders; with more specific inhalations and local diffusion of prescribed oil blends.

Regarding safety, with only one exception, all places surveyed used only electric oil vaporizers to diffuse essential oils. The survey revealed that most of the essential oils used were of high quality. Two purchased oils came with certificates of authenticity. The others were purchased from reputable suppliers who gave guarantees of quality. Essential oils most often used were: *Citrus aurantium* var. *amara*, *C. sinensis*, *C. limon* and *C. paradisi*, *Lavandula angustifolia*, *Rosmarinus officinalis*, *Zingiber officinale*, *Eucalyptus radiata*, *Chamaemelum nobile*, *Matricaria recutita*, *Cymbopogon citratus*, *Pelargonium graveolens*, *Piper nigrum*, *Salvea sclarea*, *Cupressus sempervirens*, *Mentha* × *piperita*, *M. spicata*, *Melaleuca alternifolia*, *Leptospermum scoparium* and *Juniperus communis*.

Conditions treated include nausea, insomnia, respiratory problems, constipation, digestive problems, wound management, sleeping problems, terminal illness, depression, skin problems, poor circulation, muscular pain and anxiety. In one institution the aromatherapist has used lotions containing *L. scoparium* [MANUKA] with success in cases of chronic skin problems. *M. alternifolia* [TEA TREE] in cream base has also been found to be efficacious.

Training

Those who assisted in the compilation of information on aromatherapy in New Zealand are trained aromatherapists (some are also nurses) who have an input to programmes and training in healthcare institutions. Sarah Wallacy, an aromatherapist presently working at Te Omango hospice, developed an in-house basic training at the hospice where she had worked previously, covering, in addition to massage and diffusion techniques, extraction methods, safety precautions and a detailed study of a minimum of six essential oils. She says 'to avoid aromatherapy remaining on the fringe, it is vital that a programme like this be set up in the most professional manner'. In this she has the enthusiastic support of trained practitioners in New Zealand.

The Mary Potter hospice in Wellington has its own in-house training programme currently being developed for nursing and medical staff by the director of complementary therapies, Katrina Lloyd. An in-house training programme set up by Anne Bennett (aromatherapy consultant, tutor and practitioner) at the War Veterans Services home at Levin will begin shortly and will be funded by a special grant from a local service organization. Training will include the history of aromatherapy and its uses today, safety issues, in-depth study of eight oils, how to use them and how they work; using and cleaning the vaporizers; basic massage techniques for feet, hands, neck and shoulders, keeping records of treatments and a holistic approach to health. Treatments will be under the supervision of the consulting aromatherapist who will make up the blends of oils for each client. It will be the aromatherapist's responsibility to administer the programme, monitor it and evaluate it.

Only six to eight essential oils are studied on the basic courses above, as it is felt to be sensible to consider only the few oils which will be used at that level.

It is true to say that after modest and hesitant beginnings, most training courses offered in various parts of the country today have syllabi and standards that will equip practitioners to offer a professional service. The number of essential oils studied in these is naturally much greater than those studied above.

As an example of the increased demand and recognition for adequate training, a 2 year full-time diploma in professional aromatherapy is now being offered, which is about 1200 classroom hours. This has developed over the last 4 years from an initial 250 hour course. The first year Manawatu polytechnic ran this diploma course there were four full-time students; this year there are 40.

New Zealand is fortunate in that it has only one professional body for aromatherapy, which means that there is some degree of consistency in training.

The way ahead

Although aromatherapy in New Zealand lags behind the level of development in the UK, where it is widely accepted in traditional health areas and institutions, it appears that it is well on the way to following that model. It is being enthusiastically received in various health institutions and much effort is being made right now to develop policies and protocols, high standards and professionalism.

Books such as 'Aromatherapy for health professionals' are a great asset and resource and certainly help to increase the professional profile.

SOUTH AFRICA

In South Africa the field of complementary health care in general—and aromatherapy in particular—has grown considerably over the past few years. The Association of Aromatherapists of South Africa (AAOSA) began 6 years ago with some 30 members and now has, at the time of

writing (August 1997), over 500 members. One of its main aims has always been to inform and educate the public regarding the use of essential oils.

The association has remained active within the community during its existence, running a successful voluntary service within hospice and hospital situations through its Aroma Care Plan, as well as in other areas where nurses and aromatherapists have been using essential oils, e.g. in midwifery, independently of the association.

Aroma Care Plan

The Aroma Care Plan provides a weekly service of aromatherapy at the haematology unit, Groote Schuur Hospital, Cape Town. This is a large government-funded teaching hospital and the haematology unit provides care for patients receiving chemotherapy and radiotherapy, mainly for the treatment of leukaemia and other bone marrow diseases.

Although no formal studies at the hospital have been carried out, this service to the patients has become increasingly valued by doctors and nurses there, the weekly aromatherapy treatments being considered to be positively beneficial to patients, helping to reduce stress levels and muscular tension as well as providing relaxation and a feeling of well-being. Sessions mainly consist of foot and hand or back and shoulder massage.

At the nursing college attached to Groote Schuur Hospital there is increasing interest in aromatherapy among the nurses, shown by requests for lectures to postbasic students. At St Luke's Hospice, Cape Town, where Aroma Care therapists first began working at the beginning of 1993, the demand for their services has grown considerably. Here, all aromatherapists in the Aroma Care Plan are required to do the hospice counselling course before having contact with the patients. The aromatherapists make weekly visits to St Luke's, working on the wards and in the daycare centre, where a number of patients come specifically for aromatherapy. Many of them come for massage of oedematous limbs, and some for the easing of specific aches and pains associated with bone metastasis. Shoulder massage is of great relief to those suffering from lung cancer and the associated dyspnoea and many come just for the benefits of the touch therapy itself.

The essential oils which appear to be used most often on the wards are: benzoin, lavender, frankincense and rose otto. This service has been extended successfully to include house calls.

Aroma Care Plan therapists in Cape Town are also active in the field of AIDS, where a weekly sevice is provided within a centre for people living with AIDS and HIV.

The fourth area where aromatherapists work in Cape Town is at a school for children with cerebral palsy, where therapists achieve exciting results with both mobile and wheelchair-bound children of all ages up to 18 years. Teachers and physiotherapists have commented on the reduced limb spasticity and reduced anxiety rate following sessions.

Outside of Cape Town, the Aroma Care Plan is active in Kwazulu Natal, where aromatherapists work with patients on a daily basis at the Highway Hospice. In Gauteng, aromatherapists are carrying out a pilot study on aromatherapy and stress management in a group of police volunteers.

In terms of recognition of the profession, a great deal of work has been done within the national committee over the past 2 years. At the time of writing, the submission is with the Minister of Health, and results are awaited.

TAIWAN

There are three main medicine systems in Taiwan: orthodox or Western medicine (which is almost the same as in Western countries), Traditional Chinese Medicine and complementary health care. Complementary health care is very popular in Taiwan, the favoured disciplines being acupuncture, reflexology, osteopathy, shiatsu and qigong (chikung) (meditation of mind for relaxation and good circulation, and physical exercise) and recently, aromatherapy. Traditional Chinese Medicine has a different philosophy towards the maintenance of human health, using a vast number of natural substances, plant, animal, mineral, etc. As both Western style and traditional Chinese doctors

are legally recognized by the government Health Department, Taiwanese people may choose between the two, which means that someone with a cold who does not wish to take synthetic medication could consult a Chinese medical doctor, who would prescribe either dry herbs for cooking or ready-mixed herb powders. Although it is easy to find a Chinese doctor, even in a small town, it is rare to find a qualified aromatherapist.

Essential oil use

There are many shops selling essential oils or aromatherapy products, most essential oils being imported by private trading companies from Europe, Australia and the USA (except for some locally distilled oils such as camphor, Hinoki wood and lemongrass, though the quantities of these are small). The essential oils available are of differing qualities, some being adulterated or standardized, and labelling is incomplete. Many do not indicate how to blend and use them for improving health safely and correctly. Unfortunately, if someone is introduced to essential oils to alleviate his problems and he is supplied with poor quality oils, he will lose his confidence and have a negative view about the effectiveness of aromatherapy.

So far there are no rules or regulations regarding the sales, methods of use or storage of essential oils. They are viewed in Taiwan as a commercial commodity related to healthcare and many people know neither the nature nor the definition of an essential oil unless they have participated in an aromatherapy seminar.

The main methods of aromatherapy used are application, massage, vaporization and inhalation. Owing to the wet and hot climate of Taiwan, many elderly people frequently get muscle aches, arthritis and influenza. Many also suffer with sinus and lung problems as a result of air pollution and are helped by essential oil mixes.

Training

Universities and colleges do not have aromatherapy courses, neither is there an organization, association or society for aromatherapy as in the UK. The introduction of aromatherapy in Taiwan relies upon private companies who represent or sell essential oils of various brands, or on independent individuals who are interested in this natural way of personal care.

Because aromatherapy has grown rapidly during the last few years, people are going to England or Australia to study aromatherapy, returning to promote the knowledge they have learnt. One of the difficulties encountered in trying to promote aromatherapy in Taiwan is the lack of books printed in Chinese.

One company has good contacts with beauty salons and also cooperates with beauty therapy colleges; its director, Jeong Yeong, has also initiated the following to promote the fundamentals of aromatherapy, having had 17 years' experience in the research, development, manufacture and marketing of skincare products:

- writing and publishing in Chinese of a book entitled 'Aromatherapy and essential oils— how to use essential oils to enhance vitality and health'
- conducting a series of training seminars related to essential oils and aromatherapy in major cities
- translating Shirley Price's Aromatherapy workbook into Chinese (Price 1999).

UNITED STATES OF AMERICA

A national survey carried out on 1539 adults in 1990 revealed that 34% had used at least one unconventional therapy in the past year; projection of figures to the total US population suggested that, in that year, 425 million visits were made by Americans to an unconventional therapist (Eisenberg et al 1993).

As there is no National Health Service in the USA, healthcare is paid for by private health insurance. Only a few insurance companies cover the use of complementary therapies, which makes it difficult for hospitals to provide these services. However, there is an increasing awareness amongst those working in the health field of the value, both therapeutic and financial, of com-plementary forms of medicine, so the insurance situation is expected to improve.

One complementary therapy which is gaining ground is massage (which is covered by several insurance companies). This is due in part to dramatic research findings, such as those from the University of Miami School of Medicine's Touch Research Institute. Research begun there in the early 1980s looked at the effects of massage on premature babies. The results from over 10 years' study show that premature babies who are massaged have a 47% greater weight gain and 6 day shorter stay in hospital than do babies who are not massaged. This represents a cost saving of $3000 per baby (Cohen 1994).

The National Association of Nurse Massage Therapists, founded in 1987 by a small Atlanta group of nurse massage therapists, was officially recognized by the National Federation for Specialty Nursing Organisations in 1992. As has been shown by Passant (1990) in Britain, it is a comparatively easy step for massage therapists to enhance the techniques they have already mastered by the introduction of essential oils. It is probable therefore that these nurses will be the ones who, having studied essential oil use, will go on to introduce aromatherapy into mainstream hospitals in the USA.

Aromatherapy is believed to have made its first US appearance in the state of California, where many workshops and seminars were held from the mid 1980s. California housed most, if not all, of the companies selling essential oils, mainly by mail order, although The Essential Oil Company started in Oregon in 1976. During the 1980s interest in aromatherapy grew nationally— the authors, for example, introduced aromatherapy to a number of states including Pennsylvania, Colorado, Montana and Delaware.

Professional organizations

A national association was set up in California in the late 1980s, which showed great promise, holding a world conference in 1990 in Los Angeles. Unfortunately, administration difficulties led to its early demise and it was replaced by the strong and well-represented National

Association for Holistic Aromatherapy (NAHA), founded in 1990 in Boulder, Colorado. The NAHA:

- offers a quarterly journal called Scentsitivity
- publishes a directory of its professional members
- gives information on aromatherapy courses
- offers an educational scholarship every 2 years
- is involved with the Steering Committee (set up at the San Francisco conference in 1996) to set national standards of aromatherapy education
- is establishing a Code of Ethics for teachers, practitioners, manufacturers and students
- creating a True Aromatherapy Product (TAP) registered certification mark for manufacturers who can demonstrate that their product is 'true aromatherapy'
- supports an aromatic plant project (founded by Jeanne Rose)
- hosts international conferences and trade shows.

A world conference on aromatherapy was held in New York in 1994 and several are now being held in different states. One or two schools in states as far apart as California and Oregon have now obtained liability insurance for graduates of aromatherapy through the Associated Bodywork and Massage Professionals and courses in Oregon and New York have been accredited by the Institute of Aromatic Medicine (formerly the Institute of Aromatic Therapists).

Essential oil use in healthcare settings

The use of essential oils in healthcare settings is already beginning, albeit in isolated instances. Many US-based aromatherapists estimate the development of aromatherapy in their country to be approximately 5 years behind the UK in its level of integration into the clinical healthcare setting, though they are rapidly catching up. Professional aromatherapy practice standards, for example, are now being developed by a group of educators belonging to NAHA, which includes the Steering Committee. The steering committee is focused on this goal and is working

as a special committee within NAHA's education committee.

In Colorado, a nurse massage therapist and teacher, Laraine Kyle, is working with several nurse colleagues writing protocols for the use of aromatherapy in their facility. 'Aromatherapy is still considered a "cutting edge" treatment methodology, yet it is gaining acceptance in the care of the chronically and terminally ill' she says. On her Alzheimer unit Kyle is using lavender, which has also been shown to be effective as an intervention for sundowning effect (a form of dementia in which the symptoms are worse at night); patients are now rarely given hypnotics to regulate sleep patterns. Another aromatherapist, working on an acute care psychiatric unit, has developed a stress management module using essential oils. The same nurse prepared a blend for the staff psychiatrist to assist him with mental alertness during the day. Ixchel Leigh, another nurse therapist in Colorado, whose courses have been accredited by the State of Colorado Department of Higher Education, says that, over the 2 years that nurses in Durango have been using essential oils on the elderly, there has been a noticeable reduction in the need for antipsychotic drugs: 'Patients are sleeping more soundly, smile more and occasionally recognize individual nurses when they arrive.'

In Indiana, a Nurse Practitioner Program has begun implementing complementary therapies, including aromatherapy, and the medical profession are beginning to show some acceptance. The Australasian College in Oregon now offers registered nurses in California continuing educational units in aromatherapy by distance learning. In 1997, the Massachusetts State Board of Nursing voted to write aromatherapy into their nurse practice act (the first state to do this). In Illinois recent approval has been given to implement a study of the effectiveness of aromatherapy care in the psychiatric unit. In Texas aromatherapy is being used to aid stress and minor discomforts such as sore muscles, bruises and vein relief.

Kaiser, a prominent educator and acknowledged authority on the changing healthcare system, states that leading healthcare institutions are now using the power of aromatherapy to promote patient healing (Kaiser 1993). His Healing

Health Care Network newsletter gives the following vision of the future:

> Picture a nurse preparing to pass daily medications. Next to each dispensing cup she places a cartridge filled with natural essential oils. She heads down to Mr Scott's room, hands him his oral medicine and places the cartridge into an atomizer which disperses a therapeutic lavender aroma into the air to help Mr Scott's migraine. Next door, three year old Stephanie's atomizer will be filled with peppermint oil to help her asthma and Mrs Roth will receive the scent of orange blossom to help alleviate stress and anxiety the night before her open heart surgery.
>
> (Horzely 1993)

Synthetic aromas

The use of synthetic aromas in place of genuine essential oils is growing in the USA, and is a cause for concern in some circles. In 1991 for instance, a so-called 'aromatherapy' trial was conducted at the Sloane Kettering Cancer Center using a synthetic heliotrope. The aim of the trial was to establish whether the heliotrope's fragrance could reduce anxiety levels in patients before and whilst they were undergoing a—very stressful—MRI scan. Spielberger test results, and the patients' own reports, indicated that this was indeed the case (Taylor 1993).

Another use of synthetic aromas is in environmental fragrancing, which is becoming popular in hospitals and other public buildings. But experts disagree about the effects of synthetic aromas. Many chemists believe that a synthetic copy of an essential oil will have identical effects to those of the genuine essential oil. All professional aromatherapists disagree vehemently, arguing that synthetic aromas can produce side-effects such as headaches, breathing problems and nausea. No research which could resolve this difference of opinion has been carried out. Until it has been, it is important to be able to distinguish between synthetic aromas and the genuine essential oils used in aromatherapy. This might best be achieved by reserving the terms 'fragrancing' and 'fragrance' for synthetic aromas.

Summary

It is clear that interest in the use of aromatherapy in a healthcare setting is growing rapidly worldwide. There is scope in all countries for the introduction of both the French model—i.e. aromatherapy as a branch of medicine—and of the UK model—i.e. aromatherapy as the therapeutic use of essential oils by trained non-medical and interested medical personnel. In order that both these models develop according to the best possible practice it is vital that aromatherapists in different countries communicate with each other, sharing their experience and expertise to the benefit of all.

ACKNOWLEDGEMENTS

The people who helped the authors compile this chapter have been acknowledged at the beginning of this book.

REFERENCES

Anon 1997 On the front line in nursing and complementary therapies. The Lamp (Journal of the NSW Nurses' Association) 54(6): 3–6

Barrett S 1993 Aromatherapy incare. Simply Essential 10 (October): 16

Cadwallader 1997 Aromatherapy in a hospital setting. Lecture at Monash University, Gipsland, Australia

Cohen J 1994 The healing touch. Longevity January: 26

Eisenberg D M, Kessler R C, Foster C, Norlock F E, Calkins D R, Delbanco T 1993 Unconventional medicine in the United States. New England Journal of Medicine 328: 246–252

George M 1996 Complementary therapies come to the coronary centre. Nursing Review (Melbourne) November: 14

Horzely J M 1993 The art of aromatherapy: an olfactory map toward healing and wellbeing. Healing Healthcare 4(1): 3–5

Kaiser L 1993 Follow your nose. Healing Healthcare 4(1): 2

Nursing Board of Victoria 1995 Guidelines for the use of complementary therapies in nursing practice. Nursing Board of Victoria, Melbourne

Passant H 1990 A holistic approach in the ward. Nursing Times 86(4): 26–28

Price S 1993 Aromathérapie guide pratique. Amrita, Plazac-Rouffignac

Price S 1994 L'aromathérapie au quotidien. Amrita, Plazac-Rouffignac

Price S 1999 Aromatherapy workbook (Chinese trans.). Jong Yeong Cosmetic Co Ltd, Taiwan

Roberts L 1996 Widespread acceptance in treatment of the elderly. Nursing Review (Melbourne) November: 1

Taylor L 1993 Aromas and anxiety at Memorial Sloan-Kettering. Healing Healthcare 4(1): 1

Appendices, Glossary and Useful addresses

SECTION CONTENTS

Appendix A

OILS CONTAINED IN APPENDIX A

Botanical name [COMMON NAME]

Achillea millefolium herb. [YARROW]
Aniba rosaeodora fol. [ROSEWOOD, BOIS DE ROSE]
Boswellia carteri res. dist. [FRANKINCENSE, OLIBANUM]
Cananga odorata flos [YLANG YLANG]
Carum carvi fruct. [CARAWAY]
Cedrus atlantica lig. [ATLAS CEDARWOOD, SATINWOOD]
Chamaemelum nobile (= Anthemis nobilis) flos
  [ROMANCHAMOMILE]
Chamomilla recutita (= Matricaria chamomilla, M.
  recutita) flos [GERMAN CHAMOMILE]
Citrus aurantium var. *amara* flos [NEROLI BIGARADE]
Citrus aurantium var. *amara* fol. [PETITGRAIN BIGARADE]
Citrus aurantium var. *amara* per. [ORANGE BIGARADE]
Citrus bergamia per. [BERGAMOT]
Citrus limon per. [LEMON]
Citrus reticulata per. [MANDARIN]
Commiphora myrrha var. *molmol (= C. molmol,*
Balsamodendron myrrha) res. dist. [MYRRH]
Coriandrum sativum fruct. [CORIANDER]
Cupressus sempervirens fol., strob. [CYPRESS]
Eucalyptus citriodora fol. [LEMON-SCENTED GUM]
Eucalyptus dives (ct. piperitenone) fol.
  [BROAD-LEAVED PEPPERMINT]
Eucalyptus globulus fol. [TASMANIAN BLUE GUM]
Eucalyptus radiata subsp. *radiata (= E. numerosa,*
  E. lindleyana) fol. [BLACK PEPPERMINT, NARROW-LEAVED
  PEPPERMINT]
Eucalyptus smithii fol. [GULLY GUM]
Foeniculum vulgare var. *dulce* fruct. [SWEET FENNEL]
Helichrysum angustifolium (= H. italicum) flos
  [EVERLASTING, IMMORTELLE]
Hyssopus officinalis flos, fol. [HYSSOP]
Juniperus communis fruct. [JUNIPER BERRY]
Juniperus communis ram. [JUNIPER TWIG]
Lavandula angustifolia (= L. officinalis, L. vera) flos
  [LAVENDER]
Lavandula × *intermedia* 'Super' flos [LAVANDIN]
Melaleuca alternifolia fol. [TEA TREE]

Melaleuca leucadendron (= M. cajuputi) fol. [CAJUPUT]
Melaleuca viridiflora (= M. quinquenervia) fol. [NIAOULI]
Melissa officinalis fol. [MELISSA]
Mentha × *piperita* fol. [PEPPERMINT]
Myristica fragrans sem. [NUTMEG]
Nardostachys jatamansi (= N. grandiflora) rad.
  [SPIKENARD]
Nepeta cataria var. *citriodora* flos, fol. [CATNEP]
Ocimum basilicum fol. [EUROPEAN BASIL]
Origanum vulgare subsp. *viride (= O. heracleoticum),*
  [GREEK OREGANO, GREEN OREGANO]
Origanum majorana flos, fol. [SWEET MARJORAM]
Ormenis mixta flos [MOROCCAN CHAMOMILE]
Pelargonium graveolens fol. [GERANIUM]
Pimpinella anisum fruct. [ANISEED]
Pinus sylvestris fol. [PINE]
Piper nigrum fruct. [BLACK PEPPER]
Pogostemon patchouli fol. [PATCHOULI]
Ravensara aromatica fol. [AROMATIC RAVENSARA]
Rosa damascena, R. centifolia flos (dist.) [ROSE OTTO]
Rosmarinus officinalis (ct. cineole, ct. camphor) fol.
  [ROSEMARY]
Rosmarinus officinalis (ct. verbenone) fol. [ROSEMARY]
Salvia officinalis fol. [SAGE, DALMATIAN SAGE]
Salvia sclarea flos, fol. [CLARY]
Santalum album lig. [SANDALWOOD]
Satureia hortensis fol. [SUMMER OR GARDEN SAVORY]
Satureia montana fol. [WINTER OR MOUNTAIN SAVORY]
Syzygium aromaticum (= Eugenia caryophyllata) flos
  [CLOVE BUD]
Tagetes minuta (= T. glandulifera, T. patula, T. erecta)
  flos [TAGET, FRENCH MARIGOLD]
Thymus mastichina flos, fol. [SPANISH MARJORAM]
Thymus satureioides [MOROCCAN THYME, BORNEOL THYME]
Thymus vulgaris (population) herb. [THYME]
Thymus vulgaris (ct. geraniol, ct. linalool) herb.
  [SWEET THYME]
Thymus vulgaris (ct. thujanol-4) herb. [SWEET THYME]
Thymus vulgaris (ct. thymol, ct. carvacrol) herb. [THYME]
Vetiveria zizanioides rad. [VETIVER]
Zingiber officinale rhiz. [GINGER]

ESSENTIAL OILS FOR GENERAL USE IN HEALTHCARE SETTINGS

This appendix is not intended to be a comprehensive list of essential oils and their properties. It is designed with healthcare situations in mind, and includes enough information to cover most eventualities where treatment with essential oils is appropriate. Several essential oils mentioned in the text of this book which do not appear here are shown in the chart in Appendix B9.

It is not possible in a general list such as this to give precise figures for the presence of a component in a given essential oil, particularly when the essential oils used in aromatherapy are not standardized but are taken directly from the still and used without any further treatment. The percentages shown for the constituents are aggregated and show the highs and lows for given compounds, and thus the variation, sometimes remarkably wide, in these. A common misinterpretation of aggregated data is that a species might appear to be high in two closely related compounds, e.g. thymol and carvacrol. It must be borne in mind that there is often compensation between the two compounds so that when the quantity of one is raised another is lowered (Beckstrom-Sternberg & Duke 1996). The factors which affect the variability of components have been discussed in Section 1, Essential oil science. Authors also give widely varying information—and sometimes fail to identify accurately the plant being discussed. It cannot be ruled out that some sources may be referring to standardized or adulterated oils.

Asterisks (*) are used to indicate where the authors have found essential oils to be particularly effective.

ACHILLEA MILLEFOLIUM herb. [YARROW] ASTERACEAE

Representative constituents

Hydrocarbons
monoterpenes α-pinene 1.5–3.5%, β-pinene 6–12.3%, camphene < 2.5%, sabinene 7.5–41.5%, myrcene 0.6–2%, α-terpinene 0.5–1.1%, limonene 0.4–1%, γ-terpinene 1.3–3.6%, terpinolene 0.2–0.6%, *p*-cymene 0.1–1.2%
sesquiterpenes chamazulene 5–33.2%, dihydroazulenes, caryophyllene 2.7–4.9%, germacrene D 9.3–13.6%

Alcohols
monoterpenols terpinen-4-ol 2.1–5.6%, borneol 0.2–9.5%
sesquiterpenols cadinols 0.4–1.1%

Oxides
1,8-cineole 1.9–11%, caryophyllene oxide 0.4–1.7%

Ketones
monoterpenones isoartemisia ketone 9%, camphor < 2.9%, thujone

Esters
bornyl acetate < 2.2%

Lactones
achilline

Phenols
eugenol

Properties and indications

analgesic	neuralgia, sprained ankle, sprains
anticatarrhal*	colds, catarrh
antiinflammatory*	prostatitis, neuritis, rheumatism
antiseptic	urinary infections
choleretic*	hepatobiliary deficiency, poor digestion
cicatrizant*	
decongestant	dysmenorrhoea
digestive stimulant	
diuretic	
emmenagogic*	oligomenorrhoea, amenorrhoea
expectorant	
febrifuge	fevers
hypotensor	hypertension
litholytic	kidney stones
vulnerary	varicose ulcers

Observations

- not normally used for babies, children and pregnant women
- neurotoxic and abortive (Franchomme & Pénoël 1990)
- yarrow contains little or no thujone (Leung 1980)
- some individuals show positive patch test reactions to yarrow
- cross-sensitivity between other Asteraceae members and yarrow has been demonstrated (Duke 1985)
- yarrow oil is obtained from the *A. millefolium* complex, a group of hardly separable species or subspecies of Asteraceae found throughout the temperate and boreal zones of the northern and southern hemispheres; the taxonomic problem is extensive and confusing (Lawrence 1984) and what is known as yarrow oil may come from one of several species
- at least 14 different chemical races have been identified in Europe (Mills 1991)
- yarrow has been universally used for the treatment of rheumatism, colds, catarrh, fevers, hypertension and amenorrhoea (Wren 1988)
- yarrow is diaphoretic, a peripheral vasodilator (Mills 1991)
- persons known to be allergic to ragweeds should be cautious about drinking chamomile or yarrow teas (Tyler 1982)
- isoartemisia ketone 9% is listed by Franchomme & Pénöel (1990) for this oil, but not by Lawrence; according to Guenther (1948–1952) it is found in *Artemisia annua*
- camphor chemotype should be used with caution; when taken orally camphor causes convulsions if sufficient quantity is taken (Craig 1953)
- antiinflammatory properties are associated with azulenes (Chandler, Hooper & Harvey 1982)
- CNS-depressant activity in mice has been documented (Kudrzycka-Bieloszabska & Glowniak 1966)

ANIBA ROSAEODORA fol.
[ROSEWOOD, BOIS DE ROSE] LAURACEAE

Representative constituents

Hydrocarbons
monoterpenes   α-pinene 0.15%, camphene 0.03%,
β-pinene 0.5%, myrcene 0.04%, limonene 0.6%, *p*-cymene,
β-phellandrene
sesquiterpenes   caryophyllene 0.03%,
α-selinene, β-elemene, γ-cadinene

Alcohols
monoterpenols   linalool 82–95%, geraniol, terpinen-4-ol 0.4%,
α-terpineol 3.5%
other (C8)   methyl heptenol

Aldehydes
neral, geranial, benzaldehyde

Esters
geranyl acetate 0.14%

Ketones
methyl heptenone

Oxides
cis-linalool oxide 1.5%, *trans*-linalool oxide 1.3%,
1,8-cineole 0.2–2.3%

Properties and indications

antifungal*	candida
antiinfectious	respiratory infections*, coughs
antiparasitic	
antiseptic	skin problems
antiviral*	colds
astringent	
bactericidal*	
cicatrizant	
stimulating*	general debility, overwork, sexual debility
tonic	nervous depression, stress-related headaches

Observations
- no known contraindications to aromatherapy use
- potent antibacterial agent (Lis-Balchin, Deans & Hart 1994)
- non-toxic when applied externally (Opdyke 1978a)
- linalool was found to have weak tumour-promoting properties in mice (Homburger & Boger 1968, Opdyke 1975a)
- anticonvulsant activity in mice and rats; spasmolytic activity on isolated guinea pig ileum and antimicrobial properties have been reported (Opdyke 1975)
- maximum level allowed in perfumes is 1.0% (Opdyke 1978a)

BOSWELLIA CARTERI res. dist.
[FRANKINCENSE, OLIBANUM] BURSERACEAE

Representative constituents

Hydrocarbons
monoterpenes (40%)   α-pinene 21%, α-thujene 24%,
limonene 8%, *p*-cymene 6%, sabinene 6%, camphene,
myrcene, α-terpinene, β-pinene, caryophyllene, γ-terpinene,
terpinolene
sesquiterpenes   α-gurjunene, α-guaiene,
α- and β-phellandrene, copaene

Alcohols
monoterpenols   borneol, terpinen-4-ol, *trans*-pinocarveol
sesquiterpenols   farnesol

Ketones
verbenone

Esters
octyl acetate

Properties and indications

analgesic	rheumatism, sports injuries
anticatarrhal*	asthma, bronchitis*
antidepressive*	nervous depression*
antiinfectious	respiratory tract
antiinflammatory	rheumatism
antioxidant	combats ageing process
cicatrizant	scars, ulcers, wounds
energizing	
expectorant	
immunostimulant*	immunodeficiency*

Observations
- no contraindications yet known for this gentle, effective, distilled oil
- olibanum absolute produces no skin irritation or sensitization reactions at 8% dilution when tested on humans, no phototoxic effects when undiluted (Opdyke 1978b)
- antibacterial action including *Listeria monocytogenes* (Lis-Balchin, Deans & Hart 1994)
- mild antifungal activity (Maruzzella 1960)
- the leaf oil of *Boswellia serrata* has antifungal effects (Garg 1974)

CANANGA ODORATA flos [YLANG YLANG] ANONACEAE

Representative constituents
(Percentage composition figures are given as a rough guide—ylang ylang is an oil of variable make-up.)

Hydrocarbons
monoterpenes   α-pinene, β-pinene
sesquiterpenes   α-farnesene and γ-cadinene 6.5–17.4%,
β-caryophyllene 15–22%, germacrene D 15–25%,
δ-cadinene 2–4.7%, α-humulene 0.9–2.5%

Alcohols
monoterpenols   linalool 11.6–30%, geraniol, nerol
sesquiterpenols   farnesol
aromatic   benzyl alcohol

Phenols
eugenol, isoeugenol

Esters (15%)
geranyl acetate 5–10%, benzyl acetate 3–8%,

benzyl benzoate 5–12%, methyl benzoate 1–5.5%,
methyl salicylate 1–10%, methyl anthranilate,
cresyl acetate, farnesyl acetate 1–7%,
benzyl salicylate

Phenyl methyl ethers
paracresyl methyl ether 15%, safrole, isosafrole, methyl
eugenol

Properties and indications

antidiabetic	diabetes
antiseptic	intestinal infections
antispasmodic*	cramp,colic
balancing*	
calming	tachycardia*, hyperpnoea, insomnia
hypotensor*	hypertension
tonic	scalp, hair growth
reproductive stimulant	frigidity, impotence
sedative	

Observations

- no contraindications known to normal aromatherapy use
- ylang ylang oil has been recognized as an allergen and removed from certain cosmetics (Mitchell & Rook 1979)
- no sensitization reactions at 10% dilution (Draize 1959)
- no irritation when tested at 10% dilution on humans (Opdyke 1974a)
- no phototoxic effects reported (Opdyke 1974a)
- can produce dermatitis in sensitized individuals (Duke 1985)
- the oil has been suggested as a possible substitute for quinine in malaria (Burkhill 1966)
- an essential oil is also prepared from the leaves
- stimulant when applied as a mask or by spraying (Rovesti & Colombo 1973)
- a folk remedy for asthma, boils, diarrhoea, headache, malaria, ophthalmia, rheumatism, stomach ailments (Duke & Wain 1981)

CARUM CARVI fruct. [CARAWAY] APIACEAE

Representative constituents

Hydrocarbons
monoterpenes (38–45%)   limonene 10–45%, carvene 30%, caryophyllene 0.1%, terpinolene 0.2%, myrcene, *p*-cymene

Alcohols
monoterpenols (2–6%)   *cis*-carveol 5.5%, *cis*-perillyl alcohol 0.1%, dihydrocarveol, cuminyl alcohol

Ketones
monoterpenones (50–60%) carvone 45–80%, dihydrocarvones 0.7%

Aldehydes
cuminaldehyde 0.1%

Coumarins
herniarin trace

Properties and indications

antibacterial	see Table 4.4
antihistaminic	hay fever
antispasmodic*	gastric spasm*, large intestine spasm, intestinal problems
aperitive	loss of appetite
calming	anger, vertigo
carminative*	flatulence*, aerophagy*
cholagogic, choleretic	insufficient bile, indigestion
diuretic	
emmenagogic	
larvicidal	
mucolytic*	bronchitis*
stimulant	scalp problems

Observations

- although caraway oil contains a substantial proportion of carvone, tests have proved that the whole oil is safe in normal use; however, it is best not used on infants under 3 years or expectant mothers
- in excessive dose it is neurotoxic and abortive
- no irritation or sensitization when tested at 4% dilution on humans (Opdyke 1973a)
- has a low level of phototoxicity (Opdyke 1973a)
- carvone and limonene have recently been shown to have an experimental cancer chemopreventative effect (Zheng, Kenney & Lam 1992)
- the seeds are chewed to relieve toothache and for carminative effect (Foster 1993b p. 59)
- it is a well-known digestive stimulant and this property is made use of in drinks such as Benedictine, Grand Chartreuse and Izarra
- caraway seeds have been found in 3000-year-old Egyptian tombs
- caraway and peppermint oils combined in enteric coated capsules (Enteroplant®) were found to improve non-ulcer dyspepsia (May et al 1996)
- the oil exhibits antibacterial and larvicidal activities (Oishi et al 1974; Ramadan et al 1972a)
- has antispasmodic and antihistaminic activities (Debelmas & Rochat 1967)
- carvone induces the detoxifying enzyme glutathione S-transferase (GST) in mouse tissue. Compounds that induce increased GST detoxification are considered potential inhibitors of carcinogenesis (Zheng, Kenney & Lam 1992)

CEDRUS ATLANTICA lig. [ATLAS CEDARWOOD, SATINWOOD] ABIETACEAE

Representative constituents

Hydrocarbons
sesquiterpenes (50%)   cedrene

Alcohols
sesquiterpenols (30%)   atlantol, α-caryophyllene alcohol, epi-β-cubenol

Ketones
sesquiterpenones (20%)   α-atlantone, γ-atlantone

Other
α-ionone, epoxy-β–himachalene and its epimer deodarone

Properties and indications

antibacterial	see Table 4.4
antiseptic	skin problems, scalp (with cade oil), urinary tract, eczema, pruritus (with bergamot oil)
arterial regenerator*	arteriosclerosis*
cicatrizant	skin problems, wounds
lipolytic*	cellulite*
lymph tonic*	cellulite*, lymph circulation problems, water retention
mucolytic	bronchitis*
stimulant	scalp problems

Observations

- it is important to specify this oil accurately: the term cedarwood oil has little meaning, because many oils are sold under this name, many of them from the Cupressaceae family
- considered in France to be neurotoxic and abortive, and not normally used there for pregnant women and infants
- Duraffourd (1982) recommends leaving internal use of this oil to a doctor
- the Moroccan oil *C. atlantica*
  — showed no irritation or sensitization at 8% dilution when tested on humans (Opdyke 1976a)
  — has no phototoxic effects reported, although the use of toilet preparations containing unspecified cedarwood oils followed by exposure to various wavelengths sometimes causes dermatitis (Winter 1984)

CHAMAEMELUM NOBILE (= *ANTHEMIS NOBILIS*) flos [ROMAN CHAMOMILE] ASTERACEAE

Representative constituents

Hydrocarbons
monoterpenes   α-terpene 0–10%, α-pinene 0–10%, β-pinene 0–10%, sabinene 0–10%, camphene, myrcene, γ-terpinene, *p*-cymene
sesquiterpenes   sabinene 0–10%, caryophyllene 0–10%, chamazulene, copaene, β-copaene, δ-cadinene

Alcohols
monoterpenols   *trans*-pinocarveol 5%
sesquiterpenols (5–6%)   farnesol, nerolidol

Aldehydes
myrtenal 0–10%

Ketones
monoterpenones   pinocarvone 13%

Esters (75–80%)
2-methylbutyl 2-methyl propionate 0.5–25%,
2-methylpropyl butyrate 0.5–10%,

2-methylbutyl 2-methylbutyrate 0.5–25%,
2-methylpropyl 3-methylbutyrate 0–10%,
propyl angelate 0.5–10%, 2-methylpropyl angelate 0.5–25%,
butyl angelate 0.5–10%, 3-methylpentyl angelate 0–10%
(Nano, Sacco & Frattini 1974).
Also given: isobutyl angelate 36–40%,
isobutyl isobutyrate 4%, 2-methylbutyl methyl-2-butyrate 3%,
isoamyl methyl-2-butyrate 3%, propyl angelate 1%,
hexyl acetate 0.5–10%

Oxides
1,8-cineole 0–25%

Coumarins
scopoletin-7-β-glucoside

Properties and indications

antianaemic	anaemia
antiinflammatory*	eczema, gout, inflamed skin, rheumatic pain, urticaria, skin irritation after shaving, cracked nipples, inflamed gums, neuritis
antineuralgic	
antiparasitic*	
antispasmodic*	migraines, headaches, (relaxes neuromuscular tension), infantile diarrhoea
calming, sedative	insomnia*, irritability, migraine, nervous depression*, nervous shock*
carminative	gas, intestinal colic
digestive	indigestion, loss of appetite
emmenagogic	nervous menstrual problems
menstrual	menopause, amenorrhoea, dysmenorrhoea
ophthalmic	conjunctivitis, sore tired eyes
stimulant	
sudorific	
vulnerary	boils, burns, wounds

Observations

- no contraindications known
- no irritation or sensitization at 4% dilution when tested on humans (Opdyke 1974b)
- no phototoxic effects reported (Opdyke 1974b)
- chamomile tea may cause anaphylaxis, contact dermatitis or other hypersensitivity reactions in allergic individuals; persons known to be allergic to ragweeds should be cautious about drinking chamomile or yarrow teas (Tyler 1982)
- the oil mixed with flour is a folk remedy for indurations of the liver, stomach and spleen (Duke 1985)
- oil used in 'Kamillosan' ointment at 0.5% to treat cracked nipples and nappy rash
- included in shampoos and for rinsing blond hair (Reynolds 1972)
- the oil is considered antispasmodic, carminative, cordial and sudorific (Duke 1985 p 111)
- generally non-toxic when applied externally (Food and Drug Administration 1978)

- oil is active against *Staphylococcus aureus* and *Candida albicans* and is used as an inhalant (Bartram 1995 p 106)
- in animals large dose produced sedation with drop in body temperature (Rossi et al 1988)
- the oil has antiinflammatory activity, antidiuretic and sedative effects following intraperitoneal administration in rats (Melegari et al 1988)

CHAMOMILLA RECUTITA (= MATRICARIA CHAMOMILLA, M. RECUTITA) flos [GERMAN CHAMOMILE] ASTERACEAE

Representative constituents

Hydrocarbons
monoterpenes α-terpinene trace, limonene, *p*-cymene, ocimene 1.7%
sesquiterpenes chamazulene 1–35%, bisabolenes, *trans*-β-farnesene 2–13%, *trans*-α-farnesene 27%, δ-cadinene 5.2%, α-copaene 0.2%, caryophyllene 0.5%, γ-muurolene 1.3%, α-muurolene 3.4%

Alcohols
sesquiterpenols α-bisabolol 2–67%, spathulenol, farnesol

Oxides
α-bisabol oxide A 0–55%, α-bisabolol oxide B 4.3–19%, epoxybisabolol, bisabolone oxide A 0–64%, 1,8-cineole

Coumarins
herniarin (7-methoxycoumarin), umbelliferone (7-hydroxycoumarin)

Ethers
en-yn-dicycloether 0.7%

Properties and indications

antiallergic	
antifungal	see Table 4.5
antiinflammatory*	eczema, gastritis, skin problems, rheumatism
antispasmodic	gastric spasm
cicatrizant	infected wounds, ulcers
decongestant	dysmenorrhoea
digestive tonic	duodenal ulcers, gastric ulcers, indigestion, morning sickness, nausea
hormone-like	amenorrhoea, PMS

Observations

- no known contraindications
- there are several chemotypes of this plant, hence the wide limits for the constituents quoted
- no irritation or sensitization at 4% dilution when tested on humans (Opdyke 1974c)
- no phototoxic effects reported (Opdyke 1974c)
- bisabolol-type chamomile extracts have low sensitizing activity but there are reports of allergenic properties perhaps due to a linear sesquiterpene lactone (anthecotulide) (Hausen, Busker & Carle 1984)
- the azulenes and bisabolol are antiinflammatory and antispasmodic, reducing histamine-induced reactions such as anaphylaxis and hay fever, allergic asthma and eczema (Mills 1991): the oil has antiinflammatory activity (Reynolds 1972)
- (–)-α-bisabolol possesses low acute toxicity after oral administration in mice, rats, dogs and rhesus monkeys (Habersang et al 1979)
- the sesquiterpenol (–)-α-bisabolol has been found to possess ulcer protective (Szelenyi & Thiemer 1979), spasmolytic (Achterrath-Tuckermann et al 1980), antiphlogistic (Jakovlev et al 1983) and antiinflammatory (Tubaro et al 1984) properties
- Foster (1991, 1993a) says that it is now generally believed that the chief pharmacological benefits are primarily due to α-bisabolol
- bisabolol has been shown to reduce the amount of proteolytic enzyme pepsin secreted by the stomach without any change occurring in the amount of stomach acid (Szelenyi & Thiemer 1979); it has also shown antiinflammatory action on granulomas, and shortens the healing time of cutaneous burns (Isaac 1979)
- chamazulene is anodyne, antispasmodic, antiinflammatory and antiallergenic (Foster 1993b)
- chamazulene is active against *Staphylococcus aureus* (Bartram 1995)
- azulenes reduce histamine-induced tissue reactions, calm the nervous system both peripherally as in visceral tension and centrally as in anxiety, nervous tension and headaches; their activity also extends to reducing the anaphylaxis due to the allergic response and so are indicated for hay fever, allergic asthma and eczema (Mills 1991)
- included in the pharmacopoeia of 26 countries (Salamon 1992)
- it has been shown that the use of the herbicide Propyzamide caused an increase in essential oil content; it has also been stated that the use of herbicides over extended periods could readily affect the plant's metabolism and it is recommended that all medicinal and essential oil plants be screened against a number of herbicides to see if there is any long term effect on secondary product metabolism; it is noteworthy that the effects under discussion were found in plants in which residual amounts of the herbicide were absent (Reichling, Becker & Drager 1978, Vömel et al 1977)
- the tea induced deep sleep (Reynolds 1972)
- antioxidant action and weak antibacterial, antifungal action (Lis-Balchin, Deans & Hart 1994)
- used externally for neuralgia (Bartram 1995)
- azulene components of the oil are thought to inhibit histamine release and prevent allergic seizures in guinea pigs (Mann & Staba 1986)
- azulenes have the ability to regenerate liver tissue in partially hepatectomized rats (Mann & Staba 1986)
- the oil reduced serum urea concentration in rabbits with induced uraemic conditions (Grochulski & Borkowski 1972)

CITRUS AURANTIUM VAR. AMARA flos
[NEROLI BIGARADE] RUTACEAE

Representative constituents

Hydrocarbons
monoterpenes (35%)   α-pinene 0.84%, β-pinene 13–14.3%,
limonene 12–18%, sabinene 0.73%, myrcene 1.62%,
trans--β-ocimene 3.65%

Alcohols
monoterpenols (40%)   linalool 30–36.4%, α-terpineol 2–5%,
geraniol 2–3%, nerol 1–3%
sesquiterpenols (6%)   *trans*-nerolidol 3–6%, farnesol 1.7%
aromatic   phenyl ethyl alcohol, benzyl alcohol

Esters (7–21%)
linalyl acetate 4–8.9%, neryl acetate 0.8–3%,
geranyl acetate 1–1.8%, methyl anthranilate B

Aldehydes (2.5%)
2.5-dimethyl-2-vinyl-hex-4-enal (Corbier & Teisseire 1974)
and others (unspecified)

Ketones
jasmone

Oxides
cis-linalool oxide

Other
cis-heptadec-8-ene (Corbier & Teisseire 1974)

Properties and indications

antibacterial	see Table 4.4
antidepressive*	nervous depression, neurasthenia, lightly tranquillizing
antiinfectious	colitis
antiparasitic*	
antitumoral	
digestive	liver and pancreas (diabetes)
hypotensor	hypertension
neurotonic*	fatigue, aids sleep, sympathetic nervous system imbalance, spasms, cardiovascular erethism, sustains uterus tone
phlebotonic	haemorrhoids, varicose veins
unspecified	bronchitis
unspecified	tuberculosis

Observations

- no known contraindications
- no irritation or sensitization at 4% dilution when tested on humans (Opdyke 1976b); devoid of irritating properties (Peterson & Hall 1946)
- it is essential to use the genuine version of this much adulterated and simulated oil. Neroli portugal, the oil distilled from the flowers of the sweet orange tree, is of a lesser quality
- the vapour of neroli showed strong antibacterial activity in vitro against one of five bacteria (Maruzzella & Sicurella 1960)

- a 1 : 50 dilution of neroli oil exhibited antifungal activity against all of a group of eight phytopathogenic fungi (Rao & Joseph 1971)
- no phototoxic effects reported (Opdyke 1976b)
- Huang et al (1981) showed that myrcenol and nerol possessed antiasthmatic activity
- bactericidal action five times greater than that of phenol (Reynolds 1972)
- some antifungal action (Maruzzella 1960)

CITRUS AURANTIUM VAR. AMARA fol.
[PETITGRAIN BIGARADE] RUTACEAE

Representative constituents

Hydrocarbons
monoterpenes (10%)   myrcene 1–6%,
cis-and-*trans*-β-cymenes 3–5%, *p*-cymene 1–3%,
β-pinene 0.7–1.7%, sabinene < 0.4%,
α-phellandrene trace–0.2%, limonene 0.7–1.1%,
cis-ocimene trace–1.1%, γ-terpinene 0.5–1.1%,
trans-ocimene trace–3.3%, terpinolene trace–0.1%,
α-pinene trace, α-terpinene trace

Alcohols
monoterpenols (30–40%)   linalool 20–27.9%,
α-terpineol 4.6–7.6%, nerol 1–2%, geraniol 2–4%,
terpinen-4-ol 0.5–0.8%, citronellol trace–0.2%

Esters (50–70%)
linalyl acetate 44–55%, neryl acetate 0.55–2.6%,
geranyl acetate 2–3%, α-terpinyl acetate 0.2–2.2%

Aldehydes
decanal trace, neral trace, geranial trace

Phenols
thymol trace

Coumarins
citropten, bergapten

Properties and indications

antibacterial	see Table 4.4
antiinfectious	boils, infected acne*, respiratory infections
antiinflammatory	acne
antispasmodic*	
balancing*	calming, energizing to sympathetic nervous system

Observations

- no known contraindications
- no irritation at 5% dilution when tested on humans (Fujii, Furukawa & Suzuki 1972)
- no irritation at 8% dilution when tested on humans (Ford, Api & Letizia 1992a)
- no phototoxic effects when tested on mice (Forbes, Urbach & Davies 1977)
- strong antibacterial and antifungal action (Lis-Balchin, Deans & Hart 1994, Maruzzella 1960, Maruzzella & Sicurella 1960, Maruzzella & Liguori 1958)

- the common name 'petitgrain' is used as a general term for oils distilled from the leaves of citrus trees, and so should be qualified to indicate from which tree the oil was obtained—orange (bitter or sweet), lemon, mandarin, etc.

CITRUS AURANTIUM VAR. *AMARA* per. [ORANGE BIGARADE] RUTACEAE

Representative constituents

Hydrocarbons
monoterpenes (90–98%)   limonene 98%, myrcene 1–2%, terpinolene, α-pinene 0.1–1%, camphene
sesquiterpenes   caryophyllene, copaenes, farnesene, α-humulene

Alcohols (0.3–0.5%)
citronellol, α-terpineol, nerol, linalool, nerol

Aldehydes (0.9–3%)
geranial, neral, undecanal, sinensal

Esters (2%)
linalyl acetate 1%; geranyl acetate, neryl acetate, citronellyl acetate

Coumarins (< 1%)
osthol (7-methoxy-8-isopentenoxycoumarin), auraptenol (7-methoxy-8-(2-hydroxy-3-methyl-3-butenyl) coumarin), bergapten (5-methoxpsoralen), 7-geranoxycoumarin, 7-hydroxycoumarin, 5-isopentenoxypsoralen

Properties and indications

antiinflammatory	
anticoagulant	poor circulation
calming*	gastric spasm, nervousness, sympathetic nervous system, vertigo, palpitations
cholagogic	
digestive	constipation*, liver stimulant, indigestion*
sedative*	anxiety
tonic*	tonic for the gums, mouth ulcers

Observations

- no irritation or sensitization at 10% dilution when tested on humans (Opdyke 1974d); cutaneous irritation has been reported (Schwarz, Tulipan & Peck 1947)
- a case of dermatitis has been reported in a girl employed to peel bitter orange (Murray 1921)
- phototoxic effects have been reported (Opdyke 1974d)
- it is lightly hypnotic (P Collin personal communication)
- the majority of the compounds in this oil are present at less than 1%
- orange oil spray had an antidepressant effect on patients (Rovesti & Colombo 1973)
- dried orange peel is used commonly by Puerto Ricans to treat sleep disorders, gastrointestinal disorders, respiratory ailments and raised blood pressure (Reynolds 1972)

CITRUS BERGAMIA per. [BERGAMOT] RUTACEAE

Representative constituents

Hydrocarbons
monoterpenes   α-pinene 0.5–1%, camphene trace–0.03%, limonene 26.7–42.5%, β-pinene 2.9–5.1%, sabinene 0.6–0.7%, myrcene 0.4–1.4%, δ-3-carene 0–2%, *p*-cymene 0.1–3.6%, γ-terpinene 1.2–4.8%
sesquiterpenes   β-bisabolene 0.02–0.9%

Alcohols
monoterpenols (45–65%)   linalool 11–22%, nerol, geraniol 0–5.6%, α-terpineol
aromatic alcohols   dihydrocumin alcohol

Esters
linalyl acetate 30–60%, geranyl acetate 0.6–1.3%, neryl acetate 0.5–0.9%

Aldehydes
geranial 0.1–0.5%, neral 0.04–0.4%

Coumarins, furanocoumarins
bergamottin, bergamottin 5% (5-methoxyfurano-2, 3, 6, 7-coumarin)

Properties and indications

antibacterial	see Table 4.4
antiinfectious	wounds
antiseptic*	intestinal, gas, colic, gargles for mouth and throat
antispasmodic*	colic, indigestion
antiviral	herpes simplex I
calming*	insomnia
cicatrizant	burns
photosensitizer	vitiligo
sedative	agitation
stomachic*	loss of appetite
tonic	digestive system, central nervous system
unspecified	psoriasis

Observations

- not normally used prior to exposure to ultraviolet (UV) light because it is phototoxic to human skin on account of the bergamottin and bergapten compounds, which accelerate suntanning (Musajo, Rodighiero & Caporale 1953, 1954, Pathak & Fitzpatrick 1959, Zaynoun, Johnson & Frain-Bell 1977)
- for the same reason some perfumes (e.g. eau de Cologne) should be used with care
- there is a melanoma risk associated with sun creams containing bergamot oil, but thought to be so because people who use these creams are more likely to spend more time in the sun
- in 1995 the EU limited furanocoumarins to 1 ppm in sun products
- a rectified oil did not exhibit any phototoxic effects; berloque dermatitis is due to bergapten (5-methoxypsoralen) and this must be reduced to 0.001% to obviate bergapten dermatitis (Marzulli & Maibach 1970)

- no sensitization at 30% dilution when tested on humans (Opdyke 1973b)
- undiluted oil is slightly irritating to skin
- distilled oil is obtained from the residue of cold extraction and small, unripe fruits which cannot be cold extracted
- bergamot oil is used in most perfumes as a natural fixative
- there are three cultivars of bergamot, namely Castagnaro, Feminello, Fantastico (by far the most popular (80%))
- natural bergamot is 60% of consumption, but reconstituted oils are often found
- there are approximately 350 constituents in bergamot essential oil
- in the presence of UVA, 5-methoxypsoralen is mutagenic in vitro (Averbeck et al 1990) and was carcinogenic when tested on mice (Young et al 1990, Zajdela & Bisagni 1981), but Mezzadra et al (1981) found no increase in cutaneous carcinogenesis in Calabrian workers in contact with bergamot oil and fruits
- Berloque dermatitis, or bergapten dermatitis, is caused by exposure to UV light following bergapten application (Young et al 1990)
- the non-volatile residue of the cold-pressed oil has a CNS depressant action in rats (Occhiuto et al 1995)
- bergamottin has antiarrhythmic and antianginal effects on guinea pigs (Occhutio & Circosta 1996)
- it has sedative action (Manley 1993)

CITRUS LIMON per. [LEMON] RUTACEAE

Representative constituents

Hydrocarbons

monoterpenes (90–95%)   limonene 55–80%, α-pinene 1.9–2.4%, β-pinene 10–17%, γ-terpinene 3–10%, sabinene 2%, α-thujene 0.01–0.4%, myrcene, α-phellandrene, α-terpinene 0.2–0.4%, *p*-cymene 1%
sesquiterpenes   β-bisabolene 0.5–4%, α-bergamotene 0.4%, β-caryophyllene 0.2%

Alcohols

aliphatic alcohols   hexanol, *N*-heptanol, octanol, nonanol, decanol
monoterpenols   linalool 0.1%, terpinen-4-ol 0.05%, α-terpineol 0.1–0.2%

Aldehydes

geranial 0.9–1.6%, neral 0.5–1%, citronellal 0.1%, nonanal, octanal, decanal 0.05%

Esters

neryl acetate 0.5%, geranyl acetate 0.5%, α-terpinyl acetate 0–0.7%

Coumarins, furanocoumarins

bergamottin 0.2%, citropten, bergaptol trace, phellopterin, bergapten 0.6%, oxypeucedanin, imperaterin, isoimperaterin

Properties and indications

antianaemic	anaemia
antibacterial*	see Table 4.4

anticoagulant	hypertension, phlebitis, poor circulation, thrombosis, varicose veins
antifungal	thrush
antiinfectious	respiratory system
antiinflammatory	boils, gout, insect bites, rheumatism
antimelanistic	brown skin spots
antisclerotic	combats ageing process
antiseptic* (air)	crêches, burns units, hospital wards
antispasmodic	diarrhoea
antiviral	colds, herpes, veruccas, warts
astringent	diarrhoea, nosebleeds, seborrhoea (scalp and face), skin, broken capillaries
calming	headache, insomnia, nightmares
carminative	flatulence
digestive	nausea, painful digestion, aerophagy, loss of appetite
diuretic	obesity, oedema
expectorant	respiratory system
immunostimulant	white cell deficiency
litholytic*	gall stones, urinary stones
pancreatic stimulant*	diabetes
phlebotonic	
stomachic	gastritis, stomach ulcers

Observations

- no irritation or sensitization at 10% dilution when tested on humans (Opdyke 1974e)
- no phototoxic effects reported for distilled lemon oil (Opdyke 1974f)
- the expressed oil is phototoxic (Opdyke 1974e), therefore exposure to sunlight is to be avoided for 1 hour after skin application
- in the case of expressed oils it is very important to ensure that the fruits have not been sprayed with chemicals
- non-volatile constituents make up about 2% of expressed lemon oil
- weak antibacterial and antifungal activity (Deans & Ritchie 1987)
- (+)-limonene preparation used to dissolve gall stones (Reynolds 1972)
- lemon oil spray relieved depression of patients (Rovesti & Colombo 1973)
- oil of lemon was found to have expectorant activity in guinea pigs (Boyd & Pearson 1946)
- lemon oil exhibits antimicrobial activity (Poretta & Casolari 1966, Subba et al 1967)

CITRUS RETICULATA per. [MANDARIN] RUTACEAE

Representative constituents

Hydrocarbons

monoterpenes   limonene 65–77%, α-pinene 1.5–3%, β-pinene 1.3–2.5%, myrcene 1.6–2.2%, γ-terpinene 13.7–20.9%, terpinolene 0.6–1%, *p*-cymene 1.2–3.6%, α-phellandrene 0.05–0.1%

Alcohols

aliphatic alcohols   nonanol, octanol 1%

monoterpenols   citronellol, linalool 1–5%, α-terpineol 0.1–0.25%

Aldehydes (1%)

decanal 0.05–0.17%, α-sinensal 0.15–0.3%, perillaldehyde < 0.1%, octanal 0.1%

Phenols

thymol < 0.1%

Esters

methyl *N*-methyl anthranilate 0.1–0.7%, benzyl acetate

Properties and indications

antiepileptic	
antifungal	
antispasmodic	hiccoughs, stomach cramp, spasm
calming*	insomnia, nervous tension, cardiovascular erethism, excitability
cholagogic	
eupeptic	indigestion, constipation
hepatic	
stomachic	stomach pains

Observations

- because mandarin oil may be phototoxic, exposure to sunlight should be avoided for 1 hour after skin application
- no irritation or sensitization at 8% dilution when tested on humans (Ford, Api & Letizia 1992b)
- no coumarins were detected in mandarin oil by Shu, Waradt & Taylor (1974) but Franchomme & Pénoël (1990) identify a presence

COMMIPHORA MYRRHA VAR. *MOLMOL* (= *C. MOLMOL, BALSAMODENDRON MYRRHA*) res. dist. [MYRRH] BURSERACEAE

Representative constituents

Hydrocarbons

monoterpenes   furanoeudesma-1,3-diene 12.5%, *cis*-ocimene 1.9%, *p*-cymene 1.51%, *trans*-ocimene 1.27%, α-thujene 0.76%, myrcene 0.45%, limonene 0.42%, isoallo-ocimene 0.03%, α-pinene, dipentene

sesquiterpenes   δ-elemene 28.79%, α-copaene 10.02–11.9%, β-elemene 6.19%, bourbonene 4.9%, α-bergamotene 4.9%, α-muurolene 0.14%, γ-cadinene 0.12%, curzerene (iso-furanogermacrene) 0.09–11.9%, α-caryophyllene 0.08%, heerabolene, σ-elemene, lindestrene 3.5%

Ketones

curzerenone 11.7%, methyl isobutyl ketone 5.68%, 3 methoxy-10 (15)-dihydrofuranodien-6-one 1.5%, 1, 10 (15)-furanodien-6-one 1.2%, dihydropyrocurzerenone (dihydrofuranoeudesmadiene) 1.1%, 3 methoxy-10-methylenefuranogermacra-1-en-6-one 0.9%, furanodien-6-one 0.4%, 6-methyl-5-hepten-2-one 0.23%, 3 methoxy-4,5-dihydrofuranodien-6-one 0.2%, 3 methoxyfuranoguaia-9-en-8-one 0.1%

Aldehydes

5-methylfurfural 1.66%, furfural 1.44%, benzaldehyde 0.53%, cuminaldehyde, cinnamaldehyde

Phenols

eugenol, *m*-cresol

Alcohols

aromatic alcohols   cuminyl alcohol

Acids

acetic acid, formic acid, palmitic acid

Other

2-methyl-5-isopropenylfuran 4.63%, xylene 2.84%, 2 methyl furan 1.93%, 2-methyl-5-isopropylfuran 1.18%, 4,4-dimethyl-2-butenolide 1.04%, methyl anisole 0.14%, 2-phenyl-2-methylbutane 0.14%, rosefuran 0.09%, tridecane 0.09%

Properties and indications

antiinflammatory	
antiseptic	urinary tract, cleansing sores, wounds, ulcers
antispasmodic	
astringent	
cardiac tonic	
carminative	
cicatrizant	wounds, skin diseases, mouth ulcers
emmenagogic?	
expectorant	bronchitis, laryngitis, influenza
sedative	
stomachic	
tonic	

Observations

- the oil was not irritating when applied to the backs of hairless mice and pigs (Urbach & Forbes 1973); 5% in petrolatum was not irritating and 8% in petrolatum was non-sensitizing (Epstein 1973)
- no phototoxicity on mice and swine has been noted (Urbach & Forbes 1973)
- acute oral toxicity LD$_{50}$ 1.65 g/kg in rats (Moreno 1973)
- a flavour component of foods; a fragrance component or fixative in soaps, detergents, creams and lotions; used in perfumes (0.8% max.) (Opdyke 1976c)
- a leukocytogenic agent (increases number of white cells in blood: bacteriostatic against *Staphylococcus aureus* and other Gram positive bacteria; perhaps the most widely used herbal antiseptic (Bartram 1996 p 304)
- myrrh was always present in the coffins and as salve on the bodies in ancient Egypt
- Dioscorides mentioned myrrh as warming, astringent and 'numbing'; it was to some extent used as an anaesthetic in operations.
- the condemned Christ was offered wine spiced with myrrh to diminish his suffering on the cross (Mark 15: 23).

This use of wine containing myrrh or incense at the Flagellation and Crucifixion seems to have been customary in ancient times in order to diminish to some extent the sufferings of martyrdom (Storp 1996)

- *Bisabol myrrh* is believed by some to be the myrrh of the Bible (Holmes 1916)

CORIANDRUM SATIVUM fruct. [CORIANDER] APIACEAE

Representative constituents

Hydrocarbons
monoterpenes (10–20%)   γ-terpinene 1–8%, *p*-cymene trace–3.5%, limonene 0.5–4%, α-pinene 0.2–8.5%, camphene trace–1.4%, myrcene 0.2–2%

Alcohols
monoterpenols (60–80%)   linalool 60–87%, geraniol 1.2–3.3%, terpinen-4-ol trace–3%, α-terpineol < 0.5%

Ketones (7–9%)
camphor 0.9–4%

Esters
geranyl acetate 0.1–4.7%, linalyl acetate 0–2.7%

Coumarins, furanocoumarins
umbelliferone trace, bergapten trace

Properties and indications

analgesic	osteoarthritis, rheumatic pain
antibacterial*	see Table 4.4
antiinfectious*	cystitis, influenza
antiinflammatory	gastroenteritis
antispasmodic	digestive, uterine
carminative*	flatulence, aerophagy
euphoric*	sadness
larvicidal	
neurotonic*	anorexia, debility, general fatigue, mental fatigue
stomachic	indigestion, sluggish digestion

Observations

- no irritation or sensitization at 6% dilution when tested on humans (Opdyke 1973c)
- weakly cytotoxic
- the linalool content depends upon the ripeness of the fruits and the geographical source, as do the proportions of the constituents
- coriandrol is a synonym for (+)-linalool (Foster 1993b)
- the leaf oil has the fragrance of decylaldehyde and other fatty aldehydes (Prakash 1990)
- experimentally coriander is antiinflammatory and hypoglycaemic (Foster 1993b)
- a Chinese remedy for measles, of value in diabetes (hypoglycaemic), gastroenteritis, also used for schistosomiasis (Bartram 1995 p. 128)
- coriander oil is larvicidal, bactericidal and cytotoxic (Abdullin 1962, Silyanovska et al 1969)

CUPRESSUS SEMPERVIRENS fol., strob. [CYPRESS] CUPRESSACEAE

Representative constituents

Hydrocarbons
monoterpenes   α-pinene 35–55%, β-pinene 3%, δ-3-camphene 0.5%, δ-3-camphene 15–25%, limonene 2.5–5%, terpinolene 2.4–6%, *p*-cymene 0.2–1.5%, sabinene 0.1–3%, γ-terpinene 0.3%
sesquiterpenes   α-cedrene 0.4%, δ-cadinene 1.5–3%, ocimenes 0.4%, β-cedrene 0.3%

Alcohols
monoterpenols   terpinen-4-ol, α-terpineol 1–2%, borneol 1–8.7%, linalool 0.8%, sabinol
sesquiterpenols   cedrol 5.3–21%
diterpenols (trace)   manool, abienols, pimarinols, totarol

Oxides
1,8-cineole 0.3%, manoyl oxide 0.5%

Esters
α-terpenyl acetate 4–5%, terpinen-4-yl acetate 1–2%

Other
sandaracopimara-8(14), 15-diene 1.3%

Properties and indications

antibacterial	see Table 4.4
antiinfectious	bronchitis, influenza
antispasmodic	cramp
antisudorific	excessive perspiration
antitussive	whooping cough, bronchitis
astringent	broken capillaries
calming	regulates sympathetic nervous system, irritability
deodorant	sweaty feet
diuretic	oedema, rheumatic swelling
hormone-like	ovary problems
neurotonic*	debility
phlebotonic*	varicose veins, haemorrhoids, poor venous circulation, protects capillary circulation

Observations

- no contraindications known
- has a very remarkable astringent action, much superior to that of witch hazel (Duraffourd 1982)
- oil of cypress is a homologue of the ovarian hormone (Valnet 1980)
- no irritation or sensitization at 5% dilution when tested on humans (Opdyke 1978c)
- no phototoxic effects reported (Opdyke 1978c)

EUCALYPTUS CITRIODORA fol. [LEMON-SCENTED GUM] MYRTACEAE

Representative constituents

Hydrocarbons
monoterpenes (1–1.2%)   isopropylhexane 0.3%, α-pinene 0.2–1.9%, camphene trace, *p*-cymene 0.1–0.9%,

β-pinene 0.4–1.5%, α-phellandrene limonene < 7.1%, γ-terpinene < 0.9%, p-mentha-3,8-diene 0.2%, terpinolene 0.1–0.8%, myrcene < 0.6%
sesquiterpenes caryophyllene 0.3–3.9%, α-humulene 0.1%, β-cubebene 0.1%, α-elemene 0.1%, aromadendrene

Alcohols
monoterpenols (12–18%) citronellol 4.6–14.4%, geraniol < 5%, α-terpineol 0.1%, nerol trace, spathulenol 0.1%, linalool 0.3–1.5%, *trans*- and *cis-p*-menthan-3,8-diols, *trans*-pinocarveol
sesquiterpenols (2–4%)

Phenols
isopulegol 0.3–29.8%, eugenol

Aldehydes
citronellal 26.7–90.1%, geranylcitronellal trace, 2,6-dimethyl-5-heptenal 0.2%, hydroxycitronellal

Esters
citronellyl acetate 0.4–3.1%, citronellyl butyrate, citronellyl citronellate

Ketones
carvone, menthone trace

Oxides
1,8-cineole 0.4–17.9%, *cis*-rose oxide 0.4%, linalool oxide 0.4%

Other
1,8-terpin hydrate 0.8%, methyl-*cis*-9-octadecenoate trace, 1-methyl-4-isopropyl-cyclohexane trace

Properties and indications:

analgesic*	
antifungal	see Table 4.5
antiinflammatory	arthritis, cystitis, vaginitis, pericarditis, coronaritis
antirheumatic*	rheumatoid arthritis
antiinfectious	shingles
antispasmodic	
antidiabetic	diabetes (some)
bactericidal	*Staphylococcus aureus*
calming, sedative	hypertension

Observations

- *trans*- and *cis-p*-menthan-3,8-diols are allelopathic substances
- no known contraindications
- makes a synergistic mix with copaiba balsam, wintergreen and *Helichrysum italicum* (Roulier 1990)
- the tree is grown in many tropical areas for its wood and as a source of citronellal.
- four forms have been identified (Penfold & Willis 1961):
  1. citronellal 65–85%, citronellol 15–20%, esters
  2. citronellal 1–14%, citronellol, esters
  3. citronellal 10–50%, guaiol
  4. hydrocarbons.
- Bacteriostatic properties are due to natural synergism between citronellal and citronellol. The oil is active

against *S. aureus* and has a minimal inhibitory concentration of 1:32. Tests on the individual components of this oil showed them to be relatively inactive but a combination of the three major components in the ratio found in the natural oil produced a fourfold increase in antimicrobial activity (Low, Rawal & Griffin 1974)
- inhibits *Trichophyton mentagrophytes* and *Microsporum audonil* (Yadav & Dubey 1994); active antibacterial agent (Asre 1994)
- effective against *Candida* and other fungi (Asre 1994)

EUCALYPTUS DIVES CT. PIPERITENONE fol.
[BROAD-LEAVED PEPPERMINT] MYRTACEAE

Representative constituents

Hydrocarbons
monoterpenes α-phellandrene 30%
sesquiterpenes α-cubebene, β-caryophyllene, longifolene, γ-elemene, δ-cadinene

Alcohols
α-terpineol, linalool, terpinen-1-ol-4, piperitol

Ketones
piperitone 40–50%

Properties and indications:

antibacterial	
anticatarrhal	
antifungal	
antiinfectious	sinusitis, otitis, bronchitis, nephritis, vaginitis (leukorrhoea)
antiviral	
cicatrizant	wound healing
diuretic	
lipolytic	
mucolytic	

Observations

- contraindicated for babies and pregnant women (Franchomme & Pénoël 1990)
- generally regarded as safe in normal aromatherapy use
- this species is not generally cultivated therefore the oil comes from wild plants (Weiss 1997 p. 279)
- there are at least four distinct chemotypes of *E. dives* (Boland, Brophy & House 1991) including a cineole type (up to 75%) closely related to *E. radiata* and a phellandrene type (up to 80%) used in industrial perfumery and insecticides
- piperitone is antiasthmatic and insectifuge (Beckstrom-Sternberg & Duke 1996 p. 411)

EUCALYPTUS GLOBULUS fol.
[TASMANIAN BLUE GUM] MYRTACEAE

Representative constituents

Hydrocarbons
monoterpenes α-pinene 3–27%, p-cymene 1.2–3.5%, limonene 1.8–9%, camphene 0.2–0.4%

sesquiterpenes   aromadendrene 0.1–6%, α-phellandrene 0.2%

Alcohols
monoterpenols   α-fenchyl alcohol 1–2%, α-terpineol 0.1–0.6%, myrtenol 1.3%
sesquiterpenols   globulol 0–6%, ledol 1–2%, *trans*-pinocarveol 0.8–4.5%, viridiflorol, epi-globulol

Ketones
monoterpenones   pinocarvone 1–2%, carvone 0.1%, fenchone 0.4%

Oxides
1,8-cineole 60–85%, α-pinene epoxide 0.2%

Aldehydes
myrtenal, geranial, valeric aldehyde, butyric aldehyde, caproic aldehyde

Esters
α-terpenyl acetate 0.1–2%

Properties and indications

antibacterial	see Table 4.4
anticatarrhal	coughs, sinusitis
antifungal	candida see Table 4.5
antiinfectious	acute bronchitis, coughs, influenza, pneumonia, respiratory tract infections, sinusitis, laryngitis
antiinflammatory	pleurisy, bronchitis, sinusitis, laryngitis, cystitis
antimigraine	migraine
antiseptic*	cystitis, urinary tract infection
antiviral	colds, influenza
balsamic	combats fever and acts like a balm
decongestant	asthma, headaches, migraine
expectorant*	bronchitis, cough, catarrh, cold
insect repellent	gnats, mosquitoes
mucolytic	cough, sinusitis
rubefacient	subcutaneous infection, arthritis

Observations

- contraindicated for very young children and babies because of the high cineole content: several cases of poisoning in children have been reported (Craig 1953, Foggie 1911, Kirkness 1910, McPherson 1925, Neale 1893, Patel & Wiggins 1980, Sewell 1925)
- as with many essential oils in excessive dose, eucalyptus oil has caused fatalities from intestinal irritation (Morton 1981); death is reported from ingestion of 4–24 ml of essential oil, but recoveries are also reported for the same amount (Reynolds 1972)
- eliminated from the body via the respiratory tract
- it may be necessary to rid certain eucalyptus oils of some short chain aldehydes (e.g. valerian aldehyde, butyraldehyde, capronaldehyde), which are irritant and tussigenic (Belaiche 1979, Wagner, Bladt & Zgainski 1984)
- no irritation or sensitization at 10% dilution when tested on humans (Opdyke 1975b)
- hypersensitivity has been reported (Goodman & Gilman 1942, Löwenfeld 1932, Schwartz & Peck 1946, Schwartz, Tulipan & Peck 1947)
- no phototoxic effects reported (Opdyke 1975b)
- there is a difference between the oils from the young leaves and those from the old leaves
- *E. globulus* oil is used in catarrhal conditions, given orally on a lump of sugar or as an emulsion with olive oil (Reynolds 1972)
- found to increase output of respiratory tract fluid in guinea pigs (Boyd & Pearson 1946)
- the oil is used in cough drops as antiseptic, rubefacient and stimulant (Morton 1981)
- used in Cuba for bronchitis, bladder and liver infections, lung ailments, malaria and stomach trouble (Morton 1981)
- the oil has antibacterial and expectorant properties (Maruzella & Henry 1958, Pizsolitto 1975, Prakash et al 1972)
- strongly antibacterial against several *Streptococcus* strains (Benouda, Hasser & Benjilali 1988)
- oil is used as an antiseptic, febrifuge and expectorant (Bisset 1994, Wren 1988)
- the oil is taken orally for catarrh and applied as a rubefacient (Reynolds 1989)

EUCALYPTUS RADIATA SUBSP. *RADIATA* (= *E. NUMEROSA, E. LINDLEYANA*) fol.
[BLACK PEPPERMINT, NARROW-LEAVED PEPPERMINT]
MYRTACEAE

Representative constituents

Hydrocarbons
monoterpenes   α-pinene 3.7%, β-pinene 1.0%, myrcene 2.0%

Alcohols
monoterpenols   linalool 0.4%, geraniol 2.6%, α-terpineol 14.0%, isoterpineol-4 2.0%, borneol

Aldehydes
monoterpenals   geranial, neral, citronellal, myrtenal

Oxides
1,8-cineole 62–72%, caryophyllene oxide (an epoxycyclic monoterpene)

Properties and indications

anticatarrhal	
antiinfectious	acute and chronic respiratory infections, influenza*
antiinflammatory	rhinitis, rhinopharyngitis, otitis, bronchitis, conjunctivitis, vaginitis, acne
antiseptic	strong antiseptic
antiviral	
energizing*	chronic fatigue, immune deficiency
expectorant	
mucolytic	coughs, powerful expectorant and fluidification properties (especially when blended with *Eucalyptus smithii*)

Observations

- long lasting action, quick penetration
- particularly indicated for children (Roulier 1990)
- no contraindications known
- it is important to blend with a terpene rich oil for best results
- Weiss (1997 p. 294) gives phellandrene as a major constituent at up to 40%

EUCALYPTUS SMITHII fol. [GULLY GUM] MYRTACEAE

Representative constituents

Hydrocarbons
monoterpenes (20%)   limonene 9–10%, α-pinene 7%, *p*-cymene

Alcohols
monoterpenols   terpineol, terpineol-4, geraniol, linalool
sesquiterpenols   eudesmol

Oxides
1,8-cineole 70–80%

Esters
small quantities

Aldehyde
isovaleraldehyde

Properties and indications

analgesic	painful joints and muscles
anticatarrhal	bronchitis, coughs
antiinfectious	respiratory system
antiviral	colds, influenza
balancing	calming (evening use), stimulant (morning use)
decongestant	asthma, headaches
digestive stimulant	sluggish digestion
expectorant	bronchitis, coughs
prophylactic	colds, influenza

Observations

- no contraindications known
- the oil has great synergistic and quenching properties (Pénoël 1993)
- an effective chest rub; may be used undiluted

FOENICULUM VULGARE VAR. *DULCE* fruct. [SWEET FENNEL] APIACEAE

Representative constituents

Hydrocarbons
monoterpenes   α-pinene 1.4–10%, limonene 1.4–17%, α-phellandrene 0.2–4%, α-thujene 0.2%, camphene 0.2%, β-pinene 0.3–1%, sabinene 2%, myrcene 0.5–3%, α-terpinene 0.5–1%, β-phellandrene 0.4–2.6%, γ-terpinene 10.5%, *cis*-ocimene 12%, terpinolene trace–3.3%, *p*-cymene 0.4–4.7%

Alcohols
monoterpenols   fenchol 3–4%

Ketones
fenchone trace–22%

Phenolic ethers
methyl chavicol 2–12%, *cis*-anethole trace–1.7%, *trans*-anethole 50–90%

Aldehydes
anisaldehyde trace–0.5%

Oxides
1,8-cineole 1–6%

Coumarins, furanocoumarins
bergaptene, umbelliferone

Properties and indications

analgesic	backache, gout, painful menstruation
antibacterial	see Table 4.4
antifungal	see Table 4.5
antiinflammatory	cystitis, gout
antiseptic	urinary tract infections
antispasmodic	gastric enteritis
cardiotonic	heart palpitations
carminative*	flatulence
cholagogic	
circulatory stimulant	
decongestant	breast engorgement, bruises
digestive	indigestion, loss of appetite
diuretic	cellulite, oedema
emmenagogic	lack of, irregular or scanty menstruation*
hormone-like	
lactogenic*	lack of milk in breastfeeding mothers*
laxative	constipation
litholytic	urinary stones
oestrogen like*	ovary problems, PMS, menopause
respiratory tonic	rapid breathing

Observations

- must be well diluted for young children and is best avoided in pregnancy until last 2 months
- if the oil is given in excessively high dose it may cause disturbance of the nervous system, but is safe when used in the amounts normally employed in aromatherapy
- no irritation or sensitization at 4% dilution when tested on humans (Opdyke 1974g)
- no phototoxic effects reported (Opdyke 1974g)
- large doses of oil reduced the body weight of mice
- has an epileptic action at high dose (Roulier 1990)
- special consideration must be given to the amount used when treating young children (note: it is an ingredient of gripe water); fennel oil is used as a carminative for children (Reynolds 1972)
- has caused pulmonary oedema, respiratory problems, and seizures in quantities of 1–5 ml; for this reason, self-

medication with fennel should be restricted to moderate use of the fruits (seeds), and the volatile oil should not be used (Tyler 1982)

- anethole is reported to have allergenic and toxic properties; its structural similarity to catecholemines (adrenaline, noradrenaline, dopamine) may help to explain its ephedrine-like bronchodilator action and amphetamine-like facilitation of weight loss; similarity of anethole to the psychoactive compounds mescaline, asarone and myristicin has been noted (Mills 1991); fennel oil is oestrogen like (Albert-Puleo 1980; Zondek et al 1938)
- therapeutic doses of the distilled oil of fennel occasionally induced epileptiform madness and hallucinations; dill, anise and parsley (plants) all have similar oils, and it has been demonstrated that in vivo amination of these ring-substituted oils can result in a series of three hallucinogenic amphetamines (Emboden 1972)
- due to anethole content it is best avoided in liver disease and when taking paracetamol
- the oil is recommended for hookworm (Council of Scientific and Industrial Research 1948–1976)
- best avoided in alcoholism, liver disease, and if taking paracetamol owing to anethole content
- exhibits antibacterial activities (Ramadan et al 1972a)
- potentially carcinogenic depending on dosage, assumed owing to estragole content, oral dose not recommended (Drinkwater et al 1976, Swanson et al 1981, Zangouras et al 1981)
- the essential oil of fennel is used as a lactogenic in cases of deficiency of milk in nursing mothers, but puerperal lactation may be suppressed by the use of the flowers and inhalation of *Jasminum sambac* (Abraham et al 1979, Shrivastav et al 1988)

HELICHRYSUM ANGUSTIFOLIUM (= H. ITALICUM) flos
[EVERLASTING, IMMORTELLE] ASTERACEAE

Representative constituents

Hydrocarbons
monoterpenes   α-pinene, camphene, β-pinene, myrcene, limonene, *cis*-ocimene, *trans*-ocimene

Alcohols
linalool, terpinen-4-ol, nerol, geraniol

Phenols
eugenol

Ketones
4,7-dimethyloct-6-en-3-one
diones   italidiones 15–20%, beta-diketones, 2,5,7-trimethyldec-2-en-6,8-dione, 2,5,7,9-tetramethyldec-2-en-6,8-dione, 2,5,7,9-tetramethylundec-2-en-6,8-dione, 3,5-dimethyloctan-4,6-dione, 2,4-dimethylheptan-3,5-dione

Esters
neryl acetate 75%

Oxides
1,8-cineole

Properties and indications

antiallergic	asthma, hay fever, eczema
anticoagulant	
antidiabetic	
antifungal	Candida albicans
antiinfectious	
antiinflammatory	arthritis, polyarthritis (with wintergreen or sweet birch), dermatitis, salivary gland inflammation, rhinitis, sinusitus, whooping cough, gastritis, colitis
antispasmodic	coughs
antiviral	colds, influenza
cicatrizant	bruises, skin regeneration, acne, burns, scars, ulcers, open wounds
digestive	aerophagy
hepatic	stimulates liver function
lipolytic	
mucolytic	bronchitis, pulmonary cleanser
neurotonic	solar plexus, nervous depression
phlebotonic	red veins (couperose), haematoma (even old), thromboses, prevention of bruises

Observations

- the oil from Corsica was found to contain 64% esters (Zola & LeVanda 1975)
- everlasting oil is used as a source of nerol, which is found in its free state and esterified (Guenther 1949)
- sometimes called the super arnica of aromatherapy (Pénoël 1991)
- isovaleric aldehyde, furfurol have also been mentioned as compounds sometimes present in *H. angustifolium*
- RIFM monograph 1979 Food Cosmetics & Toxicology 17 p. 821 refers to immortelle absolute
- in case of trauma can be applied to the skin neat or diluted 10–50% in a carrier oil (Roulier 1990 p. 272)

HYSSOPUS OFFICINALIS flos, fol.
[HYSSOP] LAMIACEAE

Representative constituents

Hydrocarbons
monoterpenes (25–30%)   β-pinene 8.8–22.9%, phellandrene, limonene 0.7–1%, α-pinene 0.7–1.4%, camphene 0.1–0.4%, α-phellandrene 0.03–0.3%, sabinene 1.5–2%, myrcene 0.7–2%, *cis*-ocimene 0.1–3.6%, *trans*-ocimene 0.3–0.5%, *p*-cymene 0.1–0.9%
sesquiterpenes (12%)   β-caryophyllene 0.4–3.2%, germacrene D 0.4–2.8%, allo-aromadendrene 0.5–0.8%, δ-cadinene 0.1%, calamenene trace, α-humulene

Alcohols
monoterpenols (5–10%)   nerolidol 0.1–1%, spathulenol 0.7–2.2%, borneol, geraniol, terpinen-4-ol 0.1%, α-terpineol 1–1.8%, myrtenol 0.4–2.2%, linalool
sesquiterpenols   elemol 0.4–1.7%
other   1-octen-3-ol 0.1%

Esters
bornyl acetate, methyl myrtenate 2%

Ketones
monoterpenones (45–58%) α-thujone trace–0.08%, β-thujone 0.1–0.3%, camphor, pinocamphone 12–58%, iso-pinocamphone 25–32.6%, 2-hydroxy-isopinocamphone 0.3–0.7%

Phenols
carvacrol trace

Phenolic ethers (4%)
myrtenyl methyl ether 0.8–3.9%, methyl chavicol 0.1–1.3%, methyl eugenol 0.1–0.5%

Oxides
1,8-cineole 0.6%, caryophyllene oxide 0.2%

Properties and indications

antibacterial	see Table 4.4
anticatarrhal	bronchitis, coughs
antiinfectious	colds, coughs, influenza
antiinflammatory	bronchitis, rhinopharyngitis, sinusitis, emphysema, cystitis, rheumatism
antitussive	coughs, influenza
astringent, styptic	
cicatrizant	wounds, bruises*, scars, eczema
decongestant	
digestive	loss of appetite, dyspepsia, sluggish digestion
diuretic	
emmenagogic	scanty periods, irregular periods
expectorant	
hypertensor	hypotension
lipolytic	
litholytic	urinary stones
mucolytic*	bronchitis, coughs, sinusitis, pneumonia, asthma*, hay fever, dyspnoea
sudorific	
tonic	asthenia
vermifuge	intestinal parasites
unspecified	multiple sclerosis
unspecified	leukorrhoea

Observations

- hyssop essential oil can be neurotoxic and abortive in overdose
- not normally used on babies, children, pregnant women and the elderly
- no irritation or sensitization at 4% dilution on humans (Opdyke 1978d)
- no phototoxic effects reported (Opdyke 1978d)
- makes a synergistic mix together with *Eucalyptus globulus, Ravensara aromatica* and *Melaleuca viridiflora* for respiratory problems (Roulier 1990)
- maximum dose is four drops per day for a 70 kg adult
- may cause epileptic attack in those so predisposed (Valnet 1980)

- high dose of hyssop essential oil can cause muscular spasm (Bunny 1984); hyssop is a convulsant, owing to pinocamphone and iso-pinocamphone (Millet 1979, Millet et al 1981)
- eliminated via the lungs
- the essence neutralizes the tuberculosis bacillus at 0.2 parts per 1000 (Valnet 1980)
- extracts of hyssop have had antiviral effects against herpes virus (unspecified) (Foster 1993b)
- also mentioned for leprosy and scrofula (Gattefossé 1937)
- plant extracts and the essential oil, used in minute amounts as commercial flavourings in foods, are generally recognized as safe
- the essential oil is used to flavour Benedictine and Grand Chartreuse

JUNIPERUS COMMUNIS fruct.
[JUNIPER BERRY] CUPRESSACEAE

Representative constituents

Hydrocarbons
monoterpenes (60–80%) α-pinene 26.5–70%, β-pinene 1.7–13.6%, limonene 2.5–40%, camphene 0.3–0.8%, α-thujene 1.2–3%, sabinene 0.3–8.8%, myrcene 2.6–9.5%, γ-terpinene 0.3–4%, α-terpinene 0.1–2.2%, *p*-cymene 1.3–2.4%, δ-3-carene 0.03%, terpinolene 0.3–1.8%, α-phellandrene 0.3%, β-phellandrene 0.7%, 2-*p*-tolylpropene 0.3%, α-cubebene 0.4%, α-*p*-dimethylstyrene 0.2%
sesquiterpenes β-caryophyllene trace-2%, α-copaene 0.1–0.4%, δ-cadinene 0.2–2.9%, α-humulene 1.9%, germacrene D 2.7%

Alcohols
monoterpenols terpinen-4-ol 2.1–9.5%, α-terpineol 0.5%, borneol 0.08%, geraniol 0.1%
sesquiterpenols elemol, α-eudesmol, α-cadinol 0.7%

Oxides
caryophyllene oxide 0.1%

Esters
bornyl acetate, terpinyl acetate

Coumarins
umbelliferone

Properties and indications

analgesic	articular pain
antidiabetic	diabetes, pancreatic stimulant
antiseptic	cystitis
depurative	skin affections, articular pain
digestive tonic*	cirrhosis, loss of appetite
diuretic*	cellulite, oedema
litholytic	bladder and kidney stones
soporific	insomnia

Observations

- not to be used where there is inflammation of the kidneys; 4-terpineol and terpinen-4-ol are diuretic principles, and excessive doses may produce kidney irritation

- the diuretic action is due to a direct irritation of the urinary tubule wall by terpineol (Mills 1991)
- this oil has a general augmenting action on mucous secretions; elimination by all natural paths; aids active elimination of unwanted material, which then cannot be deposited in the joints
- juniper and extracts should not be used by expectant mothers
- symptoms of external poisoning caused by the essential oil on the skin include burning, redness, inflammation with blisters and swelling; internal overdoses cause pain in or near the kidney, strong diuresis, albuminuria, hematuria, accelerated heartbeat and blood pressure elevation (Duke 1985, List & Horhammer 1969–1979)
- undiluted oil when patch tested on 20 subjects showed two irritant reactions (Opdyke 1976d)
- no irritation or sensitization at 8% dilution when tested on humans (Opdyke 1976d)
- no phototoxic effects reported (Opdyke 1976d)
- makes a synergistic mix with rosemary
- juniper berry oil imparts to the urine a smell of violets (Mabey 1988)
- juniper berry oil is commonly adulterated; care in procurement is necessary
- terpinen-4-ol increases glomerular filtration rate, responsible for the diuretic activity (Tyler 1993) and may produce kidney irritation (Tyler 1982)
- the oil is carminative, cephalic, deobstruent, depurative, diaphoretic, digestive, diuretic, emmenagogic, stimulant and sudorific (Duke & Wain 1981, Tierra 1980, Watt & Breyer-Brandwijk 1962)
- uterine-stimulating activity has been reported (Farnsworth 1975)
- oil is used in folk remedies for cancer, indurations, polyps, swellings, tumours and warts (Hartwell 1967–1971)

JUNIPERUS COMMUNIS ram.
[JUNIPER TWIG] CUPRESSACEAE

Representative constituents

Hydrocarbons
monoterpenes   α-pinene 35%, β-pinene, limonene 3–40%, camphene 0.3%, thujene 3%, sabinene 5%, myrcene 9%, γ-terpinene 4%
sesquiterpenes   β-caryophyllene 2%

Alcohols
monoterpenols   terpinen-1-ol-4

Properties and indications

analgesic	
anticatarrhal*	bronchitis, rhinitis
antiinflammatory	
antiseborrhoeic	greasy scalp
antiseptic*	acne, cystitis, weeping eczema
depurative	kidneys, digestive system, urinary stones

diuretic*	gout, rheumatism* (uric acid excretion)
expectorant	
neurotonic	debility, fatigue
unspecified	arteriosclerosis

Observations
- no known contraindications
- see also notes under *J. communis* fruct. [JUNIPER BERRY]

LAVANDULA ANGUSTIFOLIA
(= *L. OFFICINALIS*, *L. VERA*) flos
[LAVENDER] LAMIACEAE

Representative constituents

Hydrocarbons
monoterpenes (4–5%)   α-pinenes 0.02–1.1%, *cis*-ocimene 1.3–10.9%, *trans*-ocimene 0.8–5.8%, limonene 0.2–7%, β-pinene 0.1–0.2%, camphene 0.1–0.3%, δ-3-carene 0.5%, allo-ocimene < 1%
sesquiterpenes   β-caryophyllene 2.6–7.6%, β-farnesene 1%

Alcohols
monoterpenols   linalool 26–49%, terpinen-4-ol 0.03–6.4%, α-terpineol 0.1–1.4%, borneol 0.8–1.4%, geraniol 1%, lavandulol 0.5–1.5%
aliphatic   *cis*-3-hexen-1-ol trace

Esters (40–55%)
linalyl acetate 36–53%, lavandulyl acetate 0.2–5.9%, terpenyl acetate 0.5%, geranyl acetate 0.5%, 2,6-dimethyl-3,7-octadiene-2-ol-6-yl acetate

Oxides (2%)
1,8-cineole 0.5–2.5%, linalool oxide, caryophyllene oxide

Ketones (4%)
camphor < 1%, octanone-3 0.5–3%, *p*-methyl-acetophenone

Aldehydes (2%)
myrtenal 0.1%, cuminal 0.4%, benzaldehyde 0.2%, neral and geranial 0.4%, *trans*-22-hexanal 0.4%

Lactones, coumarins (0.3%)
herniarin trace, butanolides trace, coumarin 0.04%, umbelliferone, santonin

Properties and indications

analgesic*	arthritis, muscular aches and pains, rheumatism
antibacterial	see Table 4.4
antifungal	candida, tinea pedis (including infection of the nails) see Table 4.5
antiinflammatory	eczema (dry), insect bites, phlebitis, sinusitis, otitis, cystitis, bruises, sprains, acne, herpes, pruritus
antiseptic	acne, bronchial secretions, cystitis, otitis, infectious skin complaints, influenza, sinusitis, tuberculosis, pityriasis
antispasmodic	cramp, spasmodic coughing

calming, sedative	headaches*, migraines, insomnia, sleep problems, anxiety, nervous system regulator (opposite effect at high dose)
cardiotonic	tachycardia
carminative	flatulence, colic
cicatrizant*	burns, scabs, scars, varicose ulcers, wounds
emmenagogic	scanty periods
hypotensor*	hypertension
tonic	debility, melancholy
unspecified	leukorrhoea

Observations

- no known contraindications
- a remarkable balancing effect on the CNS (Duraffourd 1982)
- no irritation or sensitization at 16% dilution when tested on humans (Opdyke 1976e)
- the oil can cause dermatitis (Duke 1985)
- no phototoxic effects reported (Opdyke 1976e)
- fine lavender oils have ketones belonging to the amyl group, while in the hybrids and lavender species other than *L. angustifolia* the ketones take on the form of camphor (Foster 1993b)
- there are more than 30 different types of lavender oils traded on commercial markets; buying a high quality one is an art known only to a few experienced specialists (Foster 1993b)
- Prager & Miskiewicz (1979) came to the conclusion that two oils imported as lavender oils were in fact blends of lavender oils and lavandin oils, while one further sample was found to be a blend of spike lavender oil and lavender oil
- Bulgarian lavender oils have 35.2–37.6% linalyl acetate (Ognyanov 1984)
- used as an insect repellent (Hartwell 1967–1971, Reynolds 1972)
- maximum acceptable daily intake of the components linalool and linalyl acetate is 500 µg/kg body weight per day (Reynolds 1972)
- found to be sedative in mice (Buchbauer et al 1991) and humans (Buchbauer et al 1993)
- sedative influence of lavender oil and the excitatory effects of jasmine oil on human behaviour was clearly shown (Karamat et al 1992)
- oil has antimicrobial activities (Uzdenikov 1970)

LAVANDULA × INTERMEDIA 'SUPER' flos [LAVANDIN] LAMIACEAE

Representative constituents

Hydrocarbons

monoterpenes α-pinene 0.05–0.5%, β-pinene 0.05–0.4%, myrcene 0.4–2.5%, limonene 0.2–1.6%, camphene 0.2%, sabinene 0.06%, δ-3-carene 0.02%, *cis*-ocimene 1.3%, γ-terpinene 0.02%, *p*-cymene 0.7%, terpinolene 0.1%
sesquiterpenes caryophyllene 0.6–1.7%

Alcohols

monoterpenols linalool 23–48%, lavandulol 0.2–1%, α-terpineol 0.5–6.3%, nerol 0.05–0.6%, geraniol 0.2–1.3%, 1-octen-3-ol 0.2%, terpinen-4-ol 0.4%, borneol 2.27%

Esters (25%)

linalyl acetate 32–52%, neryl acetate 0.1–0.5%, geranyl acetate 0.4–2%, hexyl isobutyrate 0.1%, 1-octen-3-yl acetate 0.5%, hexyl butyrate 0.6%, lavandulyl acetate 1.5%

Oxides

1,8-cineole 1.8–10.8%, *trans*-linalool oxide 0.2%, *cis*-linalool oxide 0.08%

Ketones

camphor 5–14.8%

Coumarins

coumarin, dihydrocoumarin, 7-methoxycoumarin and others

Properties and indications

anticatarrhal	bronchitis, pharyngitis
antifungal	athlete's foot, candida
antimigraine	chronic migraine
antiviral*	enteritis
expectorant	bronchitis, coughs
neurotonic	nervous debility, listlessness
sedative	postcardiac surgery (Buckle 1993)

Observations

- no known contraindications
- no irritation or sensitization at 5% dilution when tested on humans (Opdyke 1976f)
- no phototoxic effects reported (Opdyke 1976f)
- see notes on *Lavandula angustifolia*: *L. × intermedia* 'Super' is a lavandin clone which is close to *L. angustifolia* in its constituents, and therefore in its properties and effects

MELALEUCA ALTERNIFOLIA fol. [TEA TREE] MYRTACEAE

Representative constituents

Hydrocarbons

monoterpenes (25–40%) α-pinene 0.8–3.6%, β-pinene 0.1–1.6%, α-terpinene 4.6–12.8%, γ-terpinene 9.5–28.3%, *p*-cymene 0.4–12.4%, limonene 0.4–2.77%, terpinolene 1.6–5.4%, α-thujene 0.1–2.1%, sabinene 0–3.2%, myrcene 0.1–1.8%, α-phellandrene 0.1–1.9%, β-phellandrene 0.4–1.6%, terpinolene 3%
sesquiterpenes β-caryophyllene 1%, aromadendrene 0.1–6.6%, viridiflorene 0.3–6.1%, δ-cadinene 0.1–7.5%, allo-aromadendrene 0.3%, α-muurolene 0.1%, bicyclogermacrene 0.1%, α-gurjunene 0.2%, calamenene 0.1%

Alcohols

monoterpenols terpenen-4-ol 28.6–57.9%, α-terpineol 1.5–7.6%
sesquiterpenols globulol 0.1–3.0%, viridiflorol 0.1–1.4%, cubenol 0.1%

Oxides

1,8-cineole 0.5–17.7%, 1,4-cineole trace

Properties and indications

analgesic	
antibacterial	see Table 4.4
antifungal	candida* see Table 4.5
antiinfectious*	abscesses, skin infections, intestinal infections, bronchitis, genital infections
antiinflammatory	abscesses (including dental), pyorrhoea, vaginitis, sinusitis, otitis
antiparasitic	lamblias, ascaris, ankylostoma
antiviral	viral enteritis
immunostimulant	low immunoglobulin A and immunoglobulin M
neurotonic	debility, depression, PMS, anxiety
phlebotonic	haemorrhoids, varicose veins, aneurism

Observations

- no known contraindications
- no irritation or sensitization at 1% dilution when tested on humans (Ford, Api & Letizia 1988)
- no phototoxic effects reported (Ford, Api & Letizia 1988)
- said to prevent postoperative shock due to anaesthetic (Franchomme & Pénoël 1990)
- tea tree oil has a low cineole content and is non-irritant to the skin or the mucous surfaces
- in a single-blind randomized study on 124 patients with mild to moderate acne, tea tree oil was compared with benzoyl peroxide: both treatments produced a significant improvement, while fewer patients using the tea tree oil reported unwanted effects (Bassett, Pannowitz & Barnetson 1990)
- see observation under *Melaleuca viridiflora* concerning possible radioprotective property
- tea tree oil may be useful in removing transient skin flora owing to its ability to penetrate the outer layers of the skin giving a residual effect, while suppressing but maintaining resident flora. *Staphylococcus aureus* and Gram negative bacteria were susceptible to tea tree oil (Hammer, Carson & Riley 1996)
- excellent antimicrobial and antifungal action including *Listeria monocytogenes, Candida albicans, Pityrosporum ovale* and *Trychophyton* (Asre 1994, Lis-Balchin, Deans & Hart 1994, Maruzzella 1960, Millet et al 1981); this is probably due to *p*-cymene content
- in vitro tests on *S. aureus* suggest tea tree oil may be useful in the treatment of MRSA carriage (Carson, Hammer & Riley 1995, Carson et al 1995); of 66 isolates tested, 64 were methicillin resistant and 33 were mupirocin resistant; all were susceptible to *M. alternifolia* essential oil
- tea tree has been used to treat skin conditions such as acne and furunculosis (boils); vaginal thrush; foot problems; coughs and colds (Mayo 1992)
- tea tree oil is as effective as clotrimazole as an antifungal agent (Anon 1994a)

MELALEUCA LEUCADENDRON (= *M. CAJUPUTI*) fol. [CAJUPUT] MYRTACEAE

Representative constituents

Hydrocarbons

monoterpenes   α-pinene 4%, β-pinene 35%, limonene 7%
sesquiterpenes   β-caryophyllene 5.9%

Alcohols

monoterpenols   (–)-α-terpineol 6.4%
sesquiterpenols   (+)-viridiflorol, nerilodol

Oxides

1,8-cineole 50–75%

Aldehydes

valeric, butyric, benzoic aldehydes

Esters

terpineol acetate

Properties and indications

analgesic	earache, gout, painful periods, rheumatism, toothache, earache, painful joints, neuralgia, arthritis, gout
antibacterial	see Table 4.4
antifungal	see Table 4.5
antiinfectious	bronchitis, colds, coughs, enteritis
antiseptic	intestines, urinary tract, cystitis, respiratory tract, cholera, pityriasis, psoriasis
antispasmodic	gastroenteritis, colic
decongestant	haemorrhoids, varicose veins
expectorant	bronchitis, coughs, lungs
hormone-like	
insect repellent	mosquitoes, lice, fleas
phlebotonic	varicose veins, haemorrhoids
sudorific	helps influenza

Observations

- no known contraindications, but care is advisable with pregnancy
- no irritation or sensitization at 4% dilution when tested on humans (Opdyke 1976g)
- no phototoxic effects reported (Opdyke 1976g)
- see observation under *Melaleuca viridiflora* concerning possible radioprotective property
- widely used in the East; Indochina—arthritis, rheumatism, colds, rhinitis; Indonesia—burns, cramp, colic, earache, headache, skin disease, toothache; New Guinea—malaria; Malaya—pain relief, stomachic, cholera, colic (Perry 1980)
- very good antibacterial action (Maruzzella & Sicurella 1960)
- used internally as a carminative and externally as a rubefacient (Reynolds 1972)

MELALEUCA VIRIDIFLORA (= *M. QUIN-QUENERVIA*) fol. [NIAOULI] MYRTACEAE

Representative ingredients

Hydrocarbons

monoterpenes α-pinene 7.5%, β-pinene 3%, 1-limonene 4–8%
sesquiterpenes β-caryophyllene 2%, aromadendrene, allo-aromadendrene, viridiflorene, α-humulene, δ-cadinene

Alcohols

monoterpenols linalool, α-terpineol 9–14%, terpinen-1-ol-4 2%
sesquiterpenols viridiflorol 6–15%, globulol, nerolidol 1–7%

Aldehydes

isovaleraldehyde, benzaldehyde < 1%

Oxides

1,8-cineole 38–65%, epoxycaryophyllene

Other

sulphur constituents

Properties and indications

analgesic	labour
antibacterial	see Table 4.4
anticatarrhal	chronic catarrh
antiinfectious	respiratory infections, skin fungal infections, insect bites, boils
antiinflammatory	sinusitis*, rhinopharyngitis, bronchitis*, blepharitis, vulvovaginitis, urethritis, prostatitis, inflammation of coronary arteries
antiparasitic	
antipruritic	insect bites
antirheumatic	rheumatoid arthritis
antiseptic	infected wounds, respiratory
antitumoral	breast cancer (non-hormonal), rectal cancer, fibroma (some)*
antiviral*	viral hepatitis*, viral enteritis, genital herpes*
digestive	aerophagy, gastritis, gastric and duodenal ulcers, diarrhoea
expectorant*	bronchitis*, coughs, colds
febrifuge	fevers
hepatic stimulant	
hormone-like	amenorrhoea, oligomenorrhoea, irregular menses
hypotensor	atherosclerosis, hypertension
immunostimulant	activates defences and augments leukocytes and antibodies in infected areas
litholytic	gall stones
phlebotonic	varicose veins*, haemorrhoids*
skin tonic	psoriasis, boils, wrinkles, fungal infections
tonic	postviral nervous depression
unspecified	leukorrhoea

Observations

- no known contraindications but care is advised for pregnant women and children
- used in New Caledonia to purify air (Duraffourd 1982)
- procuring the genuine natural oil is not easy
- the French pharmacopoeia lists natural niaouli and purified niaouli; only the latter can be used in anticatarrhal preparations or for applications for use on burns or on wounds (Belaiche 1979)
- niaouli is thought by some to act as a radioprotective, i.e. as a preventative for radiotherapy burns by attenuating the effects of burning of the epidermis. The neat essential oil may be applied before irradiation sessions, and afterwards may be applied as a mixture consisting of 50% niaouli oil and 50% of either *Rosa mosquetta* [ROSE HIP OIL] or *Hypericum perforatum* [ST JOHN'S WORT] macerated oil (Roulier 1990 p. 230). This same characteristic has been attributed also to *Melaleuca alternifolia* and *M. leucadendron* (Franchomme & Pénoël 1990 pp. 369–370)

MELISSA OFFICINALIS fol. [MELISSA] LAMIACEAE

Representative constituents

Hydrocarbons

monoterpenes *trans*-ocimene 0.2%, β-bourbonene 0.3%, limonene 0.2%
sesquiterpenes β-caryophyllene 8–10%, α-copaene 4–5%, β-elemene < 1%, α-humulene < 1%, δ-cadinene 1%, γ-cadinene 1%

Alcohols

monoterpenols linalool 0.4–1.3%, nerol < 1%, geraniol < 1%, citronellol < 1%, isopulegol < 1%
sesquiterpenols α-cadinol 0.3%, elemol < 1%, (Z)-3-hexanol 0.1%, 1-octen-3-ol 1.3%

Ketones

6-methyl-5-hepten-2-one 4.5%, hexahydrofarnesyl-acetone 0.2%

Esters

geranyl acetate < 0.5%, neryl acetate, citronellyl acetate

Oxides

1,8-cineole, caryophyllene oxide 2.5–3.6%

Aldehydes

neral 22–24%, geranial 32–37%, citronellal 0.7–2.2%

Coumarins

aesculetine

Other

3-octanone 0.6%, methyl heptanone 0.6%

Properties and indications

antiinflammatory	
antispasmodic	stomach cramp
antiviral	herpes simplex 1
calming	hysteria, palpitations, headaches, vertigo*, erethism

choleretic	regularizes secretions (bile, stomach)
digestive	indigestion*, nausea, morning sickness*, sluggish liver
hypotensor*	hypertension
sedative	insomnia, calming to CNS
vasodilator (capillaries)	palpitations, angina

Observations

- no known contraindications, but care may be necessary in sunlight
- often adulterated or reconstructed: caution is advised when procuring it, because the properties given above relate only to the true oil; melissa is frequently adulterated by mixing with lemongrass or citronella to increase its bulk, but is more usually totally simulated; these reconstructed oils have a similar 'lemony' aroma and contain some of the compounds found in natural melissa oil, e.g. citral, citronellal
- citronellal is the terpene to which sedative action is primarily attributed (Foster 1993b)
- skin allergies and respiratory problems are often made worse if not treated with a suitably low concentration of melissa oil (usually less than 1%)
- a powerful choleretic which triples the volume of bile in 30 min (Duraffourd 1982)
- the hydrosol is useful for regulating fever in children (Roulier 1990)
- studies have indicated that a cream with lemon balm (available in Germany) reduces the healing time of herpes simplex type I lesions and lengthens the time before recurrence (Tyler 1992)
- two chemotypes of melissa are known to exist: citral (as above) and citronellal (Lawrence 1989)
- melissa oil was found to be a strong antioxidant (Lis-Balchin, Deans & Hart 1994) and a relaxant (Torii et al 1988)
- citral can cause an increase in ocular tension (Leach & Lloyd 1956)
- the oil has antibacterial (Wagner & Sprinkmeyer 1973) and antifungal activity (Mulkens et al 1985)

MENTHA × *PIPERITA* fol. [PEPPERMINT] LAMIACEAE

Representative constituents

Hydrocarbons

monoterpenes (3–18%)   α-pinene 0.2–2%, β-pinene 0.3–4%, limonene 0.6–6%, menthene, phellandrene, sabinene < 1%, myrcene < 1%, *cis*-ocimene trace–1.5%, *p*-cymene trace–0.5%, terpinolene trace–0.2%, α-terpinene < 1%, γ-terpinene < 1%
sesquiterpenes   β-caryophyllene < 1%, *trans*-β-farnesene trace–0.5%, α-muurolene trace–0.5%, germacrene D 2.1–4.3%, γ-cadinene trace–0.7%, β-bourbonene < 1%

Alcohols

monoterpenols (50%)   menthol 28–46%, isomenthol, neomenthol 2–7.7%, piperitol, piperitenol, isopiperitenol, α-terpineol 0.1–1.9%, linalool < 1%, terpinen-4-ol 0–2.4%
sesquiterpenols   viridiflorol 0.5–1.3%, 10-α-cadinol trace–0.3%

Other

3-octanol < 1%

Ketones

menthone 16–36%, iso-menthone 4–10.4%, neomenthone 2–3%, piperitone 0.5–1.2%, isopiperitone, pulegone < 1%, piperitenone trace–0.7%

Oxides

1,8-cineole 3–7.4%, menthofuran < 3%, *trans*-piperitonoxide 0.5–3.1%, caryophyllene oxide trace–0.5%

Esters

menthyl acetate 1.6–10%, neomenthyl acetate, isomenthyl acetate, menthyl butyrate, menthyl isovalerate

Coumarins

aesculetine

Other

menthofuran 0.1–5.7% *trans*-sabinene hydrate 0.2–1.4%, *cis*-sabinene hydrate trace–0.8%

Properties and indications

analgesic	migraine, neuralgia, sciatica
antibacterial	see Table 4.4
antifungal	ringworm, skin infections see Table 4.5
antiinfectious	
antiinflammatory	bronchitis, colitis, cystitis, eczema*, enteritis, gastritis, hepatitis, laryngitis, sinusitis, urticaria*
antilactogenic	prevents milk forming
antimigraine	headache, migraine
antipyretic	fever
antispasmodic	colic, gastric spasm
antiviral	herpes, viral hepatitis
carminative	flatulence
decongestant	cirrhosis
digestive	indigestion, nausea, painful digestion, digestive problems, irritable bowel syndrome
expectorant	bronchial asthma, bronchitis
hepatic stimulant	cirrhosis, jaundice
hormone-like	irregular periods (ovarian stimulant)
hypertensor	hypotension
insect repellent	gnats, mosquitoes
mucolytic	bronchial asthma, bronchitis
neurotonic	apathy, nervous vomiting, travel sickness, palpitations, vertigo, (excites the motor nerves but damps the excitation of sensor nerves)
reproductive stimulant	impotence

soothing   skin irritation, rashes, redness
uterotonic   facilitates delivery

Observations

- contraindicated for babies and young children, where it can produce reflex apnoea or laryngospasm; an ointment containing menthol applied to the nostrils of infants for the treatment of cold symptoms has been reported to cause instantaneous collapse (Tester-Dalderup 1980)
- may cause allergic reactions such as contact dermatitis, flushing and headache in some individuals
- skin irritations may be made worse unless used in suitably low concentration
- should not be used externally in high concentration (i.e. low dilution) as in certain adults it may result in sleep disturbance
- peppermint oil is reported to be effective as an analgesic when used in conjunction with *Ravensara aromatica* (Roulier 1990)
- helps local circulation in the head
- there is a consensus of opinion that peppermint should not be used concurrently with homoeopathic treatment, although the reasons given vary
- menthol is cooling and anaesthetic when applied to the skin, increasing bloodflow to the area to which it is applied (Mabey 1988)
- whole peppermint has more antispasmodic effect than menthol alone (Trease & Evans 1983)
- oil of peppermint is antispasmodic (Leung 1980); studies have shown peppermint oil to inhibit gastrointestinal smooth muscle spasms and reduce colonic motility (Duthie 1981, Leicester & Hunt 1982, Sigmund & McNally 1969, Taylor, Luscombe & Duthie 1983)
- *M. × piperita* is a hybrid of *Mentha spicata* [SPEARMINT] and *Mentha aquatica* [WATERMINT]
- local anaesthetic and counterirritant for muscular aches and pains (Dew, Evans & Rhodes 1984, Rees 1979, Reynolds 1972)
- peppermint and caraway oils combined in enteric-coated capsules (Enteroplant®) were found to improve non-ulcer dyspepsia (May et al 1996)
- the oil is reported to have antimicrobial (Abdullin 1962, Pizsolitto 1975, Ramadan et al 1972b, Sanyal and Varma 1969) and antiviral activity (Hermann and Kucera 1967)
- reported to have cytotoxic properties (Silyanovska et al 1969)

MYRISTICA FRAGRANS sem. [NUTMEG] MYRISTICACEAE

Representative constituents

Hydrocarbons
monoterpenes (70–75%) α-pinene 14–25%, β-pinene 10–15%, myrcene 2%, sabinene 14–35%, α-terpinene 2–4%, γ-terpinene 1.9–7.7%, limonene 3.7–4%, β-phellandrene, camphene < 1%, α-phellandrene 0.7–1%, *p*-cymene 1.1–3.1%, terpinolene 0.9–1.7%

sesquiterpenes β-caryophyllene 0–1%

Alcohols
monoterpenols terpinen-4-ol 4–8.2%, α-terpineol 0.4–1.2%

Phenolic ethers
safrole 0.7–1.7%, myristicin 2.9–10.4%, elemicin 0.4–2.1%, eugenol 0.2%, methyl eugenol 0.6%

Oxides
1,8-cineole 2–3%

Other
trans-sabinene hydrate < 1%, *cis*-sabinene hydrate < 1%

Properties and indications

analgesic   aches and pains, rheumatism, sprains, toothache, neuralgia
antibacterial   see Table 4.4
antiseptic   chronic diarrhoea
carminative   flatulence
circulatory stimulant
digestive stimulant   loss of appetite, sluggish digestion, difficulty with starches and heavy meals, speeds up intestinal transit
emmenagogic   scanty periods
neurotonic   debility
psychoactive
reproductive stimulant impotence, frigidity
uterotonic   facilitates delivery

Observations

- requires great care in use on account of the myristicin content (a hallucinogen); ingestion of an overdose may produce epileptiform convulsions, coma and death (Åkesson & Wålinder 1965, Dale 1909)
- doses exceeding 5 ml take effect within 2–5 hours, producing time–space distortions and sometimes visual hallucinations accompanied by dizziness, headache, illness and rapid heartbeat (Duke 1985)
- it has been hypothesized that myristicin and elemicin can readily be modified in the body to amphetamines (Duke 1985)
- no irritation or sensitization at 2% dilution when tested on humans (Opdyke 1976h)
- Valnet (1980) lists the monoterpenols linalool, geraniol and borneol as constituents of this oil
- inhibits prostaglandin synthesis (Reynolds 1972) and platelet aggregation (Shafran, Maurer & Thomas 1977)
- used to treat diarrhoea owing to eugenol content (Bennett et al 1988)
- myristicin has been shown to cross the placenta causing an increase in the fetal heartbeat (Lavy 1987)
- oral doses of the oil together with pethidine is not advisable as myristicin has been shown to inhibit monoamine synthesis (Reynolds 1993)
- oil is recommended for inflammation of the bladder and urinary tract
- nutmeg oil has larvicidal activity (Oishi et al 1974)

NARDOSTACHYS JATAMANSI (= *N. GRANDI-FLORA*) rad. [SPIKENARD] VALERIANACEAE

Representative constituents

Hydrocarbons
monoterpenes α-pinene 0.1%, β-pinene 0.1%, limonene 0.1%
sesquiterpenes aristolene 5%, dihydroazulenes, α-gurjunene 0.6%, β-gurjunene 29%, α-patchoulene 29%, β-patchoulene 0.7%, seychellene 1.7%, β-maaliene

Alcohols
sesquiterpenols calarenol, nardol, valerianol, patchouli alcohol 6%, maaliol

Aldehydes
sesquiterpenals valerianal

Ketones
sesquiterpenones valeranone, β-ionone 1.4%, 3,4-dihydro-β-ionone trace, 1-hydroxyaristolenone 6%, aristolenone 0.7%

Oxides
1,8-cineole 0.2%

Coumarins
coumarin

Properties and indications

antiepileptic	
antifungal	see Table 4.5
antispasmodic	convulsions, intestinal colic
calming	tachycardia, epilepsy, hysteria
cardiotonic	arrhythmia
phlebotonic	varicose veins, haemorrhoids
unspecified	anaemia, ovarian insufficiency, psoriasis*

Observations
- no known contraindications
- it is sometimes used in place of valerian
- a history of religious use; used in meditation
- in tests *N. jatamansi* inhibited the growth of *Aspergillus flavus*, *A. niger* and *Fusarium oxysporum*; it was also active against a wide range of other fungi (Mishra et al 1995)

NEPETA CATARIA VAR. *CITRIODORA* flos, fol. [CATNEP] LAMIACEAE

Representative constituents

Hydrocarbons
monoterpenes myrcene trace–1.5%, limonene trace–0.4%, ocimenes trace–0.7%
sesquiterpenes β-caryophyllene 1.1–6.8%, α-humulene trace–4.3%

Alcohols
monoterpenols geraniol 13.7%, citronellol 48.3%

Esters
acetates, valerates, butyrates

Aldehydes
neral 4.9%, geranial 5.6%

Lactones
nepetalactone 9.4%, epinepetalactone 1.6%, dihydronepetalactone 1.2%

Properties and indications

antiinfectious	urinary infections
antiinflammatory*	irritable bowel syndrome, rheumatism*, arthritis
antiviral*	herpes
calming*	anxiety
litholytic	gall stones
neurotonic*	nervous depression

Observations
- no known contraindications
- the nepetalactone chemotype is described as diaphoretic and expectorant (Secondini 1990)
- the chemical structure of nepetalactone is similar to the valepotriates, the sedative principle in valerian

OCIMUM BASILICUM fol. [EUROPEAN BASIL] LAMIACEAE

Representative constituents

Hydrocarbons
monoterpenes (2%) α-pinene, β-pinene, camphene, limonene, *cis*-ocimene, *p*-cymene, γ-terpinene
sesquiterpenes socaryophyllene, β-caryophyllene 2–3%, β-elemene

Alcohols
monoterpenols linalool 40–55%, α-fenchyl alcohol 3–12%, terpinen-4-ol 1.6%, α-terpineol 2%, citronellol 1.5%, geraniol 1.2%

Esters
linalyl acetate, α-fenchyl acetate < 1%, methyl cinnamate 0.1–7%, α-terpinyl acetate trace

Phenols
eugenol 1–19%, iso-eugenol 2%

Phenolic ethers
methyl chavicol 3–31%, methyl eugenol 1–9%

Oxides
1,8-cineole 2–8%

Ketones
camphor 0.1%

Other
cis-3-hexanol

Properties and indications

analgesic	gout, migraine, rheumatoid arthritis
anthelminthic	threadworms

antibacterial coliform cystitis see Table 4.4
antifungal* see Table 4.5
antiinflammatory* gout, wasp stings
antiseptic intestinal infections, gastritis
antispasmodic gastric spasm, muscle cramp
antiviral viral hepatitis
cardiotonic arrhythmia, arteriosclerosis, tachycardia
carminative, eupeptic flatulence, sluggish digestion
digestive tonic stimulates digestive secretions, ulcers
fungistatic
hypertensor hypotension
insecticidal housefly, mosquito
liver stimulant hepatobiliary deficiency
nervous system anxiety*, epilepsy, nervous
  regulator insomnia, nervousness, travel sickness, vertigo
neurotonic debility, mental strain, convalescence, depression
reproductive uterine and prostatic
  decongestant congestion
unspecified dry eczema

Observations

- no known contraindications
- no irritation or sensitization at 4% dilution when tested on humans (Opdyke 1973d)
- no phototoxic effects reported (Opdyke 1973d)
- this oil may be used with safety when the methyl chavicol content is low; methyl chavicol causes liver cancer when fed to mice; no tests have been carried out on the application to the skin of humans and subsequent metabolization. There are no reports of cancer ever having been caused in humans owing to the use of essential oils (Tisserand & Balacs 1995)
- a prolonged daily intake of five drops would be ill advised (Caldwell 1991)
- the fact that it is a uterine decongestant does not mean that it is emmenagogic
- there is a natural variation in the chemical constituents of this essential oil both between plants and according to where the plant is grown
- oil has insecticidal and insect repellent properties, effective against house flies and mosquitoes (Deshpande & Ripnis 1977); out of 250 insects of *Allocophora foveicollis* tested, basil oil repelled 134, attracted 59 and 57 were non-reactive (Dube, Upadhyay & Tripathi 1988); also bactericidal against *Salmonella typhi*
- estragole is metabolized to 1-hydroxyestragole in humans (Sangster et al 1987) but small amounts are detoxified easily (Anthony et al 1987, Zangouras et al 1981)
- *O. basilicum* essential oil inhibited the mycelial growth of 22 species of fungi (Dube, Upadhyay & Tripathi 1988)
- the oil is a stimulant (Manley 1993)

ORIGANUM VULGARE SUBSP. *VIRIDE* (= *O. HERACLEOTICUM*)
[GREEK OREGANO, GREEN OREGANO] LAMIACEAE

Representative constituents

Hydrocarbons
monoterpenes p-cymene 7–10%, α-terpinene 0.8–1%, γ-terpinene 3.6%, α-thujene and α-pinene 0.95%, camphene 0.14%, β-pinene 0.1%, myrcene 0.93%, limonene 0.1%
sesquiterpenes caryophyllene 1.05%, β-bisabolene

Alcohols
monoterpenols linalool 0.2%, pentyl alcohol trace, terpinen-4-ol 0.85%, borneol 0.74%

Phenols
carvacrol 50–75%, thymol trace–7%

Esters
linalyl acetate 3.5%

Oxides
4,5-epoxy-p-menth-l-ene, 1,8-cineole 0.2%

Ketones
carvone trace

Other
cis-sabinene hydrate 0.1%

Properties and indications

antiinfectious*** | wide range of action, infections of the respiratory tract, digestive tract, genitourinary system
antiparasitic***
immunostimulant
tonic** | asthenia

Observations

- no known contraindications
- prudence should be exercised in dermal application because of the high phenol content

ORIGANUM MAJORANA flos, fol.
[SWEET MARJORAM] LAMIACEAE

Representative constituents

Hydrocarbons
monoterpenes (40%) sabinene 2–10%, myrcene 1–9%, p-cymene 1–6%, terpinolene 1–7%, α-pinene 1–5%, β-pinene 0.2–2.5%, ocimene 6.4%, cadinene 4.2%, 3-carene 6.2%, α-terpinene 6–8%, γ-terpinene 14–20%, α-phellandrene, β-phellandrene 0.9%, myrcene, limonene 0.6%
sesquiterpenes β-caryophyllene 2–4.6%, α-humulene 0.1%

Alcohols
monoterpenols (50%) terpinen-1-ol-4 14–20%, *cis*-thujanol-4 4–13%, *trans*-thujanol-4 1–5%, linalool 2–9.5%,

α-terpineol 7–27%, *cis-p*-menth-2-en-1-ol 2%,
trans-p-menth-2-en-ol 2%, *cis*-piperitol 0.5%

Esters
terpenyl acetate 0–3%, geranyl acetate 1–7.8%,
linlyl acetate 0.1%

Aldehydes
citral 5.4%

Other
trans-sabinene hydrate 1%, *cis*-sabinene hydrate 4%

Properties and indications

analgesic*	arthritis*, migraine, muscular pain*, rheumatism*, toothache
antibacterial	see Table 4.4
antiinfectious	whooping cough, bronchitis, headaches, respiratory infections, rhinitis, sinusitis
antispasmodic	colic, muscles, respiratory spasm, nervous spasm
calming	ether addiction, psychoses, agitation, anxiety, epilepsy, insomnia, migraine, sexual obsessions, vertigo
digestive stimulant	flatulence, gastroduodenal ulcers, indigestion
diuretic	
expectorant	catarrh, coughs, bronchitis
hormone-like	hyperthyroidism
hypotensor	hypertension, tachycardia, palpitations, fainting
neurotonic	debility*, mental instability, nervous spasm (by balancing the parasympathetic nervous system), anguish, agitation, nervous depression
respiratory tonic	nervous breathing
stomachic	diarrhoea, enteritis
vasodilator	

Observations

- no known contraindication at normal dose
- marjoram oil stimulates the vagus (parasympathetic) nerve and does not act on the sympathetic nerve, therefore its action is tranquillizing and lightly narcotic, a nervous sedative (Duraffourd 1982)
- no irritation or sensitization at 6% dilution when tested on humans (Opdyke 1976i)
- used in Vermouth
- the naming and correct identification of this group of herbs presents difficulties even to the expert: there are some 30 species of marjoram with the generic name *Origanum*
- has antiviral activities against herpes simplex (Herrmann & Kucera 1967)

ORMENIS MIXTA flos [MOROCCAN CHAMOMILE] ASTERACEAE

Representative constituents

Hydrocarbons
monoterpenes α-pinene 15%, camphene 0.4%, limonene 8%, γ-terpinene 0.1%, terpinolene 0.25%
sesquiterpenes germacrene 5%, β-caryophyllene 1.5%, bisabolene 2.5%, δ-elemene 0.7%

Alcohols
α-terpineol, santalina alcohol 32%, yomogi alcohol 2.4%, artemisia alcohol 2.3%, linalool 0.3%, borneol 1%, ormenol, *trans*-pinocarveol 3%

Ketones
camphor, pinocarvone 0.5%

Oxides
1,8-cineole

Esters
bornyl acetate 2.2%, bornyl butanoate 1.3%

Properties and indications

antibacterial*	see Table 4.4
antiinfectious	acne, cysts
antiinflammatory	dermatitis, eczema, rheumatism, colitis, cystitis
antiirritant	pruritus
hepatobiliary tonic sluggish	gall bladder and pancreas, liver
neurotonic*	nervous depression*

Observations

- no known contraindications

PELARGONIUM GRAVEOLENS fol. [GERANIUM] GERANIACEAE

Representative constituents

Hydrocarbons
monoterpenes (1–2%) α-phellandrene trace, β-phellandrene, α-pinene 1%, β-pinene 0.2%, myrcene 0.2%, limonene 0.2%, *cis*-ocimene 0.2%
sesquiterpenes (1–2%) guaia-6,9-diene 3.9–5.3%, guaiazulene, α-copaene, δ-cadinene, γ-cadinene, α-bourbonene, β-bourbonene, caryophyllene 0.7%

Alcohols
monoterpenols (55–65%) citronellol 21–45%, geraniol 17–25%, linalool 1–13%, nerol 1.2%, α-terpineol 0.7%
sesquiterpinols 10-epi-γ-eudesmol 1%
aromatic phenyl ethyl alcohol < 1%

Esters (15%)
citronellyl formates 8–18%, geranyl formates 1–6%, citronellyl proprionates 1–3%, geranyl proprionates 0–1%,

geranyl tiglates 1–2%, geranyl acetate 0.4%, citronellyl butyrate 1.3%, geranyl butyrate 1.3%, phenyl ethyl isobutyrate, phenyl ethyl tiglate

Aldehydes (Bourbon variety) (0–10%)
neral, geranial 0–9%, citronellal 0–1%

Ketones (1–8%)
menthone 0.6–3%, isomenthone 4–8.4%, piperitone, methyl heptanone, furopelargone 0.4%

Oxides (only in Chinese variety) (2–3%)
cis-rose oxide 2–25%, trans-rose oxide 1%, cis-linalool oxide 0.6%, trans-linalool oxide 0.2%

Properties and indications

analgesic	facial neuralgia, osteoarthritis, rheumatism
antibacterial*	see Table 4.4
antidiabetic	sluggish pancreas, diabetes
antifungal*	athlete's foot and other skin and nail fungi, candida
antiinfectious	infectious colitis, acne, cuts, wounds, impetigo, infectious skin diseases
antiinflammatory	arthritis, colitis, pruritus, rheumatism, tonsillitis
antiseptic	
antispasmodic	colic, cramp, gastroenteritis, painful menstruation
astringent	diarrhoea, haemorrhoids, varicose veins
cicatrizant	burns, cuts, ulcers, uterine haemorrhage, stretch marks, wounds
decongestant	breast congestion, lymph congestion
digestive stimulant	jaundice, sluggish liver
haemostatic, styptic	burns, cuts, ulcers, uterine haemorrhage, wounds
insect repellent	gnats, mosquitoes
phlebotonic* (lymph*)	haemorrhoids, varicose ulcers, varicose veins
relaxant*	agitation, anxiety, debility, nervous fatigue

Observations

- no known contraindications
- to be used with care on the skin of hypersensitive individuals (Winter 1984)
- no irritation or sensitization at 10% dilution when tested on humans (Opdyke 1974h)
- no phototoxic effects reported (Opdyke 1974h)
- contact with the leaves of the plant has been reported to cause vesicular dermatitis
- maximum acceptable daily intake of 500 µg/kg body weight of citral, geranyl acetate, citronellol and linalool is recommended (Reynolds 1972)

PIMPINELLA ANISUM fruct. [ANISEED] APIACEAE

Representative constituents

Hydrocarbons
sesquiterpenes γ-himachalene trace, β-caryophyllene

Alcohols (0.5–4%)
monoterpenols anisol 0.5–4%, linalool < 1.5%, α-terpineol < 1.5%

Phenols (0.5%)
isochavibetol 0.5%

Phenolic ethers (90–95%)
cis-anethole 0–1%, trans-anethole 90–93%, methyl chavicol 0–2%, myristicin trace

Aldehydes
aniseed aldehyde 1–2%

Ketones
p-methoxyphenylacetone

Coumarins, furanocoumarins
umbelliferone, scopoletine

Properties and indications

analgesic	arthritis, backache, nauseous migraine, period pains, rheumatism, sciatica, vertigo
antispasmodic	bronchial spasm, colic, enteritis, flatulence, indigestion, infantile colic, vomiting (of nervous origin), painful periods
aperitive	stimulates digestive juices
cardiotonic	cardiovascular erethism, palpitations, tired heart
carminative*	flatulence, indigestion
diuretic	oliguria
emmenagogic	amenorrhoea, oligomenorrhoea*
expectorant*	catarrh
lactogenic	lack of milk
narcotic (gentle)	
oestrogen like*	menopause, PMS
psychoactive*	
respiratory tonic	asthma, bronchitis, congestion in lungs, nervous breathing
sexual tonic	frigidity, impotence
uterotonic	facilitates delivery

Observations

- not normally used on babies, young children and pregnant women
- like fennel oil, anise oil contains compounds that can be aminated in vivo resulting in a series of three dangerous hallucinogenic amphetamines (Emboden 1972)
- the major component of aniseed oil, anethole, can cause dermatitis (erythema, scaling and vesiculation) in some individuals

- anethole has two isomers, the *cis* isomer being 15 to 38 times more toxic than the *trans* isomer (Leung 1980)
- several cases of sensitization have been reported (Loveman 1938, Schwarz 1934, Tulipan 1938), and attributed to the presence of anethole (Schwarz, Tulipan & Peck 1947)
- no irritation or sensitization at 4% dilution when tested on humans (Opdyke 1973e); not a primary irritant to normal skin (Harry 1948)
- *trans*-anethole and its derivatives are oestrogen like; avoid oral intake during pregnancy and breastfeeding (Albert-Puleo 1980, Zondek et al 1938)
- found to be a most effective expectorant in guinea pigs (Boyd & Pearson 1946)
- anethole, anisaldehyde, (+)-carvone and myristicin have mild insecticidal properties (Carter 1976); anethole inhibits also the growth of toxin-producing *Aspergillus* species (Hitokoto et al 1980)
- anethole is considered to be an oestrogenic agent; however, research suggests that dianethole and photoanethole (polymers of anethole) are the active oestrogenic compounds (Albert-Puleo 1980)
- anethole is structurally related to the hallucinogenic compound myristicin (Reynolds 1989)
- anethole is responsible for contact dermatitis reactions (Chandler & Hawkes 1984, Mitchell & Rook 1979)
- ingestion of 1–5 ml of the oil can cause nausea, vomiting, seizures and pulmonary oedema (Chandler & Hawkes 1984)

PINUS SYLVESTRIS fol. [PINE]
ABIETACEAE

Representative constituents

Hydrocarbons
monoterpenes (60–70%)   α-pinene 22–43%, β-pinene 3–33%, limonene 0.7–4.1%, δ-3-carene 0.4–31%, β-caryophyllene 0.7–5.5%, camphene 1.6–3.3%, sabinene 0.2–0.6%, γ-terpinene 0.1–0.5%, *trans*-ocimene 0.7–1.4%, β-phellandrene 1–2.7%, *p*-cymene 0–0.2%, terpinolene 0.3–3%
sesquiterpenes   longifolene, γ-cadinene 0.5–5.4%, α-copaene 0–0.2%, δ-elemene trace, α-ylangene trace, longifolene 0–0.2%, β-guaiene 0.2–0.7%, β-farnesene trace, γ-muurolene trace–0.4%, α-humulene trace–0.5%, γ-patchoulene 0–0.2%, γ-cadinene trace–0.3%, α-muurolene trace–1%, cubenene trace, calemenene trace

Alcohols
monoterpenols   borneol 2%, terpinen-4-ol 1%
sesquiterpenols   epi-α-cadinol < 1%, epi-α-muurolol < 1%, α-cadinol 0–0.2%

Aldehydes
citronellal 0–0.2%

Esters (1–10%)
bornyl acetate 0–3%

Properties and indications

analgesic	gastralgia, intestinal pains, arthritis, rheumatism
antibacterial	see Table 4.4
antifungal	see Table 4.5
antiinfectious*	antiseptic (air), respiratory infections, asthma*, bronchitis*, colds, influenza, pneumonia, sinusitis*, tracheitis, tuberculosis, urinary infections (cystitis, prostatitis, pyelitis)
antiinflammatory	inflammatory and allergic conditions, arthritis, gall bladder inflammation, gout, rheumatism
antisudorific	hyperhidrosis of the feet
balsamic	
cortisone-like	stimulates suprarenal cortex
decongestant	congested lymph, uterine or ovarian congestion, breaks down bronchial secretions
expectorant	respiratory tract
hypertensor*	hypotension*
insulin-like	pancreatic diabetes
litholytic	gall stones
neurotonic*	debility*, fatigue, insufficient semen (nervous origin), multiple sclerosis
rubefacient	arthritis, rheumatism
testosterone-like	impotence

Observations

- no known contraindications
- in patch tests on 21 patients with essential oil dermatoses, positive reactions to full-strength or diluted oils including *P. sylvestris* oil were attributed to 3-carene (a major component of pine oil), α-phellandrene and eugenol (Woeber & Krombach 1969)
- no irritation or sensitization at 12% dilution when tested on humans (Opdyke 1976j)
- no phototoxic effects reported (Opdyke 1976j)
- limonene, dipentene and bornyl acetate are responsible for antiviral and antibacterial activity (Joubert & Gattefossé 1968)

PIPER NIGRUM fruct. [BLACK PEPPER]
PIPERACEAE

Representative constituents

Hydrocarbons
monoterpenes   α-pinene 2–9%, β-pinene 5–14%, α-thujene 0.5–3.5%, sabinene 9–19%, α-terpinene 0.4–2.8%, δ-3-carene 1–15%, myrcene 1.6–2.5%,(–)-limonene 17%, α-phellandrene 5–9%, δ-elemene 2.6%, *p*-cymene 1–2.8%, γ-terpinene 0.5–3.9%, terpinolene 0.5–1.5%, camphene *sesquiterpenes*   β-caryophyllene 9–29%, α-humulene 1–2%, α-guaiene, α- and β-cubebene 0.2–1.6%, α- and β-selinenes 0.5–7.7%, α- and β-elemene 0.3–2.4%, β-bisabolene 2–5%,

calamenene, α-copaene 0.5–1.5%, β-farnesene 1–3%, zingiberene trace, bergamotene 0.5%, ar-curcumene 0.5%

Alcohols
monoterpenols terpinen-4-ol < 1%, α-terpineol 0.1%, linalool < 1%, *trans*-pinocarveol, *trans*-carveol, elemol 0.5%, α-bisabolol 0.1%

Phenolic ethers
p-cymene methyl ether, carvacrol methyl ether trace, myristicin trace, safrole trace

Ketones (1–8%)
di-hydrocarvone 0.05%, piperitone < 1%

Aldehydes
piperonal

Oxides
caryophyllene oxide 0.6%

Properties and indications

analgesic*	rheumatic pain, toothache*
antibacterial	see Table 4.4
anticatarrhal	chronic bronchitis, laryngitis, colds
antiseptic	urinary system
eupeptic	sluggish liver, pancreas and digestion
expectorant	bronchitis, coughs
febrifuge	fevers
sexual tonic	frigidity, general

Observations

- no known contraindications to *P. nigrum*
- no irritation or sensitization at 4% dilution when tested on humans (Opdyke 1978e)
- low level (insignificant) phototoxic effects (Opdyke 1978e)
- myristicin and elemicin can be readily modified in the body to amphetamines (Buchanan 1978, Duke 1985)
- it is mutagenic with *Leptospira*; in large doses it has a bactericidal effect and has an inhibiting effect on *Lactobacillus plantarum*, *Escherichia coli* and *Streptococcus faecalis* (Duke & Ayensu 1985)
- smoking withdrawal symptoms are lessened by the inhalation of the vapour from an extract of black pepper (Rose & Behm 1994)

POGOSTEMON PATCHOULI fol. [PATCHOULI] LAMIACEAE

Representative constituents

Hydrocarbons
monoterpenes α-pinene 0.5–1%, β-pinene 0.5–1%, limonene trace
sesquiterpenes (40–50%) α-bulnesene 10–19.6%, β-bulnesene 14–16%, α-guaiene 6–15%, β-guaiene, α-patchoulene 3–5.3%, β-patchoulene 1.9–6.6%, seychellene 5–12%, cyclo-seychellene < 1%, β-caryophyllene 2–4.2%, δ-cadinene 1–2.8%,

aromadendrene 10.8–20.9%, 1,5-epoxy-α-guaiene 0.1%, 1,10-epoxy-α-bulnesene 0.2–0.6%

Alcohols
sesquiterpenols (35–45%) patchoulol 23.6–45.9%, pogostol 1–3%, bulnesol 1%, guaiol, norpatchoulenol < 1%

Ketones
patchoulenone trace–2.2%, isopatchoulenone 1%

Oxides
α-guaiene oxide 1%, α-bulnesene oxide 4%, caryophyllene oxide 0.5–1%

Properties and indications

antifungal	
antiinfectious	enteritis
antiinflammatory	acne*, allergies, inflamed skin, seborrhoeic eczema
cicatrizant	cracked skin, scar tissue, abnormal epidermis
decongestant	
immunostimulant	low natural defences
insect repellent	
phlebotonic*	haemorrhoids*, varicose veins*

Observations

- no known contraindications
- no irritation was produced by the oil on humans at 20% in petroleum jelly or in an ointment, or at 0.1% in a non-irritant cream base in subjects with dermatoses (Fujii, Furukawa & Suzuki 1972)
- no irritation or sensitization at 10% dilution when tested on humans (Opdyke & Letizia 1982a)
- no phototoxic effects reported (Opdyke & Letizia 1982a)

RAVENSARA AROMATICA fol. [AROMATIC RAVENSARA] LAURACEAE

Representative constituents

Hydrocarbons
monoterpenes α-pinene, β-pinene, sabinene 13.5–15%
sesquiterpenes β-caryophyllene

Alcohols
monoterpenols α-terpineol 6–7%, terpinen-4-ol 2%

Esters
terpenyl acetate

Oxides
1,8-cineole 61%

Properties and indications

antibacterial	
antifungal	
antiinfectious*	glandular fever, bronchitis, influenza*, sinusitis, whooping cough
antiinflammatory	rhinopharyngitis

antiviral* — chicken pox, dendritis*, herpes zoster*, viral enteritis, viral hepatitis*

detoxicant
expectorant* — bronchitis, coughs
neurotonic — insomnia*, muscle fatigue, neuromuscular problems

Observations

- no contraindications known
- well tolerated on the skin
- relaxing when massaged over the vertebral column

ROSA DAMASCENA, R. CENTIFOLIA flos (dist.) [ROSE OTTO] ROSACEAE

Representative constituents

Hydrocarbons (25%)
monoterpenes stearoptene 16–22%, α-pinene, β-pinene, α-terpinene, limonene, myrcene, ocimene, *p*-cymene, camphene
sesquiterpenes β-caryophyllene 0.3%
other octadecane 0.2%, nonadecane and nonadecene 2–15%

Alcohols
monoterpenols geraniol 15.8–22.2%, citronellol 22.5–60?%, nerol 8.5%, linalool 1.5–2.7%, iso-borneol 0.4%, α-terpineol < 1%
sesquiterpenols farnesol 0.2–2%
aromatic phenyl ethyl alcohol 0.9–3%

Aldehydes
neral 0.5%

Esters (2–6%)
citronellyl acetate 0.5%, geranyl and neryl acetate 1.2%

Phenolic ethers
methyl eugenol 1.4%

Oxides
rose oxide 0.3%

Other
damascenone 0.2–1.6%, eicosane 1%, heneicosane, docosane 0.1–0.4%, tricosane 0.04–0.9%, tetracosane 0.2%, pentacosane 0.4%

Properties and indications

antibacterial	see Table 4.4
antiinfectious	acute and chronic bronchitis, asthma, mouth ulcers
antiinflammatory	blotchy skin, gingivitis, conjunctivitis
astringent	
cicatrizant	mouth ulcers, skin problems, sprains, wounds
general tonic	chronic bronchitis
neurotonic*	debility, depression
sexual tonic	frigidity, sexual debility
styptic	wounds

Observations

- no known contraindications
- no irritation or sensitization at 2% dilution when tested on humans (Opdyke 1974i, 1975c)
- no phototoxic effects reported (Opdyke 1974i, 1975c)
- rose absolute is produced in a different way from rose otto and has a different chemical composition
- French rose absolute produced one sensitization reaction in a test on 25 individuals (Opdyke 1975d)

ROSMARINUS OFFICINALIS CT. CINEOLE, CT. CAMPHOR fol. [ROSEMARY] LAMIACEAE

NB. The cineole and camphor chemotypes have almost the same constituents, properties and indications. They are therefore considered together here.

Representative constituents

Hydrocarbons
monoterpenes (30–37%) α-pinene 1.4–12%, β-pinene 3–9%, camphene 3–22%, myrcene 1–2%, α-phellandrene, β-phellandrene, α-terpinene, γ-terpinene, limonene 1.9–2.4%, *p*-cymene 1.1–2%
sesquiterpenes β-caryophyllene 0.9–3%, α-humulene 0.6–1.2%

Alcohols
monoterpenols linalool 0.6–2%, α-terpineol 1–4.5%, borneol 3.4–12%, isoborneol, terpenen-4-ol 0.6–1.5%, *cis*- and *trans*-thujanol-4, *p*-cymene-8-ol, verbenol

Esters
iso-bornyl acetate trace–1.2, α-fenchyl acetate

Oxides
1,8-cineole 30–55%, caryophyllene oxide, humulene epoxides

Ketones
monoterpenones α-thujone, β-thujone, camphor 6.4–30%, verbenone trace, carvone 1%
aliphatic 3-hexanone, methyl heptanone

Properties and indications

analgesic	migraine, painful digestion
antibacterial	see Table 4.4
antifungal	see Table 4.5
antiinfectious	chills, diarrhoea, enteritis, influenza
antiinflammatory	cystitis, gout, muscular pains, otitis, rheumatism, inflamed gall bladder
antispasmodic	muscle cramp
antitussive	coughing, whooping cough
antiviral	
cardiotonic	palpitations, weak heart
carminative	flatulence
choleretic*	insufficient bile
cicatrizant	burns, wounds
decongestant (venous)	migraine, headache, poor circulation, arteriosclerosis, bruises

detoxicant	hepatitis, jaundice, cirrhosis, enlarged liver, gall bladder malfunction
digestive	indigestion, sluggish digestion, colitis, constipation, painful digestion
diuretic	liver*, gall bladder*
emmenagogic	amenorrhoea, oligomenorrhoea
hyperglycaemic	
hypertensor (high dose)	hypotension
hypotensor (low dose)	hypertension
litholytic	gall stones
lowers cholesterol	high cholesterol
mucolytic*	chronic bronchitis, sinusitis
neuromuscular action*	multiple sclerosis, painful muscles, epilepsy, neuralgia, rheumatism
neurotonic	fainting, general debility, general fatigue, hysteria, loss of memory, vertigo
sexual tonic	impotence
stimulant	adrenal cortex
unspecified	enuresis (bedwetting)

Observations

- usually regarded as having no contraindications
- there are conflicting opinions regarding the use of rosemary oils in pregnancy and epilepsy:
  — some cite it as an oil to avoid in the first 4 months of pregnancy
  — Roulier (1990) warns against its use in pregnancy but does not give this warning for the verbenone chemotype
  — Franchomme & Pénoël (1990) warn against using the verbenone chemotype on pregnant women, but do not mention the cineole and camphor chemotypes
  — some contraindicate its use on people prone to epilepsy
  — Valnet (1980) recommends its use on epileptics
  — thought to induce epileptic fits in epileptic patients receiving massage with the oil (Betts 1994)
- bath preparations containing the oil can cause erythema (Duke 1985)
- toiletries containing the oil can cause dermatitis in hypersensitive individuals (Mitchell & Rook 1979)
- the essential oil in wine is said to help cancers (Hartwell 1967–1971)
- no irritation or sensitization at 10% dilution when tested on humans (Opdyke 1974j)
- stimulating action in humans and mice (Buchbauer et al 1991)
- neurotoxic due to camphor content, which can cause convulsions in oral use (Craig 1953); some oils have low camphor level
- tests suggest that the volatile oil of *R. officinalis* has hyperglycaemic and insulin release inhibitory effects in the rabbit (Al-Hader, Hasan & Aqel 1994)
- carminative and a mild irritant (Reynolds 1972)
- potent antibacterial action (Aureli, Constantini & Zolea 1992, Deans & Ritchie 1987, Lis-Balchin, Deans & Hart 1994, Maruzzella 1960, Maruzzella & Sicurella 1960), poor

antifungal action (Lis-Balchin, Deans & Hart 1994, Maruzzella 1960, Maruzzella & Liguori 1958)
- active against *Staphylococcus aureus*, *S. albus*, *Vibrio cholerae*, *Escherichia coli* and *Corynebacterium* (Opdyke 1974j)

ROSMARINUS OFFICINALIS CT. VERBENONE fol. [ROSEMARY] LAMIACEAE

Representative constituents

Hydrocarbons
monoterpenes α-pinene 15–34%, β-pinene, camphene, myrcene, limonene, α-terpinene, terpinolene
sesquiterpenes β-caryophyllene

Alcohols
monoterpenols borneol trace–7%

Esters
bornyl acetate

Ketones
monoterpenones verbenone 15–37%, camphor 1–15%

Oxides
1,8-cineole trace–20%

Properties and indications

antibacterial	
antiinfectious	leukorrhoea, vaginitis, candida
anticatarrhal	bronchitis, sinusitis
antispasmodic	digestive, cardiovascular
antiviral*	viral colic*, viral hepatitis
cardiotonic	angina pectoris, arrhythmia, tachycardia
cicatrizant	
detoxicant	liver and bilious affections [but see Observations]
expectorant	bronchitis, coughs
hormone regulator	ovaries and testicles
mucolytic	bronchitis, coughs, sinusitis
nervous system regulator	fatigue, nervous depression, nervous digestive*, sexual problems

Observations

- not normally used on those inclined to liver problems, children and in pregnancy (except where necessary)
- the oil is neurotoxic and abortive (Franchomme & Pénoël 1990); not to be used in pregnancy (Roulier 1990)

SALVIA OFFICINALIS fol. [SAGE, DALMATIAN SAGE] LAMIACEAE

Representative constituents

Hydrocarbons
monoterpenes (3–15%) α-pinene 3.2–6.4%, β-pinene 1.9%, camphene 1–5.4%, myrcene 0.4–1.1%, limonene 0.9–4%, *p*-cymene 1–2%, terpinolene, salvene, α-phellandrene 0.1%,

β-phellandrene 0.1%, α-thujene trace, sabinene 0.2%, α-terpinene 0.2%, γ-terpinene 0.3%
sesquiterpenes β-caryophyllene 1–7%, aromadendrene, α-humulene 4–5%, α-cadinene, β-cadinene, β-copaene

Alcohols
monoterpenols (3–38%) linalool 0.4–12%, terpinen-4-ol 0.2–4%, α-terpineol trace–9%, borneol 1.5–14%, salviol, *trans*-sabinol trace
sesquiterpenols viridiflorol 0–10%

Esters
bornyl acetate 0.1–3%, linalyl acetate 1–2%, sabinyl acetate, linalyl and methyl isovalerates

Phenols
thymol trace

Oxides
1,8-cineole 5–14%, caryophyllene oxide 0.4–2.1%

Ketones
monoterpenones (20–70%) α-thujone 12–35.7%, β-thujone 2–33%, camphor 4.1–26%, fenchone 0.2%

Aldehydes
3-hexanal trace

Coumarins
aesculetine trace

Phenolic ethers
methyl chavicol 0.4%

Other
trans-sabinene hydrate 0.2%, tricyclene 0.3%, *cis*-2-methyl-3-methylene-5-heptene 0.7%, *trans*-2-methyl-3-methylene-5-heptene 0.1%, *cis*-sabinene hydrate trace

Properties and indications

analgesic	angina, rheumatism, toothache
antibacterial	see Table 4.4
anticancer	malignant conditions
anticatarrhal	asthma, bronchitis, coughs
antifungal*	Candida albicans*
antiinfectious	influenza, gingivitis, insect bites, intermittent fevers, leukorrhoea, sore throat
antilactogenic	see Observations
antipyretic	hot flushes
antispasmodic	dysmenorrhoea
antisudorific	excessive hand and armpit hyperhidrosis, night sweating
antiviral	genital herpes, thrush, viral enteritis, viral meningitis, viral neuritis
choleretic	insufficient bile*
cicatrizant	
circulatory regulator	poor circulation, rheumatism, congestion
digestive (low dose)	indigestion, loss of appetite, sluggish digestion
diuretic	oliguria, urinary disorders
drains biliary canal	
emmenagogic	amenorrhoea, irregular periods, scanty periods
expectorant	bronchitis, coughs
hormone-like	conducive to conception, facilitates delivery, sterility, menopause, premenopause*
hypertensor	hypotension
hypoglycaemiant	prediabetes
insecticidal	
lipolytic*	cellulite
mucolytic	coughs, sinusitis
neurotonic	alopecia, general debility, nervous debility, tremors, vertigo

Observations

- not normally used for breastfeeding mothers and young children
- antilactogenic: halts lactation in nursing mothers (Roulier 1990, Valnet 1980)
- neurotoxic and abortive (may cause malformed heart in babies if used throughout pregnancy (Franchomme & Pénoël 1990)
- because of its potential toxicity, sage oil, like all essential oils, should be used only in very small quantities (Foster 1993b)
- no irritation or sensitization at 8% dilution when tested on humans (Opdyke 1974k)
- German authorities recommend an internal dosage level of one drop of the essential oil per cup of water in infusion, perhaps taken up to three times per day
- although sage has more thujone than wormwood it seems a far safer plant: but the tea should only be taken for a week or two at a time because of the potentially toxic effects of thujone (Mabey 1988)
- cheilitis and stomatitis follow some cases of sage tea ingestion (Duke 1985)
- the distilled oil is said to be a violent epileptiform convulsant, resembling the essential oils of absinth, nutmeg and wormwood (Duke 1985)
- the Flavourings and Food Regulations 1992 allow 0.5 mg/kg food of α- and β-thujone
- salvin and salvin monomethyl ether (phenolic acids) have antimicrobial activities especially against *Staphylococcus aureus* (Alimkhodzhaeva & Khazanovich 1972, Dobrynin et al 1976)
- thujone is responsible for the antimicrobial activity (Jalsenjak et al 1987)
- antimicrobial activity of the oil was demonstrated against *Escherichia coli*, *Shigella sonnei*, *Salmonella* species, *Klebsiella ozanae*, *Bacillus subtilis*, *Candida albicans* and *Cryptococcus neoformans* (Recio et al 1989)
- reported to show anticonvulsive activity in animals (Atanasova-Shopova & Rusinov 1970)
- is a relaxant (Kubota et al 1992)
- has antifungal activities (Dikshit & Husain 1984)

SALVIA SCLAREA flos, fol. [CLARY] LAMIACEAE

Representative constituents

Hydrocarbons

monoterpenes (2–3%)   α-pinene 0.1–0.25%, β-pinenes 0.3%, sabinene trace, camphene, myrcene 0.1–1.7%, terpinolene, *p*-cymene trace, α-terpinene trace, limonene 0.1–0.8%
sesquiterpenes (5%)   β-caryophyllene 0.8–3%, germacrene D 1.6–4%, curcumene, *trans*-calamene, *trans*-ocimene 0.4–1%, terpinolene 0.1–0.4%, α-cubebene trace, α-copaene 0.1–0.5%, β-bourbonene 0.1%

Alcohols

monoterpenols (15%)   linalool 5–26%, α-terpineol 1%, citronellol, nerol trace–1%, geraniol 0.1–3.2%, borneol, isoborneol, thujol, terpinen-4-ol trace–0.1%
sesquiterpenols   α-bisabol, junerol
diterpenols (5–7%)   sclareol 1–7%
other cis-3-hexanol trace–0.3%, *trans*-2-hexanol 0.2%, 1-octen-3-ol trace, spathulenol trace

Aldehydes

trans-2-hexanal trace–0.1%, caryophyllenals

Esters

linalyl acetate 49–75%, citronellyl acetate, geranyl acetate 0.3–3.2%, neryl acetate 0.2–1.7%, butyrates, valerates, bornyl acetate 0.2%, α-terpinyl acetate trace–0.1%

Oxides

1,8-cineole, *trans*-linalool oxide trace, caryophyllene oxide 0.2–0.5%, sclareol oxide, *cis*-linalool oxide trace

Ketones

α- and β-thujones

Coumarins

coumarin

Properties and indications

antifungal	dermal fungal conditions
antiinfectious	genital infections (connected with hormone deficiency)
antispasmodic	
antisudorific	hyperhidrosis
decongestant	dysmenorrhoea
detoxicant	
hormone (oestrogen-like)	amenorrhoea*, oligomenorrhoea, premenopause
neurotonic	epilepsy, nervous fatigue, calming to parasympathetic nervous system, alopecia
phlebotonic	circulatory problems, haemorrhoids, varicose veins, venous aneurism, cholesterol
regenerative	cellular ageing, poor hair growth, alopecia

Observations

- no known contraindications, but is not normally used on people with cancers or tumours
- no irritation or sensitization at 8% dilution when tested on humans (Opdyke & Letizia 1982b)
- there are in excess of 250 constituents in clary oil
- contains a diterpenol, which is rare in distilled oils

SANTALUM ALBUM lig. [SANDALWOOD] SANTALACEAE

Representative constituents

Hydrocarbons

sesquiterpenes   α- and β-santalene 10%, epi-β-santalene 6%, α- and β-curcumene, farnesene

Alcohols

sesquiterpenols   α-santalol 46–60%, β-santalol 20–30%, epi-β-santalol 4–5%, *trans*-β-santalol 1–2%, *cis*-lanceol 1.5%, *cis*-nuciferol 1%, a monocyclic sesquiterpenol 5%, a tricyclic sesquiterpenol 1%

Aldehydes

sesquiterpenals   teresantalal

Properties and indications

antiinfectious	pulmonary: chronic bronchitis, colibacillosis; urinary: cystitis, gonorrhoea, urinary tract infections
astringent	diarrhoea
cardiotonic*	tired heart, haemorrhoids, varicose veins
decongestant*	pelvic congestion*, acne, skin problems
dilator (bronchial)	restricted bronchioles
diuretic	
moisturizer	dry skin
nerve relaxant	lumbago, neuralgia, sciatica, meditation
sedative	
sexual tonic	impotence
tonic	

Observations

- no known contraindications
- regarded as a general and sexual tonic
- does not irritate the mucous linings of the stomach or intestine
- no irritation or sensitization at 10% dilution when tested on humans (Opdyke 1974l)
- no phototoxic effects reported (Opdyke 1974l)
- approved for food use (Duke 1985)
- isolated santalol can cause dermatitis in sensitive individuals (Claus 1961, Reynolds 1972, Lewis & Elvin-Lewis 1977, Leung 1980)
- the oil has diuretic and urinary antiseptic properties (Leung 1980)

SATUREIA HORTENSIS fol.
[SUMMER OR GARDEN SAVORY] LAMIACEAE

Representative constituents

Hydrocarbons
monoterpenes (34%)   α-thujene < 1%, α-pinene < 1%,
β-pinene trace, myrcene 1–2.8%, α-terpinene 1–3.1%,
γ-terpinene 20–24%, *p*-cymene 3.7–15.3%, cymene ?–25%,
camphene trace, δ-3-carene, δ-4-carene, α-phellandrene,
β-phellandrene trace, limonene trace, sabinene trace
sesquiterpenes (3–4%)   β-caryophyllene 2–4%,
β-bisabolene 1%, δ-cadinene 3%, calacorene and γ-cadinene
3.6%

Alcohols
monoterpenols   linalool, terpinen-4-ol, borneol, α-terpineol,
nerol trace, geraniol trace

Phenols (39–40%)
thymol, carvacrol 35–40%, eugenol

Ketones
camphor trace

Aldehydes
piperonal

Oxides
1,8-cineole

Other
damascenone 1%

Properties and indications

antibacterial	see Table 4.4
antifungal	see Table 4.5
antiinfectious*	wide range of action
antioxidant	
antiparasitic	
antiseptic	respiratory tract infections
antiviral	
cardiotonic	
choleretic	
digestive tonic	indigestion, facilitates elimination, carminative, sluggish bile
expectorant	
general tonic/stimulant	debility*
nervous system balancer	
revitalizing	
sexual tonic	

Observations

- no irritation or sensitization at 6% dilution when tested on humans (Opdyke 1976k)
- no phototoxic effects reported (Opdyke 1976k)
- two species of *Satureia*—*S. hortensis* and *S. montana*—have a pronounced thyme-like odour and flavour, and the oils of the two plants are closely related in chemical composition (Guenther 1949)
- carvacrol has antidiuretic properties

SATUREIA MONTANA fol.
[WINTER OR MOUNTAIN SAVORY] LAMIACEAE

Representative constituents

Hydrocarbons
monoterpenes (40–50%)   α- and γ-terpinenes 2–20%,
p-cymene 10–25%, α-pinene, β-pinene, camphene, sabinene,
myrcene, limonene, α-phellandrene
sesquiterpenes   β-caryophyllene, α-humulene,
aromadendrene, β-bisabolene, α-cadinene, γ-cadinene,
calacorene

Alcohols
monoterpenols   linalool 9–54%, *cis*-thujanol-4,
trans-thujanol-4, terpinen-4-ol trace–7%, α-terpineol 6–9%,
geraniol, borneol

Esters
linalyl acetate, terpinen-4-yl acetate, geranyl acetate,
α-terpinyl acetate

Phenols (25–50%)
carvacrol 25–50%, eugenol, thymol 1–5%

Phenolic ethers
carvacrol methyl ether

Oxides
1,8-cineole 1%, caryophyllene oxide

Ketones
camphor, damascenone

Properties and indications

analgesic*	rheumatoid arthritis*
antibacterial	see Table 4.4
anticatarrhal	bronchitis, coughs
antifungal	Candida albicans, fungal infections of the mouth
antiinfectious*	wide range of action, colitis, enteritis, tonsillitis, sore throat, tuberculosis, diarrhoea, cystitis, malaria*, skin infections, abscesses, impetigo, lichen
antiparasitic*	oxyurids, ascaris, taenia, amoebiasis*
antispasmodic	intestinal spasm, colic, muscle spasms
antiviral	
carminative	flatulence
cicatrizant	insect bites, sores
digestive stimulant	painful digestion
expectorant	asthma, bronchitis, catarrh
general tonic*	general debility
hypertensor	hypotension*
immunostimulant	repetitive infections
mental stimulant	mental debility
neurotonic	lymph ganglion inflammation*, debility, nervous fatigue*, depression

Observations

- possible skin irritant and therefore to be used in low concentration
- savory oil is an efficient antidiuretic because of the carvacrol present (Duke 1985 p. 432)
- winter savory is used for catarrh, colic, otitis, sclerosis and spasms (Duke 1985 p. 432)
- Winter savory has diuretic activity in rats (Stanic & Samarzija 1993)

SYZYGIUM AROMATICUM (= *EUGENIA CARYOPHYLLATA*) flos [CLOVE BUD] MYRTACEAE

Representative constituents

Hydrocarbons
monoterpenes   pinene
sesquiterpenes   α- and β-caryophyllene 5–13%, α- and β-humulene 0.5–1.5%, α-cubebene 0.01–0.3%, α-copaene 0.01–0.2%, calamenene 0.2–0.5%

Phenols (60–90%)
eugenol 36–85%, isoeugenol 0.1–0.25%, acetoeugenol 11–21.8%

Esters (20–25%)
eugenyl acetate 0.5–12%, 2-nonanyl acetate trace, α-terpinyl acetate 0.1–0.2%, benzyl acetate trace, methyl benzoate 0.04–0.13%

Oxides
humulene epoxide trace, caryophyllene oxide trace–1.8%

Properties and indications

analgesic	rheumatoid arthritis, toothache, neuralgia*
antibacterial	see Table 4.4
antifungal	see Table 4.5
antiinfectious	abscesses, gum infections, infected acne, ulcers, wounds
antiinflammatory	bronchitis, salpingitis, sinusitis, arthritis, bursitis
antiseptic	prevention of disease, cystitis, diarrhoea, sinusitis
antispasmodic	diarrhoea, intestinal spasm
antiviral*	enteritis*, influenza, hepatitis, herpes, tuberculosis*
carminative	flatulence
cicatrizant	infected acne, ulcers, wounds
hormone-like	thyroid imbalance
hypertensor	hypotension
immunostimulant	low immunity
insect repellent	mosquitoes, clothes moths
mental stimulant*	memory loss, mental fatigue
neurotonic*	debility, fatigue*
sexual tonic	impotence
unspecified	stimulates secretion of saliva
uterotonic*	difficult labour, long labour

Observations

- should not be applied undiluted to skin because clove oils may cause irritation at high dosage levels
- considered non-toxic at normal usage levels
- 20% dilution of clove bud oil on humans produced erythema in two of the 25 tested; no irritation or sensitization occurred at 2%, or at 0.2% on subjects with dermatoses (Fujii, Furukawa & Suzuki 1972)
- no irritation or sensitization at 5% dilution when tested on humans (Opdyke 1975e)
- no phototoxic effects reported for any of the clove oils (Opdyke 1975e)
- is used as an antiseptic mouthwash
- eugenol sensitizes some people causing contact dermatitis (Duke 1985)
- clove bud oil and savory oil create a synergistic mix (Duraffourd 1982)
- used externally in patented treatments of bone degeneration, joint inflammation, bursitis and treatment of sinuses
- antiviral due to eugeniin, present in buds; eugeniin has strong antiviral activity against herpes simplex virus (Takechi & Tanaka 1981)
- oil is used widely for toothache
- the oil is an irritant and stimulates peristalsis; used as an expectorant in bronchitis and phthisis (Duke 1985)
- eugenol is responsible for the anodyne and mild antiseptic properties; exhibits broad antimicrobial activities against Gram positive, Gram negative and acid fast bacteria as well as fungi (Anon 1977, Martinez Nadal et al 1973, Ramadan et al 1972b)
- also has larvicidal and anthelminthic properties (Oishi et al 1974)

TAGETES MINUTA (= *T. GLANDULIFERA*), *T. PATULA*, *T. ERECTA* flos [TAGET, FRENCH MARIGOLD] ASTERACEAE

Representative constituents

Hydrocarbons
monoterpenes   (+)-limonene 3–7.3%, *cis*-β-ocimene and *trans*-β-ocimene 30–59%

Ketones
tagetone 40–60%, 2,6-dimethyl-7-octene-4-one, 2 and E-ocimenones 26%, 2 and E-tagetones 9%, dihydrotagetones 9.1–13%, *cis*-tagetone 5.5%

Coumarins

Properties and indications

anthelminthic	parasitic enteritis
antifungal	candida, tinea pedis, ungueal infections, see Table 4.5
antiinfectious	catarrhal infections
cicatrizant	scratches, burns, chronic skin lesions, bruises, slow healing wounds
emmenagogic	amenorrhoea
mucolytic	bronchitis, coughs
phototoxic	

Observations

- avoid use on babies, children and in pregnancy because of ketone content; tagetone may be harmful (Arctander 1960)
- phototoxic when used inappropriately; IFRA recommends not more than 0.05% in preparations for use on skin exposed to sunlight (IFRA 1992)
- given as photosensitizing by Franchomme & Pénoël (1990)
- stated to be non-toxic, not phototoxic, non-irritant, not a sensitizer (Opdyke 1982)
- hypotensive in rats (Chandhoke & Ghatak 1969)
- has tranquillizing, hypotensive, bronchodilatory, spasmolytic and antiinflammatory properties in experimental animals (Bye 1986, Chandhoke & Ghatak 1969)
- (5E)-Ocimenone has larvicidal activity against mosquito larvae (Maradufu et al 1978)

THYMUS MASTICHINA flos, fol.
[SPANISH MARJORAM] LAMIACEAE

Representative constituents

Hydrocarbons
monoterpenes terpinolene 4%, limonene 2–2.8%, α-pinene 2.6%, β-pinene 2–3%, *p*-cymene 1.3–3.4%, sabinene 0.8–1.1%, α-thujene 0.2–0.5%, myrcene 0.2–1%, camphene 0.2–1.4%, γ-terpinene < 1%
sesquiterpenes β-caryophyllene 0.1%, β-gurjunene 0.3%, allo-aromadendrene 0.2–1%, γ- and δ-cadinene 0.1%, β-bourbonene 0.1%, caryophyllene 1–1.5%

Alcohols
monoterpenols borneol trace–3.5%, linalool 8.5–43%, α-terpineol 8%, geraniol 0.2%, *cis*- and *trans*-thujanol-4 0.2%, *trans*-pinocarveol 1%, 3-terpinen-l-ol 0.2%, terpinen-4-ol 0.1–0.7%

Phenols
thymol 0–5%

Ketones
camphor trace–4%

Oxides
1,8-cineole 41–75%, caryophyllene oxide trace

Esters
linalyl acetate 1–1.5%, 3-terpinen-l-yl acetate 0.2%, bornyl acetate 0.2%, *trans*-pinocarveol acetate 1.5%, α-terpinyl acetate 3%, geranyl acetate 0.1%

Other
trans-sabinene hydrate 0.2%

Properties and indications

antibacterial	see Table 4.4
antifungal	see Table 4.5
antiinfectious	sinusitis, catarrhal bronchitis*, viral and bacterial infections

Observations

- no contraindications known at normal dose
- no irritation or sensitization at 6% dilution when tested on humans (Opdyke 1976l)
- no phototoxic effects reported (Opdyke 1976l)

THYMUS SATUREIOIDES [MOROCCAN THYME, BORNEOL THYME] LAMIACEAE

Representative constituents

Hydrocarbons
monoterpenes α-pinene 0.1–5.6%, γ-terpinene 0–4.2%, *p*-cymene 0–9.9%, camphene 0.1–11.2%, β-pinene 0–1.3%, α-thujene 0–0.8%, sabinene 0–0.2%, β-pinene 0–1.3%, myrcene 0–1%, α-phellandrene 0–0.1%, α-terpinene 0–0.7%, limonene 0.1–1.1%, terpinolene 0–0.3%
sesquiterpenes β-caryophyllene 1.8–7.0%, δ-cadinene 0.1–1.3%, α-copaene 0–0.6%, β-bourbonene 0–0.1%, aromadendrene 0–0.3%, α-humulene 0–0.5%, allo-aromadendrene 0–0.2%, γ-muurolene 0–0.2%, α-muurolene 0–0.3%, β-guaiene 0–1%

Alcohols
monoterpenols borneol 13.0–77.6%, α-terpineol 4.7–21%, terpinen-4-ol 0.7–4.8%, linalool 0.4–12.3%, ρ-cymen-8-ol 0.1–0.7%, *trans*-pinocarveol 0–0.4%
other 3-octanol 0–0.8%

Aldehydes
campholenic aldehyde 0–0.4%

Phenols
thymol 0–21.3%, carvacrol 0.5–49.5%, methyl carvacrol 0–7.1%

Phenol ethers
methyl thymol 0–0.1%, methyl carvacrol 0–7.1%

Ketones
dihydrocarvones 0.2–3%, verbenone 0–0.1%, camphor 0.1–2.6%

Esters
bornyl acetate 0.1–5.4%, linalyl acetate 0–0.2%

Oxides
caryophyllene oxide 0.4–3.7%, 1,8-cineole 0–0.16%, *cis*-linalool oxide 0–0.1%

Other
tricyclene 0–0.5%, α-irone 0–0.5%, *cis*-sabinene hydrate 0–0.5%, *p*-mentha-1(7), 2-dien-8-ol 0–0.1%

Properties and indications

antibacterial	tuberculosis*
antiinfectious	acne, chronic sinusitis, cystiitis, infections (viral and bacterial)
antiinflammatory	tonsillitis, arthritis*, cystitis
general tonic	gall bladder malfunction, gall stones, hepatic deficiency
immunostimulant*	autoimmune deficiency
neurotonic*	debility*, general fatigue*

sexual tonic*	sexual apathy*
uterotonic	lack of uterine muscle tone

Observations

- no known contraindications at normal dose
- possible skin irritant

THYMUS VULGARIS (POPULATION) herb. [THYME] LAMIACEAE

Representative constituents

Hydrocarbons

monoterpenes   p-cymene 2.2–42.8%, γ-terpinene 0.3–12.4%, α-pinene 0.9–3.7%, camphene 0.5–2.4%, myrcene trace–2.6%, α-terpinene 0.8–1.5%, limonene 0.4–2.1%, terpinolene trace–2%, α-thujene 0.5%, δ-3-carene 0.1%, sabinene 0.6%, α-phellandrene 0.1–0.2%, β-pinene trace
sesquiterpenes   β-caryophyllene 0.2–2.9%

Phenols

thymol 30–48.2%, carvacrol 0.5–5.5%, methoxy carvacrol trace

Alcohols

monoterpenols   borneol trace–1.8%, linalool 1.3–12.4%, terpinen-4-ol 0.3–9.5%, α-terpineol 0.4–9.4%, geraniol 0.1–0.2%, β-terpineol 0.6–0.9%
sesquiterpenols   nerolidol 0–0.8%

Ketones

camphor 2.3–16.3%, α-thujone 0.2%

Esters

linalyl acetate 0.9%, α-terpinyl acetate 0.7–1.4%, geranyl acetate 0–0.5%

Oxides

1,8-cineole 0.4–7.4%, *trans*-linalool oxide 0.5%, *cis*-linalool oxide 1%

Properties and indications

antibacterial	see Table 4.4
antifungal	see Table 4.5
antioxidant	
antiseptic	acne, boils, skin problems, etc.
antispasmodic	
capillary stimulant	anaemia, circulatory disorders, hair loss
carminative	flatulence
cicatrizant	
digestive tonic	sluggish digestion
diuretic	
expectorant	bronchial secretions, bronchitis, sinusitis, asthma
general tonic	general fatigue
hypertensor	hypotension
mental stimulant	depression, exam nerves
neurotonic	anxiety, debility
parasiticide	

stomachic	
sudorific	
vermifuge	intestinal parasites
warming	rheumatism, stiff joints
unspecified	leukorrhoea

Observations

- irritant to the skin
- the volatile oil is toxic in any quantity and internal use should be restricted to professionals (Mabey 1988)
- oil of thyme is largely eliminated through the alveoli of the lung (Weiss 1988)
- the German Bundes Gesundsheitamt (BGA) publishes monographs on acceptable labelling for herb products and permits thyme to be designated for symptoms of bronchitis, whooping cough and catarrh of the upper airways (Foster 1993b)
- carvacrol stimulates mucosal secretory activity (Mills 1991)
- thyme oil has been shown to be antispasmodic owing to its phenols
- thyme plants grown from seed (known as population thyme) yield an essential oil with a rich variety of components
- there is wide variation of constituents in oils from *T. vulgaris*, hence the broad limits given above
- like many of the herbaceous members of the Lamiaceae family that have achieved economic importance, there are nomenclatural and botanical authenticity problems associated with thyme (Lawrence 1979); there are about 400 species—or 100 species with 400 names (Foster 1993b). (Phillips 1989, 1991) has attempted to sort out the confusion of species occurring in the USA
- at least nine naturally occurring chemotypes are known
- *T. vulgaris* ct. thymol and *T. vulgaris* ct. carvacrol have thymol and carvacrol respectively as major components
- *T. vulgaris* ct. geraniol has geraniol 60–80%; *T. vulgaris* ct. linalool has linalool 60–80%
- see observations under other types of *T. vulgaris*
- has antispasmodic, expectorant and carminative properties as well as antimicrobial activities, owing to thymol and carvacrol (Patakova & Chladek 1974, Pizsolitto 1975, Simeon de Bouchberg et al 1976, Van Den Broucke & Lernli 1981, Vincenzi & Dessi 1991)
- reported to be lethal to mosquito larvae (Novak 1968)

THYMUS VULGARIS CT. GERANIOL, CT. LINALOOL herb.[SWEET THYME] LAMIACEAE

Properties and indications

antifungal*	see Table 4.5
antiinfectious	bronchitis, sinusitis, tuberculosis
antiinflammatory	bronchitis, cystitis, muscular rheumatism, otitis, urethritis, vaginitis, dry eczema, psoriasis, weeping eczema

antiseptic	sore throat, tonsillitis, colitis, infected acne
antispasmodic (ct. linalool)	bronchiole spasm
antiviral*	veruccae, viral enteritis*, people prone to repeated viral attacks*
cardiotonic (ct. geraniol)	tired heart
choleretic	
diuretic (ct. linalool)	
immunostimulant (ct. linalool)	
neurotonic*	fatigue, insomnia
ophthalmic	eye problems (informed use only)
sexual tonic (ct. linalool)	
uterotonic*	facilitates delivery

Observations

- no known contraindications
- sweet thyme oils do not contain the aggressive elements of the red thymes
- preferred for general use, children and the elderly (Price 1993)

THYMUS VULGARIS CT. THUJANOL-4 herb. [SWEET THYME] LAMIACEAE

Representative constituents

Hydrocarbons

monoterpenes   myrcene, γ-terpinene

Alcohols

monoterpenols   (+)-*trans*-thujanol-4, (+)-terpinen-4-ol, *cis*-myrcenol-8, (−)-linalool

Properties and indications

antiinfectious	influenza, bronchitis, sinusitis, rhinopharyngitis, otitis, urethritis, cystitis
antiinflammatory	dermatitis, arthritis, tendonitis
bactericide	*chlamydia**
hepatic	inadequate liver function
hormone like	diabetes
immunostimulant	increase IgA
neurotonic	balancing to CNS, asthenia*
viricide	

Observations

- no contraindications known at normal aromatherapeutic dose
- this clone does not survive well under cultivation and therefore the oil is rare today, making caution necessary when procuring it; strenuous efforts are being made to overcome this problem and it is hoped to be resolved in the near future (Lamy personal communication 1997)
- due to this fact, reliable information on ct. thujanol-4 is hard to find
- said to be useful for warming by improving the circulation (Franchomme & Pénoël 1990 p. 403)

THYMUS VULGARIS CT. THYMOL, CT. CARVACROL herb. [THYME] LAMIACEAE

Properties and indications

anthelminthic*	
antibacterial*	tuberculosis
antidiuretic (ct. carvacrol)	enuresis
antifungal	see Table 4.5
antiinfectious	influenza, general infections*, head colds, infectious diseases, sinusitis
antiparasitic	
mental stimulant	mental strain, depression
mucolytic*	asthma, emphysema, pulmonary diseases
warming*	rheumatism of joints and muscles, sciatica, lumbago

Observations

- red thymes are powerful antiseptic and antibacterial agents
- to be used with care because of the high phenol content
- no irritation or sensitization at 8% dilution when tested on humans; can be irritating at full strength (Opdyke 1974m)
- thymol is a dermal and mucous membrane irritant (Anon 1994b, Tisserand & Balacs 1995)
- no phototoxic effects reported (Opdyke 1974m)
- it is to be avoided in pregnancy as the carvacrol content stimulates the mucosal secretory systems (Mills 1991)
- thymol is an antiseptic 20 times stronger than phenol, yet, unlike phenol, does not irritate or corrode the skin or mucosa
- thymol can be highly toxic; it is strongly fungicidal, antibacterial, antioxidant and toxic to the hookworm (Foster 1993b)
- thymol is a starting material for synthetic menthone and is used in embalming fluids
- thymol is an effective antifungal agent and anthelminthic: it is poorly absorbed into body fluids, so finds its main use within the gut or on the surface of the body; it is ideal for toothpastes and mouthwashes (Mills 1991)
- thymol has caused dermatitis in dentists, and (in toothpaste) has caused glossitis (Duke 1985)
- the oil of thyme used in bath preparations has caused hyperaemia and inflammation (Rook 1979)
- effective in vitro against *Salmonella typhimurium* and *Staphylococcus aureus* (Juven et al 1993)

VETIVERIA ZIZANIOIDES rad. [VETIVER] POACEAE

Representative constituents

Hydrocarbons

sesquiterpenes   vetivene, vetivazulene, tricyclovetivene

Alcohols

sesquiterpenols   vetiverol, bicyclovetiverol 12.1%, tricyclovetiverol 3.3%

Esters

sesquiterpenic   vetiverol acetate

Ketones

sesquiterpenones   α-vetivone 3.9%, β-vetivone 3%

Acids

vetivenic acid, palmitic acid, benzoic acid

Properties and indications

antiinfectious	general infections, skin infections, acne
circulatory tonic*	inflamed coronary artery
emmenagogic	amenorrhoea, oligomenorrhoea
glandular tonic	insufficient pancreatic secretion, liver congestion
immunostimulant	low immunity
unspecified	arthritis
unspecified	urticaria

Observations

- no known contraindications
- no irritation or sensitization at 8% dilution when tested on humans (Opdyke 1974n)
- no phototoxic effects reported (Opdyke 1974n)

ZINGIBER OFFICINALE rhiz. [GINGER] ZINGERBERACEAE

Representative constituents

Hydrocarbons

monoterpenes (20%)   α-pinene 0.4–4.2%, β-pinene 0.1–2.3%, camphene 1.1–8%, myrcene 0.1–1%, limonene 1.2–3%, β-phellandrene 1.3–4%
aromatic   p-cymene 0.2–10.8%, toluene decanes
sesquiterpenes (55%)   zingiberene 11.3–50.9%, β-sesquiphellandrene 1.6–9%, ar-curcumene 0.1–32.9%, cis-γ-bisabolene 7%, copaene, sesquithujene, β-ylangene, β-elemene, β-farnesene 19.8%, β-caryophyllene, calamenene, β-bisabolene 0.2%, α-selinene 1.4%

Alcohols

monoterpenols   citronellol 6%, linalool 1–5.5%, 2-butanol, 2-nonanol 2.1–7.8%, 2-heptanol trace
sesquiterpenols   nerolidol trace–8.9%, elemol, β-bisabol, zingiberol, *trans*-β-sesquiphellandrol, δ-borneol 1.3%

Aldehydes

monoterpenals   citronellal, myrtenal, phellandral, neral, geranial

Ketones

acetone, 2-hexanone, 2-heptanone, methyl-heptanone, 2-nonanone, cryptone, carvotanacetone, gingerone

Oxides

1,8-cineole 1.3%

Properties and indications

analgesic*	angina, painful indigestion, rheumatism, toothache
anticatarrhal	chronic bronchitis
carminative*	flatulence
digestive stimulant	constipation, loss of appetite, sluggish digestion, nausea
expectorant	chronic bronchitis
general tonic	fatigue, impotence
sexual tonic	impotence
stomachic	diarrhoea

Observations

- no known contraindications at normal dose
- gingerols and shogaols do not appear in the distilled essential oil
- no irritation or sensitization at 4% dilution when tested on humans (Opdyke 1974o)
- low level insignificant phototoxic effects reported (Opdyke 1974o)

Appendix B

1. UTEROTONIC OILS WHICH FACILITATE DELIVERY

The percentage figure given for toxic components is the average or a typical range.

Cymbopogon martinii fol. [PALMAROSA]: alcohols 80–90% (geraniol).
Foeniculum vulgare var. *dulce* fruct. [SWEET FENNEL]: phenolic ether 70%.
Mentha × piperita fol. [PEPPERMINT]: ketones 20–30%.
Myristica fragrans sem. [NUTMEG]: terpenes 40%, myristicin 2–3%.
Pimenta racemosa fol. [BAY]: phenol 90%. Difficult deliveries.
Pimpinella anisum fruct. [ANISEED]: phenolic ether 90%.
Syzygium aromaticum flos [CLOVE BUD]: phenol 70–80%. Difficult deliveries.
Thymus vulgaris ct. geraniol, herb. [SWEET THYME]: alcohol 60–80%.

2. EMMENAGOGIC ESSENTIAL OILS

The percentage figure given for toxic components is an average. See also Chapter 10.

Achillea millefolium flos [YARROW, MILFOIL]: combined ketone and oxide 30%. Not generally considered to be toxic.
Cinnamomum zeylanicum cort. [CINNAMON]: phenolic ether 60%.
Foeniculum vulgare var. *dulce* fruct. [SWEET FENNEL]: phenolic ether 60%. Also hormone-like, diuretic and lactogenic; facilitates delivery.
Melaleuca viridiflora fol. [NIAOULI]: oxide 50%. Contains the hormone-like sesquiterpenol viridiflorol.
Myristica fragrans sem. [NUTMEG, MACE]: phenolic ether 6%. Large dose produces narcosis, delirium and death—see also Appendix A. Also facilitates delivery.
Petroselinum sativum fruct. [PARSLEY SEED]: phenolic ether 55%.
Pimpinella anisum fruct. [ANISEED]: phenolic ether 83%. Also hormone-like; facilitates delivery.
Salvia officinalis fol. [SAGE]: ketone 35%. Also hormone-like.

351

3. DISPUTED EMMENAGOGIC OILS

Essential oils not yet mentioned, which some books suggest are emmenagogic and need care during pregnancy, although there is no research to support or reject these suggestions. See also Chapter 10.

Commiphora molmol (= *C. myrrha*) [MYRRH]: hormone-like.
Juniperus communis fruct. [JUNIPER BERRY]: diuretic.
Juniperus communis ram. [JUNIPER]: no known toxic component.
Levisticum officinale rad. [LOVAGE]: diuretic.
Chamomilla recutita flos [GERMAN CHAMOMILE]: hormone-like.
Melaleuca leucadendron fol. [CAJUPUT]: hormone-like.
Mentha × piperita fol. [PEPPERMINT]: hormone-like.
Ocimum basilicum fol. [BASIL].
Origanum majorana fol. [MARJORAM].
Rosa damascena, R. centifolia flos [ROSE OTTO]: hormone-like.
Rosmarinus officinalis ct. camphor [ROSEMARY].
Salvia sclarea [CLARY]: hormone-like.
Vetiveria zizanioides rad. [VETIVER].

4. TOXIC, NEUROTOXIC AND ABORTIVE OILS NOT USED IN AROMATHERAPY

This list comprises toxic, neurotoxic and abortive essential oils used by the medical profession in France. Whether or not they are known to aromatherapists, they are not normally used by them. The percentage figure given for toxic components is an average unless otherwise qualified. Common names are given where known.

Acorus calamus [CALAMUS]: phenolic ether 75%.
Agathosma betulina [BUCHU]: ketone 60%.
Artemisia absinthium [WORMWOOD]: ketone 35%. Also emmenagogic.
Artemisia afra: ketone 40%.
Artemisia annua: ketone 28%. Also hormone-like.
Artemisia arborescens: ketone 55%.
Artemisia herba alba: ketone 65%.
Artemisia pallens [DAVANA]: ketone 40%.
Artemisia vulgaris [MUGWORT]. Also emmenagogic.
Brassica nigra [MUSTARD]: allylisothiocyanate up to 99%.
Calamintha nepeta [WILD BASIL]: ketone 65%.
Calamintha sylvatica [CALAMINT]: ketone 65%.
Cedrus deodora [HIMALAYAN CEDARWOOD]: ketone 50%.
Chenopodium ambrosioides [WORMSEED]: oxide 60%.
Chrysanthemum balsamita: ketone 75%.
Cinnamomum camphora lig. [BROWN CAMPHOR, BLUE CAMPHOR]: safrole 60%.
Cochlearia armoracia [HORSERADISH]: allylisothiocyanate 90%.
Cupressus arizonica [BLUE CYPRESS]: ketones > 50%.
Curcuma longa [TURMERIC]: ketone 60%.
Foeniculum vulgare var. *amara* [BITTER FENNEL]: anethole 60%.
Geranium macrorrhizum [BULGARIAN GERANIUM]: ketone 50%.
Gaultheria procumbens [WINTERGREEN]: methyl salicylate 95%.
Illicium verum [STAR ANISE]: phenolic ether 80%—also hormone-like.

Juniperus oxycedrus [OIL OF CADE, JUNIPER TAR]. Almost always a wood distillate and not an essential oil.
Juniperus sabina [SAVIN]: podophyllotoxin content in the total extract.
Lantana camara [LANTANA]: ketone > 50%. Also emmenagogic.
Lavandula stoechas [SPANISH LAVENDER]: ketone 75%.
Mentha longifolia [MINT]: oxide 65%. Also hormone-like.
Myrica gale [BOG MYRTLE]: ketone > 50%.
Ocimum canum ct. camphor [DOG BASIL]: ketone 60%.
Ocotea pretiosa [BRAZILIAN SASSAFRAS]: phenolic ether 85%.
Petroselinum sativum fruct. [PARSLEY SEED]: phenol ether (apiole)
Peumus boldus (= *Boldea fragrans*) [BOLDO]: oxide 30%.
Ruta graveolens [RUE]: ketone 65%.
Santolina chamaecyparissus [LAVENDER COTTON, SANTOLINA]: ketone 35%.
Sassafras officinale [SASSAFRAS]: phenolic ether 85%.
Tanacetum vulgare [TANSY]: ketone 75%.
Thuja occidentalis [THUJA]: ketone 55%.

5. NEUROTOXIC AND/OR ABORTIVE OILS OCCASIONALLY USED IN AROMATHERAPY

The following list comprises essential oils that are known and used by aromatherapists and are potentially neurotoxic and/or abortive (if used beyond the accepted maximum dosage).

Achillea millefolium [MILFOIL, YARROW]: ketone content variable. (See also Appendix A.)
Anethum graveolens sem. [DILL]: ketone 50%.
Artemisia dracunculus [TARRAGON]: phenolic ether 65%. Held to be non-toxic by some.
Carum carvi [CARAWAY]: ketone 50%. Usually held to be non-toxic. Also diuretic.
Cedrus atlantica [ATLAS CEDARWOOD]: ketone 20%. Considered toxic in France.
Cinnamomum camphora lig. [CAMPHOR]: ketone and oxide 70%. Camphor from the wood is usually a triple-rectified oil and unsuitable for aromatherapy. The essential oil from the leaves contains mainly alcohols and has no known contraindications.
Eucalyptus dives, E. polybractea [BROAD-LEAVED PEPPERMINT]: ketone 45%.
Hyssopus officinalis [HYSSOP]: ketone 50%. Not to be used on epileptics. See Appendix A.
Mentha pulegium [PENNYROYAL]: ketone 80%. Also emmenagogic.
Mentha spicata [SPEARMINT]: ketone 60%.
Rosmarinus officinalis ct. verbenone [ROSEMARY]: ketone 30%.
Tagetes glandulifera [TAGETTE]: ketone 45%. Also phototoxic because of coumarin content; also emmenagogic.

6. POTENTIAL SKIN IRRITANT OILS

These phenolic or aldehydic essential oils generally have no special contraindications in pregnancy. The exceptions are *Cinnamomum cassia*, which contains *trans*-cinnamic aldehyde and *Cinnamomum verum* cort., which is also emmenagogic.

Cinnamomum cassia [CASSIA]: aldehyde 78–88%; phenol 5–6% typically. Very caustic on the skin.

Cinnamomum verum cort. [CINNAMON BARK]: aldehyde 40–76%. Neurotoxic.

Cinnamomum verum fol. [CINNAMON LEAF]: phenol 70–96%.

Cuminum cyminum fruct. [CUMIN]: aldehyde 20–50%.

Cymbopogon citratus fol. [LEMONGRASS]: aldehyde 60–86%.

Origanum heracleoticum fol. [OREGANO]: phenol 51–63%.

Origanum vulgare fol. [OREGANO]: phenol 22–83%.

Syzygium aromaticum caul. [CLOVE STEM]: aldehyde 90–95%.

Syzygium aromaticum flos [CLOVE BUD]: aldehyde 60–90%.

Syzygium aromaticum fol. [CLOVE LEAF]: aldehyde 82–88%.

Thymus serpyllum herb. [WILD OR CREEPING THYME]: phenol 20–30%.

Thymus vulgaris ct. phenol herb. [RED THYME]: phenol 50–60%.

7. PHOTOTOXIC OILS

Some essential oils may render the skin hypersensitive to ultraviolet rays, producing the protective tanning reaction. Photosensitizing essential oils may contain up to approximately 2% furanocoumarins, generally found in the expressed citrus oils.

Angelica archangelica fruct., rad. [ANGELICA ROOT, SEED].

Carum carvi fruct. [CARAWAY]: low level phototoxicity.

Cinnamomum cassia fol. [CASSIA]: low level phototoxicity.

Cinnamomum verum cort. [CINNAMON BARK]: low level phototoxicity.

Citrus aurantifolia per. [LIME].

Citrus aurantium var. *amara* per. [BITTER ORANGE].

Citrus bergamia per. [BERGAMOT].

Citrus limon per. [LEMON].

Cuminum cyminum fruct. [CUMIN].

Levisticum officinale fol. [LOVAGE].

Aloysia triphylla (= *Lippia citriodora*) [LEMON VERBENA]: low level phototoxicity.

Melissa officinalis fol. [MELISSA]: low level phototoxicity.

Ruta graveolens herb. [RUE]. See also Appendix B.4.

Zingiber officinale rhiz. [GINGER]: low level phototoxicity

Generally speaking the maximum concentration of essential oils in a carrier should not exceed 5% (equivalent to 10 drops of essential oils in 10 ml of carrier). Regarding phototoxicity and sensitization, even this quantity can be too much for a few oils, as the following information (extracted from the Code of Practice of IFRA) shows.

Angelica root oil [p]	0.8% max
Bergamot oil [p+s]	0.4% max
Cassia oil [s]	0.2% max
Cinnamon bark oil [s]	0.2% max
Costus root oil [s]	0.0% (i.e. do not use at all)
Cumin oil [p]	0.4% max
Fig leaf oil [p+s]	0.0% (i.e. do not use at all)
Lemon oil [p]	2.0% max
Lime oil [p]	0.7% max
Rue oil [p]	0.8% max
Savin oil	0.0% (i.e. do not use at all)
Verbena oil [p+s]	0.0% (i.e. do not use at all)

[p] = phototoxic, [s] = sensitizer. See also Appendix B.8.

8. CONTACT-SENSITIZING OILS

Sensitization is a type of allergic reaction which can occur when a substance comes into contact with the body. A few essential oils applied to the skin may cause sensitization, perhaps only after repeated application (the amount used is not significant). The skin reaction appears as redness, irritation and perhaps vesiculation.

Cananga odorata flos [YLANG YLANG].

Cinnamomum cassia fol. [CASSIA].

Cinnamomum verum cort. [CINNAMON BARK OIL].

Costus speciosus rad. [COSTUS ROOT].

Citrus bergamia per. [BERGAMOT].

Ficus carica fol. [FIG LEAF].

Inula helenium rhiz. [ELECAMPANE].

Aloysia triphylla (= *Lippia citriodora*) [VERBENA].

Pimpinella anisum fruct. [ANISEED].

Syzygium aromaticum caul. [CLOVE STEM].

Syzygium aromaticum flos [CLOVE BUD].

Cross-sensitization

With some essential oils an allergic reaction to one oil may lead to sensitivity to other material(s). Little is known of cross-sensitization reactions, but the risk is slight. Two examples are:

- benzoin resinoid cross colophony (a resin) cross *Mentha × piperita* cross Peru balsam (not distilled) cross turpentine (a rectified oil)
- *Laurus nobilis* ram. et fol. cross *Costus speciosus* rad. cross *Cinnamomum verum* cort.

Some individuals show patch test reactions to *Achillea millefolium* [YARROW] and cross-sensitivity between this oil and other Asteraceae has been demonstrated (Duke 1985).

9. GENERAL PROPERTIES OF ESSENTIAL OILS

The following tables show general properties attributed to essential oils and to essential waters respectively. (Refer to relevant chapters in the text and to Appendix A for details.)

Table B1   General properties of essential oils

Scientific name	[Common name]	Analgesic, antineuralgic	Antibacterial	Antidiabetic	Antiepileptic	Antifungal	Antihistaminic, antiallergic	Antiinfectious	Antiinflammatory	Antiirritant	Antimigraine	Antioxidant	Antiparasitic, larvicidal	Antiseptic	Antispasmodic	Antisudorific	Antitussive	Antiviral	Cardiotonic	Carminative	Cholagogic, Choleretic	Cicatrizant, vulnerary	Circulatory stimulant	Decongestant	Detoxicant, depurative	Digestive, stomachic, eupeptic	Diuretic	Emmenagogic	Expectorant	Febrifuge, antipyretic	Hepatic	Hormone-like	Hypertensor	Hypotensor	Immunostimulant	Insecticidal, parasiticidal	Insect repellent	Lactogenic	Lipolytic	Litholytic	Mental stimulant	Mucolytic, anticatarrhal	Neurotonic, antidepressive, euphoric	Ophthalmic	Phlebotonic	Photosensitizer, phototoxic	Psychoactive	Radioprotective	Reproductive stimulant	Respiratory tonic	Rubefacient	Scalp tonic	Sedative, calming, anxiolytic	Styptic, haemostatic, astringent	Sudorific	Tonic (general), energizing	Uterotonic	Vasodilator	Vermifuge, anthelmintic
Achillea millefolium	[YARROW]	×							×					×							×	×		×		×	×	×	×	×				×						×		×																	
Aniba rosaeodora (fol.)	[ROSEWOOD]		×			×		×	×					×	×			×				×																																×		×			
Boswellia carteri (dist.)	[FRANKINCENSE]	×						×	×			×		×	×							×							×						×								×													×			
Cananga odorata (flos)	[YLANG YLANG]			×									×	×	×				×																														×			×	×						
Carum carvi (fruct.)	[CARAWAY]	×		×			×						×	×	×					×						×	×	×										×				×																
Cedrus atlantica (lig.)	[ATLAS CEDARWOOD]		×						×					×								×					×												×													×						
Chamaemelum nobile (flos)	[ROMAN CHAMOMILE]						×		×		×		×		×					×		×				×	×	×														×										×						
Chamomilla recutita (flos)	[GERMAN CHAMOMILE]					×			×						×							×				×	×	×														×		×														
Citrus aurantium var. *amara* (flos)	[NEROLI BIGARADE]						×		×				×	×	×				×							×																	×									×						
Citrus aurantium var. *amara* (fol.)	[PETITGRAIN BIGARADE]		×					×	×					×	×				×							×																	×									×						
Citrus aurantium var. *amara* (per.)	[ORANGE BIGARADE]							×	×					×	×											×						×														×							×						
Citrus bergamia (per.)	[BERGAMOT]	×	×			×		×	×				×	×	×			×			×	×				×	×	×															×			×						×						
Citrus limon (per.)	[LEMON]	×	×		×									×	×				×		×	×		×		×	×							×				×	×	×					×	×						×	×					
Citrus reticulata (per.)	[MANDARIN]		×		×										×				×							×	×									×			×													×			×			
Commiphora myrrha var. *molmol* (res. dist.)	[MYRRH]							×	×				×	×	×				×			×						?	×		×																				×							
Coriandrum sativum (fruct.)	[CORIANDER]	×	×					×	×				×	×	×				×				×	×		×													×			×	×									×		×			
Cupressus sempervirens (fol.)	[CYPRESS]	×	×					×	×					×	×	×					×		×			×			×			×										×	×		×		×			×			×			×			
Eucalyptus citriodora (fol.)	[LEMON SCENTED GUM]	×	×				×	×	×	×					×							×					×									×	×	×		×												×	×	×				×
Eucalyptus dives (fol.)	[BROAD-LEAVED PEPPERMINT]	×						×	×					×	×		×									×												×				×	×		×							×	×					
Eucalyptus globulus (fol.)	[TASMANIAN BLUE GUM]	×	×				×	×	×					×	×		×	×						×		×			×													×	×							×	×		×					

Table B1 General properties of essential oils (contd)

Species key (columns):
1 = *Eucalyptus radiata* (fol.) [NARROW-LEAVED PEPPERMINT];
2 = *Eucalyptus smithii* (fol.) [GULLY GUM, WHITE IRON BARK];
3 = *Foeniculum vulgare* var. *dulce* (fruct.) [SWEET FENNEL];
4 = *Helichrysum angustifolium* (flos.) [EVERLASTING];
5 = *Hyssopus officinalis* (flos, fol.) [HYSSOP];
6 = *Juniperus communis* (fruct.) [JUNIPER BERRY];
7 = *Juniperus communis* (ram.) [JUNIPER TWIG];
8 = *Lavandula angustifolia* (flo.) [LAVENDER];
9 = *Lavandula × intermedia* 'Super' (flos) [LAVANDIN];
10 = *Melaleuca alternifolia* (fol.) [TEA TREE];
11 = *Melaleuca leucadendron* (fol.) [CAJUPUT];
12 = *Melaleuca viridiflora* (fol.) [NIAOULI];
13 = *Melissa officinalis* (fol.) [MELISSA];
14 = *Mentha × piperita* (fol.) [PEPPERMINT];
15 = *Myristica fragrans* (sem.) [NUTMEG];
16 = *Nardostachys jatamansi* (rad.) [SPIKENARD];
17 = *Nepeta cataria* var. *citriodora* (flos, fol.) [CATNEP];
18 = *Ocimum basilicum* (fol.) [BASIL];
19 = *Origanum heracleoticum* (herb.) [GREEN ORIGANUM];
20 = *Origanum majorana* (fol.) [SWEET MARJORAM];
21 = *Ormenis mixta* (flos) [MOROCCAN CHAMOMILE];
22 = *Pelargonium graveolens* (fol.) [GERANIUM];
23 = *Pimpinella anisum* (fruct.) [ANISEED]

Property	1	2	3	4	5	6	7	8	9	10	11	12	13	14	15	16	17	18	19	20	21	22	23
Analgesic, antineuralgic	×		×		×		×	×		×	×	×		×	×			×		×		×	×
Antibacterial	×	×			×									×	×			×	×	×	×	×	
Antidiabetic				×		×																	
Antiepileptic																×		×		×			
Antifungal			×					×	×	×				×		×		×		×		×	
Antihistaminic, antiallergic				×	×		×														×		
Antiinfectious	×	×			×	×				×	×	×		×				×	×	×			
Antiinflammatory	×		×	×	×			×	×				×	×	×					×	×	×	
Antiirritant														×							×		
Antimigraine								×	×					×				×		×		×	
Antioxidant																							
Antiparasitic, larvicidal													×	×			×						
Antiseptic	×		×							×	×	×		×	×					×			×
Antispasmodic			×	×				×					×	×	×					×		×	×
Antisudorific																							
Antitussive					×																		
Antiviral	×	×			×					×	×			×			×	×					
Cardiotonic			×					×								×		×					×
Carminative			×					×						×				×		×			×
Cholagogic, choleretic			×										×										
Cicatrizant, vulnerary				×	×			×														×	
Circulatory stimulant			×													×							
Decongestant		×	×		×							×		×									×
Detoxicant, depurative						×	×																
Digestive, stomachic, eupeptic			×	×	×	×								×	×			×		×		×	×
Diuretic			×			×	×	×															
Emmenagogic			×		×											×							×
Expectorant	×	×			×	×		×			×			×						×			×
Febrifuge, antipyretic												×		×									
Hepatic					×							×		×							×	×	
Hormone-like					×						×	×		×								×	×
Hypertensor					×									×									
Hypotensor								×						×	×							×	
Immunostimulant											×	×							×				
Insecticidal, parasiticidal																	×						
Insect repellent											×			×								×	
Lactogenic			×																				×
Lipolytic			×			×		×															
Litholytic			×			×	×							×		×							
Mental stimulant																							
Mucolytic, anticatarrhal	×	×			×	×		×			×			×				×					
Neurotonic, antidepressive, euphoric					×	×		×						×			×	×		×		×	×
Ophthalmic																							
Phlebotonic				×							×	×	×				×					×	
Photosensitizer, phototoxic																							
Psychoactive															×								×
Radioprotective											×	×	×										
Reproductive stimulant																			×	×		×	×
Respiratory tonic				×																		×	×
Rubefacient																							
Scalp tonic																							
Sedative, calming, anxiolytic		×						×								×				×	×	×	×
Styptic, haemostatic, astringent					×																	×	
Sudorific					×							×											
Tonic (general), energizing	×				×					×	×			×					×		×	×	
Uterotonic															×	×							×
Vasodilator														×								×	
Vermifuge, anthelmintic					×													×					

Table B1 General properties of essential oils (contd)

Botanical name (part) [common name]	Analgesic, antineuralgic	Antibacterial	Antidiabetic	Antiepileptic	Antifungal	Antihistaminic, antiallergic	Antiinfectious	Antiinflammatory	Antiirritant	Antimigraine	Antioxidant	Antiparasitic, larvicidal	Antiseptic	Antispasmodic	Antisudorific	Antitussive	Antiviral	Cardiotonic	Carminative	Cholagogic, Choleretic	Cicatrizant, vulnerary	Circulatory stimulant	Decongestant	Detoxicant, depurative	Digestive, stomachic, eupeptic	Diuretic	Emmenagogic	Expectorant	Febrifuge, antipyretic	Hepatic	Hormone-like	Hypertensor	Hypotensor	Immunostimulant	Insecticidal, parasiticidal	Insect repellent	Lactogenic	Lipolytic	Litholytic	Mental stimulant	Mucolytic, anticatarrhal	Neurotonic, antidepressive, euphoric	Ophthalmic	Phlebotonic	Photosensitizer, phototoxic	Psychoactive	Radioprotective	Reproductive stimulant	Respiratory tonic	Rubefacient	Scalp tonic	Sedative, calming, anxiolytic	Styptic, haemostatic, astringent	Sudorific	Tonic (general), energizing	Uterotonic	Vasodilator	Vermifuge, anthelmintic
Pinus sylvestris (fol.) [SCOTS PINE]	x	x	x		x		x	x							x								x					x	x		x	x							x			x						x		x					x			
Piper nigrum (fruct.) [BLACK PEPPER]	x	x																							x			x	x																													
Pogostemon patchouli (fol.) [PATCHOULI]					x		x						x								x		x	x										x	x	x								x				x					x				
Ravensara aromatica (fol.) [RAVENSARA]	x				x		x	x									x							x				x													x	x																
Rosa centifolia R. damascena (flos) [ROSE OTTO]		x			x		x	x									x	x			x			x																		x						x					x		x			
Rosmarinus officinalis ct cineole, ct camphor [ROSEMARY]	x	x			x		x	x						x				x	x	x	x	x			x	x	x	x	x			x								x	x	x						x							x	x		
Rosmarinus officinalis ct verbenone [ROSEMARY]		x					x	x						x					x	x	x			x	x	x	x			x	x							x			x	x		x				x					x				
Salvia officinalis (fol.) [SAGE, DALMATIAN SAGE]	x				x		x	x					x	x	x						x		x				x		x		x							x			x	x						x				x	x	x	x	x		
Salvia sclarea (flos, fol.) [CLARY]														x	x			x					x	x					x		x							x				x						x				x			x			
Santalum album (lig.) [SANDALWOOD]							x	x					x				x			x	x	x	x	x	x	x												x						x									x					
Satureia hortensis (fol.) [SUMMER OR GARDEN SAVORY]	x				x		x	x			x		x					x							x			x						x	x	x																			x			
Satureia montana (fol.) [WINTER OR MOUNTAIN SAVORY]	x				x		x	x			x	x	x	x			x	x			x				x	x		x						x	x					x	x	x						x							x			
Syzygium aromaticum (flos) [CLOVE BUD]	x				x		x	x			x	x	x	x			x	x		x	x						x	x			x				x					x								x							x	x		
Tagetes glandulifera, T. minuta (flos) [TAGET, FRENCH MARIGOLD]					x		x										x				x				x	x	x														x				x			x							x	x	x	
Thymus mastichina (herb.) [SPANISH MARJORAM]					x		x						x								x				x	x		x													x																	
Thymus satureioides [MOROCCAN THYME]	x	x			x		x	x					x								x				x	x					x			x							x	x						x							x	x		
Thymus vulgaris "Population" [THYME]	x	x			x		x	x			x		x	x			x	x			x				x	x		x		x				x						x	x	x						x		x	x	x			x			
Thymus vulgaris ct linalool, ct geraniol (herb.) [SWEET THYME]	x	x			x		x	x			x	x	x	x			x			x	x				x	x								x						x	x	x										x			x			
Thymus vulgaris ct thujanol-4 (herb.) [SWEET THYME]	x				x		x	x					x	x			x	x			x	x			x					x				x							x	x						x						x				
Thymus vulgaris ct thymol, ct. carvacrol (herb.) [THYME]	x	x			x	x	x					x	x						x		x			x	x	x	x	x		x				x						x	x	x											x	x		x	
Vetiveria zizanioides (rad.) [VETIVER]	x				x	x								x								x					x			x				x							x	x		x		?		x						x				
Zingiber officinale (rhiz.) [GINGER]														x					x						x	x	x	x						x							x							?						x	x			x

Table B2 General properties and indications of essential waters

	Aerophagy	Anticancer	Antidiabetic	Antiepileptic	Antiseptic	Antispasmodic	Anxiolytic	Arthritis	Bactericidal	Blepharitis	Calming	Cardiac	Carminative	Circulation	Circulatory	Conjunctivitis	Cystitis	Dermatitis	Digestive	Diuretic	Eczema	Emmenagogue	Energizing	Euphoric	Eye problems	Gall bladder	Galactogen	Haemorrhoids	Hepatic	Hypotensor	Pancreatic	Period problems	Renal	Respiratory problems	Rheumatism	Rheumatoid arthritis	Soothing
Achillea millefolium [YARROW]														x																							
Aloysia triphylla [LEMON VERBENA]							x												x				x														
Artemisia dracunculus [TARRAGON]	x	x																																			
Calendula officinalis [MARIGOLD]					x													x			x	x				x				x							
Chamaemelum nobile [CHAMOMILE ROMAN]											x	x																									
Citrus aurantium (flos) [ORANGE FLOWER]					x						x	x						x						x													
Cupressus sempervirens [CYPRESS]																		x										x									
Eucalyptus globulus [TASMANIAN BLUE GUM]																																		x			
Foeniculum vulgare var. dulce [FENNEL]			x		x												x										x				x		x	x			
Helichrysum angustifolium [EVERLASTING]	x	x																					x	x										x			
Hypericum perforatum [ST JOHN'S WORT]	x			x																																	
Hyssopus officinalis [HYSSOP]				x																																	
Juniperus communis [JUNIPER]			x					x												x													x	x			
Lavandula angustifolia [LAVENDER]					x						x				x																						
Melissa officinalis [LEMON BALM]										x						x																					
Mentha × piperita [PEPPERMINT]					x									x			x		x																		
Myrtus communis [MYRTLE]					x																																
Ocimum basilicum [BASIL]													x						x	x																	
Origanum majorana [MARJORAM]											x			x									x?			x			x								
Origanum onites [KEKIK]												x		x																							
Pinus sylvestris [SCOTS PINE]																	x			x						x						x				x	
Rosmarinus officinalis [ROSEMARY]																						x	x			x									x	x	x
Salvia officinalis [SAGE]																						x										x					
Salvia sclarea [CLARY]															x								x														
Satureia montana [SAVORY]											x												x														
Thymus serpyllum [WILD THYME]		x			x																														x		x
Thymus vulgaris (pop.) [THYME]					x																													x	x		
Thymus vulgaris ct. alcohol [SWEET THYME]					x																				x									x			

Appendix C

ORGANIZATIONS RELEVANT TO THE PRACTICE OF AROMATHERAPY

UK COMPLEMENTARY MEDICINE ORGANIZATIONS

There are several associations representing complementary and alternative therapies as a whole—the British Complementary Medicine Association (BCMA) and the Institute of Complementary Medicine (ICM) being the largest which include aromatherapy.

BCMA

This was formed in 1990 as the National Consultative Council for Alternative and Complementary Medicine to promote complementary medicine at all levels; the name was changed to the British Complementary Medicine Association in 1992. This is a consultative body for all complementary medicine, representing around 30 therapies (26 000 practitioners in 50 organizations).

The BCMA aims to:

- encourage the diverse organizations of individual therapies to form their own umbrella group for collective action
- integrate complementary medicine into the structure of the nation's healthcare system
- act as a source of information on complementary matters
- establish a register of individual therapies and how they are practised
- consult and cooperate with other bodies in the field
- liaise with government and the EC.

ICM

The Institute of Complementary Medicine was founded in 1982 to encourage education, research and public information on complementary medicine. A major research project has been to devise a single structure, The British Register of Complementary Practitioners (BRCP), for national registration. The BRCP is working in tandem with professional registers and schools to ensure that National Occupational Standards (NOS) are established for all disciplines. The ICM is concerned to ensure that healthcare products and essential oils continue to be available at the required levels of purity to ensure that the public has access to treatments. About 20 000 enquiries are answered each year.

BCCM

The British Council of Complementary Medicine (BCCM), initiated by the ICM above, was formed to develop the standards of complementary medicine being offered through universities, colleges and individual trainers.

AROMATHERAPY ORGANIZATIONS

The associations of which therapists may become members, after qualifying to the minimum standards of the umbrella body (AOC below), are detailed in Chapter 16.

AOC

The Aromatherapy Organisations Council (AOC) was formed in 1991 as an umbrella body for aromatherapy associations, and training establishments are required to accredit their courses through one of the member professional associations. The aims of the AOC are to:

- establish common standards of training
- ensure that the associations provide appropriate standards of professional practice and conduct for their members
- initiate, support or sponsor research
- provide a collective voice through which to initiate and sustain political dialogue with government, civil and medical bodies, in order to enhance the best interests of professional aromatherapy
- to set a minimum standard for aromatherapy training.

Although most of the aromatherapy associations belong to the AOC, standards of training still vary considerably, some being higher than the AOC minimum.

OSCHSC

Responsibility for setting National Occupational Standards (NOS) (see Ch. 16) in occupational areas rests with bodies formally approved by Government called 'Occupational Standards Councils', whose role it is to promote, coordinate and evaluate the development of standards within their own sector.

The Occupational Standards Council for Health and Social Care (OSCHSC) (previously known as the Care Sector Consortium and having changed its name in June 1993) is responsible for all the health and social care in the UK, representing professional bodies, employers, trade unions, local government and criminal justice services throughout the public, private and voluntary sectors. However, development of the NOS has been delegated to member organizations through two separate committees—the Health Care Forum and the Social Care Forum.

Complementary therapists are considered to be a part of the private sector within the Health Care Forum, along with workers in nursing and residential homes, and private hospitals. The member organization representing all these interests is the Independent Care Organisations (ICO).

In 1995 the Department for Education and Employment provided funds (through the OSCHSC) to pay for consultants to oversee the establishment of NOS in four areas of complementary medicine—aromatherapy, homoeopathy, acupuncture and reflexology, along with standards for health promotion and coordination, and standards in common for professions allied to medicine. The complementary medicine project has been coordinated by the ICO.

TRADE ASSOCIATIONS

ATC

The Aromatherapy Trade Council (ATC) began in 1992 and is a self-regulating body for the aromatherapy industry, its prime concern being consumer safety. Its aims and objectives are:

- to establish guidelines for safety, labelling and packaging for the aromatherapy trade
- to promote responsible use of aromatherapy products
- to sponsor research into all aspects of essential oils and aromatherapy products
- to publish a register of current members.

EOTA

The Essential Oil Trade Association (EOTA) was established in 1987 to:

- monitor essential oil quality
- collect available research data on essential oils
- organize conferences.

The first aromatherapy conferences to be held, Aroma '88 and Aroma '90, were organized by EOTA. After a year or two of non-activity, EOTA, under the new name EOTA 95, now concentrates its efforts into oil quality, to counter the rampant spread of adulterated and false essential oils.

NORA

The Natural Oils Research Association (NORA) was formed in June 1990; it draws its membership from many different fields, including the fragrance industry, essential oil companies, universities, aromatherapy companies and individuals.

The aims of the association are:

- research
- education
- analysis: members may have oils tested and where authenticated they are given the AROMARK quality mark.
- industry–university links
- publishing.

GOVERNMENTAL BODIES

MCA

The Medicines Control Agency (MCA) is the section of the Department of Health which deals with the licensing and labelling of medicinal products. In 1995, in anticipation of a single European market in pharmaceuticals, the MCA had prepared a consultative document with a view to reconciling the UK Medicines Act 1968 with the relevant EU directives. If the document had gone ahead, under EU law all herbal medicines manufactured and sold in the UK would have to be licensed. Under the Medicines for Human Use Regulation 1994 and Medicines Act 1968 no medicinal product, unless exempt, can be placed on the market unless a marketing authorization has been granted by the licensing authority (MCA) or the EU; it is therefore an offence to sell or supply, or to advertise, a medicinal product (i.e. having a preventive or therapeutic effect) without a licence.

Although essential oils are not classified as medicines (they come under cosmetics and food), this is a grey area and therefore aromatherapists supported herbalists in their campaign to prevent sections 12 and 56 of the Act being deleted, which would have emptied the shelves of healthfood stores of all herbal products not possessing a product licence. (Section 12 (1) of the Medicines Act 1968 allows therapists in a face-to-face situation, to make, sell and supply any remedy in the course of their business. Section 56 grants exemption to herbalists from the general prohibition on sales of products other than those on the general sale list from premises other than registered pharmacies.) 'Among useful herbal medicines that would disappear would be feverfew for migraines, ginger capsules for travel sickness … and tincture of propolis for sore throats: homoeopathic mother-tinctures and essential oils of the increasingly popular aromatherapy seemed likely to go too' (Griggs 1997 p. 309).

After a national campaign The Parliamentary Secretary for Health announced in November 1994 that the position of herbal medicines had been safeguarded and was exempted from the new legislation. This 'scare' brought to the fore existing regulations regarding labelling, which before this time had not been widely known or respected by people producing therapeutic products for the aromatherapy market.

Appendix D

ESSENTIAL OIL: DEFINITION FOR AROMATHERAPEUTIC PURPOSES

Essential oils

There are only two plant extracts which should be given this name for aromatherapy purposes.

1. Essential oils: these are plant extracts which have been achieved by steam distillation of plant material from a single botanical source; nothing is involved in this process save water, heat and the plant material. The essential oil is separated from the condensed steam and nothing is added and nothing is taken away

2. Expressed oils: these are the product of citrus fruits, and they are achieved by simple pressing (expression) of the citrus peel, without heat or aid of solvents. Nothing is added and nothing is taken away.

Care is needed in the way essential oils are sold to protect both the lay public and aromatherapists. The oils for therapeutic use must be whole and unadulterated, accurately identified and labelled, and must have been correctly stored.

NB. Not all plants yield an essential oil and some yield so little that the oil would be too expensive; oils such as hyacinth, lilac, honeysuckle and jasmine do not exist in a distilled form; their fragrance is extracted by other means and it is incorrect for anyone to name extracts from these plants as essential oils in the context of aromatherapeutic use.

Aromatherapy oils

This term is widely used in the marketplace, but is a vague, almost meaningless term, which does not adequately describe the product. Products labelled thus usually consist of a 2% maximum dilution of essential oil(s) in a fixed oil. Often these inexpensive products are sold in small bottles having an integral dropper, which is misleading as droppers are not necessary for diluted oils and their presence can give the impression (sometimes intentional) that they are essential oils—they are often sold at the pure essential oil price, thus yielding an excessive profit. Oils sold under this heading usually contain standardized oils of low quality, more suited to industries other than complementary medicine.

Other ways of extracting plant components follow; none should be classed as essential oils for aromatherapy purposes.

Absolutes (not classed as essential oils)

These are aromatic liquids extracted from the plant material using solvents such as hexane, butane, etc., which is then followed by alcohol extraction; it is a complex process, yielding a liquid substance called an absolute, which is totally soluble in alcohol and important in the perfume industry.

Macerated oils

Macerated oils are made by putting plant material into a fixed vegetable oil, when those plant molecules soluble in the oil are taken up by the vegetable oil used. Examples are calendula and hypericum (St John's wort). These should not be sold in small bottles as essential oils.

Ignorance is bliss?

Much of the misnaming of oils for aromatherapy comes through ignorance on the part of the suppliers. Occasionally a supplier sells an expensive fixed oil, such as evening primrose, as an essential oil, putting it into a small bottle with an integral dropper and within an essential oil price range. Unfortunately, aromatherapy is a popular bandwagon to jump on, and the very word aromatherapy has selling power, which is used by the unscrupulous, sometimes at the expense of the unwary honest dealer. Standardized oils are cheap and easy to obtain, unlike the genuine essential oils necessary for aromatherapy.

References to Appendices and Sources

REFERENCES TO APPENDICES

Abdullin K K 1962 Uch. Zap. Kazansk. Vet. Inst. 84: 75 In: Chemical Abstracts 1964 60: 11843b

Abraham M et al 1979 Inhibiting effects of jasmine flowers on lactation. Indian Journal of Medicine Research 69: 88–92

Achterrath-Tuckerman U, Kunde R, Flaskamp O, Theimer I, Theimer K 1980 Pharmacological investigations with compounds of chamomile. V. Investigations on the spasmolytic effect of compounds of chamomile. Planta Medica, Stuttgart 39: 38–50

Åkesson H O, Wälinder J 1965 Nutmeg intoxication. Lancet i: 1271

Albert-Puleo M 1980 Fennel and anise as estrogenic agents. Journal of Ethnopharmacology 2: 337–344

Al-Hader A A, Hasan Z A, Aqel M B 1994 Hyperglycemic and insulin release inhibitory effects of *Rosmarinus officinalis*. Journal of Ethnopharmacology 43: 217–221

Alimkhodzhaeva N Z, Khazanovich R L 1972 Mater. Yubileinoi Resp. Nauchn. Konf. Farm., Posvyashch 50-Letiyu Obraz. SSSR. 37. In Chemical Abstracts 1975 82: 167491r

Anon 1977 Federal Register 42 (146): 38613

Anon 1994a Journal of Family Practice June 3: 6

Anon 1994b Herbal licensing post. Pharmaceutical Journal 253: 746

Anthony A et al 1987 Metabolism of estragole in rat and mouse and influence of dose size on excretion of the proximate carcinogen 1-hydroxyestragole. Food and Chemical Toxicology 25: 799–806

Arctander S 1960 Perfume and flavor materials of natural origin. Published by the author, Elizabeth NJ

Asre S 1994 Chemical composition and antimicrobial activity of some essential oils. MSc Thesis, Macquarie University, Sydney

Atanasova-Shopova S, Rusinov K S 1970 Izv. Acad. Nauk. Inst. Fiziol., Bulg. 13: 89 In: Chemical Abstracts 1971 74: 123533m

Aureli P, Constantini A, Zolea S 1992 Journal of Food Protection. 55(5): 344–348

Averbeck D, Averbeck S, Dubertret L, Young A R, Morliere P 1990 Gentoxicity of bergapten and bergamot oil in *Saccharomyces cervisiae*. Journal of Photochemistry and Photobiology B 7: 209–229

Bartram T 1995 Encyclopedia of herbal medicine. Grace, Christchurch

Bassett I B, Pannowitz D L, Barnetson R St C 1990 A comparative study of tea tree oil versus benzoyl peroxide in the treatment of acne. Medical Journal of Australia 153: 455–458

Beckstrom-Sternberg S M, Duke J A 1996 CRC Handbook of medicinal mints. CRC Press, Boca Raton

Belaiche P 1979 Traité de phytothérapie et d'aromathérapie. Maloine, Paris

Bennett A, Stamford I F, Tavares I A, Jacobs S, Capasso F, Mascolo N, Antore G, Romano V, Di Carlo G 1988 Phytotherapy Research 2: 124–130

Benouda A, Hasser M, Benjilali B 1988 The antiseptic properties of essential oils **in vitro** tested against pathogenic germs found in hospitals. Fitoterapia 59(27): 115–119

Betts T 1994 Sniffing the breeze. Aromatherapy Quarterly 40: 19–22

Bisset N G (ed) 1994 Herbal drugs and phytopharmaceuticals. Medpharm, Stuttgart

Boland D J, Brophy J J, House A P N 1991 Eucalyptus leaf oils. Inkata, Melbourne

Boyd E M, Pearson G L 1946 On the expectorant action of volatile oils. American Journal of Medical Science 211: 602–610

Buchanan R L 1978 Toxicity of spices containing methylenedioxybenzene derivatives: a review. Journal of Food Safety 1: 275

Buchbauer G, Jirovetz L, Jager W, Dietrich H, Plank C, Karamat E 1991 Zeitschrift Naturforschaft 46: 1067–1072

Buchbauer G, Jager W, Jirovetz L, Ilmeberger J, Dietrich H 1993 In: Teranishi et al (eds) Bioactive volatile compounds from plants. ACS Symposium Series 525

Buckle J 1993 Does it matter which lavender essential oil is used? Nursing Times 89(20): 32–35

Bunny S (ed) 1984 Illustrated book of herbs. Octopus, London

Burkhill J H 1966 A dictionary of the economic products of the Malay Peninsula. Art Printing Works, Kuala Lumpur

Bye R A 1986 Economic Botany 40(1): 103

Caldwell J 1991 Basil and methyl chavicol—statement on new data. International Journal of Aromatherapy 3(1): 6

Carson C F, Cookson B D, Farrelly H D, Riley T V 1995 Susceptibility of methicillin-resistant *Staphylococcus aureus* to the essential oil of *Melaleuca alternifolia*. Journal of Antimicrobial Chemotherapy 35: 421–424

Carson C F, Hammer K A, Riley T V 1995 Broth microdilution method for determining the susceptibility of *Escherichia coli* and *Staphylococcus aureus* to the essential oil of *Melaleuca alternifolia* (tea tree oil). Microbios 82(332): 181–185

Carter G T 1976 Dissertation Abstracts International B37: 766

Chandhoke N, Ghatak B 1969 Studies on *Tagetes minuta*: some pharmacological actions of the essential oil. Indian Journal of Medical Research 57: 864–876

Chandler R F, Hawkes D 1984 Aniseed—a spice, a flavour, a drug. Canadian Pharmaceutical Journal 117: 28–29

Chandler R F, Hooper S N, Harvey M J 1982 Ethnobotany and phytochemistry of yarrow, *Achillea millefolium*, Compositae. Economic Botany 36: 203–223

Claus E P 1961 Pharmacognosy, 4th edn. Lea & Febiger, Philadelphia

Corbier B, Teisseire P 1974 Contribution to the knowledge of neroli oil from Grasse. Recherches 19: 289–290

Craig J O 1953 Poisoning by the volatile oils in childhood. Archives of Disease in Childhood 28: 475–483

Dale H H 1909 Nutmeg. Society of Experimental Biology, New York 23: 69

Deans S G, Ritchie G 1987 International Journal of Food Microbiology 5: 165–180

Debelmas A M, Rochat J 1967 Etude pharmacologique des huiles essentielles. Activité antispasmodique étudiée sur une cinquantaine d'échantillons différents. Plantes Médicinales et Phytotherapie 1: 23–27

Deshpande R S, Ripnis H P 1977 Insecticidal activity of *Ocimum basilicum* Linn. Pesticides. 11(15): 11

De Vincenzi M, Dessi M R 1991 Botanical flavouring substances used in foods: proposal of classification. Fitoterapia 62(1): 39–63

Dew M J, Evans B K, Rhodes J 1984 Peppermint oil for the irritable bowel syndrome: a multicentre trial. British Journal of Clinical Practice 38(11–12): 394–398

Dikshit A, Husain A 1984 Fitoterapia 55: 171

Dobrynin V N et al 1976 Khimiia Prirodnykh Soedinenii 5: 686 In: Chemical Abstracts 1977 86: 117603r

Draize J H 1959 Dermal toxicity. In: Appraisal of the safety of chemicals in foods, drugs and cosmetics. Association of Food and Drug Officials of the United States, Austin, p 52

Drinkwater N R et al 1976 Hepatocarcinogenicity of estragole (1-allyl-4-methoxybenzene) and 1-hydroxyestragole in the mouse and mutagenicity of 1-acetoxyestragole in bacteria. Journal of the National Cancer Institute 57: 1323–1331

Dube S, Upadhyay D, Tripathi S C 1988 Antifungal, physicochemical and insect repelling activity of the essential oil of *Ocimum basilicum*. Canadian Journal of Botany 67: 2085–2087

Duke J A 1985 Handbook of medicinal herbs. CRC Press, Boca Raton

Duke J A, Ayensu E S 1985 Medicinal plants of China. Reference Publications, Algonac, Michigan

Duke J A, Wain K K 1981 Medicinal plants of the world. Computer Index, 3 vols, p 1654

Duraffourd P 1982 En forme tous les jours. La Vie Claire, Périgny

Duthie H L 1981 The effect of peppermint oil on colonic motility in man. British Journal of Surgery 68: 820

Emboden W A Jr 1972 Narcotic plants. Macmillan, New York

Epstein W L 1973 Report to RIFM. 30 October

Farnsworth N R 1975 Potential value of plants as sources of new antifertility agents I. Journal of Pharmaceutical Sciences 64: 535–598

Foggie W E 1911 Eucalyptus oil poisoning. British Medical Journal 1: 359–360

Food and Drug Administration 1978 Health foods business, June

Forbes P D, Urbach F, Davies R E 1977 Photo toxicity testing of fragrance raw materials. Food and Cosmetics Toxicology 15: 55–60

Ford R A, Letizia C S, Api A M 1988 Tea tree oil. Food and Chemical Toxicology 26(4): 407

Ford R A, Api A M, Letizia C S 1992a Petitgrain bigarade oil. Food and Chemical Toxicology 30 (suppl): 101S

Ford R A, Api A M, Letizia C S 1992b Mandarin oil. Food and Chemical Toxicology 30 (suppl): 69S

Foster S 1991 Chamomile, *Matricaria recutita* and *Chamaemelum nobile*. Botanical Series no 307, American Botanical Council, Austin

Foster S 1993a Chamomile. The Herb Companion December/January: 64–68

Foster S 1993b Herbal renaissance. Gibbs Smith, Layton

Franchomme P, Pénoël D 1990 L'aromathérapie exactement. Jollois, Limoges

Fujii T, Furukawa S, Suzuki S 1972 Studies on compounded perfumes for toilet goods: on the non-irritative compounded perfumes for soaps. Yukugaku 21(12): 904–908

Garg S C 1974 Antifungal effects of *Boswellia serrata* leaf oil. Indian Journal of Pharmacy 36: 46

Gattefossé R-M 1937 Aromathérapie. Girardot, Paris. (English transl 1993 Daniel, Saffron Walden)

Goodman L, Golman A 1942 The pharmacological basis of therapeutics. Macmillan, New York

Griggs B 1997 New green pharmacy. Vermilion, London

Grochulski V A, Borkowski B 1972 Influence of chamomile oil on experimental glomerulonephritis in rabbits. Planta Medica 21: 289–292

Guenther E 1949 The essential oils, 6 vols. Van Nostrand, New York

Habersang S, Leuschner O, Theimer I, Theimer K 1979 Pharmacological studies of chamomile constituents. IV. Studies on the toxicity of (–)-α-bisabolol. Planta Medica 35: 118–124

Hammer K A, Carson C F, Riley T V 1996 Susceptibility of transient and commensal skin flora to the essential oil of *Melaleuca alternifolia* (tea tree oil). Australian Journal of Infection Control 24(3): 186–189

Harry R G 1948 Cosmetic materials, vol 2. Hill, London

Hartwell J L 1967–1971 Plants used against cancer: a survey. Lloydia 30

Hausen B M, Busker E, Carle R 1984 The sensitizing capacity of Compositae plants. VII. Experimental investigations with extracts and compounds of *Chamomilla recutita* (L.) Rauschert and *Anthemis cotula* (L.). Planta Medica 229–234

Herrmann E C, Kucera L S 1967 Proceedings of the Society of Experimental Biology and Medicine 124: 865

Hitokoto H et al 1980 Applied and Environmental Microbiology 39: 818

Holmes E M 1916 Perfume Record 8: 78

Homburger F, Boger E 1968 Cancer Research 28: 2372

Huang T C, Liu P K, Chang C F, Chou C, Tseng H L 1981 Study of antiasthmatic constituents in *Ocimum basilicum* Benth. Yao Hsueh T'ung Pao 16(4): 56

IFRA 1992 Code of practice. International Fragrance Association, Geneva

Isaac O 1979 Pharmakologische Untersuchungen von Kamillen-Inhaltsstoffen I. Zur Pharmakologie des (–)-α–bisabolol und der Bisabololoxide (Übersicht). Planta Medica 35: 118–124

Jakovlev V et al 1979 Pharmacological investigations with compounds of chamomile. II. New investigations on the antiphlogistic effects of (–)-α–bisabolol and bisabolol oxides. Planta Medica 35: 125–140

Jalsenjak V et al 1987 Microcapsules of sage oil: essential oils content and antimicrobial activity. Pharmazie 42: 419–420

Joubert L, Gattefossé M 1968 Mezhdunar. Kongr. Efirnym Maslam (Mater.) 4th 1: 99 In: Chemical Abstracts 1973 78: 119653r

Juven B J, Kanner J, Schved F, Weisslowicz H 1993 Factors that interact with the antibacterial action of thyme essential oil and its active constituents. Journal of Applied Bacteriology 76: 626–631

Karamat E, Ilmberger J, Buchbauer G, Rößlhuber J, Rupp C 1992 Excitatory and sedative effects of essential oils on human reaction time performance. Chemical Senses 17: 847

Kirkness W R 1910 Poisoning by oil of eucalyptus. British Medical Journal 1: 261

Kubota M, Ikemoto T, Komaki R, Iniu M 1992 Paper given to the 12th International Congress on Flavours, Fragrances and Essential Oils. Vienna, Austria

Kudrzycka-Bieloszabska F W, Glowniak K 1966 Pharmacodynamic properties of *Oleum chamomillae* and *Oleum millefolii*. Dissertationes Pharmaceuticae et Pharmacologicae 18: 449–454

Lavy G 1987 Nutmeg intoxication in pregnancy. Journal of Reproductive Medicine 32: 63–69

Lawrence B M 1977 Progress in essential oils. Perfumer & Flavorist February/March 2(1): 3

Lawrence B M 1979 Essential oils 1976–1978. Allured, Wheaton, p 23

Lawrence B M 1984 Progress in essential oils. Perfumer & Flavorist August/September 9(4): 37

Lawrence B M 1989 Progress in essential oils. Perfumer & Flavorist 14(3): 71

Leach E H, Lloyd J P F 1956 Experimental ocular hypertension in animals. Transactions of the Ophthalmological Societies of the United Kingdom 76: 453–460

Leicester R J, Hunt R H 1982 Peppermint oil to reduce colonic spasm during endoscopy. The Lancet 30 October: 989

Leung A Y 1980 Encyclopedia of common natural ingredients used in foods, drugs and cosmetics. Wiley, New York, p 409

Lewis W H, Elvin-Lewis M P H 1977 Medical botany. Plants affecting man's health. Wiley-Interscience, New York

Lis-Balchin M, Deans S, Hart S 1994 Paper given to the 25th International Symposium on Essential Oils, Grasse

List P H, Horhammer L 1969–1979 Hager's Handbuch der pharmazeutischen Praxis. Springer-Verlag, Berlin

Loveman A B 1938 Stomatitis venenata: report of a case of sensitivity of the mucous membranes and the skin to oil of anise. Archiva Dermatologica 38: 906

Low D, Rawal B D, Griffin W J 1974 Antibacterial action of the essential oils of some of the Australian Myrtaceae with special reference to the activity of chromatic fractions of oil of *Eucalyptus citriodora*. Planta Medica 26: 184–189

Löwenfeld W 1932 Ekzematose Überempfindlichkeit gegen Eukalyptusöl. Dermatologie Wochenschrift 95: 1281

Mabey R (ed) 1988 The complete new herbal. Elm Tree Books, London

McPherson J 1925 The toxicology of eucalyptus oil. Medical Journal of Australia 2: 108–110

Manley C H 1993 Critical revue. In: Food Science and Nutrition 39(1): 57–62

Mann C, Staba E J 1986 The chemistry, pharmacology and commercial formulations of chamomile. In: Craker L E, Simon J E (eds), Herbs, spices and medicinal plants: recent advances in botany, horticulture, and pharmacology, vol 1. Oryx Press, Arizona, pp 235–280

Maradufu A et al 1978 Lloydia 41: 181

Martinez Nadal N G et al 1973 Cosmetiques et Parfumerie 88(10): 37

Maruzzella J C 1960 Soap Perfumes and Cosmetics 33: 835–837

Maruzzella J C, Henry P A 1958 Journal of the American Pharmaceutical Association 47: 294

Maruzzella J C, Liguori L 1958 Journal of the American Pharmaceutical Association 47: 250

Maruzzella J C, Sicurella N A 1960 Antibacterial activity of essential oil vapours. Journal of the American Pharmaceutical Association 49: 692

Marzulli F N, Maibach H I 1970 Perfume photo toxicity. Journal of the Society of Cosmetic Chemists 2: 695

May B, Kuntz H-D, Kieser M, Köhler S 1996 Efficacy of a fixed peppermint oil/caraway oil combination in non-ulcer dyspepsia. Arzneimittel Forschung/Drug Research 46(II): 1149–1153

Mayo W L 1992 Australian tea tree oil: a summary of medicinal, pharmacological and alternative health research and writings. International Journal of Alternative and Complementary Medicine Dec 13–16

Melegari M, Albasini A, Pecorari G, Vampa G, Rinaldi M 1988 Chemical characteristics and pharmacological properties of the essential oil of *Anthemis nobilis*. Fitoterapia (Milan) 59(6): 449–455

Mezzadra G, Guarnieri B, Grupper C, Forlot P 1981 Effects of chronic field exposure of humans to bergapten. In: Psoralens in cosmetics and dermatology. Pergamon Press, Oxford, pp 383–395

Millet Y 1979 Étude expérimentale des propriétés toxiques convulsivantes des essences de sauge et d'hysope du commerce. Revue d'Electoencephalographie et de Neurophysiologie Clinique 1: 12–18

Millet Y, Jouglard J, Steinmetz M, Tognetti P, Joanny P, Arditti J 1981 Toxicity of some essential oils. Clinical and experimental study. Clinical Toxicology 18(12): 1485–1498

Mills S Y 1991 The essential book of herbal medicine. Penguin Arkana, Harmondsworth

Mishra D et al 1995 The fungitoxic effect of the essential oil of the herb *Nardostachys jatamansi* DC. Tropical Agriculture 72(1): 48–52

Mitchell J C, Rook A 1979 Botanical dermatology. Greenglass, Vancouver

Moreno O M 1973 Report to RIFM, 21 September

Morton J F 1981 Atlas of medicinal plants of Middle America. Thomas, Springfield

Mulkens A et al 1985 Pharmaceutica Acta Helvetica 60(9–10): 276 In: Chemical Abstracts 1985 103: 211224j

Murray F A 1921 Dermatitis caused by bitter orange. British Medical Journal 1: 739

Musajo L, Rodighiero G, Caporale G 1953 The photodynamic activity of the natural coumarins. Chimica Industria (Milan) 35: 13–15

Musajo L, Rodighiero G, Caporale G 1954 The photodynamic activity of the natural coumarins. Bulletin Société de Chimie et Biologie 36: 1213–1224

Nano G M, Sacco T, Frattini C 1974 Botanical and chemical research on *Anthemis nobilis* L. and some of its cultivars. Paper no 114, Sixth International Essential Oil Congress, San Francisco

Neale A 1893 Case of death following blue gum (*Eucalyptus globulus*) oil. Australasian Medical Gazette 12: 115–116

Novak D 1968 Archives de Roumaine Pathologie et Experimental Microbiologie 27: 721 In: Chemical Abstracts 1969 71: 58264w

Occhiuto F, Circosta C 1996 Antianginal and antiarrhythmic effects of bergamottine, a furocoumarin isolated from bergamot oil. Phytotherapy Research 10: 491–496

Occhiuto F et al 1995 Effects of the non-volatile residue from the essential oil of *Citrus bergamia* on the central nervous system. International Journal of Pharmacognosy 33(3): 198–203

Ognyanov I 1984 Bulgarian lavender and Bulgarian lavender oil. Perfumer & Flavorist 8(6): 29–41

Oishi K et al 1974 Nippon Suisan Gakkaishi 40: 1241 In: Chemical Abstracts 1975 82: 84722r

Opdyke D L J 1973a Caraway oil. In: Food and Cosmetics Toxicology 11: 1051

Opdyke D L J 1973b Bergamot oil, expressed. In: Food and Cosmetics Toxicology 11: 1031

Opdyke D L J 1973c Coriander oil (*Coriandrum sativum* L.). In: Food and Cosmetics Toxicology 11: 1077

Opdyke D L J 1973d Basil oil, sweet. In: Food and Cosmetics Toxicology 11: 867

Opdyke D L J 1973e Anise oil (*Pimpinella anisum* L.). In: Food and Cosmetics Toxicology 11: 865

Opdyke D L J 1974a Ylang ylang oil. In: Food and Cosmetics Toxicology 12. Special issue I Monographs on fragrance raw materials: 1049

Opdyke D L J 1974b Chamomile oil, Roman. In: Food and Cosmetics Toxicology 12. Special issue III Monographs on fragrance raw materials: 709

Opdyke D L J 1974c Chamomile flower, Hungarian, oil (*Matricaria chamomilla* L.). In: Food and Cosmetics Toxicology 12. Special issue I Monographs on fragrance raw materials: 851

Opdyke D L J 1974d Bitter orange oil (*Citrus aurantium* L.). In: Food and Cosmetics Toxicology 12: 735

Opdyke D L J 1974e Lemon oil, expressed. In: Food and Cosmetics Toxicology 12: 725

Opdyke D L J 1974f Lemon oil, distilled. In: Food and Cosmetics Toxicology 12: 727

Opdyke D L J 1974g Fennel oil. In: Food and Cosmetics Toxicology 12. Special issue I Monographs on fragrance raw materials: 879

Opdyke D L J 1974h Geranium oil, bourbon. In: Food and Cosmetics Toxicology 12. Special issue I Monographs on fragrance raw materials: 883

Opdyke D L J 1974i Rose oil (*Rosa damascena* Mill.). In: Food and Cosmetics Toxicology 12. Special issue I Monographs on fragrance raw materials: 979, 981

Opdyke D L J 1974j Rosemary oil (*Rosmarinus officinalis* L.). In: Food and Cosmetics Toxicology 12. Special issue I Monographs on fragrance raw materials: 977

Opdyke D L J 1974k Sage Dalmatian oil (*Salvia officinalis* L.). In: Food and Cosmetics Toxicology 12. Special issue I Monographs on fragrance raw materials: 987

Opdyke D L J 1974i Sandalwood oil, East Indian. In: Food and Cosmetics Toxicology 12. Special issue I monographs on fragrance raw materials: 989

Opdyke D L J 1974m Thyme oil, red. In: Food and Cosmetics Toxicology 12. Special issue I Monographs on fragrance raw materials: 1003

Opdyke D L J 1974n Vetiver oil (*Vetiveria zizanioides* Stapf.). In: Food and Cosmetics Toxicology 12. Special issue I Monographs on fragrance raw materials: 1013

Opdyke D L J 1974o Ginger oil. In: Food and Cosmetics Toxicology 12. Special issue I Monographs on fragrance raw materials: 901

Opdyke D L J 1975a Linalool. In: Food and Cosmetics Toxicology 13. Special issue II Monographs on fragrance raw materials: 827

Opdyke D L J 1975b Eucalyptus oil (*Eucalyptus globulus* Labille). In: Food and Cosmetics Toxicology 13: 107

Opdyke D L J 1975c Rose oil (*Rosa damascena* Mill.). In: Food and Cosmetics Toxicology 13. Special issue II Monographs on fragrance raw materials: 913

Opdyke D L J 1975d Rose absolute, French. In: Food and Cosmetics Toxicology 13. Special issue II Monographs on fragrance raw materials: 911

Opdyke D L J 1975e Clove bud oil (*Eugenia* spp.) In: Food and Cosmetics Toxicology 13. Special issue II Monographs on fragrance raw materials: 761

Opdyke D L J 1976a Cedarwood oil Atlas. In: Food and Cosmetics Toxicology 14. Special issue III Monographs on fragrance raw materials: 709

Opdyke D L j 1976b Neroli oil, Tunisian. In: Food and Cosmetics Toxicology 14. Special issue III Monographs on fragrance raw materials: 813

Opdyke D L J 1976c Myrrh oil (*Commiphora* spp.). In: Food and Cosmetics Toxicology 14: 621

Opdyke D L J 1976d Juniper oil (*Juniperus communis* L.). In: Food and Cosmetics Toxicology 14: 333

Opdyke D L J 1976e Lavender oil (*Lavandula officinalis* Chaix). In: Food and Cosmetics Toxicology 14: 451

Opdyke D L J 1976f Lavandin oil (*Lavandula hybrida*). In: Food and Cosmetics Toxicology 14: 447

Opdyke D L J 1976g Cajeput oil (*Melaleuca leucadendron* L.). In: Food and Cosmetics Toxicology 14. Special issue III Monographs on fragrance raw materials: 701

Opdyke D L J 1976h Nutmeg oil, East Indian. In: Food and Cosmetics Toxicology 14: 631

Opdyke D L J 1976i Marjoram oil, sweet (*Origanum majorana*). In: Food and Cosmetics Toxicology 14: 469

Opdyke D L J 1976j *Pinus sylvestris* oil. In: Food and Cosmetics Toxicology 14. Special issue III Monographs on fragrance raw materials: 845

Opdyke D L J 1976k Savory summer oil (*Satureja hortensis* L.). In: Food and Cosmetics Toxicology 14. Special issue III Monographs on fragrance raw materials: 859

Opdyke D L J 1976l Marjoram oil, Spanish (*Thymus mastichina*). In: Food and Cosmetics Toxicology 14: 467

Opdyke D L J 1978a Bois de rose, Brazilian. In: Food and Cosmetics Toxicology 16 suppl 1. Special issue IV Monographs on fragrance raw materials: 653

Opdyke D L J 1978b Olibanum absolute. In: Food and Cosmetics Toxicology 16 suppl 1. Special issue IV Monographs on fragrance raw materials: 835

Opdyke D L J 1978c Cypress oil. In: Food and Cosmetics Toxicology 16. Special issue IV Monographs on fragrance raw materials: 699

Opdyke D L J 1978d Hyssop oil (*Hyssopus officinalis* L.). In: Food and Cosmetics Toxicology 16. Special issue IV Monographs on fragrance raw materials: 783

Opdyke D L J 1978e Pepper, black, oil (*Piper nigrum* L.) In: Food and Cosmetics Toxicology 16. Special issue IV Monographs on fragrance raw materials: 651

Opdyke D L J 1982 Tagetes oil (*Tagetes erecta* L.; *T. patula* L.; or *T. glandulifera* Schrank). In: Food and Cosmetics Toxicology 20. Special issue VI Monographs on fragrance raw materials: 829

Opdyke D L J, Letizia C 1982a Patchouli oil. Food and Chemical Toxicology 20 (suppl): 791

Opdyke D L J, Letizia C 1982b Clary oil. In: Food and Chemical Toxicology 20 (suppl): 823

Patakova D, Chladek M 1974 Pharmazie 29: 140

Patel S, Wiggins J 1980 Eucalyptus oil poisoning. Archives of Disease in Childhood 5: 405–406

Pathak M A, Fitzpatrick T B 1959 Relation of molecular configuration to the furocoumarins which increase the cutaneous responses following long wave ultraviolet radiation. Journal of Investigative Dermatology 32: 255–262

Penfold A R, Willis J L 1961 The eucalypts. Leonard Hill, London

Pénoël D 1991 Médecine aromatique, médecine planetaire. Jollois, Limoges

Pénoël D 1993 A special eucalyptus (*E. smithii*). The Aromatherapist 1(2): (insert)

Perry L M 1980 Medicinal plants of East and Southeast Asia. MIT Press, Cambridge MA, p 620

Peterson H R, Hall A 1946 Dermal irritating properties of perfume materials. Drug and Cosmetic Industry, 58 (January): 113

Phillips H F 1989 What thyme is it? A guide to the thyme taxa cultivated in the United States. In: Simon J E (ed) Proceedings of the fourth national herb growing and marketing conference. International Herb Growers and Marketers Association, Silver Spring, USA

Phillips H F 1991 The best of thymes. The Herb Companion April/May: 22–29

Pizsolitto A C 1975 Rev. Fac. Farm. Odontol. Araraquara 9: 55 In: Chemical Abstracts 1977 86: 12226s

Poretta A, Casolari A 1966 Industria Conserve (Parma) 41: 287 In: Chemical Abstracts 1967 66: 84879s

Prager M J, Miskiewicz M A 1979 Gas chromatographic-mass spectrometric analysis, identification and detection of adulteration of lavender, lavandin and spike lavender oils. Journal of the American Organization of Analytical Chemists 62: 1231–1238

Prakash S et al 1972 Indian Oil Soap Journal 37: 230 In: Chemical Abstracts 1973 79: 727y

Prakash V 1990 Leafy spices. CRC Press, Boca Raton

Price S 1993 The aromatherapy workbook. Thorsons, London

Ramadan F M et al 1972a Chemical Mikrobiology Technology Lebensmittel 2: 51

Ramadan F M et al 1972b Chemical Mikrobiology Technology Lebensmittel 1: 96

Rao B G V N, Joseph P L 1971 Die Wirksamt einiger ätherischer Öle gegenüber phytopathogenen Fungi. Riechstoffe Aromatische 21: 405

Recio M C et al 1989 Antimicrobial activity of selected plants employed in the Spanish Mediterranean area. Part II. Phytotherapy Research 3: 77

Rees W D 1979 British Medical Journal ii: 835–836

Reichling J, Becker H, Drager P-D 1978 Herbicides in chamomile cultivation. Acta Horticultiva 73: 331–338

Reynolds J E F (ed) 1972 Martindale: the extra pharmacopoeia, 26th edn. Pharmaceutical Press, London

Reynolds J E F (ed) 1989 Martindale: the extra pharmacopoeia, 29th edn. Pharmaceutical Press, London

Reynolds J E F (ed) 1993 Martindale: the extra pharmacopoeia, 30th edn. Pharmaceutical Press, London

Rook M J 1979 Botanical dermatology: plant and plant products injurious to the skin. Greengrass, Vancouver

Rose J E, Behm F M 1994 Inhalation of vapor from black pepper extract reduces smoking withdrawal symptoms. Drug and Alcohol Dependence 34: 225–229

Rossi T, Melegari M, Bianchi A, Albasini A, Vampa G 1988 Sedative, antiinflammatory and antidiuretic effects in rats by essential oils of varieties of *Anthemis nobilis*: a comprehensive study. Pharmacological Research Communications 20(5): 71–74

Roulier G 1990 Les huiles essentielles pour votre santé. Dangles, St-Jean-de-Braye

Rovesti P, Colombo E 1973 Contact Dermatitis 2: 196–200

Salamon I 1992 Chamomile production in Czecho-Slovakia. Focus on Herbs 10: 1–8

Sangster S A et al 1987 The metabolic disposition of (methoxy-C) labelled trans-anethole, estragole and *p*-propylanisole in human volunteers. Xenobiotica 17: 1223–1232

Sanyal A, Varma K C 1969 Indian Journal of Microbiology 9: 23

Schwarz L 1934 Skin hazards in American industry. Part 1. US Publication Health Bulletin no 215

Schwarz L, Peck S M 1946 Cosmetics and dermatitis. Hoeber, New York

Schwarz L, Tulipan L, Peck S M 1947 Occupational diseases of the skin. Lea & Febiger, Philadelphia

Secondini O 1990 Handbook of perfumes and flavors. Chemical Publishing, New York

Sewell J S 1925 Poisoning by eucalyptus oil. British Medical Journal 1: 922

Shafran I, Maurer W, Thomas F B 1977 New England Journal of Medicine 296: 694

Shrivastav P, George K, Balasubramaniam N, Padmini Jasper M, Thomas M, Kanagasabhapathy A S 1988 Suppression of puerperal lactation using jasmine flowers (*Jasminum sambac*). Australian and New Zealand Journal of Obstetrics and Gynaecology 28: 68–71

Shu C K, Waradt J P, Taylor W I 1975 Improved methods for bergapten determination by high performance liquid chromatography. Journal of Chromatography 106: 271–282

Sigmund C J, MacNally E F 1969 The action of a carminative on the lower oesophageal sphincter. Gastroenterology 56: 13–18

Silyanouska K et al 1969 Parfümerie and Kosmetik 50: 293

Simeon de Bouchberg M et al 1976 Rivista Italiano Esseny, Profumi, Piante Offic. Aromi, Safoni, Cosmet Aerosol 58: 527 In: Chemical Abstracts 1977 86: 84201c

Stanic G, Samarzija I 1993 Diuretic activity of *Satureia montana* ssp. *montana* extracts and oil in rats. Phytotherapy Research 7(5): 363

Storp F 1996 Harze in der Parfümerie. Drom, Baierbrunn p 38

Subba M S et al 1967 Journal of Food Science 32: 225

Swanson A B et al 1981 The side-chain epoxidation and hydroxylation of the hepatocarcinogens safrole and estragole and some related compounds by rat and mouse liver microsomes. Biochemica Biophysica Acta 673: 504

Szelenyi I, Thiemer O I K 1979 Pharmacological investigations with compounds of chamomile. III. Experimental studies of the ulcer protective effect of chamomile. Planta Medica 35: 218–227

Takechi M, Tanaka Y 1981 Purification and characterization of antiviral substance eugeniin from the bud of *Syzygium aromaticum*. Planta Medica 42(1): 69

Taylor B D, Luscombe D K, Duthie H L 1983 Inhibitory effect of peppermint oil on gastrointestinal smooth muscle. Gut 24: 992

Tester-Dalderup C B M 1980 Drugs used in bronchial asthma and cough. In: Dukes M N G (ed) Meyler's side effects of drugs, 9th edn. Excerpta Medica, Amsterdam

Thulin M, Claeson P 1991 Economic Botany 45: 487

Tierra M 1980 The way of herbs. Unity Press, Santa Cruz CA

Tisserand R, Balacs T 1995 Essential oil safety. Churchill Livingstone, New York, pp 98–99

Torii S, Fakuda H, Kanemoto H, Miyanchi R, Hamanzu Y, Kavasaki M 1988 Contingent negative variation and the psychological effects of odour. In: Van Toller S, Dodd G H (eds) 1988 Perfumery. The psychology and biology of fragrance. Chapman & Hall, London, pp 107–120

Trease G E, Evans W C 1983 Pharmacognosy, 13th edn. Baillière Tindall, Eastbourne

Tubaro A, Zilli C, Redaelli C, Della Loggia R 1984 Evaluation of antiinflammatory activity of a chamomile extract topical application. Planta Medica 50(4): 359

Tulipan L 1938 Cosmetic irritants. Archiva Dermatologica 38: 906

Tyler V E 1982 The honest herbal: a sensible guide to the use of herbs and related remedies. Stickley, Philadelphia, p 263

Tyler V E 1992 Phytomedicines in Western Europe: their potential impact on herbal medicine in the United States. Lecture delivered at the annual meeting of the American Chemical Society, San Francisco, April

Tyler V E 1993 The honest herbal: a sensible guide to the use of herbs and related remedies. 3rd edn. Stickley, Philadelphia

Urbach F, Forbes P D 1973 Report to RIFM, 16 August

Uzdenikov B N 1970 Nauchi Trudove Tyumen. Sel. Khoz. Inst. 7: 116 through Chemical Abstracts 1972 77: 8429x

Valnet J 1980 The practice of aromatherapy. Daniel, Saffron Walden

Van Den Broucke C O, Lernli J A 1981 Pharmacological and chemical investigation of thyme liquid extracts. Planta Medica 41: 129–135

Vömel A, Reichling J, Becker H, Dräger P D 1977 Herbicides in the cultivation of *Matricaria chamomilla*. 1st communication: influence of herbicides on flower and weed production. Planta Medica 31: 378–379

Wagner H, Bladt S, Zgainski E M 1984 Plant drug analysis. Springer-Verlag, Berlin, p 13

Wagner H, Sprinkmeyer L 1973 Deutsche Apotheke Zeitung 113: 1159

Watt J M, Breyer-Brandwijk M G 1962 The medicinal and poisonous plants of Southern and Eastern Africa, 2nd edn. Churchill Livingstone, New York

Weiss E A 1997 Essential oil crops. CAB International, Oxford

Weiss R F 1988 Herbal medicine. Beaconsfield Publishers, Beaconsfield

Winter R 1984 A consumer's dictionary of cosmetic ingredients. Crown, New York

Woeber K, Krombach M 1969 Zur Frage der Sensibilisierung durch Ätherische Öle (Vorläufige Mitteilung). Berufsdermatosen 17: 320

Wren R C (ed) 1988 Potter's new cyclopedia of botanical drugs and preparations, 8th edn. Daniel, Saffron Walden

Yamada K, Mimaki Y, Sashida Y 1994 Anticonvulsive effects of inhaling lavender oil vapour. Biological and Pharmaceutical Bulletin (Tokyo) 17(2): 359–360

Young A R, Walker S L, Kinley J S, Plastow S R, Averbeck D, Morliere P, Dubertret L 1990 Phototumorigenesis studies of 5MOP in bergamot oil: evaluation and modification of risk in human use in an albino mouse skin model. Journal of Photochemistry and Photobiology B 7: 231–250

Zajdela F, Bisagni E 1981 5MOP, the melanogenic additive in suntan preparations is tumerogenic in mice exposed to 365 nm UV radiation. Carcinogenesis 2: 121–127

Zangouras A et al 1981 Dose-dependent conversion of estragole in the rat and mouse to carcinogenic metabolite 1-hydroxyestragole. Biochemical Pharmacology 30: 1383–1386

Zaynoun S T, Johnson B E, Frain-Bell W 1977 A study of bergamot and its importance as a phototoxic agent. II. Factors which affect the phototoxic reaction induced by bergamot oil and psoralen derivatives. Contact Dermatitis 3: 225–239

Zheng G Q, Kenney P M, Lam K K T 1992 Anethofuran, carvone and limonene: potential cancer chemopreventative agents from dill weed oil and caraway oil. Planta Medica 58: 338–341

Zola A, LeVanda J P 1975 Quelques huiles essentielles en provenance de la Corse. Rivista Italica 57: 467–472

Zondek B et al 1938 Phenol methyl esters as estrogenic agents. Biochemical Journal 32: 641–645

SOURCES

Abdel-Malek S, Bastien J W, Mahler W F, Jia Q, Reinecke M G, Robinson W E, Shu Y, Zalles-Asin J 1996 Drug leads from the Kallawaya herbalists of Bolivia. Journal of Ethnopharmacology 50: 157–166

Adames M, Mendoza E, Ospina de Nigrinis L S 1983 Study of the essential oil of *Eucalyptus citriodora*. Bailey. Rev. Colombian Cienc. Quim. Farm. 4(1): 95–113

Agnel R, Teisseire P 1984 Essential oil of French lavender: its composition and its adulteration. Perfumer & Flavorist 9(2): 53–56

Alberto-Puleo M 1980 Fennel and anise as estrogenic agents. Journal of Ethnopharmacology 2(4): 337–344

Al-Hader A A et al 1994 Hyperglycemic and insulin release inhibitory effects of *Rosmarinus officinalis*. Journal of Ethnopharmacology 43: 217–221

Bardeau F 1976 La médecine aromatique. Robert Laffont, Paris

Bartram T 1995 Encyclopedia of herbal medicine. Grace, Christchurch

Becker H, Förster W 1984 Biologie, Chemie und Pharmakologie pflanzlicher Sedativa. Zeitschrift für Phytotherapie (Stuttgart) 5: 817–823

Benigni R, Capra C, Cattorini P E 1962 Piante medicinali: chimica farmacologia e terapia. Inverni & Della Beffa, Milan

Bernadet M 1983 La phyto-aromathérapie pratique. Dangles, St-Jean-de-Braye

Beylier M F 1979 Bacteriostatic activity of some Australian essential oils. Perfumer & Flavorist 4(2): 23–25

Boyd E M, Pearson G L 1946 On the expectorant action of volatile oils. American Journal of Medical Science 211: 602–610

Briozzo J, Nunez L, Chirife J, Herszage L, D'Aquino M 1989 Journal of Applied Bacteriology Jan. 66(1): 69–75

British Herbal Pharmacopoeia 1983 British Herbal Medicine Association, Cowling

Brunke E J et al 1996 The chemistry of sandalwood fragrance. Actes des 15émes Journées Internationales Huiles Essentielles, pp 48–83

Caldwell J et al 1990 Comparative studies on the metabolisation of food: case examples in the safety evaluation of the allylbenzene natural flavours. Nutritional Biochemistry 1: 402–409

Carson C F, Riley T V 1993 Antimicrobial activity of the essential oil of *Melaleuca alternifolia*. Letters in Applied Microbiology 16: 49–55

Carson C F, Hammer K A, Riley T V 1995 Broth microdilution method for determining the susceptibility of *Escherischia coli* and *Staphylococcus aureus* to the essential oil of *Melaleuca alternifolia* (tea tree oil). Microbios 82(332): 181–185

Chan V S W, Caldwell J 1992 Comparative induction of unscheduled DNA synthesis in cultured rat hepatocytes allylbenzenes and their 1'-hydroxy metabolites. Food and Chemical Toxicology 30(10): 831–836

Chandler R F, Hooper S N, Harvey M J 1982 Ethnobotany and phytochemistry of yarrow, *Achillea millefolium*, Compositae. Economic Botany 36(2): 203–223

Chen Y-D, Yang L, Li S-X, Jiang Z-R 1983 Study on the chemical components of essential oil from the leaves of *Eucalyptus* spp. Chemical Industries Forest Prod. 3(2): 14–31

Council of Scientific and Industrial Research 1948–1976 The wealth of India, 11 vols. New Delhi

Deans S G, Svoboda K P 1990 The antimicrobial properties of marjoram (*Origanum majorana* L.) Volatile oil. Flavor & Fragrance Journal 5(3): 187–190

Deans S G, Svoboda K P et al 1992 Essential oil profiles of several temperate and tropical aromatic plants: their antimicrobial and antioxidant properties. Acta Horticulturae 306: 229–232

Denny E F K 1981 The history of lavender oil: disturbing inferences for the future of essential oils. Perfumer & Flavorist 6: 23–25

Do Vgich N A 1971 Antimicrobial effect of essential oils. Mikrobiol. Zh. (Kiev) 33: 253–259

Duke J A 1982 Herbs as a small farm enterprise and the value of aromatic plants as economic intercrops. Research for small farms. In: Kerr H W, Knutson L (eds) Proceedings of a Special Symposium USDA miscellaneous publications no 1422 p 76

Duraffourd P 1987 Les huiles essentielles et la santé. La Maison de Bien-Etre, Montreuil-sous-Bois

Formacek K, Kubeczka K H 1982 Essential oils analysis by capillary chromatography and carbon-13 NMR spectroscopy. John Wiley, New York

Forster H B, Niklas H, Lutz S 1980 Planta Medica 40(4): 309

Franchomme P, Pénoël D 1985 Aromatherapy: advanced therapy for infectious illnesses (1). Phytoguide no 1, International Phytomedical Foundation, La Courtête

Gottlieb O R, Fineberg M, Guimasraes M L, Taveira Magalhaes M, Maravalhas N 1964 Notes on Brazilian rosewood. Perfume and Essential Oil Records 55: 253–257

Gümbel D 1986 Principles of holistic skin therapy with herbal essences. Haug, Heidelberg

Harkiss K J 1993 Eight peak index of essential oils, version 2.2. Published by the author, Bingley

Hoffman W 1979 Lavendel-Inhaltsstoffe und ausgewählte Synthesen. Seifen-Öle-Fette-Wachse 105: 287–291

Kaul V K, Nigam S S 1977 Antibacterial and antifungal studies of some essential oils. Journal of Research in Indian Medicine, Yoga and Homoeopathy 12: 132–135

Knobloch K, Pauli A, Iberl B, Weigand H, Weiss N 1989 Antibacterial and antifungal properties of essential oil components. Journal of Essential Oil Research 1: 119–128

Lahariya A K, Rao J T 1979 In vitro antimicrobial studies of the essential oil of *Cyperus scariosus* and *Ocimum basilicum*. Indian Drugs 16: 150–152

Lautié R, Passebecq A 1979 Aromatherapy. Thorsons, Wellingborough

Law D 1982 The concise herbal encyclopedia. Bartholomew, Edinburgh

Lawrence B M 1979 Essential oils 1976–1978. Allured, Wheaton

Lawrence B M 1981 Essential oils 1979–1980. Allured, Wheaton

Lawrence B M 1987/1988 Progress in essential oils. Perfumer & Flavorist 12(6): 59

Lawrence B M 1989 Essential oils 1981–1987. Allured, Wheaton pp. 187–188

Lawrence B M 1993 Essential oils 1988–1991. Allured, Wheaton

Mailhebiau P 1989 La nouvelle aromathérapie. Vie Nouvelle, Toulouse

Manitto P, Monti D, Colombo E 1972 Two new beta-diketones from *Helichrysum italicum*. Phytochemistry 11: 2112–2114

Masada Y 1976 Analysis of essential oils by gas chromatography and mass spectrometry. John Wiley, New York

May B et al 1996 Efficacy of a fixed peppermint oil/caraway oil combination in non-ulcer dyspepsia. Arzneimittel-Forschung/Drug Research 46(11): 1149–1153

Miller E C et al 1983 Structure–activity studies of the carcinogenicities in the mouse and rat of some naturally occurring and synthetic alkenylbenzene derivatives related to safrole and estragole. Cancer Research 43: 1124–1134

Merck Index 1983 An encyclopedia of chemicals and drugs, 10th edn. Merck, Rahway NJ

Miranda M, Perez Zayas J 1985 Influencia de la epoca de recoleccion sobre el rendimiento de aceite esencial la composicion quimica del *Eucalyptus citriodora* Hook. que crece in Cuba. Rev. Cub. Farm. 19: 121–127

Miranda M, Perez Zayas J, Rosado A 1983 Estudio de la composicion quimica del aceite essencial de *Eucalyptus citriodora* Hook. Rev. Cienc. Quim. 14: 211–221

Miranda Martinez M, Perez Guimeras J L, Magraner Hernandez J, Perez Zayas J R, Quintero Diaz M J, Moleyar V, Narasimham P 1992 Antibacterial activity of essential oil components. International Journal of Food Microbiology 16: 337–342

Montejo L 1986 Estudio preliminar de los aceites esenciales de esperie de eucalyptus introducidas en la region de topes de Collantes, Rev. Cub. Farm. 20: 159–168

Mwangi J W, Guantai A N, Muriuki G 1981 *Eucalyptus citriodora*—essential oil content and chemical varieties in Kenya. East African Agriculture and Forestry Journal 46(4): 89–96

Nigam I C, Levi L 1963 Essential oils and their constituents XIX. Detection of new trace components in oil of rosewood. Perfume and Essential Oil Record 54: 814–816

Nishimura H, Kaku K, Nakamura T, Fukazawa Y, Mizutani J 1982 Allelopathic substances (±)-*p*-menthan-3,8-diols isolated from *Eucalyptus citriodora* Hook. Agricultural Biological and Chemical 46: 319–320

Opdyke D L J (ed) 1979 Monographs on fragrance raw materials. Pergamon Press, Oxford

Pénoël D 1994 A staple essential oil: presentation of a new eucalyptus oil—*Eucalyptus staigeriana*—for aromatherapists. The Aromatherapist 1(3): 22–27

Pénoël D, Pénoël R-M 1992 Pratique aromatique familiale. Osmobiose, Aoûste

Perry L M 1980 Medicinal plants of East and Southeast Asia. MIT Press, Cambridge

Peyron L, Roubaud M 1971 L'essence d'imortelle del'Estorel. Parfumerie, Cosmetiques et Savons 1: 129–138

Price S 1993 The aromatherapy workbook. Thorsons, London

Renz-Rathfelder S 1986 Vom Duft der Pflanzen. Palmengarten, Frankfurt

Reynolds J E F (ed) 1993 Martindale: the extra pharmacopoeia, 30th edn. Pharmaceutical Press, London

San Martin R, Granger R, Adzet T, Passer J, Tevlade-Arbousset M G 1973 Chemical polymorphism in two Mediterranean labiates, *Satureia montana* L. and *Satureia obovata* Lag. Plantes Médicinales et Phytothérapie 7: 95

Schnaubelt K 1995 Neue Aromatherapie. vgs, Köln

Stanic G, Samarzija I 1993 Diuretic activity of *Satureia montana* ssp. *montana* extracts and oil in rats. Phytotherapy Research 7(5): 363

Stevenson C J 1994 The psychophysiological effects of aromatherapy massage following cardiac surgery. Complementary Therapies in Medicine 2: 27–35

Stewart M 1987 The encyclopedia of herbs and herbalism. Black Cat, London

Sugimoto S, Kato T 1983 Composition of eucalyptus oils. Kanzei Chuo Bunsekisho Ho 2: 31–34

Tantaoui-Elaraki A, Beraoud L 1994 Journal of Environmental Pathology, Toxicology and Oncology 13(1): 67–72

Tong M M, Altman P M, Barnetson R S 1992 Tea tree oil in the treatment of *Tinea pedis*. Australian Journal of Dermatology 33(3): 145–149

Tucker A O, Tucker S S 1988 Catnip and the catnip response. Economic Botany 42(2): 214–231

Viaud H 1983 Huiles essentielles: hydrolats. Présence, Sisteron

Weiss E A 1997 Essential oil crops. CAB International, Wallingford

Yamada K, Mimaki Y, Sashida Y 1994 Anticonvulsive effects of inhaling lavender oil vapour. Biological and Pharmaceutical Bulletin 17(2): 359–360

Yadav P, Dubey N K 1994 Screening some essential oils against ringworm fungi. Indian Journal of Pharmaceutical Sciences 56(6): 227–230

Glossary

abortifacient: inducing an abortion; causing expulsion of the fetus

adaptogenic: having a positive general effect on the body irrespective of disease condition, especially under stress

alcohols: group of hydrocarbon compounds frequently found in volatile oils

aldehydes: class of organic compounds standing between alcohols and acids

allopathy: system of medicine which uses drugs with effects opposite to the symptoms produced by the disease (in contrast to homoeopathy)

amenorrhoea: absence of menstruation outside pregnancy in premenopausal women

anaphrodisiac: of a drug, diminishing sexual drive

anodyne: relieving pain; analgesic

anthelmintic: destructive of intestinal worms

antiphlogistic: *see* antipyretic

antipyretic: counteracting inflammation or fever

antithermic: cooling; antipyretic

antitussive: relieving or preventing coughing

anxiolytic: relieving anxiety and tension

aperient: mildly laxative

aperitive: stimulating the appetite

aromatic: organic chemical compound derived from benzene; also called aromatic compound

astringent: causing contraction of living tissues (often mucous membranes), reducing haemorrhages, secretions, diarrhoea, etc.

balneotherapy: treatment by medicinal baths

bitters: botanical drugs with bitter-tasting constituents used to stimulate the gastrointestinal tract; also used as antiinflammatory agents and as relaxants

calmative: mildly sedative

cardiotonic: having a tonic effect on the heart

carminative: relieving flatulence

cathartic: strongly laxative

chemotype: visually identical plants with significantly different chemical components, resulting in different therapeutic properties; abbreviated to ct., as in *Thymus vulgaris* ct. alcohol

cholagogic: stimulating gall bladder contraction to promote the flow of bile

choleretic: stimulating the production of bile in the liver

cicatrizant: promoting formation of scar tissue and healing

cohobation: the operation of repeatedly using the water used in the distillation process; thus no water is discarded and water soluble molecules from the plant material are not lost

coumarin: a chemical compound, $C_9H_6O_2$, with a high boiling point (290°C) found within the lactones; hardly volatile with steam thus found mainly in expressed oils and sparingly in some distilled essential oils; characteristic smell of new-mown hay

cultivar: cultivated variety: a plant produced by horticulture or agriculture not normally occurring naturally; labelled by adding a 'name' to the species, as in *Lavandula angustifolia* 'Maillette'

depurative: purifying or cleansing

diaphoretic: causing or increasing perspiration; sudorific

digestive: aiding digestion

dysmenorrhoea: painful or difficult menstruation

dyspepsia: disturbed digestion

emmenagogic: inducing or regularizing menstruation; euphemism for abortifacient

enuresis: bedwetting

erethism: abnormal irritability or sensitivity

essential oil: plant volatile oil obtained by distillation

eubiotic: brings about conditions favourable to life and healing

eupeptic: aiding digestion

febrifuge: agent which reduces temperature; antipyretic

fixed oil: non-volatile oil; plant oils consist of esters of fatty acids, usually triglycerides

forma: lowest botanical rank in general use, denoting trivial differences within a species

fruit: the ripe seeds and their surrounding structures, which can be fleshy or dry

galactagogic: promoting the secretion of milk; lactogenic

genus: important botanical classification of related but distinct species given a common name; genera (pl.) are in turn grouped into families; the first word of the binomial botanical name denotes the genus

glycoside: sugar derivative found in certain plants (e.g. digoxin, used to treat heart failure)

haemostatic: checking blood flow

hallucinogen: agent affecting any or all of the senses, producing a wide range of distorted perceptions and reactions

herb: non-woody soft leafy plant; plant used in medicine and cooking

homoeopathy: system of medicine using tiny amounts of drugs which in a healthy body would produce symptoms similar to those of the disease (as distinct from allopathy)

hybrid: natural or artificially produced plant resulting from the fertilization of one species by another; indicated by '×', as in *Mentha × piperita*

hyperidrosis: excessive sweating

hypermenorrhoea: profuse or prolonged menses

hypertensor: increasing blood pressure; pressor

hypotensor: reducing blood pressure; antihypertensive

immunostimulant: stimulating the immune system

lactogenic: promoting the secretion of milk; galactagogue

laxative: loosening the bowel contents, promoting evacuation

lipid: a fat or fat-like substance insoluble in water and soluble in organic solvents

lipolytic: breaking down fat

lipophilic: having strong affinity for lipids

litholytic: breaking down stones

maceration: the extraction of substances from a plant by steeping in a fixed oil

MbOCA: symbol for methylenebis (ortho-chloroaniline); a curing agent for polyurethane and epoxy resins; believed to be carcinogenic

MDA: methylenedioxyamphetamine; has hallucinogenic effects; subject to abuse and dependence

menorrhagia: excessive periods

metrorrhagia: uterine haemorrhage occurring outside menstrual periods

narcotic: inducing insensibility (sleep) and relieving pain in small dosage, toxic in high dosage

oestrogenic: simulating the action of female hormones

officinalis: used in medicine; recognized in the pharmacopoeia

oligomenorrhoea: a condition of infrequent menstruation

organic: grown without the use of chemical fertilizers, pesticides, etc.

organoleptic: concerned with testing the effects of a substance on the senses, particularly taste and smell

parenteral: by means other than the gastrointestinal tract; the introduction of substances into an organism by an intravenous, cutaneous, intramuscular or intramedullary pathway

percutaneous: applied through the skin

pharmacokinetics: study of absorption, distribution, metabolism and elimination of drugs

photosensitization: abnormally increased sensitivity of the skin to ultraviolet radiation or natural sunlight; can follow ingestion of or contact with various substances

phytotherapy: treatment of disease by the use of plants and plant extracts; herbalism

polymenorrhoea: unusually short menstrual cycles

probiotic: favouring the beneficial bacteria in the body, while inhibiting harmful microbes; literally 'for life' as distinct from antibiotic, 'against life'

prophylactic: preventing disease

psoralens: polycyclic molecules whose structure gives them the ability to absorb ultraviolet photons

psychopharmaceutical: pertaining to drugs affecting the mind or mood

psychotropic: of a drug, affecting the brain and influencing behaviour

purgative: strongly laxative

rhizome: underground stem bearing roots, scales and nodes

rubefacient: increasing local blood circulation causing redness of the skin

spasmolytic: relieving convulsions, spasmodic pains and cramp

stomachic: agent which stimulates the secretory activity of the stomach

styptic: arresting haemorrhage by means of an astringent quality; haemostatic

subspecies: subdivision of a species, often denoting a geographic variation; structure or colour are peculiar to subspecies and are more definite than characteristics identifying varieties; subspecies can interbreed; abbreviated to subsp.

sudorific: inducing sweating

synergy: increased effect of two or more medicinal substances working together

taxonomy: scientific classification of living things

thymoleptic: antiseptic

tonic: producing or restoring normal vigour or tension (tone)

trichome: hairlike structure on the epidermis of a plant

variety: indicates a botanical rank between subspecies and forma; abbreviated to var., as in *Citrus aurantium* var. *amara*

vermifugal: expelling intestinal worms

vesicant: producing blisters (therapeutically, to induce counterirritant serosity)

vulnerary: agent promoting healing of wounds

Useful addresses

GREAT BRITAIN

Training and essential oil supplies

Shirley Price Aromatherapy Ltd
Essentia House
Upper Bond Street
Hinckley
Leics LE10 1RS
Tel: 01455 615466
Fax: 01455 615054
email: shirleypricearoma@compuserve.com

Shirley Price International College of Aromatherapy (SPICA)
See above for address.

SEED Institute
10 Magnolia Way
Fleet
Hants GU13 9JZ

Essential oil supplies:

Herbal Garden
20 Eldon Gardens
Percy Street
Newcastle upon Tyne NE1 7RA

Herbal Garden
93 Rose Street
Edinburgh EH2 3DT

Aromatology/aromatherapy associations:

Aromatherapy Organisations Council (AOC)
PO Box 19834
London SE25 6WF
Tel: 0181-251 7912

International Society of Professional Aromatherapists (ISPA)
82 Ashby Road
Hinckley
Leics LE10 1SN

Institute of Aromatic Medicine (IAM)
Aromed House
66 Upper Bond Street
Hinckley
Leics LE10 1RS

International Federation of Aromatherapists (IFA)
Stamford House
2–4 Chiswick High Road
London W4 1TH

Register of Qualified Aromatherapists (RQA)
PO Box 3431
Danbury
Chelmsford
Essex CM3 4VA

Trade associations

Aromatherapy Trade Council
PO Box 52
Market Harborough
Leics LE16 8ZX

Essential Oil Trade Association 95
Stonebridge Farmhouse
Breadsell Lane
St Leonards
Sussex TN38 8EB

Natural Oils Research Association
PO Box 2458
Reading
Berks RG30 2XU

Research Council for Complementary Medicine
60 Great Ormond Street
London WC1N 3JF

WORLDWIDE

Northern Ireland

Training:

Mary Thompson
European College of Natural Therapies
16 North Parade
Belfast
Northern Ireland BT7 2GG

Essential oil supplies:

Angela Hillis
32 Russell Park
Belfast
Northern Ireland BT5 7QW

Republic of Ireland

Training and essential oil supplies:

Mary Cavanagh
PO Box 16
Wicklow
Co. Wicklow
Republic of Ireland

Essential oil supplies:

Phil O'Flynn
1 Sunnyside
Off Barringtons Avenue
Ballintemple
Co. Cork
Republic of Ireland

Australia

Training and essential oil supplies:

Margaret Tozer
Australian School of Awareness
PO Box 187
Montrose 3765
Australia

Essential oil supplies:

House of Pan Pty Ltd
Suite 3 1st Floor
4–6 Croydon Road
Croydon 3136
Victoria
Australia

Germany

Association:

Forum Essenzia
Mäuselweg 29
81375 München
Germany

Iceland

Essential oil supplies:

Bergfell EHF
Healthcare & Medical
Skipholt 50c
105 Reykjavik
Iceland

Israel

Training:

Fern Allen
PO Box 4363
Jerusalem
Israel

Essential oil supplier:

Eden Natural Pharmacy
PO Box 21434
Tel Aviv 61214
Israel

Italy

Training:

Jenny Bird ·
Via Vigerano 43
Milan 20144
Italy

Japan

Essential oil supplies:

Oz International
Bancho Fifth Building
5-5 Nibancho
Chiyoda-Ku
Tokyo 102
Japan

Korea

Essential oil supplies:

Jung Dong Cosmetics Co Ltd
Shinhan Office Building
49-5 Chungdam Dong
Kangnam-Gu
Seoul
Korea

Norway

Training and essential oil supplies:

Margareth Thomte
SPA Norge
Nedreslottsgate 25
0157 Oslo
Norway

Singapore

Training and essential oil supplies:

Li & Low Marketing Pte Ltd
63 Hillview Avenue #09–21
Lam Soon Industrial Building
Singapore 2360

Switzerland

Associations:

VEROMA
Alte Gasse 19
CH-6390 Engelberg
Switzerland

Training and essential oil supplies:

Sara Gelzer
Eigentalstraße 552, No 14
8425 Oberembrach
Switzerland

Taiwan

Essential oil supplies:

Jong Yeong Cosmetics Co Ltd
18 Tze Chyang 3rd Road
Nan Kong Industrial Park
Nan Tou
Taiwan

USA

Training and essential oil supplies:

Hans Nordblom
Nordblom Swedish Healthcare Centre
178 Mill Creek Road
Livingstone
Montana 59047
USA

Index

Uterine inertia, 191
Uterotonic essential oils, 182–183, 351

V

Vaginal administration, 47, 93–94
Vaginal infection, 187
Valeranal, 14
Valeranone, 14
Valerian, *see Valerian officinalis*
Valerian officinalis, 20
   chemotypes, 14
    ct. cryptofouranol, 14
    ct. valeranal, 14
    ct. valeranone, 14
   insomnia, 231
   sedative effects, 81
Valerianaceae, 20
Vanilla, 10
Vaporizers, 95–96
   ethical considerations, 96
Variation, 23–24, 178
Varicose veins
   massage precautions, 126
   pregnancy, 187

Variety, 8, 373
Verbenaceae, 20
Verbenone, **14**
Vermifugal properties, 373
Vesicants, 79, 373
Vetiver, *see Vetivera zizanioides*
Vetivera zizanioides, 19, **349–350**
   antiviral properties, 74
   emmenagogic actions, **181**
Vinblastine, 2
Vincristine, 2
Virginian cedarwood, *see Juniperus virginiana*
Viridiflorol, 79
Viscosity, 99
Vitis vinifera, 104
Voluntary stress, 147
Vulnerary effects, 373

W

Water births, 101
Western red cedar, *see Thuja plicata*
Western white cedar, *see Chamaecyparis lawsoniana*

Wheatgerm, *see Triticum vulgare*
White cedar, *see Thuja occidentalis*
Wild thyme, *see Thymus serpyllum*
Winter savory, *see Satureia montana*
Wintergreen, *see Gaultheria procumbens*
Wormwood, *see Artemisia absinthium*

X

Xanthotoxin, 51

Y

Yarrow, *see Achillea millefolium*
Yield of essential oils, 16
Ylang ylang, *see Cananga odorata*

Z

Zingiber officinale, 10, 183, 278, **350**
   deodorant properties, 76
   digestive disorders, 228
   rheumatism/arthritis, 235